Communications in Computer and Information Science 3010

Rationale

The CCIS series is devoted to the publication of proceedings of computer science conferences. Its aim is to efficiently disseminate original research results in informatics in printed and electronic form. While the focus is on publication of peer-reviewed full papers presenting mature work, inclusion of reviewed short papers reporting on work in progress is welcome, too. Besides globally relevant meetings with internationally representative program committees guaranteeing a strict peer-reviewing and paper selection process, conferences run by societies or of high regional or national relevance are also considered for publication.

Topics

The topical scope of CCIS spans the entire spectrum of informatics ranging from foundational topics in the theory of computing to information and communications science and technology and a broad variety of interdisciplinary application fields.

Information for Volume Editors and Authors

Publication in CCIS is free of charge. No royalties are paid, however, we offer registered conference participants temporary free access to the online version of the conference proceedings on SpringerLink (http://link.springer.com) by means of an http referrer from the conference website and/or a number of complimentary printed copies, as specified in the official acceptance email of the event.

CCIS proceedings can be published in time for distribution at conferences or as post-proceedings, and delivered in the form of printed books and/or electronically as USBs and/or e-content licenses for accessing proceedings at SpringerLink. Furthermore, CCIS proceedings are included in the CCIS electronic book series hosted in the SpringerLink digital library at http://link.springer.com/bookseries/7899. Conferences publishing in CCIS are allowed to use our online conference service (Meteor) for managing the whole proceedings lifecycle (from submission and reviewing to preparing for publication) free of charge.

Publication process

The language of publication is exclusively English. Authors publishing in CCIS have to sign the Springer CCIS copyright transfer form, however, they are free to use their material published in CCIS for substantially changed, more elaborate subsequent publications elsewhere. For the preparation of the camera-ready papers/files, authors have to strictly adhere to the Springer CCIS Authors' Instructions and are strongly encouraged to use the CCIS LaTeX style files or templates.

Abstracting/Indexing

CCIS is abstracted/indexed in DBLP, Google Scholar, EI-Compendex, Mathematical Reviews, SCImago, Scopus. CCIS volumes are also submitted for the inclusion in ISI Proceedings.

How to start

To start the evaluation of your proposal for inclusion in the CCIS series, please send an e-mail to ccis@springer.com

Mariella Särestöniemi · Daljeet Singh ·
Erika Jarva · Jarmo Reponen
Editors

Digital Health and Wireless Solutions: Integrating AI, LLMs and Multimodal Health Data for Next-Generation Decision Support

Second Nordic Conference, NCDHWS 2026
Oulu, Finland, June 16–17, 2026
Proceedings, Part II

Springer

Editors
Mariella Särestöniemi
University of Oulu
Oulu, Finland

Daljeet Singh
University of Oulu
Oulu, Finland

Erika Jarva
University of Oulu
Oulu, Finland

Jarmo Reponen
University of Oulu
Oulu, Finland

ISSN 1865-0929 ISSN 1865-0937 (electronic)
Communications in Computer and Information Science
ISBN 978-3-032-28818-9 ISBN 978-3-032-28819-6 (eBook)
https://doi.org/10.1007/978-3-032-28819-6

This Springer imprint is published by the registered company Springer Nature Switzerland AG
The registered company address is: Gewerbestrasse 11, 6330 Cham, Switzerland

Foreword

Digital health functions as an umbrella concept encompassing a wide range of technology-enabled approaches to healthcare. It includes electronic health services traditionally referred to as eHealth, telemedicine, electronic health counselling, and the active involvement of citizens and patients in promoting their own health through the use of digital technologies. In recent years, this umbrella has expanded to include advanced computational methods, such as artificial intelligence-based analytics, and more recently, generative artificial intelligence and large language models. When combined with genomic data, large-scale health datasets, and sensor-based measurements of citizens' health status, these technologies enable the generation of precise and actionable information. Such information can be leveraged both to improve the overall quality of healthcare systems and to enhance the care of individual patients.

Digital transformation in healthcare aims to make healthcare processes more efficient through the systematic use of digital tools. Wireless technologies, in particular, enable the collection of relevant health data outside traditional clinical environments, while mobile devices allow citizens to actively participate in their own care. Together, these developments contribute to making healthcare services increasingly independent of time and place, whenever physical encounters are not strictly necessary.

The Nordic countries are at the forefront of this digital transformation of healthcare and consistently rank among the top performers in the European Union's Digital Economy and Society Index (DESI). Finland provides a prominent example: all public healthcare patient record systems have been fully electronic since 2007. National health information infrastructure components—including a nationwide electronic health record archive, electronic prescriptions, and a Health Information Exchange (HIE) connecting different healthcare service providers—have been in place since 2010. Citizen engagement is also substantial: on a monthly basis, approximately one fifth of the population regularly accesses their personal health data through the My Kanta Pages patient portal linked to the HIE. Comparable patient portals are in use across the other Nordic countries as well.

As a field of research, digital health is of particular relevance in Finland, not least due to the major administrative reform implemented in 2023. This reform merged public healthcare service providers, social welfare services, and rescue services into large regional entities known as Wellbeing Services Counties. Beyond changes in governance and financing, the reform involves extensive integration of information systems and the adoption of a "Digital First" principle in service delivery. The guiding objective is to provide services digitally and independently of location whenever face-to-face contact is not required.

At the European level, future developments and research opportunities are influenced by initiatives such as the European Health Data Space (EHDS), which aims to harmonize health data used both for primary purposes in patient care and for secondary purposes in research and innovation. At the same time, regulatory frameworks such as the EU

Artificial Intelligence Act and the EU Medical Device Regulation define the boundaries within which artificial intelligence can be deployed responsibly in healthcare. Efforts are also underway to strengthen methods for evaluating the effectiveness of digital health applications and, through Health Technology Assessment (HTA), to establish frameworks for the reimbursement of software-based health solutions. It is hoped that these regulatory developments will support, rather than constrain, Europe's ability to advance as a leading source of health innovations.

The Second Nordic Conference on Digital Health and Wireless Solutions (NCDHWS 2026) was organized by the University of Oulu's *6G Enabled Sustainable Solutions* (6GESS) and *Digital Health* (DigiHealth) research programs, in collaboration with the Profi6-Fibrobesity, Profi8-Health Dimensions, and Oulu Brain & Mind research programs. Our regional partners included Oulu University of Applied Sciences, Oulu University Hospital, the Wellbeing Services County of North Ostrobothnia (Pohde), and Business Oulu. Together, these initiatives brought multidisciplinary expertise spanning medical and health sciences, biosciences, health economics, information technology, sensor technologies, and wireless communications. Once again, we hosted an international multidisciplinary conference that provided an excellent forum for professionals, researchers, and industry leaders from diverse fields to exchange insights and discuss the latest advances in digital health and related technologies.

The conference host city of Oulu has long been at the forefront of research and development in digital health and wireless communications. Electronic health records, telemedicine, and mobile health services have been developed and deployed here for nearly three decades. Active research initiatives continue in areas such as artificial intelligence, novel sensor technologies, and edge computing. At the same time, strong emphasis is placed on the scientific evaluation of the impact of these innovations, as well as on addressing the associated educational needs.

The organization of a multidisciplinary conference of this scale—bringing together diverse academic, clinical, industrial, and societal perspectives—would not have been possible without the dedicated efforts of numerous colleagues and experts. I would like to thank the multidisciplinary Organizing Committee, my co-chair Simo Saarakkala, and our two coordinators, Chao Ding and Tuire Salonurmi, for their highly constructive collaboration. I would further like to express my special appreciation to the Chair of the Scientific Program Committee and Publication Chair, Mariella Särestöniemi, who, together with the committee members and International Reviewers, ensured the high scientific quality of the conference content.

I am also grateful to our distinguished international invited speakers for sharing their expertise in digital health and related technologies, and to the members of the International Advisory Committee for their valuable guidance. My sincere thanks go to Elina Laukka for leading the Student Volunteer Committee, and to all student volunteers whose invaluable support ensured smooth conference operations. I would also like to thank our media team, Katja Longhurst and Sallamaari Syrjä, for their excellent work in maintaining the conference's digital presence. My gratitude further extends to Minna Komu for her efforts in engaging industry partners, as well as to Oulu University Hospital and the Wellbeing Services County of North Ostrobothnia for their support in conference arrangements and for providing a rich and unique research environment.

Finally, I would like to thank all those who contributed to the success of NCDHWS 2026—whether as organizers, contributors, or participants.

June 2026

Jarmo Reponen

Preface

The Nordic Conference on Digital Health and Wireless Solutions (NCDHWS) is an international, multidisciplinary conference that brings together experts and professionals from engineering, medicine, and health sciences working at the intersection of digital health and wireless technologies. Following the successful inaugural conference in 2024, NCDHWS was organized for the second time, continuing its mission to foster interdisciplinary collaboration and advance innovative, impactful digital health solutions.

The organization of NCDHWS relies on close cooperation among multidisciplinary committees and a shared effort to harmonize the diverse scientific cultures and evaluation practices of different research fields. Consequently, the program committee chairs, organizing committee, program committee, and international advisory committee included representatives from a wide range of disciplines as well as from 32 different countries, reflecting the international and interdisciplinary nature of the conference.

The conference proceedings are published in a Springer CCIS Open Access book with three thematically organized volumes: *Volume I: Towards Trustworthy and Person-Centric Digital Health*, *Volume II: Integrating AI, LLMs and Multimodal Health Data for NextGeneration Decision Support*, and *Volume III: Connected Digital Health: Digital Twins, Wearables, Wireless Systems, and Secure Architectures.*

This Volume II focuses on AIenabled decision support and the integration of multimodal health data in digital health. The contributions examine datadriven and model-based approaches to clinical and operational decision support, multimodal data analysis, and the application of artificial intelligence, machine learning, and large language models in healthcare and social welfare settings. Several papers address clinical prediction, risk stratification, workflow optimization, and AIassisted documentation, alongside methodological advances in explainability, federated learning, and system architectures.

Emphasis is placed on tools that support healthcare professionals in clinical decisionmaking, as well as intelligent systems designed to inform, assist, and empower citizens and patients. The volume also addresses organizational, ethical, and regulatory perspectives, highlighting the importance of trustworthy, transparent, and humancentred design and deployment. Together, the contributions reflect both the transformative potential of AI in healthcare and the requirements for its responsible integration into realworld practice.

Reflecting varied publication practices across disciplines, the conference accepted three types of submissions: full papers (10–30 pages), short papers (5–9 pages), and abstracts (1–4 pages). Full and short papers are published in the main body of the Springer book and indexed, while abstracts appear in the back matter. In total, 159 submissions were received, including 90 full papers, 32 short papers, and 37 abstracts.

All submissions underwent a rigorous double-blind peer-review process involving approximately 190 international reviewers. Each full and short paper was evaluated by three to five reviewers with appropriate scientific expertise, while abstracts were reviewed by two to three reviewers. The EDAS platform was used for submission and review management, ensuring confidentiality and the automated handling of conflicts of interest. Reviewers assessed submissions using a five-point scoring scale, provided confidence levels, and offered detailed, constructive feedback. Final acceptance decisions were based on weighted average scores that incorporated reviewer confidence. Submissions with a rounded weighted average score of at least 3 ("marginally accept") were accepted, contingent upon authors revising their work in accordance with reviewers' comments. This revision requirement applied to all accepted papers. Plagiarism checks were conducted using the plagiarism detection tools integrated into EDAS, and authors were asked to take corrective action when similarity scores exceeded acceptable thresholds. EDAS also ensured confidentiality by preventing program committee chairs from accessing reviews of their own papers or from viewing reviewer identities. In total, 137 papers were accepted for publication, comprising 107 full and short papers and 30 abstracts.

We gratefully acknowledge the support of the Springer Nature team for their guidance and assistance throughout all practical aspects of the book publication process. We also extend our sincere thanks to all members of the conference committees, including the organizing committee, program committee, and international advisory committee, whose collective efforts made the organization of this multidisciplinary conference possible.

We would further like to thank the City of Oulu, European Capital of Culture 2026, for supporting the conference and for providing the opportunity to organize a get-together event at the Oulu City Hall, which greatly enriched the conference experience and facilitated informal networking and interaction among participants.

In addition, we express our deep appreciation to the keynote and invited speakers, who took time from their busy schedules to travel to Oulu and deliver inspiring presentations on their research. Finally, we sincerely thank all authors for choosing NCDHWS 2026 as a forum to present their research. Through the combination of high-quality contributed papers and excellent invited talks, this multidisciplinary gathering proved to be both productive and successful, fostering meaningful discussions and new opportunities for collaboration.

June 2026

Mariella Särestöniemi
Daljeet Singh
Erika Jarva
Jarmo Reponen

Organization

General Chairs (Conference President and Vice-president)

Jarmo Reponen	University of Oulu, Finland
Simo Saarakkala	University of Oulu, Finland

Program Committee Chairs

Mariella Särestöniemi (Chair)	University of Oulu, Finland
Daljeet Singh	University of Oulu, Finland
Erkki Harjula	University of Oulu, Finland
Minna Isomursu	University of Oulu, Finland
Miia Jansson	University of Oulu, Finland
Erika Jarva	University of Oulu, Finland
Mark van Gils	University of Tampere, Finland
Jarmo Reponen	University of Oulu, Finland
Johanna Uusimaa	University of Oulu, Finland
Johannes Kettunen	University of Oulu, Finland
Mika Martikainen	University of Oulu, Finland
Janne Hukkanen	University of Oulu, Finland
Ali Mobasheri	University of Oulu, Finland

Publication Chairs

Mariella Särestöniemi	University of Oulu, Finland
Daljeet Singh	University of Oulu, Finland
Erika Jarva	University of Oulu, Finland
Jarmo Reponen	University of Oulu, Finland

Organization Committee

Jarmo Reponen (Chair)	University of Oulu, Finland
Simo Saarakkala (Vice-chair)	University of Oulu, Finland
Chao Ding	University of Oulu, Finland
Tuire Salonurmi	University of Oulu, Finland

Mariella Särestöniemi	University of Oulu, Finland
Erkki Harjula	University of Oulu, Finland
Matti Hämäläinen	University of Oulu, Finland
Minna Isomursu	University of Oulu, Finland
Johanna Uusimaa	University of Oulu, Oulu University Hospital, Finland
Miia Jansson	University of Oulu, Finland
Salla Kangas	University of Oulu, Finland
Ritva Saastamoinen	University of Oulu, Finland
Essi Erkkilä	University of Oulu, Finland
Minna Komu	OuluHealth/BusinessOulu, Finland
Teija Kekonen	Oulu University Hospital, Finland
Elina Laukka	Oulu University of Applied Sciences, Finland
Mark van Gils	University of Tampere, Finland

Program Committee

Chew Han Shi (Jocelyn)	National University of Singapore, Singapore
Tam Wai San (Wilson)	National University of Singapore, Singapore
Raja Omman Zafar	Dalarna University, Sweden
Sarthak Acharya	University of Oulu, Finland
Ijaz Ahmad	VTT Technical Research Centre of Finland, Finland
Roni Ahola	University of Tampere, Finland
Outi Ahonen	Laurea University of Applied Sciences, Finland
Mika Alhonkoski	University of Turku, Finland
Slawomir Ambroziak	Gdańsk University of Technology, Poland
Ulla Ashorn	University of Turku, Finland
Aslak Aslaksen	Bergen University Hospital, Norway
Tunc Asuroglu	VTT Technical Research Centre of Finland, Finland
Himanshi Babbar	Chitkara University, India
Christian Becker	University of Stuttgart, Germany
Woubset Behutiye	University of Oulu, Finland
Gro Rosvold Berntsen	Norwegian Center for eHealth Research, Norway
Roberto Blanco	University of Turku, Finland
Mikael Brix	University of Oulu, Finland
Maria Bulgheroni	Ab.Acus srl, Italy
Stefano Caputo	University of Florence, Italy
Constantino Alvarez Casado	University of Oulu, Finland
Bhushan B. Chaudhari	SVKM's Institute of Technology, India

Wei Ling Chua	National University of Singapore, Singapore
Omedev Dahia	Galgotias University, India
Nils Dahlström	University of Linköping, Sweden
Livio Dalvia	Sapienza University of Rome, Italy
Aysen Degerli	VTT Technical Research Centre of Finland, Finland
Manish Deshwal	Chandigarh University, India
Satu Elo	Oulu University of Applied Sciences, Finland
Jeppe Eriksen	University of Aalborg, Denmark
Gökçe Banu Laleci Ertürkmen	Software Research & Development and Consultancy Corporation, Turkey
Shan Feng	University of Turku, Finland
Hany Ferdinando	University of Oulu, Finland
Dimitris Filos	Aristotle University of Thessaloniki, Greece
Huber Flores	University of Tartu, Estonia
Mark van Gils	University of Tampere, Finland
Heidi Gilstad	Norwegian University of Science and Technology, Norway
Guido Giunti	University of Oulu, Finland
Casandra Grundstrom	Norwegian University of Science and Technology, Norway
Ankur Gupta	Netaji Subhas University of Technology, India
Akhil Gupta	Symbiosis Institute of Technology, India
Sanaul Haque	LUT University, Lappeenranta, Finland
Erkki Harjula	University of Oulu, Finland
Nina Hautala	University of Oulu, Finland
Ying He	University of Technology Sydney, Australia
Tharaka Hewa	University of Oulu, Finland
Sari Huikko-Tarvainen	Medical Research Center Oulu, Finland
Krista Hylkilä	University of Oulu, Finland
Piia Hyvämäki	Oulu University of Applied Sciences, Finland
Matti Hämäläinen	University of Oulu, Finland
Minna Hökkä	Kajaani University of Applied Sciences, Finland
Iiris Hörhammer	Aalto University, Finland
Esa-Ville Immonen	University of Oulu, Finland
Milla Immonen	Lapland University of Applied Sciences, Finland
Antti Isosalo	University of Oulu, Finland
Erika Jarva	University of Oulu, Finland
Joel Jaskari	University of Tampere, Finland
Sara Jayousi	University of Florence, Italy
Vesa Jormanainen	University of Helsinki, Finland

Tarmo Lipping	University of Tampere, Finland
Tinja Lääveri	Aalto University, Finland
Bessie Malila	University of Johannesburg, South Africa
Andigoni Malousi	Aristotle University of Thessaloniki, Greece
Terence McSweeney	University of Oulu, Finland
Sharon Guardado Medina	University of Oulu, Finland
Heta Merikallio	University of Oulu, Finland
Nora Mickelson	University of Turku and Turku University Hospital, Finland
Kristina Mikkonen	University of Oulu, Finland
Ayan Mondal	Indian Institute of Technology Indore, India
Lorenzo Mucchi	University of Florence, Italy
Karla MunozEsquivel	Atlantic Technological University, Ireland
Joyce Mwangama	University of Cape Town, South Africa
Teemu Myllylä	University of Oulu, Finland
Vasiliki Mylonopoulou	University of Gothenburg, Sweden
Mariaana Mäki-Asiala	University of Oulu, Finland
Niko Männikkö	Oulu University of Applied Sciences, Finland
Tuija Männistö	University of Eastern Finland, Finland
My Nguyen	RMIT University, Australia
Marketta Niemelä	LAB University of Applied Sciences, Finland
Anne Oikarinen	University of Oulu, Finland
Diana Moya Osario	Linköping University, Sweden
Sofia Ouhbi	Uppsala University, Sweden
Hanna Paananen	University of Jyväskylä, Finland
Juha Pajari	University of Eastern Finland, Finland
Juha Pajula	VTT Technical Research Centre of Finland, Finland
Mika Paldanius	Oulu University of Applied Sciences, Finland
Ankur Pandley	Rajiv Gandhi Institute of Petroleum Technology, India
Egor Panfilov	University of Oulu, Finland
Lauri Parkkonen	Aalto University, Finland
Juha Partala	University of Oulu, Finland
Ella Peltonen	University of Oulu, Finland
Renu Popli	Chitkara University, India
Pawani Porambage	VTT Technical Research Centre of Finland, Finland
Tarja Pölkki	University of Oulu, Finland
Prabhat Ram	University of Oulu, Finland
Ahmad Rayani	King Saud University, Saudi Arabia
Jarmo Reponen	University of Oulu, Finland

Peeter Ross	Technical University of Tallinn, Estonia
Heidi Ruotsalainen	Oulu University of Applied Sciences, Finland
Rajkumar Saini	Luleå University of Technology, Sweden
Tuire Salonurmi	University of Oulu, Finland
Ama Samarasinghe	RMIT University, Australia
Pedro Moreno Sanchez	Tampere University, Finland
Laura Sandström	University of British Columbia, Canada
Daniel Pinto dos Santos	University Hospital of Cologne, Germany
Kaija Saranto	University of Eastern Finland, Finland
Kamran Sayrafian	National Institute of Standards and Technology, USA
Aleksi Schrey	University of Turku, Finland
Imran Shah	University of Oulu, Finland
Shallu Sharma	Bennett University, India
Stephan Sigg	Aalto University, Finland
Heidi Siira	University of Oulu, Finland
Pekka Siirtola	University of Oulu, Finland
Daljeet Singh	University of Oulu, Finland
Gurjinder Singh	Chitkara University, India
Eeva Sliz	University of Oulu, Finland
Anthony Smith	University of Queensland, Australia
Simone Soderi	IMT School for Advanced Studies Lucca, Italy
Jack Soh	University of Oulu, Finland
Mariella Säreströniemi	University of Oulu, Finland
Atthapongse Taparugssanagorn	Asian Institute of Technology, Thailand
Gianluigi Tiberi	London South Bank University, UK & UBT Srl, Italy
Jani Tikkanen	Kuura Health Ltd, Finland
Jussi-Pekka Tolonen	Oulu University Hospital, Finland
Paulus Torkki	University of Helsinki, Finland
Posco Tso	Loughborough University, UK
Annukka Tuomikoski	Northern Ostrobothnia Wellbeing Services County, Finland
Timo Tuovinen	University of Oulu, Finland
Delfin Tursin	University of Oulu, Finland
Shingo Ueki	Kyushu University, Japan
Johanna Uusimaa	University of Oulu, Finland
Minna Vanhanen	Oulu University of Applied Sciences, Finland
Sampsa Vanhatalo	University of Helsinki, Finland
Antti Vehkaoja	University of Tampere, Finland
Paula Veikkolainen	University of Oulu, Finland
Märt Vesinurm	Aalto University, Finland

Gillian Vesty	RMIT University, Australia
Johanna Viitanen	Aalto University, Finland
Sidsel Villumsen	University of Aalborg, Denmark
Mari Virtanen	Metropolia University of Applied Sciences, Finland
Anna-Leena Vuorinen	University of Tampere, Finland
Alpo Värri	University of Tampere, Finland
Fan Wang	University of Oulu, Finland
Zhou Wentao	National University of Singapore, Singapore
Brigitte Woo	National University of Singapore, Singapore
Xiaoting Wu	University of Oulu, Finland
Miyae Yamakawa	Osaka University, Japan
Rameem Zahra	Netaji Subhas University of Technology, India
Yingchun Zeng (Chloe)	National University of Singapore, Singapore
Aleksandra Zienkiewicz	University of Oulu, Finland
Ece Üreten	Delft University of Technology, Netherlands

International Advisory Committee

Najeeb Al-Shorbaji	eHealth Development Association, Jordan
Slawomir Ambroziak	Gdańsk University of Technology, Poland
D. K. Arvind	University of Edinburgh, UK
Rimma Axelsson	Karolinska Institutet, Sweden
Gro Rosvold Berntsen	Norwegian Centre for E-health Research, Norway
Paolo Bifulco	University Federico II of Naples, Italy
Paola Buedo	University of Munich, Germany
Filipe Cardonso	Polytechnic Institute of Setúbal, Portugal
Jessica Centracchio	University Federico II of Naples, Italy
Akshay Chaudhari	Stanford University, USA
Luis M. Correia	University of Lisbon, Portugal
Georg Dorffner	Medical University of Vienna, Austria
Sandra Dudley	London South Bank University, UK
Osama Elhassan	UAE Health Informatics Society, UAE
Flavio Esposito	Saint Louis University, USA
Simone Farah	UNIFASE/Petrópolis Faculty of Medicine, Brazil
Vahid Farrahi	TU Dortmund University, Germany
Michael Fuchsjäger	Medical University Graz, Austria
Mohammad Ghvami	London South Bank University, UK
Hassan Ghazal	Moroccan Society for Telemedicine and eHealth, Morocco

Michele Y. Griffith	International Society for Telemedicine and eHealth, USA
Ingfrid S. Haldorsen	Haukeland University Hospital, Norway
Clayton Hamilton	World Health Organization, Denmark
Manami Hori	Tokai University, Japan
Lars Hulbæk	MedCom, Denmark
Michael Inouye	University of Cambridge, UK
Vesa Jormanainen	Ministry of Social Affairs and Health, Finland
Dipak Kalra	European Institute for Innovation through Health Data, Belgium
Ulla-Mari Kinnunen	University of Eastern Finland, Finland
Hiroshi Kondoh	Tottori University, Japan
Ilkka Korhonen	University of Tampere, Finland
Elisabeth A. Krupinski	Emory University, USA
Line Helen Linstad	Norwegian Centre for E-health Research, Norway
Anthony Maeder	Flinders University, Australia
Janne Martikainen	University of Eastern Finland, Finland
Lorenzo Mucchi	University of Florence, Italy
Miika Nieminen	University of Oulu, Finland
Jérôme Noailly	University of Pompeu Fabra, Spain
Aud Uhlen Obstfelder	Norwegian University of Science and Technology, Norway
Peter van Ooijen	University Medical Center Groningen, Netherlands
Kaija Saranto	University of Eastern Finland, Finland
Kamran Sayrafian	National Institute of Standards and Technology, USA
Päivi Sillanaukee	Ministry of Social Affairs and Health, Finland
Piotr H. Skarzynski	Institute of Physiology and Pathology of Hearing, Poland
Anthony Smith	University of Queensland, Australia
Attaphongse Taparugssanagorn	Asian Institute of Technology, Thailand
Rosanna Tarricone	Bocconi University, Italy
Gianluigi Tiberi	Umbria Bioengineering Technologies, Italy
Paulus Torkki	University of Helsinki, Finland
Yoshito Tsushima	Gunma University, Japan
Gillian Vesty	RMIT University, Australia
Johanna Viitanen	Aalto University, Finland
Anssi Ylimaula	OunasHealth, Finland

Contents

Abstracts

Data-Driven and Modelling-Based Decision Support and Multimodal Health Data Analysis

A Multi-filter and Multi-scale U-Net for Cone-Beam Computed Tomography

Mustafa Al-Rubaye[1(✉)], Andreas Hauptmann[2,3], Miika T. Nieminen[1,4], and Mikael A. K. Brix[1,4]

[1] Research Unit of Health Sciences and Technology, University of Oulu, Oulu, Finland
Mustafa.Al-Rubaye@oulu.fi
[2] Research Unit of Mathematical Sciences, University of Oulu, Oulu, Finland
[3] Department of Computer Science, University College London, London, UK
[4] Department of Diagnostic Radiology, Oulu University Hospital, Oulu, Finland

Abstract. Efficient 3D cone-beam computed tomography (CBCT) reconstructions typically demand substantial hardware capabilities for both training and execution. This paper introduces a multi-filter and multi-scale U-Net (mU-Net) architecture designed for post-processing CBCT images by incorporating multiple input channels, each processed with distinct frequency filters or reconstruction resolutions. We present a detailed comparison between the mU-Net and a baseline U-Net for low-dose and clinical dose denoising scenarios, reporting key metrics such as Peak Signal-to-Noise Ratio (PSNR), Structural Similarity Index Measure (SSIM), and inference time. The mU-Net showed only marginal quantitative differences compared with the baseline U-Net: it performed slightly better in the clinical dose scenario, while the baseline U-Net performed better in the low-dose scenario. The mU-Net required approximately 13% more time per epoch during training and 13.08 s per volume for FDK reconstruction and inference, compared with 10.43 s per volume for the baseline U-Net. In the clinical dose scenario, the mU-Net showed slightly improved visual noise texture and artifact suppression, but these observations were not supported by dedicated texture or observer-study metrics. Notably, the mU-Net and baseline U-Net approaches placed 3rd in the ICASSP 2024 3D-CBCT grand challenge, demonstrating that a properly trained U-Net remains competitive. This study shows that multi-filter and multi-scale inputs can be used for CBCT post-processing under limited computational resources, but the gains over a baseline U-Net were modest.

Keywords: Cone-beam Computed Tomography · Deep Learning · U-Net · Denoising · Learned Reconstruction

1 Introduction

Cone-beam computed tomography (CBCT) is widely used in clinical and research settings for 3D imaging. However, CBCT images often suffer from noise

M. Särestöniemi et al. (Eds.): NCDHWS 2026, CCIS 3010, pp. 3–18, 2026.
https://doi.org/10.1007/978-3-032-28819-6_1

and artifacts, which are further exacerbated by the geometry of the cone-beam, subsequently degrading the image quality. CBCT reconstruction is modeled as a three-dimensional problem, leading to higher memory requirements and computation times compared to helical CT reconstruction [22], which can typically be treated two-dimensionally through z-interpolation [11]. Full statistical iterative reconstruction (IR) methods include repeated forward and backprojection operations, which necessitate more computational power, *i.e.*, more graphics processing unit (GPU) memory and clock speed, for CBCT as the forward model simulates a three-dimensional acquisition geometry. Consequently, the use of IR for CBCT is still limited [22], and the computationally inexpensive analytical Feldkamp-Davis-Kress (FDK) algorithm is commonly used [4]. Owing to this inherent challenge with CBCT reconstruction, projection data preprocessing or post-processing methods are investigated to achieve enhanced noise reduction and diagnostically feasible computation times [14,22]. A comprehensive review of the latest commercially used techniques is available in [10].

In the context of the FDK algorithm, the initial reconstruction of CBCT projection data (y) is achieved using:

$$x_{\text{rec}} = \mathcal{F}y. \tag{1}$$

where $\mathcal{F} : y \mapsto x$ represents the FDK algorithm.

If y is undersampled or noisy, the reconstructions x_{rec} will exhibit artifacts. Additionally, the cone-beam geometry introduces further artifacts in areas where only a partial set of rays passes through the target. Hence, improving the reconstructions obtained by (1) is essential. One effective method is to use a post-processing network Λ_θ, such as a convolutional neural network (CNN) with parameters θ, trained to enhance the initial reconstructions x_{rec} by mitigating artifacts and noise.

The U-Net architecture [16] has been particularly successful for this task. Instead of using a basic U-Net that learns features independently, guiding the network's learning with inputs processed by multiple frequency-level filters may be more effective. This approach involves applying different frequency cut-offs to the initial FDK reconstructions, offering a richer set of features for the network. Processing inputs with multiple frequency-level filters can enhance the network's ability to capture a broader range of image features, potentially improving reconstruction quality. This method leverages frequency-domain information to distinguish between different types of artifacts and noise. In contrast, a basic U-Net might be simpler to implement but may not fully utilize the information in multi-frequency inputs. Guiding the U-Net with pre-processed inputs could streamline learning and improve efficiency.

In this paper, we propose an approach to enhance network performance by providing a more informative input to the post-processing network, inspired by [5]. We achieve this by performing a multi-filter FDK reconstruction using several frequency cut-offs for the frequency filter. Additionally, we leverage the discretisation invariance of the ray transform to create initial reconstructions on multiple scales, similar to [5]. This approach should provide richer information to the network, simplifying the learning task.

In summary, our contributions are the development of a multi-filter and multi-scale U-Net approach for CBCT image denoising, evaluation of the approach under memory constraints using a single GPU workstation, and demonstration of slight improvements in reconstruction quality when applied for denoising clinical dose image data.

The proposed multi-filter and multi-scale U-Net (mU-Net) and a baseline U-Net were submitted to the reconstruction challenge and achieved 3rd place.

1.1 Related Work

Denoising and artifact reduction in CBCT images have been extensively studied, with various approaches proposed to enhance image quality. Traditional methods often rely on iterative reconstruction techniques, such as those based on total variation minimization [18]. While effective, these methods can be computationally expensive and time-consuming.

Recent advances in deep learning have led to the development of CNNs for image denoising and enhancement. The U-Net architecture [16], originally designed for biomedical image segmentation, has been adapted for denoising tasks due to its ability to capture multi-scale features through its encoder-decoder structure. Variants of U-Net, including residual U-Net and 3D U-Net [3], have shown promise in medical image processing.

Multi-scale approaches have been explored to improve network performance by incorporating information at different resolutions. For instance, [7] proposed a multi-scale residual learning framework for image denoising, which demonstrated enhanced performance by leveraging features at various scales.

Additionally, multiple reconstructions have been employed to provide richer input representations. Hauptmann et al. [5] introduced a multi-scale iterative approach for tomographic reconstruction, utilizing reconstructions on different scales and iterations to improve image quality. Inspired by this method, we obtain multiple reconstructions by utilizing different frequency filters to create multi-filter and multi-scale inputs to train a more effective post-processing network.

The use of low-dose imaging has been a focus of several studies due to the need to optimize radiation exposure. Techniques such as transfer learning and domain adaptation have been employed to enhance low-dose image reconstructions by leveraging high-dose data [12].

Our work builds upon these advancements by integrating multi-filter and multi-scale techniques within a U-Net architecture to address the challenges of CBCT image denoising under memory constraints. By providing a comprehensive evaluation and comparison with baseline methods, we aim to compare the effectiveness of our approach against a baseline U-Net in improving image quality while maintaining computational efficiency.

2 Materials and Methods

We proposed a multi-filter and multi-scale U-Net (mU-Net) architecture to enhance the reconstruction of 3D cone-beam computed tomography (CBCT) images. The post-processing network was trained on initial reconstructions using a combination of multiple inputs processed with different frequency filters and scales.

2.1 Description of the Data

The dataset utilized in this study comprised 1008 patient examinations derived from the Lung Image Database Consortium image collection (LIDC-IDRI) [13] dataset, which features chest fan beam computed tomography (CT) scans focused on lung nodule analysis. These images were used as ground truth for the simulation of Cone Beam Computed Tomography (CBCT) sinograms, generated using the ASTRA toolbox [19]. It is important to note that the term "ground truth" in this context refers to an over-sampled, high-dose reconstruction.

The data used in this study were obtained from the ICASSP-2024 3D-CBCT challenge [2]. These datasets were generated by the challenge organizers. To accommodate the dataset size requirements, the challenge organizers produced simplified simulations. These simulations, together with a basic flat-field correction and scatter simulator, included photon, electronic, and quantification noise models to approximate real scanner noise. The dataset contained data corresponding to two dose levels: one at 100% clinical dose and the other at 10% of the clinical dose.

The dataset was divided into three subsets: 799 samples for training, 100 samples for validation, and 109 samples for testing. The training and validation datasets were used to set the hyperparameters, and the test data were then used to test the performance of the model on new unseen data. Each dataset included three types of images: Ground Truth, which are over-sampled, high-dose reconstructions; Clinical Dose, consisting of reconstructions with noise levels typical of clinical settings; and Low Dose, featuring reconstructions with 10% of the clinical dose noise levels.

2.2 Data Pre-processing

The data pre-processing step was crucial for preparing the CBCT scans for training the U-Net. This process involved defining the geometry of the CBCT scan, creating reconstruction operators, and generating multiple reconstructions with various frequency filters. This step was computed in advance to save GPU memory usage during the U-Net training. In total, 360 projections were simulated with a constant angular increment from a range of 0 to 2π. The volume and cone-beam geometries were created using the Tomosipo library (0.6.0) [6] in Python (3.11.5) [20]. The Python environment was compiled with GCC 11.2.0 and executed on a Linux operating system. Operators for full ($256 \times 256 \times 256$) and half-resolution ($128 \times 128 \times 128$) volumes were defined. For each projection data, the FDK algorithm was applied using the defined operators to generate initial reconstructions. The Ram-Lak filter was adjusted to create multiple frequency cut-offs, which were then used to generate different reconstructions. These reconstructions were concatenated to form multi-scale inputs. Specifically, the filter was adjusted to produce 10 different frequency cut-offs as follows.

The frequency cut-offs were created by progressively zeroing out parts of the Ram-Lak filter to limit the frequency range. For example, the filter range was divided into 10 equal segments, and progressively higher segments were set to zero. This resulted in a set of reconstructions that captured different frequency bands of the original data.

We selected four specific cut-offs from these 10 different filters corresponding to indices 1, 6, 8, and 10. These indices were chosen because the resulting images were the most distinct from each other, providing the network with a diverse and informative set of different inputs. This multi-scale input was structured as a $256 \times 256 \times 256 \times 4$ tensor for full-scale and $128 \times 128 \times 128 \times 4$ for downscaled reconstructions, where the first three dimensions represented the spatial dimensions of the reconstruction, and the fourth dimension represented the number of different reconstructions with various filters. The model took input images at two scales: full-scale and downscaled. These reconstructions allowed the network to utilize the diverse information from the multiple scales and filters. The processed reconstructions were saved in the specified directory for later use in training.

For the baseline U-Net, the input was a single FDK reconstruction without frequency cutoff in the reconstruction filter. The input was structured as a $256 \times 256 \times 256 \times 1$ tensor. This tensor represented the spatial dimensions of the reconstruction and provided the baseline network with the same volume dimensions as the multi-scale inputs but without the additional multi-frequency filter information.

2.3 Network Architecture

Both U-Nets in this study comprised several convolutional layers, group normalization, and ReLU activations (Fig. 1). The network included downsampling and upsampling layers to capture and reconstruct high-resolution features effectively. Specifically, the network was structured as follows:

- The initial layer performed a double convolution on the input, followed by group normalization with group size 8 and ReLU activation. This setup ensured that the initial features were extracted effectively and normalized for stable training.
- The downsampling path included multiple stages, each consisting of double convolutions with increasing filter sizes. After each convolutional block, a max-pooling layer was applied to reduce the spatial dimensions and retain important features while discarding redundant information.
- The upsampling path mirrored the downsampling path but in reverse. It utilized 3D transposed convolution operators for upsampling, which increased

the spatial dimensions of the feature maps. After each upsampling operation, double convolution layers were applied to refine the features and enhance the reconstruction.
- The final layer combined the upsampled features and performed a convolution to generate the output. This layer synthesized the high-resolution output from the refined features obtained through the upsampling path.

Baseline U-Net. The baseline U-Net followed the structure mentioned above with the following specifics:

- The input was a single FDK reconstruction structured as a $256 \times 256 \times 256 \times 1$ tensor. This tensor represented the spatial dimensions of the reconstruction and provided the baseline network with the necessary volume dimensions.
- The downsampling path included stages with filter sizes 16, 64, 128, and 256. Each stage was followed by a max-pooling layer to reduce the feature map size.
- The upsampling path used 3D transposed convolution operators with filter sizes decreasing from 256, 128, 64, to 32. After each upsampling operation, double convolution layers were applied to refine the features.
- The final convolutional layer generated the output by combining the upsampled features.
- During the forward pass, the input was processed through the downsampling path, and the extracted features were then upsampled and refined to produce the final output.
- A learnable parameter called `stepsize` adjusted the step size during the update process, allowing for fine-tuning of the final output.

Multi-filter and Multi-scale U-Net. The multi-filter and multi-scale U-Net (mU-Net) extended the baseline U-Net by incorporating multiple scales and filters to provide a richer set of features:

- Similar to the baseline U-Net, the initial layer performed a double convolution on the input, followed by group normalization and ReLU activation.
- The downsampling path included stages with filter sizes 16, 64, 128, and 256. Each stage was followed by a max-pooling layer to reduce the feature map size.
- In addition to the standard downsampling path, the mU-Net concatenated inputs processed through different frequency cut-offs. This allowed the network to leverage a diverse set of features from multiple scales and filters.
- The upsampling path mirrored the downsampling path, utilizing 3D transposed convolution operators to increase the spatial dimensions of the feature maps, followed by double convolution layers to refine the features.
- The final layer combined the upsampled features and performed a convolution to generate the output.

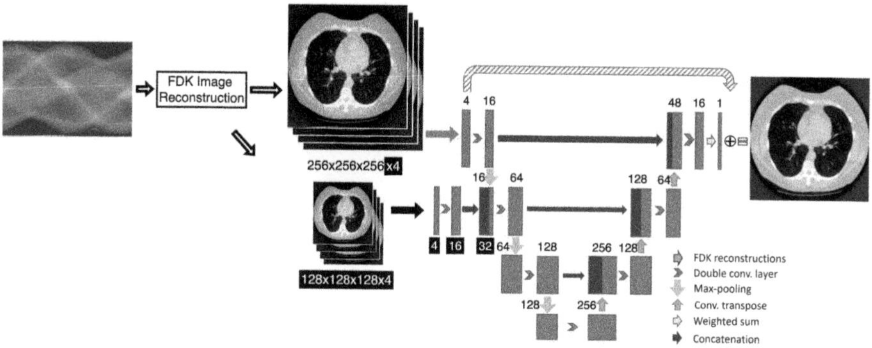

Fig. 1. Projection data are reconstructed using the FDK algorithm with four different frequency cut-offs. The multi-filter and multi-scale U-Net (shown in white font) processes input images at both full-scale ($256 \times 256 \times 256$) and downscaled ($128 \times 128 \times 128$) resolutions. The baseline U-Net uses a single reconstruction ($256 \times 256 \times 256$).

- During the forward pass, the input was processed through the downsampling path, and additional inputs processed through different frequency cut-offs were concatenated. The combined features were then upsampled and refined to produce the final output.
- A learnable parameter called `stepsize` adjusted the step size during the update process, allowing for fine-tuning of the final output.

The network was designed to handle multiple scales and filters by using concatenated inputs processed through different frequency cut-offs. This approach allowed the network to utilize a richer set of features, potentially improving reconstruction quality.

2.4 Training Procedure

The networks were trained on a single 24 GB GPU using the Adam optimizer with a learning rate of 1×10^{-4} (Table 1). The training and validation datasets included ground truth images, initial reconstructions, and additional reconstructions processed with different frequency filters. The mean squared error (MSE) loss was used to measure the difference between the network output and the ground truth. The network parameters were optimized using the Adam optimizer with a cosine annealing learning rate schedule. The GradScaler was employed for mixed-precision training to improve computational efficiency. The network was trained for 100 epochs, with each iteration involving forward and backward passes, gradient updates, and loss computation.

Table 1. Summary of the trained networks.

Experiment	Description
1	mU-Net: low-dose → high-dose
2	mU-Net: clinical-dose → high-dose
3	Baseline U-Net: low-dose → high-dose
4	Baseline U-Net: clinical-dose → high-dose

2.5 Validation and Evaluation

The validation process involved evaluating the trained network on a separate validation dataset. Key metrics such as Peak Signal-to-Noise Ratio (PSNR), Structural Similarity Index Measure (SSIM), and the MSE loss function were computed to assess the reconstruction quality. The network performed inference on the validation data, generating reconstructed images. These metrics were used to adjust hyperparameters, ensuring optimal performance.

An early stopping mechanism was implemented at epoch 43 after the values of PSNR, SSIM, and the loss did not improve for 5 consecutive epochs. Once the hyperparameters were fixed based on the validation data, the final evaluation was conducted using the test dataset to determine the network's performance. The results from the test data were compared with the ground truth to evaluate the effectiveness of the mU-Net.

3 Results

This section presents the quantitative and qualitative results of our mU-Net architecture for 3D CBCT reconstruction. We compared the performance of our proposed method with the baseline U-Net across different metrics and dose levels.

3.1 Low-Dose to High-Dose Comparison

The mU-Net architecture yielded slightly inferior PSNR and MSE values compared to the baseline U-Net, as shown in Table 2. Based on visual assessment, the noise grain size increased with the mU-Net, and the resolution was slightly poorer compared to the baseline U-Net.

Table 2. Results for the baseline U-Net and the multi-filter and multi-scale U-Net when using low-dose input.

Metrics	Baseline U-Net (Low)	mU-Net (Low)
mean PSNR	37.40 ± 2.12	36.40 ± 2.03
min PSNR	31.59	30.77
max PSNR	45.82	44.56
mean SSIM	0.92 ± 0.03	0.91 ± 0.03
min SSIM	0.81	0.81
max SSIM	0.97	0.97

The visual assessment (Fig. 2) indicated that the baseline U-Net produced clearer images with finer noise grain compared to the mU-Net. The differences were subtle, but the baseline U-Net consistently showed better resolution and artifact suppression.

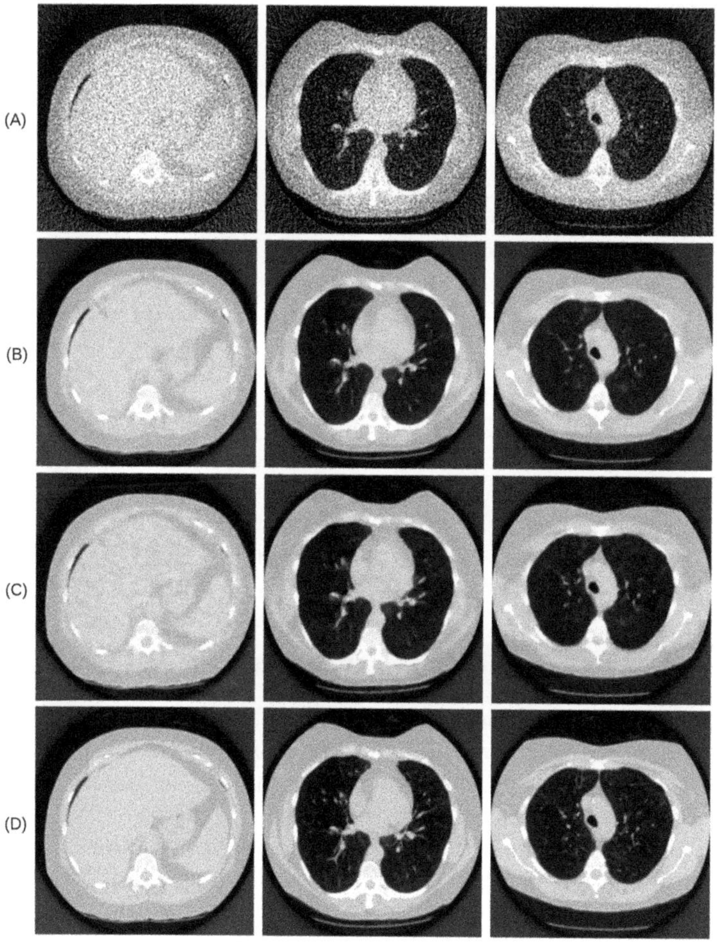

Fig. 2. Comparison of reconstructed (A) low-dose input images, (B) baseline U-Net, (C) mU-Net, and (D) ground truth. The arrow indicates a region where the difference in noise texture between the networks is observable.

3.2 Clinical-Dose to High-Dose Comparison

The mU-Net architecture produced slightly higher mean PSNR and SSIM values than the baseline U-Net when using clinical-dose input (Table 3); however, no statistical significance testing was performed. The mean PSNR and SSIM values were marginally higher for the mU-Net, indicating better structural preservation in the reconstructions.

Table 3. Results for the baseline U-Net and the multi-filter and multi-scale U-Net when using clinical-dose input.

Metrics	Baseline U-Net (Clinical)	mU-Net (Clinical)
mean PSNR	39.82 ± 2.31	39.98 ± 2.29
min PSNR	34.07	33.93
max PSNR	48.59	48.72
mean SSIM	0.94 ± 0.02	0.95 ± 0.18
min SSIM	0.85	0.89
max SSIM	0.99	0.99

The visual comparison in Fig. 3 highlighted the ability of the mU-Net to reduce artifacts and noise more effectively than the baseline U-Net. At the clinical dose setting, the mU-Net reconstructions exhibited reduced noise in the liver region (both with regards to noise magnitude and smaller grain size), overall clearer anatomical structures, and fewer artifacts, corroborating the quantitative improvements observed. When evaluated subjectively, the visibility of lung nodules was comparable for both U-Nets.

3.3 Comparison of Computation Time and Memory Usage

In addition to evaluating the reconstruction quality, it was crucial to compare the computation time and memory usage of the baseline U-Net and the proposed mU-Net. These factors are particularly important in clinical settings where computational resources may be limited.

The computation time for both networks was measured during the training and inference phases. Training time included the time taken for forward and backward passes over the entire training dataset per epoch, while total processing time was measured as the combined time required for both the FDK reconstruction and inference. Table 4 presents the average computation times for the baseline U-Net and the mU-Net.

The results indicated that the mU-Net required approximately 12.93% more time per epoch during training compared to the baseline U-Net. However, the total processing time for the mU-Net was nearly 25.3% higher than the baseline U-Net due to the additional reconstruction time needed for the multiple FDK inputs.

Memory usage is a critical factor, especially when operating under hardware constraints. The memory consumption of both networks was measured during the training and inference phases. The mU-Net exhibited only slightly higher

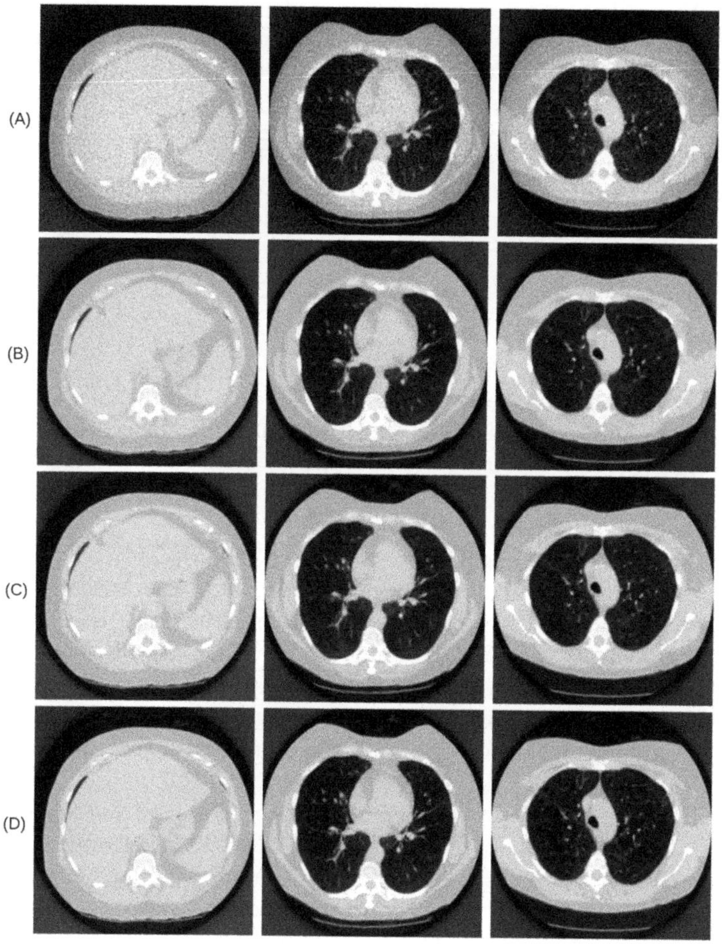

Fig. 3. Comparison of reconstructed (A) clinical-dose input images, (B) baseline U-Net, (C) mU-Net, and (D) ground truth. The arrow indicates a region where the difference in noise texture between the networks is observable.

memory footprint compared to the baseline U-Net, with an increase of approximately 5.37% during training and 1.39% during inference (Table 4).

4 Discussion

The results highlighted that a well-trained multi-filter and multi-scale U-Net (mU-Net) could deliver comparable or improved results to a baseline U-Net. While the proposed U-Net architecture achieved competitive results, particularly in the clinical dose scenario, the differences in performance compared to the baseline were quite minimal. Our proposed mU-Net architecture demonstrated

Table 4. Comparison of computation time and memory usage. Training time is reported per epoch. Total time includes FDK reconstruction and inference per volume. The baseline U-Net requires one FDK reconstruction, while the mU-Net requires multiple (N = 8).

Method	Training (s/epoch)	Total Time (s/volume)	Training Memory (GB)	Inference Memory (GB)
Baseline U-Net	6516.40	10.43	22.35	8.64
mU-Net	7359.81	13.08	23.55	8.76

slightly inferior performance in terms of PSNR and MSE values compared to the baseline U-Net when using low-dose input data. However, the architecture showed slightly higher mean PSNR and SSIM values than the baseline U-Net when using clinical-dose input data, although the practical and statistical significance of these differences remains unclear.

The visual assessment highlighted that while the mU-Net could reduce artifacts and noise more effectively in clinical dose scenarios, the baseline U-Net performed better in low-dose scenarios, with the differences being more pronounced. A properly trained U-Net and the multi-scale variant are still competitive, as indicated by the challenge, where our implementation achieved 3rd place. Given the higher computational cost and memory usage, the marginal gains may not justify the implementation of the multi-filter and multi-scale approach in all clinical settings.

Several factors might have contributed to the observed outcomes. Primarily, the mU-Net exhibited slightly inferior PSNR and MSE values compared to the baseline U-Net when using low-dose input data. This may be related to the high-noise regime of the low-dose input, where concatenating multiple filtered and multi-scale inputs may also propagate noise patterns that the network cannot fully suppress with the current channel capacity. The limited channel size in the full-resolution scales likely restricted the network's ability to fully utilize the increased information provided by the multi-filter approach. This constraint suggested that while the mU-Net could process more diverse input features, it might require more extensive channel capacity to leverage these features effectively at higher resolutions.

The comparison of computation time and memory usage revealed that the mU-Net required approximately 12.93% more time per epoch during training compared to the baseline U-Net, with a slightly higher memory footprint during both training and inference. The increased training time could be attributed to the additional complexity introduced by the multi-scale and multi-filter inputs. Similarly, the inference time for the mU-Net was higher due to the additional processing required for the enhanced input features. As the multi-scale method required several FDK reconstructions, the total reconstruction and denoising time of the mU-Net exceeded that of the baseline U-Net, which required only one input reconstruction with a sharp reconstruction filter. The comparison highlighted the trade-offs between reconstruction quality and computational efficiency. While the mU-Net might incrementally improve image quality in some scenarios, it came at the cost of increased computation time and memory usage. These factors underscored the importance of optimizing network architecture to balance performance improvements with computational efficiency.

These investigative results indicated only incremental differences between the mU-Net and a traditional U-Net. Future work should focus on exploring these aspects in greater detail, potentially adjusting the network's channel sizes and other hyperparameters to better harness the multi-scale information. Additionally, conducting comprehensive ablation studies at full resolution would be crucial for understanding the potential performance gains and optimizing the architecture accordingly. This would involve fine-tuning the network to effectively handle the increased information from multiple frequency filters, thus enhancing image quality while maintaining feasible computation times and memory usage in clinical applications.

Additionally, evaluating other metrics than SSIM and PSNR could provide a more comprehensive assessment of the network's performance. These additional evaluations could help in identifying subtle differences in reconstruction quality that might not be detected by the aforementioned metrics alone. In particular, the larger noise grain size, reported for mU-Net in the low dose scenario and baseline U-Net for the clinical dose, could be quantitatively characterized using noise power spectrum (NPS) assessment. The NPS is routinely used in CT quality assurance, and it captures the frequency distribution of noise and thus changes in texture [9,21]. Additionally, evaluating the modulation transfer function (MTF) or task-transfer function (TTF) [8,15,17] would provide quantitative information on the observed sharpness and resolution. These metrics (NPS, MTF, TTF) would bridge the quantitative image quality results closer to qualitative image quality preferences and towards actual observer models [1,21].

The proposed approach also opened up avenues for further optimization and application across various medical imaging challenges. Investigating the scalability of the mU-Net to other imaging modalities and different clinical scenarios could prove beneficial, given the promising results observed in the CBCT domain. Future work should focus on further optimizing the mU-Net to reduce computational overhead without compromising reconstruction quality. In addition, because the present evaluation was performed on simulated challenge data derived from CT scans, validation on real CBCT data is needed before drawing stronger conclusions about clinical applicability. Exploring techniques such as model pruning, quantization, and more efficient network architectures could help achieve this balance, making the approach more feasible for clinical applications with limited resources.

5 Conclusion

In this paper, we compared the use of a baseline U-Net and a mU-Net architecture aimed at enhancing 3D CBCT image reconstructions under hardware constraints. Our approach demonstrated that the mU-Net provided slightly different (and in some cases better) performance than the baseline U-Net, particularly in the clinical dose scenario. However, it is important to consider whether the performance difference is significant enough to counterbalance the increased computation time.

The key findings from our study were as follows:

- The mU-Net architecture could effectively enhance reconstruction quality when operating under limited GPU memory conditions, showing competitive performance with the baseline U-Net in clinical dose scenarios.
- The architecture demonstrated slightly inferior performance in terms of PSNR and MSE values compared to the baseline U-Net when using low-dose input data, likely due to increased noise grain size and slightly poorer resolution.
- At full resolution, the baseline U-Net slightly outperformed the mU-Net, indicating the need for further optimization of the network's architecture to fully leverage the multi-scale inputs.
- The mU-Net required approximately 12.93% more time per epoch during training compared to the baseline U-Net, with a slightly higher memory footprint during both training and inference.
- Inference times were crucial in clinical applications. The mU-Net required approximately 13.08 s per volume during inference and FDK reconstruction, which was slower than the baseline U-Net's 10.43 s per volume.

Despite these constraints, the mU-Net architecture showed only modest potential for improving image quality, mainly in the clinical-dose scenario, under limited computational resources.

Future work will focus on optimizing the full-resolution network architecture, conducting extensive ablation studies, and exploring additional metrics such as NPS, MTF, or TTF for a more nuanced evaluation. We also plan to extend this approach to other medical imaging modalities and clinical scenarios, aiming to generalize the benefits observed in CBCT reconstructions.

In conclusion, the mU-Net presented a viable solution for improving 3D CBCT reconstructions, especially in resource-constrained environments, and may hold promise for broader applications in medical imaging.

Acknowledgements. The author thanks Professor Tristan van Leeuwen, Dr. Alexander Skorikov, and Dr. Richard Schoonhoven for their technical support and invaluable guidance during a research visit to Centrum Wiskunde & Informatica (CWI). Their expertise and assistance greatly contributed to the progress of this work.

This work was supported by Business Finland (Project No. 8095/31/2022) and by the Research Council of Finland (Flagship of Advanced Mathematics for Sensing, Imaging and Modelling (FAME), Project No. 359186).

Disclosure of Interests. The authors have no competing interests to declare that are relevant to the content of this article.

References

1. Beutel, J., et al.: Handbook of medical imaging. volumes 1 3. Physics Today - PHYS TODAY **54** (2001)
2. Challenge, I..S.D.C.: Icassp-2024 3d-cbct challenge (2024). https://sites.google.com/view/icassp2024-spgc-3dcbct/home. Accessed 24 July 2024
3. Çiçek, Ö., Abdulkadir, A., Lienkamp, S.S., Brox, T., Ronneberger, O.: 3D U-Net: learning dense volumetric segmentation from sparse annotation. In: Ourselin, S., Joskowicz, L., Sabuncu, M.R., Unal, G., Wells, W. (eds.) MICCAI 2016. LNCS, vol. 9901, pp. 424–432. Springer, Cham (2016). https://doi.org/10.1007/978-3-319-46723-8_49
4. Feldkamp, L., Davis, L., Kress, J.: Practical cone-beam algorithm. Josa a **1**(6), 612–619 (1984)
5. Hauptmann, A., Adler, J., Arridge, S., Öktem, O.: Multi-scale learned iterative reconstruction (2020)
6. Hendriksen, A., et al.: Tomosipo: fast, flexible, and convenient 3D tomography for complex scanning geometries in Python. Optics Express (2021). https://doi.org/10.1364/oe.439909
7. Hu, X., Mu, H., Zhang, X., Wang, Z., Li, Z., Tan, T.: Multi-scale residual network for image super-resolution. In: Proceedings of the IEEE Conference on Computer Vision and Pattern Recognition Workshops. IEEE (2018). https://doi.org/10.1109/CVPRW.2018.00009
8. Juntunen, M., Kotiaho, A., Nieminen, M., Inkinen, S.: Optimizing iterative reconstruction for quantification of calcium hydroxyapatite with photon counting flat-detector computed tomography: a cardiac phantom study. J. Med. Imaging **8** (2021). https://doi.org/10.1117/1.JMI.8.5.052102
9. Juntunen, M.A.K., Rautiainen, J., Hänninen, N.E., Kotiaho, A.O.: Harmonization of technical image quality in computed tomography: comparison between different reconstruction algorithms and kernels from six scanners. Biomed. Phys. Eng. Express **8**(3), 037002 (2022). https://doi.org/10.1088/2057-1976/ac605b
10. Kaasalainen, T., Ekholm, M., Siiskonen, T., Kortesniemi, M.: Dental cone beam ct: An updated review. Physica Medica **88**, 193–217 (2021). https://doi.org/10.1016/j.ejmp.2021.07.007, https://www.sciencedirect.com/science/article/pii/S1120179721002519
11. Kalender, W.: Computed Tomography: Fundamentals, System Technology, Image Quality, Applications, vol. 33 (2005)
12. Kang, E., Min, J., Ye, J.C.: A deep convolutional neural network using directional wavelets for low-dose x-ray CT reconstruction. Med. Phys. **45**(12), e360–e373 (2018). https://doi.org/10.1002/mp.13036
13. Mader, K.S.: The lung image database consortium image collection (lidc-idri) (2021). https://doi.org/10.21227/zce3-jp96
14. Planmeca: Planmeca aino (2024). https://www.planmeca.com/fi/kuvantaminen/kktt-kuvaus/planmeca-aino. Accessed 24 July 2024
15. Richard, S., Husarik, D., Yadava, G., Murphy, S., Samei, E.: Towards task-based assessment of CT performance: system and object MTF across different reconstruction algorithms. Med. Phys. **39**, 4115–22 (2012). https://doi.org/10.1118/1.4725171
16. Ronneberger, O., Fischer, P., Brox, T.: U-Net: convolutional networks for biomedical image segmentation. In: Navab, N., Hornegger, J., Wells, W.M., Frangi, A.F. (eds.) MICCAI 2015. LNCS, vol. 9351, pp. 234–241. Springer, Cham (2015). https://doi.org/10.1007/978-3-319-24574-4_28

17. Samei, E., et al.: Performance evaluation of computed tomography systems: Summary of AAPM task group 233. Med. Phys. **46** (2019). https://doi.org/10.1002/mp.13763
18. Sidky, E.Y., Pan, X.: Image reconstruction in circular cone-beam computed tomography by constrained, total-variation minimization. Phys. Med. Biol. **53**(17), 4777–4807 (2008). https://doi.org/10.1088/0031-9155/53/17/021
19. van Aarle, W., et al.: The astra toolbox: a platform for advanced algorithm development in electron tomography. Ultramicroscopy **157**, 35–47 (2015). https://doi.org/10.1016/j.ultramic.2015.05.002,https://www.sciencedirect.com/science/article/pii/S0304399115001060
20. Van Rossum, G., Drake Jr, F.L.: Python reference manual. Centrum voor Wiskunde en Informatica Amsterdam (1995)
21. Verdun, F., et al.: Image quality in CT: from physical measurements to model observers. Physica Medica **31**(8), 823–843 (2015). https://doi.org/10.1016/j.ejmp.2015.08.007, https://www.sciencedirect.com/science/article/pii/S1120179715003294
22. Ylisiurua, S., Sipola, A., Nieminen, M.T., Brix, M.A.: Deep learning enables time-efficient soft tissue enhancement in CBCT: proof-of-concept study for dentomaxillofacial applications. Physica Medica **117**, 103184 (2024). https://doi.org/10.1016/j.ejmp.2023.103184, https://www.sciencedirect.com/science/article/pii/S1120179723012127

Computer Vision-Based Breast Volume Quantification Using Digital Mammography Data with Manual Measurement Validation

Katariina Kilpivaara[1,2](✉), Antti Isosalo[3,4], Pasi Ohtonen[1,2,5], Pieta Ipatti[1,2,6], Miika T. Nieminen[2,3,6], Terhi Piltonen[7], and Tero Rautio[1,2]

[1] Oulu University Hospital, P.O. BOX 21, 90029 OYS Oulu, Finland
katariina.kilpivaara@oulu.fi
[2] Medical Research Center, University of Oulu, University of Oulu, P.O. BOX 8000, 90014 Oulu, Finland
[3] Research Unit of Health Sciences and Technology, University of Oulu, Oulu, Finland
[4] Centre for Wireless Communications, University of Oulu, Oulu, Finland
[5] Research Service Unit, University of Oulu, Oulu, Finland
[6] Department of Diagnostic Radiology, Oulu University Hospital, Oulu, Finland
[7] Department of Obstetrics and Gynecology, Research Unit of Clinical Medicine, Oulu University Hospital, University of Oulu, Oulu, Finland

Abstract. Mammographic images are commonly used in cancer screening protocols, yet there is a lack of automated tools evaluating breast volume from the images, which could help preoperative planning of breast surgery or epidemiological research. The study aimed at creating and validating an automated workflow utilizing computer vision for quantifying breast volume from a large dataset of digital mammographic images. The study was conducted in two phases. First, an automated workflow for analyzing breast volume was developed using Python-based computer vision libraries. This was followed by the validation and analysis of the method by utilizing seventy-three mammographic images of women undergoing preoperative mammography. The performance of the automated volume calculation method was evaluated and validated with manually measured breast dimensions. In a retrospective register study, a total of seventy-three mammograms from 41 females ages 35–82 years (mean 60 years) were analyzed showing effective analysis process and excellent accuracy of the automated computer vision approach in estimating breast volume from mammographic data. The mean difference (bias) between manually measured and computer vision approach volumes was minimal (0.01 cm^3) resulting in an excellent correlation ($R = 1.0$, $p < 0.001$) between the techniques. The proposed automated method provides an accurate, fast, and cost-effective solution for obtaining breast volume measurements from large-scale mammography datasets, and it could be useful for preoperative planning and research on breast health.

Keywords: Breast · Organ size · Digital mammography · Computer Vision System

M. Säreстöniemi et al. (Eds.): NCDHWS 2026, CCIS 3010, pp. 19–30, 2026.
https://doi.org/10.1007/978-3-032-28819-6_2

1 Introduction

Mammography is a pivotal breast cancer detection tool that employs low-dose x-rays to image breast tissue and is widely used in breast cancer screening protocols [1, 2]. The improved survival of breast cancer cases has benefitted both from rapid development in treatment modalities but also developmental steps in diagnostic mammographic imaging. Indeed, recent technological advancements, including digital mammography and tomosynthesis, have enhanced its diagnostic capabilities by making the interpretation of images technically more feasible [3].

While primarily used for breast cancer screening, mammography derived images and data can also be utilized in assessing other conditions such as breast hypertrophy preoperatively [4]. In fact, mammography imaging has not been typically used for evaluating breast volume despite its potential value in preoperative assessment and resection planning.

Various other methods for breast volume assessment have been presented in the literature, ranging from direct physical measurement to advanced imaging-based techniques. Traditional anthropometric measuring approaches, such as water displacement, are accurate but impractical in clinical workflows and impossible in retrospective setting [1, 2]. More advanced techniques such as magnetic resonance imaging (MRI) and three-dimensional surface scanning deliver accurate breast volume estimates [3, 4]. However, the above-mentioned are resource demanding, costly, and not routinely available for all patients.

Automated breast density assessment systems can also be used to derive approximate breast volume metrics, as they compute fibroglandular and total breast tissue volumes based on mammographic image data. Among these, Quantra™ produces volumetric breast density estimates by applying machine learning analysis to 2D and tomosynthesis images, yielding standardized measures of tissue composition as part of its clinical workflow [5]. Volpara™ generates similarly volumetric breast density measurements by analyzing mammograms and estimating both fibroglandular and total tissue volume through its algorithm [6, 7].

The aim of this study is to introduce an automated method for calculating breast volume from mammograms, using computer vision techniques, and utilizing readily available information from the Digital Imaging and Communications in Medicine (DICOM) files. This approach seeks to provide an efficient, cost-effective, and extra-radiation-free solution for obtaining breast volume measurements from existing mammography datasets. The present study aims to develop a method for handling high-volume mammography datasets, with the goal of demonstrating its effectiveness through validation data and analysis. Despite being validated with a relatively small set of 73 images, due to the labor-intensive nature of the manual measurements used as the reference standard, the method is theoretically designed for mammography datasets containing a sizeable number of mammograms.

2 Materials and Methods

2.1 Breast Volume Approximation

Digital mammograms were analyzed using an automated computer vision workflow developed specifically for breast volume measurement. Python programming language and supplemental software libraries such as Pydicom for handling DICOM files (pixel data and associated metadata) and Open Source Computer Vision Library (OpenCV) for image analysis [8–10] were used in the development. The formula for breast volume approximation was obtained from the literature [11, 12]. It is defined as.

$$v = \frac{\pi}{4} HWC, \tag{1}$$

where H is the height of the breast in the craniocaudal projection, W is width, and C is the thickness of the compressed breast as seen in Fig. 1a. The height and width can be obtained from the images and the imaging parameter C from the study metadata.

First, pixel data and study metadata were read from the DICOM file header [13, 14]. In preparation of the image analysis phase, the pixel data was passed through a windowing operation by utilizing the values in the DICOM header. For the breast volume calculations, body part thickness (i.e., compression thickness) and pixel pitch (i.e., physical distance of the centers of each pixel in the image) must be present in the DICOM header.

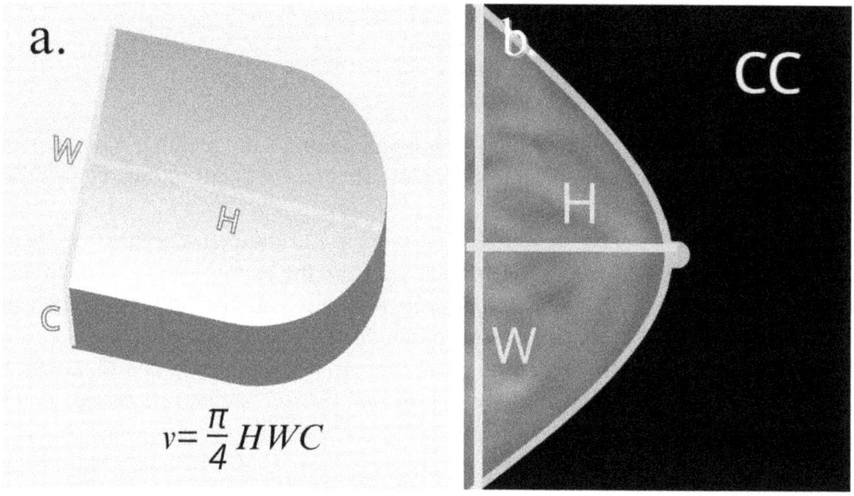

Fig. 1. Dimensions needed in volume calculation; H = height, W = width, C = compression thickness (from DICOM data), a) foundation of the formula, b) dimensions in mammogram, CC refers to craniocaudal projection.

Digital mammograms used in the experiments originated from devices by several manufacturers: Hologic, Inc. (Marlborough, MA, United States), GE Healthcare (Chicago, IL, United States), Siemens (Erlangen, Germany), Fujifilm Corporation (Tokyo, Japan), and Planmed Oy (Helsinki, Finland).

2.2 Workflow

The breast region was identified and extracted from mammography images using OpenCV functions incorporated in the workflow, including:

Thresholding: A binary mask of the mammogram image is generated using a thresholding function with a fixed threshold value, isolating the breast region from the surrounding background.

Erosion: Consequently, the binary mask undergoes morphological erosion to eliminate minimal noise and small artifacts, attempting to exclude areas not in region of interest.

Connected Component Analysis and Largest Combined Component Selection: Next, the connected component analysis and identifying of the largest foreground component (by area) within the eroded mask is performed.

Dilation: The selected largest combined component was dilated to restore its original size and shape, which may have been reduced during the erosion phase.

Contour Detection and Bounding Box: Finally, contours were identified, and a bounding rectangle was drawn around the largest connected component. This bounding rectangle provides the height H, and width W of the craniocaudal (CC) projection of the breast (Eq. 1), as shown in Fig. 1b. Furthermore, the calculated height and width of the breast can be translated to real dimensions using the pixel spacing information.

All computations were performed on a Lenovo laptop with an Intel® Core™ i5-1135G7 CPU (4 cores, 8 threads, 2.40 GHz base frequency), 16 GB of RAM, SSD disk (NVMe), and running Microsoft Windows 11 operating system.

2.3 Validation Setup and Test Set

To facilitate a comprehensive evaluation and validation of the method, a comparative study was conducted between the measurements obtained with the automated workflow and manual measurements.

An experienced surgeon (K.K.) manually measured the breast area twice (height and width of the breast) from the CC projection from the mammograms to form mean measurements (Fig. 1b). The same dimensions were also automatically measured using the automated workflow. The measurement conducted by the specialist was set as the gold standard for annotations. A statistical comparison was performed to assess the performance of machine vision relative to manual measurement with paired samples t-test.

2.4 Patient Data Source

After the method development, a total of 193 patients with preoperative mammographic images were selected from the university hospital patient registry, corresponding to patients who underwent mastectomy in the years 2021–2022. The method was developed for (direct) digital mammograms, thus other modalities had to be excluded, patient inclusions and exclusions are presented in Fig. 2.

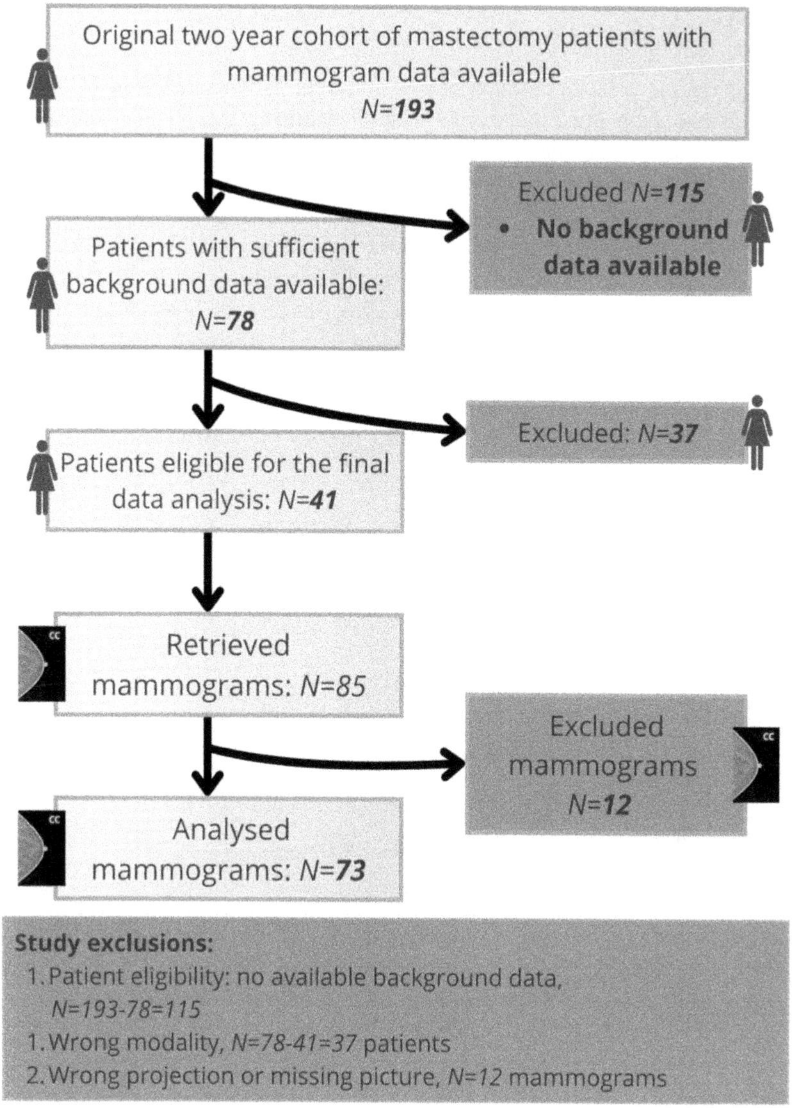

Fig. 2. Flowchart of the study.

2.5 Statistical Analysis

Summary measurements are presented as a mean with standard deviation, unless otherwise stated. The mean difference (bias) with 95% confidence interval (95% CI) between the two techniques was calculated using paired samples t-test. The Bland-Altman plot [15] with limits of agreement was created for visual assessment between the techniques. Spearman correlation coefficient (ρ) was calculated between human and computer-based volume calculation.

3 Results

The final analytical cohort consisted of seventy-eight patients, selected from an initial pool of 193 based on predefined criteria applied during the method validation process. A portion of the unassorted images were transferred from different organizations, and images utilizing imaging modalities other than Digital Mammography (DM), such as Computed Radiography (CR), were excluded. This process ultimately resulted in a cohort of forty-one patients with seventy-three craniocaudal (CC) projection mammogram images. The data comprised females aged 35 to 82 years (mean age 60, SD 12) with a BMI range of 19.5 to 54.3 (mean BMI 29.6, SD 7.1), the body surface area (BSA) range of 1.50 to 2.4 (mean 1.9, SD 0.2). Descriptive data is presented in Table 1. The mean glandular dose varied from 0.0037 to 0.0536 dGy with a mean (±SD) of 0.0131 (±0.0078) dGy, which is within the expected range for diagnostic-quality mammography. The execution times ranged from 0.058 s to 0.493 s, with a mean elapsed time of 0.187 s.

Table 1. Descriptive Statistics

	N	Mean (SD)	Minimum	Maximum
Age	41	60.3 (11.8)	35.0	82.0
BMI	41	29.61 (7,06)	19.50	54.30
Body surface area, m^2	41	1.85 (0.22)	1.50	2.40
Lean body mass, kg	41	48.6 (6.70)	37.0	77.0
Manual volume cm^3	41	1215.74 (654.77)	381.27	3503.41
Automatic volume cm^3	41	1215.68 (654.75)	381.27	3503.42

SD, standard deviation

The paired samples t-test showed only a minimal bias of 0.01 cm^3 (95% CI –0.05 to 0.07 cm^3) with an excellent Spearman correlation coefficient of 1.00 ($p < 0.001$) between the methods, as seen also in Fig. 3.

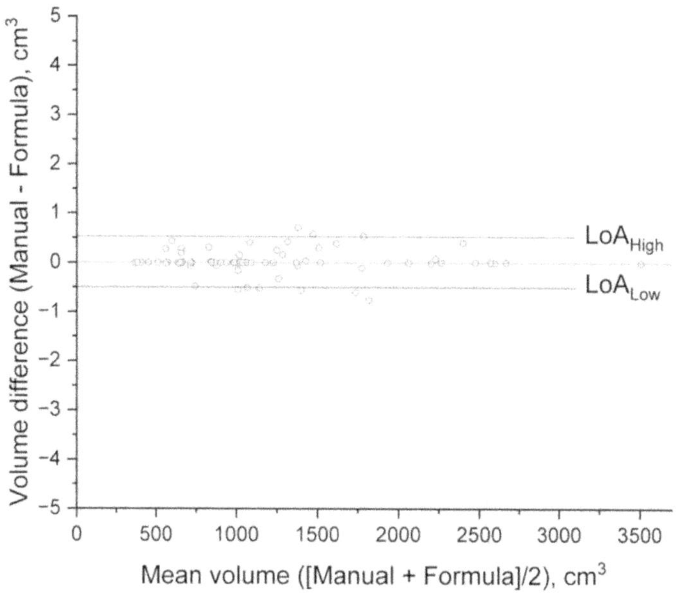

Fig. 3. The Bland-Altman plot of measured breast volumes: difference (cm3) (Manual-Formula) between manual or formula-based mean breast volume with 95% limit of an agreement LoA) between the measurement types.

4 Discussion

An accurate breast volume assessment is crucial for plastic surgery planning and epidemiological studies linked to breast health. While several automated volumetric breast density systems (e.g., Quantra™, Volpara™) exist, which can also produce breast volume, these tools focus on density estimation and rely on proprietary models [5, 7]. There is a scarcity of openly documented, fully transparent workflows for anatomical breast volume estimation based solely on two-dimensional mammography. We present a sophisticated image processing workflow that rapidly analyzes digital mammograms to estimate breast volume. The proposed workflow is computationally effective and was seamlessly integrated into the analysis of existing mammography data. This practical computer vision workflow utilizes widely accessible tools, including Python, OpenCV, and DICOM metadata. This tool was developed for accurate breast volume evaluation in clinical practice and for epidemiological breast health research [16].

A similar kind of procedure for region of interest extraction has been introduced as a post-processing step Wu et al., which investigated a screening mammography exam classification [17]. In that work, mammograms were cropped to reduce image background and, consequently, computational overhead.

Various breast volume measurement methods exist. Mammography is a reasonably accurate method for volume measurements across all size ranges [12]. Each method has unique strengths and limitations [18]. Digital mammography has largely replaced traditional film-screen/analog mammography, presenting improved image quality, easy digital transfer, and image analysis. Also, it offers the ability to manipulate and enhance images digitally [19]. The industry standard DICOM plays a crucial role in mammography imaging, facilitating standardized storage, communication, and management of medical images [13]. The DICOM standard has been instrumental in transforming medical imaging over the last three decades, including mammography [20]. In mammography, the DICOM standard enables the capture and storage of valuable auxiliary information such as mean glandular dose, exposure indices, compression force/thickness, and field of view [21]. Based on our results analysis, the method described appears to be highly accurate and well-suited for processing large mammography datasets. This approach is reasonable if the intention is to conduct mammography, as it does not bring any extra burden on patients or nursing staff, and has minimal additional cost if automated.

On the other hand, the developed automated method also has limitations. At the moment, the measurement approach is not suitable for older analog mammogram images or damaged pictures. There are methods for skin-line estimation and breast boundary segmentation from analog and digital mammograms proposed in the literature [22, 23]. Moreover, the mathematical approximation using a half-elliptic cylinder may not accurately represent the actual breast shape, and the breast is more likely to have a smaller area than the model suggests [12, 24]. Currently, this method analyzes digital mammograms with Standard Operating Procedure Class Unique Identifier 1.2.840.10008.5.1.4.1.1.1.2 and can be adapted to all full-field digital mammography data in DICOM format that includes the necessary metadata.

The limitations of this study include the relatively small sample size of seventy-three mammogram images, which may not fully represent the diverse range of breast characteristics or imaging challenges present in the broader population. However, it is important to acknowledge that the data still covers a substantial portion of breasts images with a typical range of breast sizes. The limited sample size may not capture the emerging image interpretation issues that could arise when applying this automated method to a more diverse set of mammography data. Also, regarding the manual measurements, only one person conducted the mammography measurements, thus accuracy may vary between different measures giving an advantage to automated measuring. The involvement of a single measurer could introduce observer bias and undermine the research's reliability. Supplementary validation on a larger and more representative dataset may help assess the performance and generalizability of the method across different patient demographics and imaging conditions.

A further possible limitation distresses the method's generalizability across different mammography devices. Exposure-differences in image contrast may also affect threshold-based segmentation, further highlighting the need for adaptive advances. Imaging systems vary in detector characteristics and manufacturer-specific processing [25, 26], which can modify intensity distributions and the visual appearance of breast boundaries. As the current workflow relies on a fixed global threshold and predefined image-processing parameters, its performance may vary across mammography systems with differing detector characteristics and manufacturer-specific processing. Our study, however, indicates that the method described is feasible with various mammography devices. Nonetheless, future work could include validation across multiple imaging systems.

Finally, the developed method can present problems with low quality mammograms, for example images with extra tissue, other than breast tissue, or images with distortions (noise, defective pixel rows, grid lines) (Fig. 4). To improve the prototype, the algorithm could be further optimized to ignore extra tissue outside the breast borders, such as flank area (Fig. 4a) or interference in the picture (Fig. 4b), which would enhance the accuracy of the method. Potential improvements could also involve more sophisticated segmentation algorithms or machine learning techniques to identify breast borders more precisely.

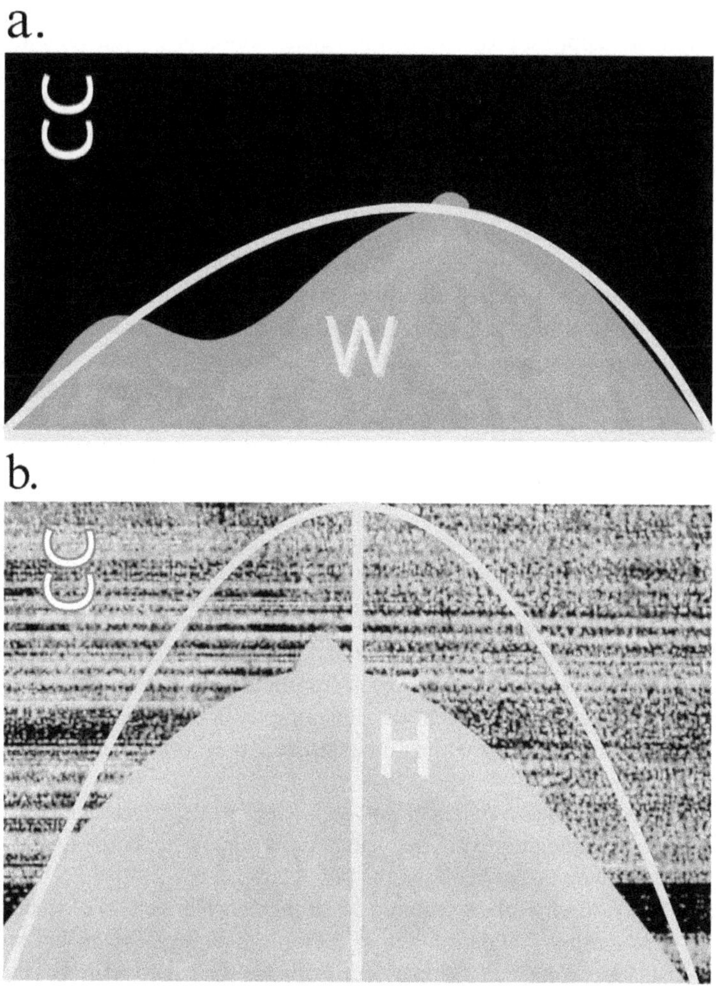

Fig. 4. Error sources of measuring, a) The width is excessively broad due to the inclusion of soft tissue from the flank in the image. b) The height is excessively elevated because of the distortion present in the image.

Despite these limitations, the strengths of our study include the use of a well-established "gold standard" of manual measurements by an experienced surgeon, providing a reliable benchmark for evaluating the accuracy of the automated method. Additionally, the comparative approach, i.e., examining the performance of the computer vision workflow compared to manual measurements, offers valuable insights into the feasibility and potential of this automated breast volume estimation approach. The results demonstrate a high correlation between manual measurements and measurements obtained through image processing and computer vision techniques, suggesting that the developed method could help streamline the workload in healthcare settings and enable more efficient breast health research and diagnostics.

This automated approach for breast volume estimation offers practical advantages, including faster and more consistent measurements and a reduced need for manual assessment. Although the image processing steps themselves rely on established computer vision operations, the novelty of this work lies in the integration of these components into a transparent, metadata driven workflow that enables reproducible and anatomically grounded volume estimation from routine mammograms. In contrast to existing proprietary tools, the method provides an openly documented and lightweight workflow that can be applied at scale, supporting large datasets. This enables streamlined workloads in both clinical and research environments. Such automation has the potential to enhance diagnostic planning, support breast and plastic surgery, and strengthen population level studies on breast health. To further validate and refine this workflow, additional research is necessary, particularly involving comparison with volume of actual mastectomized breast. Such validation would strengthen confidence in the method's accuracy and clinical utility, paving the way for broader adoption and integration into routine practice.

5 Conclusions

In conclusion, the present study determines that a transparent, metadata assisted computer vision workflow can provide accurate and reproducible breast volume estimates from digital mammograms. By combining geometric measurements extracted from the craniocaudal projection with DICOM derived compression thickness, the method can offer quantitative volume assessment without the need for additional measuring, imaging or commercial software.

The workflow provides a practical and accessible strategy that can be effectively utilized for large mammography datasets, potentially supporting both clinical decision-making and research on breast health at the population level.

Nevertheless, further work is required to strengthen the method's generalizability and clinical applicability. Validation across multiple imaging devices and larger, heterogeneous datasets, as well as comparisons with volumes derived from mastectomy specimens, would provide important evidence regarding the robustness and accuracy of the workflow.

Acknowledgments. We thank Aleksi Penttilä for the practical contributions to the experimental setup. Antti Isosalo would like to acknowledge the financial support of the Jenny and Antti Wihuri Foundation (grant no. 220106).

Disclosure of Interests. The authors have no competing interests to declare that are relevant to the content of this article.

References

1. Nicosia, L., Gnocchi, G., Gorini, I., et al.: History of Mammography: Analysis of Breast Imaging Diagnostic Achievements over the Last Century. Healthcare 2023, Vol 11, Page 1596 11:1596. https://doi.org/10.3390/HEALTHCARE11111596
2. Nyström, L., Wall, S., Rutqvist, L.E., et al.: Breast cancer screening with mammography: overview of Swedish randomised trials. Lancet **341**, 973–978 (1993). https://doi.org/10.1016/0140-6736(93)91067-V
3. Sardanelli, F., Fallenberg, E.M., Clauser, P., et al.: Mammography: an update of the EUSOBI recommendations on information for women. Insights Imaging **8**, 11 (2016). https://doi.org/10.1007/S13244-016-0531-4
4. Thulkar, S., Hari, S.: Present role of mammography/digital mammography in breast cancer management. PET Clin **4**, 213–225 (2009). https://doi.org/10.1016/j.cpet.2009.09.006
5. Kim, J.S., Bae, K., Lee, E.J., Bang, M.: Mammography with a fully automated breast volumetric software as a novel method for estimating the preoperative breast volume prior to mastectomy. Ann. Surg. Treat Res. **100**, 313 (2021). https://doi.org/10.4174/ASTR.2021.100.6.313
6. Highnam, R., Brady, M., Yaffe, M.J., et al.: Robust breast composition measurement - VolparaTM. Lecture Notes in Computer Science (including subseries Lecture Notes in Artificial Intelligence and Lecture Notes in Bioinformatics), vol. 6136, pp. 342–349. Springer, Cham (2010)https://doi.org/10.1007/978-3-642-13666-5_46
7. Sartor, H., Lång, K., Rosso, A., et al.: Measuring mammographic density: comparing a fully automated volumetric assessment versus European radiologists' qualitative classification. Eur. Radiol. **26**, 4354–4360 (2016). https://doi.org/10.1007/S00330-016-4309-3
8. Mason, D.: SU-E-T-33: Pydicom: an open source DICOM library. Med. Phys. **38**, 3493 (2011). https://doi.org/10.1118/1.3611983
9. Pulli, K., Baksheev, A., Kornyakov, K., Eruhimov, V.: Mobile computer-vision technology will soon become as ubiquitous as touch interfaces. Commun. ACM **55**, 61–69 (2012). https://doi.org/10.1145/2184319.2184337
10. Bradski, G.: The OpenCV Library. Dr Dobb's J. Softw. Tools **120**, 122–125 (2000)
11. Itsukage, S., Sowa, Y., Goto, M., et al.: Breast volume measurement by recycling the data obtained from 2 routine modalities, mammography and magnetic resonance imaging. Eplasty. 2017 Dec 20;17:e39 (2017)
12. Kalbhen, C.L., McGill, J.J., Fendley, P.M., et al.: Mammographic determination of breast volume: comparing different methods. Am. J. Roentgenol. **173**, 1643–1649 (1999). https://doi.org/10.2214/AJR.173.6.10584814
13. Mustra, M., Delac, K.: Overview of the DICOM standard. In: ELMAR, 50th International (2008)
14. Best, D.E., Horii, S.C., Bennett, W.C., et al.: Update of the ACR-NEMA digital imaging and communications in medicine standard. SPIE **1654**, 356–361 (1992). https://doi.org/10.1117/12.60322
15. Bland, J.M., Altman, D.G.: Measuring agreement in method comparison studies. Stat. Methods Med. Res. **8**, 135–160 (1999). https://doi.org/10.1177/096228029900800204
16. Artificial Intelligence Guided Diagnostics in Medical Imaging: Oulu Dataset of Screening Mammography (versio 1) (2021)

17. Wu, N., Phang, J., Park, J., et al.: Deep neural networks improve radiologists' performance in breast cancer screening. IEEE Trans. Med. Imaging **39**, 1184–1194 (2020). https://doi.org/10.1109/TMI.2019.2945514
18. Kayar, R., Civelek, S., Cobanoglu, M., et al.: Five methods of breast volume measurement: a comparative study of measurements of specimen volume in 30 mastectomy cases. Breast Cancer (Auckl) **5**, 43–52 (2011). https://doi.org/10.4137/BCBCR.S6128
19. Pisano, E.D., Gatsonis, C., Hendrick, E., et al.: Diagnostic performance of digital versus film mammography for breast-cancer screening. N. Engl. J. Med. **353**, 1773–1783 (2005). https://doi.org/10.1056/NEJMOA052911
20. Larobina M (2023) Thirty Years of the DICOM Standard. Tomography 2023, Vol 9, Pages 1829–1838 9:1829–1838. https://doi.org/10.3390/TOMOGRAPHY9050145
21. Bidgood, W.D., Horii, S.C., Prior, F.W., Van Syckle, D.E.: Understanding and using DICOM, the data interchange standard for biomedical imaging. J. Am. Med. Inform. Assoc. **4**, 199 (1997). https://doi.org/10.1136/JAMIA.1997.0040199
22. Shi, P., Zhong, J., Rampun, A., Wang, H.: A hierarchical pipeline for breast boundary segmentation and calcification detection in mammograms. Comput. Biol. Med. **96**, 178–188 (2018). https://doi.org/10.1016/J.COMPBIOMED.2018.03.011
23. Casti, P., Mencattini, A., Salmeri, M., et al.: Estimation of the breast skin-line in mammograms using multidirectional Gabor filters. Comput. Biol. Med. **43**, 1870–1881 (2013). https://doi.org/10.1016/J.COMPBIOMED.2013.09.001
24. Shanley, E., Johnston, A., Hillick, D., et al.: Digital breast volume estimation (DBVE)—a new technique. Br. J. Radiol. **91**, 20180406 (2018). https://doi.org/10.1259/BJR.20180406
25. Wang, Y., Keller, B.M., Zheng, Y., et al.: A phantom study for assessing the effect of different digital detectors on mammographic texture features. In: Breast Imaging. IWDM 2012. Lecture Notes in Computer Science, vol. 7361. Springer, Heidelberg (2012).https://doi.org/10.1007/978-3-642-31271-7_78
26. Wessling, D., Männlin, S., Schwarz, R., et al.: Background enhancement in contrast-enhanced spectral mammography (CESM): are there qualitative and quantitative differences between imaging systems? Eur. Radiol. **33**, 2945–2953 (2023). https://doi.org/10.1007/s00330-022-09238-9

Multimodal Machine Learning Approach for Timed-Up-and-Go Test Score Prediction from Wearable Gait Data

Nabid Faiem[1(✉)], Tunc Asuroglu[1,2], Koray Acici[3], Antti Kallonen[1], and Mark van Gils[1]

[1] Faculty of Medicine and Health Technology, Tampere University, 33720 Tampere, Finland
nabid.faiem@tuni.fi

[2] VTT Technical Research Centre of Finland, 33101 Tampere, Finland

[3] Department of Artificial Intelligence and Data Engineering, Ankara University, 06830 Ankara, Turkey

Abstract. Falls are a major cause of injury and disability in older adults and people with Parkinson's disease (PD). The Timed-Up-and-Go (TUG) test assesses mobility and falls risk but requires supervised clinical testing, limiting its regular use. We investigated whether TUG time can be estimated from two-minute walking data captured using in-shoe vertical ground reaction force (GRF) sensors, which are easy to use during daily life and provide detailed gait information. While prior studies have estimated TUG from wearable sensors, how different input modalities such as gait representations and demographics contribute individually and in combination has received little attention.

Using the PhysioNet GRF dataset, we analyzed 100 participants (62 PD, 38 controls) with demographics (age, sex, height, and weight) and 16-channel GRF recordings. A Perceiver-based multimodal framework was trained to estimate TUG time from raw GRF timeseries, GRF-derived summary features, and demographics in unimodal and multimodal configurations and benchmarked against conventional feature-based regressors trained on extracted features. Models were evaluated using ten-fold subject-wise cross-validation with mean absolute error (MAE), root mean square error (RMSE), and Pearson correlation coefficient (CC).

Combining raw timeseries and features (MAE 0.80 $\pm$ 0.34 s, RMSE 1.27 $\pm$ 0.85 s, CC 0.93 $\pm$ 0.07) achieved best performance, outperforming unimodal models, conventional regressors, and prior GRF-based TUG results. PD participants showed higher prediction errors (MAE 0.97 s) than controls (MAE 0.41 s), with accuracy decreasing in older age groups. Adding demographics provided no consistent benefit.

These findings suggest that steady-walking vertical GRF can approximate TUG time and could support continuous mobility assessment in PD.

Keywords: Parkinson's disease · Fall-risk assessment · Timed-Up-and-Go (TUG) · Gait analysis · GRF sensors · In-shoe wearable sensors · Perceiver architecture · Multimodal deep learning

M. Säreströniemi et al. (Eds.): NCDHWS 2026, CCIS 3010, pp. 31–50, 2026.
https://doi.org/10.1007/978-3-032-28819-6_3

1 Introduction

Functional mobility is essential for independent living and safe performance of daily activities. Impaired mobility not only complicates health-related issues but also diminishes quality of life. Poor balance, gait impairment, and reduced functional mobility significantly increase the risk of falls among older adults [1] and in patients with neurological disorders, such as Parkinson's disease (PD) [2]. The risk further increases in advanced PD stages, where fall-related injuries may cause severe disabilities or even death. Epidemiological studies suggest that roughly one-third of individuals aged 65 years or older fall at least once per year [3], and fall-related mortality has risen in many countries over recent decades. The Global Burden of Disease study reported an age-standardized mortality rate of 9.2 per 100,000 in 2017 [1]. Deaths due to falls have also steadily increased across Europe since 1990 [1]. These events impose not only a personal burden but also a substantial economic cost. In the USA alone, healthcare spending attributes to non-fatal falls in adults aged 65 years and older were estimated at US$ 80 billion in 2020 [4], and average treatment costs per fall-related hospitalization can exceed US$ 18.000 [5]. Falls also impose major costs on European health systems. The cost of treating fall-related injuries in the EU is estimated to be about 25 billion Euros per year [6].

The Timed-Up-and-Go (TUG) test is one of the most widely used tools for assessing mobility and fall risk. Podsiadlo and Richardson formalized the timed version of "Get-Up-and-Go" [7] in 1991 and showed that the time taken to rise from a chair, walk 3 m, turn, walk back and sit down is a reliable and valid measure of functional mobility that correlates strongly with balance, gait speed and activities of daily living [8]. Longer completion times are associated with greater fall risk. In community-dwelling older adults, a cut-off of 13.5 s is often cited, with high sensitivity and specificity for fall prediction [9], although alternative thresholds between approximately 8 to 16 s have been reported [10]. For PD patients specifically, a threshold of 11.5 s has been associated with increased fall risk and disease severity [2]. Despite this utility, TUG assessment has limitations. It requires a supervised and task-specific protocol. The notion of a "comfortable pace" is subjective and may vary between raters and patients. TUG time exhibits test-retest variability. Clinical physiotherapy guidance in PD report minimal detectable change (MDC) values of approximately 3.5–11 s [11]. Most critically, TUG time compresses complex movement into a single scaler outcome, providing no direct insight into which specific gait components or transitions are most impaired.

Quantitative gait analysis offers a more detailed assessment of mobility by capturing spatiotemporal dynamics and biomechanical patterns relevant to fall risk. Wearable sensors such as inertial measurement units (IMUs), accelerometers, and ground reaction force (GRF) sensors have enabled continuous and non-invasive gait monitoring [12]. GRF sensors are particularly informative because they reflect how forces are distributed across the feet and thus indirectly, joint mechanics and muscle activity. Previous studies have shown that gait signals can be used to estimate PD symptoms' severity [13–15] and support fall risk prediction through spatiotemporal gait features [14]. However, many approaches rely solely on sensor data or extracted features, overlooking clinically relevant factors such as demographic characteristics (e.g., age, sex, height, weight) which may provide complementary predictive value.

In our previous work [13], we demonstrated the feasibility of predicting Unified Parkinson's Disease Rating Scale (UPDRS) scores from raw multichannel GRF time-series signals combined with expert-derived features using the Perceiver architecture from Google DeepMind [16]. While promising, both modalities originated from the same data sources (in-shoe GRF sensors), and the outcome focused on overall motor severity rather than functional mobility and fall risk. Moreover, the impact of including additional modalities beyond gait-derived signals, such as demographics, on prediction performance was not systemically examined. This highlights a key gap in the present study context, specifically the absence of a unified multimodal framework for TUG prediction that integrates GRF recordings and demographic covariates on the same dataset.

In this study, we extend our previous GRF-based work in two directions. First, we target TUG completion time as a proxy for functional mobility and fall risk, and we investigate whether it can be estimated from two-minute walking recording without administering the TUG test itself. Second, we explicitly consider demographics as an additional modality and systemically compare unimodal and multimodal configurations to quantify the impact of combining demographics with GRF-derived features and GRF timeseries signals.

The major contributions of this paper can be summarized as follows:

1. Evaluate the feasibility of estimating TUG completion time from vertical GRF-based gait signals acquired during two-minute walking tests in people with PD and healthy controls and examine how prediction performance varies across diagnostic status and age groups.
2. Compare unimodal and multimodal using raw GRF timeseries signals, GRF-derived summary features, and demographics covariates to quantify the contribution of each input modality and their combinations.
3. Benchmark a Perceiver-based multimodal architecture, using both unimodal and multimodal input configurations, against standard machine-learning (ML) regressors (KNN, SVR, Decision Tree and Random Forest) trained on the same hand-crafted feature set.

The rest of the paper is organized as follows. Section 2 discusses related work on TUG assessment, wearable-based gait analysis and multimodal modelling in PD. Section 3 describes the dataset, preprocessing and component of the proposed framework. Section 4 presents the results of the performance evaluation of the model configurations. Section 5 discusses the findings, strengths and limitations, challenges, and implications for future research. Section 6 concludes the paper.

2 Related Work

The TUG test is a standard clinical tool for assessing basic functional mobility and fall risk, particularly in older adults and people with neurological conditions. Podsiadlo and Richardson reported that TUG test is reliable (inter-rater and intra-rater) and shows a good correlation with gait speed, balance and activities of daily life in frail older adults [8]. Subsequent studies and reviews have shown its prognostic value for falls [9, 10].

A major limitation of conventional TUG is that it compresses complex movement into a single scalar outcome. This has motivated the development of instrumented TUG (iTUG) protocols using wearable sensors, which can quantify spatiotemporal gait characteristics and postural transition beyond raw completion time [17–20]. Recent reviews conclude that iTUG provides more sensitive fall-risk and mobility metrics than conventional TUG [21].

Beyond iTUG, several studies have investigated whether TUG time can be estimated from gait outside formal TUG trials. Choi et al. used IMU-based 3D accelerometers on the pelvis and both feet during outdoor walking in 37 older adults, extracting 120 step-based gait features [22]. Elastic-net regression was applied for feature reduction, followed by ridge regression to predict TUG time. Across repeated train-test splits, the model achieved small mean absolute prediction errors (MAPE) of approximately 0.865 s for the foot configuration, 0.918 s for the combined foot-pelvis configuration, and 0.921 s for the pelvis configuration. This study therefore illustrates how feature-based regression can leverage wearable gait data collected in real-world community settings to approximate conventional TUG assessments [22].

GRF and planer-pressure sensors are less commonly used for TUG prediction than IMUs, but they are important in PD gait research. Systematic reviews of wearable-based digital biomarkers [23] highlight the PhysioNet vertical GRF database [24], which uses in-shoe vertical GRF sensors in people with PD and healthy controls, and show that GRF-derived spatiotemporal and kinetic features support accurate PD diagnosis and severity assessment. Complementary to these GRF-based studies, Hao et al. proposed a sensor-agnostic ML pipeline that predicts TUG time from day-to-day, unscripted walking rather than controlled TUG tests [25]. They used 303 participants in three cohorts (healthy older adults, PD patients and individuals with mild cognitive impairment or dementia) and three wearable setups (lower-back accelerometer, wrist-accelerometer and in-sole GRF sensors). A random forest model evaluated with leave-one-subject-out validation achieved errors (MAE of 1.7 ± 1.7 s), within the minimal detectable change for most predictions, supporting the feasibility of using heterogeneous wearable signals collected in free-living conditions as a passive proxy for TUG-related mobility biomarker.

Mostafavi et al. [26] applied a Gramian Angular Field (GSF) and convolutional neural network (CNN) pipeline to the PhysioNet vertical GRF dataset [24]. Raw gait signals from eight in-shoe sensors under each foot (16 channels) were segmented into overlapping 10–60 s windows, and each window was converted into a 2D GAF image that encodes temporal correlations. These images were then used as input to CNNs for PD versus healthy control classification and for regression of continuous clinical scores (Hoehn and Yahr, UPDRS, UPDRS motor and TUG time). Predictions from multiple windows were averaged to obtain a single TUG estimate per participant. With this framework, the authors achieved 98.6% accuracy for the classification task and an R^2 of 0.80 for TUG regression with a MAE of 1.32 s and RMSE of 1.75 s (TUG range 7.27–36.34 s) [26]. This work demonstrated that transformed GRF signals combined with CNNs can support continuous TUG prediction.

Our previous work on the same dataset [24] proposed a Perceiver-based multimodal framework to estimate UPDRS scores from raw 16-channel vertical GRF signals and GRF-derived time- and frequency- domain features [13]. Using gait data from 93 PD patients and 73 controls, the multimodal Perceiver achieved MAE of 2.23 ± 1.31, an RMSE of 5.75 ± 4.16 and correlation coefficient of 0.93 ± 0.08, for UPDRS prediction, outperforming earlier GRF-based approaches in terms of MAE and correlation [13]. This supports the idea that combining raw sensor signals with engineered features in a single architecture can improve PD severity estimation. These findings are consistent with observations that multimodal architectures can improve biomedical prediction. Acosta et al. reviewed multimodal biomedical AI and concluded that integrating heterogeneous data sources such as image, electronic health records and wearable data often yields more accurate and robust models than single-modality design [27]. Recent PD-focused multimodal frameworks, such as MultiParkNet, which fuses speech, drawing, neuroimaging and cardiovascular signals [28], and the model of Li et al., which combines structural MRI, wearable accelerometry, genetic risk scores and lifestyle neurodegenerative disease prediction [29], also report clear gains over unimodal baselines.

Taken together, these studies suggest that TUG can be approximated from wearable gait signals using both classical and deep learning methods. However, most existing work either focuses on IMUs and free-living accelerometry, or, in the case of GRF-based approaches, relies on image-like transformations and CNNs. The relative contribution of raw GRF timeseries, GRF-derived features and demographic factors within a unified multimodal architecture remains largely unexplored, and direct comparisons of unimodal versus multimodal models on a common GRF-based dataset are uncommon. In this context, we investigate how different GRF representations and demographics relate to TUG prediction performance and how multimodal fusion behaves compared with unimodal designs in PD and health controls.

3 Materials and Methods

This study proposes a multimodal machine learning framework based on the Perceiver architecture to estimate TUG scores in individuals with PD and healthy controls. The pipeline consists of data curation, signal preprocessing and feature extraction, model architecture and evaluation protocol.

3.1 Dataset Description

The publicly available Parkinson's gait dataset from PhysioNet [24] was used which includes recording from three independent research groups [30–32]. This dataset includes gait recordings from 93 patients with idiopathic PD and 73 healthy subjects.

Researchers measured gait signals using eight GRF sensors positioned under each foot. These sensors measured the force signal in Newtons at a sampling rate of 100 Hz. Recordings were acquired under two walking conditions:

- **Single-task gait:** walking at a self-selected comfortable pace.
- **Dual-task gait:** walking while performing a concurrent cognitive task (serial subtraction by sevens from a pre-defined number).

Both single-task and dual-task gait recordings were used when available: otherwise, only the available recording was included. In addition to raw gait signals, demographic metadata were available: sex, age, height, weight, UPDRS score, and TUG completion time. Figure 1 presents the distribution of TUG scores across the cohort and their variation with age. For the present study, we included only participants with complete demographics profiles (age, sex, height and weight) and valid TUG scores. Recordings shorter than two minutes were excluded to maintain a consistent minimum signal duration. After applying these criteria, 100 participants (62 PD, 38 controls) were retained for analysis. Figure 2 illustrates typical GRF sensors outputs over a single gait cycle, highlighting stance and swing phases.

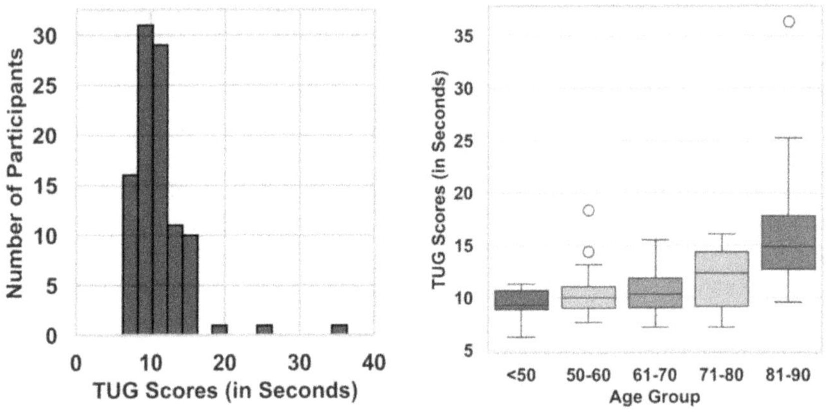

Fig. 1. (Left) Histogram of TUG scores distribution. Most participants completed the test within 5–16 s. (Right) Box plot of TUG scores distribution among participants across different age groups. The data show a gradual increase in median TUG scores with age.

3.2 Pre-Processing and Feature Extraction

To minimize the end-of-trial artifacts and to obtain fixed length for the Perceiver implementation, we extracted 10,025 samples segments from each GRF recording, corresponding to approximately 100 s of continuous walking at 100 Hz. Recordings that did not contain at least this duration of usable data were discarded. This procedure ensured that all measurements had the same number of time points and allowed the GRF signals to reshape into matrices size of 10025×16 (samples $\times$ sensors) for model input.

Signal denoising was performed using a median filter of length three to suppress spikes while preserving gait dynamics. Feature extraction was then conducted to complement raw gait signals with interpretable descriptors. Both time- and frequency-domain features were derived for each GRF sensor over the 100-s segment and are presented in Table 1. These features, validated in prior PD studies [13–15], capture the variability, and spectral properties of the GRF signals.

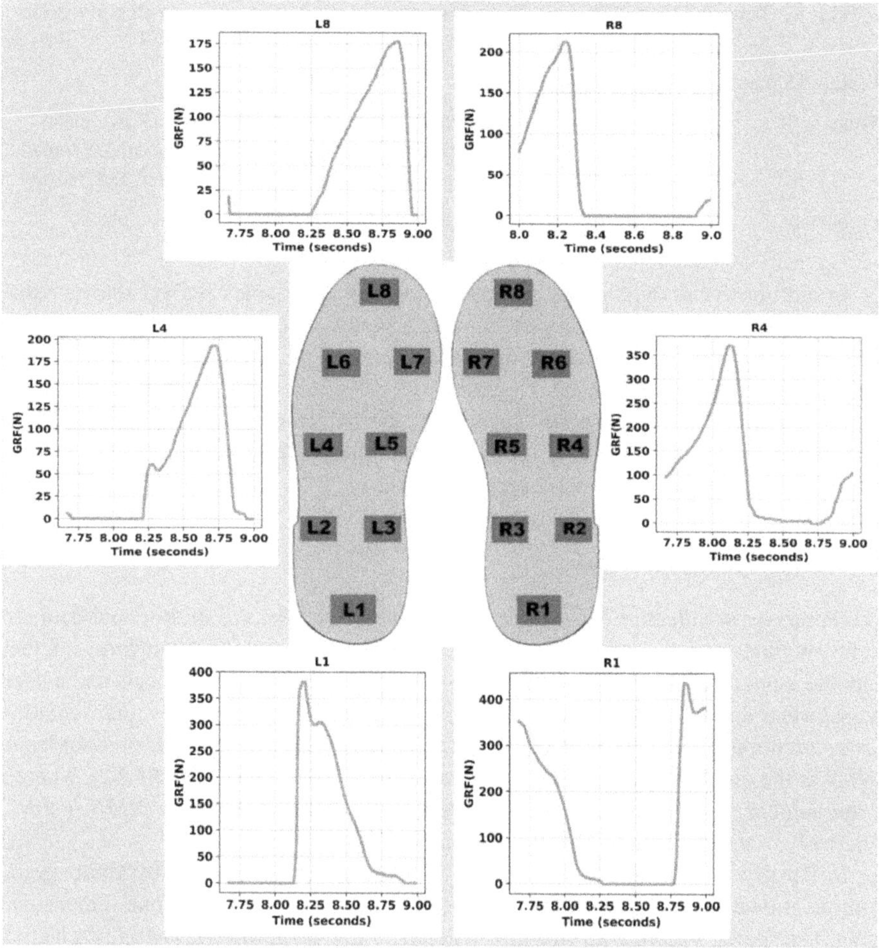

Fig. 2. This figure illustrates the force data measured by GRF sensors placed on the participant's left (L) and right (R) feet, numbered from 1 to 8 to indicate their positions on the feet. Timeseries plots depict the force exerted during a gait cycle. Signal variations from these sensors provide insights into the distinct gait characteristics, reflecting dynamic changes across the stance and swing phases of the gait cycle.

All features were z-score standardized according to Eq. 1 using the mean and standard deviation estimated from the full cohort.

$$z = \frac{x - \mu}{\sigma} \quad (1)$$

In this equation, $\boldsymbol{x}$ denotes the feature value, $\boldsymbol{\mu}$ the cohort mean and $\boldsymbol{\sigma}$ the standard deviation.

Table 1. Time and Frequency based features extracted from each sensor of all participants

Feature Domain	Features calculated from each GRF sensor
Time	mean, harmonic mean, median, range, interquartile range (IQR), mean absolute deviation, maximum amplitude and minimum/maximum spread, skewness, kurtosis, root mean square (RMS), energy, power, and entropy
Frequency	mean, minimum, maximum, normalized, energy, power, and phase

In addition to gait signals, we used four demographic variables as a separate modality: age, sex, height and weight. Sex encoded as a binary categorical variable (male = 1, female = 2). After preprocessing, demographic attributes were reshaped to for each subject were represented as a 4 x 1 vector.

In this study, ***raw timeseries*** denote the original 16-channel GRF signals, ***summary features*** refer to handcrafted features computed from the GRF segment, and ***demographics*** represent subject-level covariates.

3.3 Perceiver Architecture

The Perceiver architecture was selected for its ability to process multimodal data efficiently without introducing domain-specific biases [16]. A learnable latent array interacts with the input through cross-attention to form a fixed-size latent bottleneck, and a latent Transformer applies self-attention only over latent indices to refine this representation. Cross-attention scales approximately as $O(MN)$, where M is the number of input length and N is the number of latent vectors. Latent self-attention scales as $O(LN2)$, where L is the number of latent self-attention layers. The overall complexity is $O(MN + LN2)$, where $O(\cdot)$ denotes asymptotic (Big-O) complexity.

In Perceiver networks, each modality is represented as an array of input vectors with positional information added to preserve temporal structure for one-dimensional inputs and spatial structure for two-dimensional inputs. In multimodal settings, a learned modality-specific embedding is concatenated to each input vector prior to attention. All input vectors from a given modality shares the same embedding. This embedding identifies the modality and can be sized to align channel dimensions across modalities. This input formulation preserves a modality-agnostic nature of the architecture and supports learned fusion across heterogenous inputs.

Despite its strengths, the design has a clear trade-off. Computation and memory still include a quadratic term in the latent vectors N and using a large N or many latent self-attention layers L can become computationally expensive. The latent bottleneck may miss fine details unless inputs are re-queried. Adding additional cross-attention layers allows the latent array to re-query the inputs and can improve accuracy, but it increases the number of input-linear operations and therefore raises computing and latency (Fig. 3).

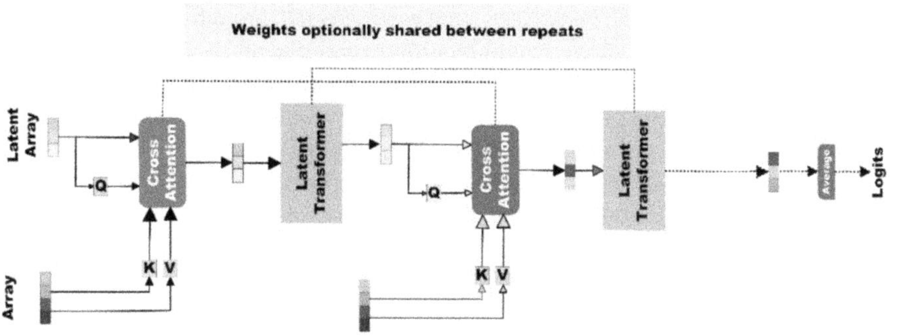

Fig. 3. The Perceiver architecture uses an iterative approach that alternates between cross-attention layers and several latent self-attention blocks. By alternating between these two types of blocks, the model can receptively attend to the input data and find patterns between the input and output layers more effectively. This mechanism allows the model to reduce the dimensionality of the input data while preserving the most critical information. The weight sharing strategy of architecture can also improve predictive performance.

3.4 Proposed Framework

The multimodal Perceiver was employed to estimate TUG scores as a continuous outcome. The open-source PyTorch implementation [33] was used in its standard form, configuring only the input modalities and a single-unit regression output. Following preprocessing, GRF timeseries were reshaped to 10025×16 (samples $\times$ sensors), extracted features to 368×1 and demographic attributes to 4×1. Each modality was flattened into a one-dimensional vector to conform to the PyTorch Multimodal Perceiver implementation [33]. Thus, the model operated on three modalities: raw GRF timeseries, GRF-derived features and demographics.

Inside a Perceiver block, positional encodings and modality identifiers are concatenated to each input vector, producing modality-aware arrays as described in Sect. 3.3. These inputs are jointly processed in a single forward pass. A learnable latent array queries the full set of input vectors via cross-attention, forming a fixed-size latent bottleneck. This latent representation is refined through several latent-only self-attention blocks. When enabled, re-entrant cross-attention allows the latent re-query the inputs, acquiring additional detail without reprocessing the entire sequence.

After refinement, latent states are averaged across latent indices to produce a global summary vector. A lightweight linear projection head maps this summary to the predicted TUG score. Because the model operates on pooled latent representations, it returns a single prediction per sample in each forward pass.

3.5 Experimental Setup

The cohort included an unequal number of PD and control participants (62 PD vs 38 controls). Although our objective was regression, this group imbalance could bias training if the TUG time distribution differed between groups. We, therefore, used PyTorch's weighted random sampler to balance PD and control representation in mini batches, so that both groups contributed more evenly to the optimization.

Hyperparameters for the Perceiver model were selected through iterative experimentation. Initial values were chosen based on prior experience and adjusted incrementally to minimize prediction errors. This process led to the selection of a network depth of 4, with 6 layers each for cross-attention and latent self-attention. Weight sharing was enabled between the cross-attention and the latent blocks.

Training was conducted with a mini-batch size of six due to GPU memory constraints. The model was optimized using the Adam optimizer with a learning rate of 1×10^{-4}, and a combined regression loss defined as the sum of MAE and MSE. Validation loss and evaluation metrics were computed on the entire held-out validation fold without rebalancing to simulate the real-world data distribution.

The framework was developed in Python using the PyTorch library and executed within a JupyterLab environment. All experiments were run on a workstation equipped with an AMD Ryzen 5 5600X 6-Core Processor, 16 GB RAM, and a 12 GB NVIDIA GeForce RTX 3060 GPU. CUDA support was utilized to accelerate training. Typical training sessions for processing either multimodal data or timeseries input configurations required approximately 50 h. Once trained, the model requires only a single forward pass and can provide predictions quickly on a standard laptop CPU.

3.6 Evaluation

Model performance was assessed by comparing predicted TUG scores against ground truth values using three matrices: Mean Absolute Error (MAE), Root Mean Square Error (RMSE), and Pearson Correlation Coefficient (CC). These metrics quantify the average deviation, squared error and linear relationship between predicted and actual scores, respectively.

$$MAE = \frac{|p_1 - a_1| + \cdots + |p_n - a_n|}{n} \tag{2}$$

$$RMSE = \sqrt{\frac{(p_1 - a_1)^2 + \cdots + (p_n - a_n)^2}{n}} \tag{3}$$

Here $\boldsymbol{n}$ denotes the number of samples, $\boldsymbol{p}$ the predicted value, and $\boldsymbol{a}$ the actual value.

To obtain robust estimation of generalization performance and to avoid information leakage between training and validation sets, we employed ten-fold cross validation (CV) with subject-wise splits. The 100 participants were randomly divided into ten disjoint folds at the subject level. In each iteration, nine folds ($\approx 90\%$ of subjects) were used for training and one-fold ($\approx 10\%$ of subjects) for validation. All recordings (both walking conditions) from a given subject were kept within the same fold, to prevent any information leakage during training and validations sets. Pearson CC was computed between predicted and actual TUG scores across all subjects in the validation fold for each CV run. This process was then repeated ten times, and the final performance was reported as the mean and standard deviation (SD) of MAE, RMSE, and CC across all folds.

The best-performing model was identified based on the lowest mean and SD in MAE and RMSE, and the highest mean with lowest SD in CC. Comparative analysis was conducted between multimodal and unimodal models to determine the most effective configuration. Scatter plots of actual versus predicted TUG scores were used to visually illustrate model performance.

In addition to overall performance, subgroup analyses were performed by diagnostic group (PD vs healthy controls) and age range using subject-level out-of-fold predictions from the ten-fold subject-wise CV. For participant with multiple measurements, observed and predicted TUG scores were average within each subject before subgroup analysis. Subjects were then grouped into predefined age categories for the age-based analysis. We also examined model performance near the clinically relevant 11.5 s TUG threshold in participants with PD. Specifically, we assessed whether subjects with observed TUG values within ± 1.0 s and ± 1.5 s of this cut-off were placed on the correct side of the threshold based on predicted TUG values.

For benchmarking, conventional regressors including KNN, SVR, Decision Tree and Random Forest were implemented using scikit-learn library. Hyperparameters for these benchmark regressors were selected through iterative experimentation, starting from standard defaults and adjusting key settings incrementally to minimize prediction error. These models were trained and evaluated under the same ten-fold CV protocol as the proposed framework. Since these algorithms cannot directly handle raw timeseries signals, they were applied only to the handcrafted extracted features.

4 Results

Table 2 summarizes the accuracy across input configurations. Among unimodal models, the GRF-derived summary features model achieved low prediction error (MAE of 0.82 ± 0.42 s, RMSE of 1.38 ± 1.06 s and CC of 0.92 ± 0.07). The raw GRF timeseries model performed similarly (MAE of 0.87 ± 0.31 s, RMSE of 1.34 ± 0.80 s and CC of 0.94 ± 0.05). In contrast, the demographics-only model produced substantially higher errors and a lower correlation (MAE: 1.80 ± 0.63 s, RMSE: 2.63 ± 1.63 s, and CC: 0.55 ± 0.37), indicating that gait information captured by the GRF signals contributes most to prediction accuracy.

The Multimodal (Summary features + raw GRF timeseries signal) configuration yielded the best overall performance (MAE 0.80 ± 0.34 s, RMSE 1.27 ± 0.85 s and CC 0.93 ± 0.07). In contrast, the three-modality setting (Summary features + raw GRF timeseries + demographics) produced similar but slightly inferior results (MAE of 0.87 ± 0.32, RMSE of 1.29 ± 0.73, and CC of 0.94 ± 0.05). The modestly lower CC for the summary features and raw timeseries configuration is largely driven by a single outlier participant with a time of 36.34 s, for whom all models under-predict. Overall, these findings indicate that adding demographic data does not systematically improve prediction accuracy, whereas fusing raw GRF timeseries signal with handcrafted features offers a consistent, though modest advantage over unimodal inputs.

Figure 4 visualizes the relationship between actual and predicted TUG scores across the three main configurations (Feature, Timeseries and Multimodal data). Predictions cluster closely around the reference line (y = x), indicating strong agreement across all models.

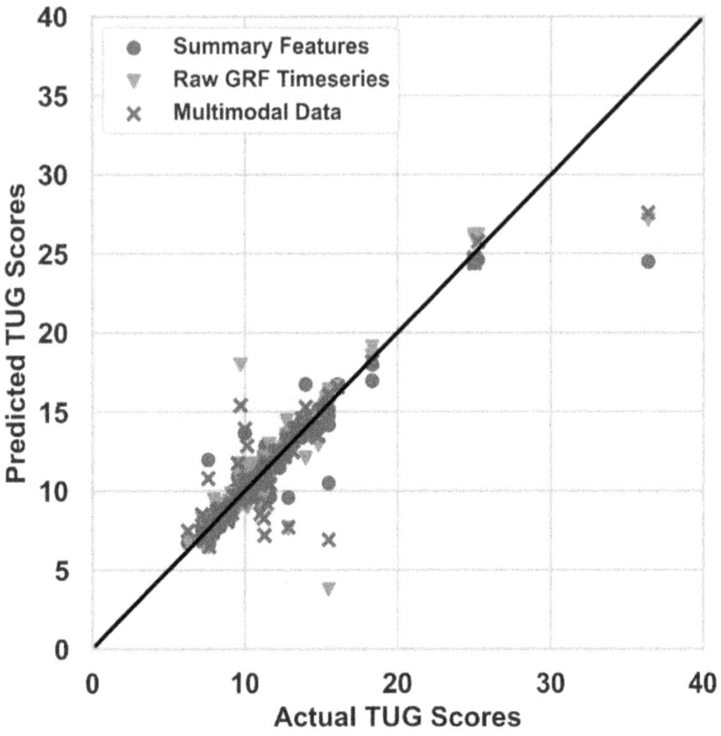

Fig. 4. Scatter plot showing the predicted versus the actual TUG scores for three main Perceiver configurations: GRF-derived summary features (blue circles), raw GRF timeseries signals (pink down-pointing triangle) and Multimodal Data (purple cross). The black dashed line represents the ideal prediction (y = x). Here "Multimodal Data" refers to the combination of GRF-derived summary features and raw GRF timeseries signals.

Table 2. Performance comparison across input modalities

Input Modality	MAE Mean ± SD	RMSE Mean ± SD	CC Mean ± SD
Demography	1.80 ± 0.63	2.63 ± 1.63	0.55 ± 0.37
Features	0.82 ± 0.42	1.38 ± 1.06	0.92 ± 0.07
Timeseries	0.87 ± 0.31	1.34 ± 0.80	0.94 ± 0.05
Multimodal Data (Features + Timeseries)	0.80 ± 0.34	1.27 ± 0.85	0.93 ± 0.07
Multimodal Data (Features + Timeseries + Demographics)	0.87 ± 0.32	1.29 ± 0.73	0.94 ± 0.05

For the best performing model (Multimodal: Summary features + Raw timeseries signal), errors were lower in healthy controls (MAE 0.41 s, RMSE 0.57 s and CC 0.93) than in participants with PD (MAE 0.97 s, RMSE 2.15 s and CC 0.86), consistence with the broader range and higher variability of TUG times in PD (Table 3).

Table 3. Diagnostic-group performance of the best performed model Multimodal Data (GRF summary features + raw GRF timeseries). N denotes unique participants in each group

Diagnostic-group	N	MAE(s)	RMSE (s)	CC
Control	38	0.41	0.57	0.93
PD	62	0.97	2.15	0.86

Errors were lowest in the 50–70 years ranges (MAE $\approx$ 0.53–0.67 s) and increased in older participants, with the largest error in the 81–90 age group (MAE 1.88 s and RMSE 4.59 s), reflecting largest variability in gait and mobility. The $<$ 50 years bin contains only two participants and should be interpreted cautiously (Table 4).

Table 4. Age-stratified performance of the best performed model Multimodal Data (GRF summary features + raw GRF timeseries). N denotes unique participants in each group

Age bins	N	MAE (s)	RMSE (s)
$<$ 50 years	2	0.64	0.70
50–60 years	34	0.53	0.76
61–70 years	42	0.67	1.24
71–80 years	14	0.95	1.79
81–90 years	8	1.88	4.59

Using the PD-specific cutoff, 15 of 19 subjects (78.9%) within $\pm$ 1.0 s and 26 out of 32 subjects (81.3%) within $\pm$ 1.5 s of the threshold was placed on the correct side of the cutoff based on predicted TUG values.

Table 5 summarizes representative studies that predict continuous TUG time from wearable or clinical data. Direct numerical comparison is difficult because cohorts, sensing modalities and protocols differ, but several patterns emerge. Choi et al. IMU-based accelerometers on the pelvis and feet during outdoor walking in 37 older adults and obtained MAPE of approximately 0.87–0.92 s, depending on sensor configuration [22].

The sensor-agnostic random forest pipeline [25], trained on heterogenous free-living accelerometer and GRF data from 303 participants, reported a substantially larger MAE of 1.7 $\pm$ 1.7 s. On the same PhysioNet GRF dataset Mostafavi et al. [26] applied a GAF + CNN model and achieved MAE 1.32 s and RMSE of 1.75 s for TUG regression. Other heterogenous wearable or clinical-variable models typically report MAE $\geq$ 1.7 $\pm$ 1.7 s. In this context, our Multimodal Data (Summary features + Raw timeseries) configuration attains a lower MAE (0.80 ± 0.34 s) and comparable or higher correlations (CC 0.93 ± 0.07), with an RMSE (1.27 ± 0.85 s) below the GRF-based GAF + CNN results and broadly in line with IMU-based regression. These findings suggest that vertical GRF, when modelled with multimodal Perceiver architecture, is comparable with more commonly used IMU setups for TUG predictions.

Table 5. Comparison with previous studies on TUG score estimation

Study	Modality	Method	Reported Metrics
Choi et al. [22]	IMU-based 3D accelerometers on pelvis and both feet during outdoor walking	Elastic-net feature selection + ridge regression	MAPE ≈ 0.865 s (feet), 0.918 s (feet + pelvis), 0.921 s (pelvis only) RMSE/CC not reported
Hao et al. [25]	Lower-back and wrist accelerometers plus in-shoe vertical GRF (16 sensors)	Random Forest regression	MAE: 1.7 ± 1.7 s other metrics not reported
Mostafavi et al. [26]	In-shoe vertical GRF (16 sensors)	GAF transformation + CNN	MAE: 1.32 s; RMSE: 1.75 s; R^2: 0.80
Multimodal Data	**In-shoe vertical GRF (16 sensors)**	**Perceiver-based multimodal regression**	**MAE: 0.80 ± 0.34; RMSE: 1.27 ± 0.85; CC: 0.93 ± 0.07**

The Perceiver-based framework consistently outperforms traditional machine learning models. Conventional regressors applied to extracted features showed substantially higher errors rates and weaker correlations compared to the Perceiver-based approach as shown in Table 6. For example, KNN produced an MAE of 2.01 ± 0.62 s, RMSE of 2.82 ± 1.47 s and CC of 0.51 ± 0.21, while Decision Tree performed worst overall (MAE: 2.65 ± 1.29 s, RMSE: 3.51 ± 1.22 s, and CC: 0.28 ± 0.29).

Table 6. Performance of Conventional regressors

Input Modality	Hyperparameters	MAE Mean ± SD	RMSE Mean ± SD	CC Mean ± SD
Features		0.82 ± 0.42	1.38 ± 1.06	0.92 ± 0.07
Multimodal Data		0.80 ± 0.34	1.27 ± 0.85	0.93 ± 0.07
KNN	n_neighbors = 23	2.01 ± 0.62	2.82 ± 1.47	0.51 ± 0.21
SVR	C = 10.0, gamma =" scale", epsilon = 0.1	2.04 ± 0.66	2.80 ± 1.43	0.47 ± 0.29
Decision Tree	min_samples_leaf = 3	2.65 ± 0.69	3.51 ± 1.22	0.28 ± 0.29

(*continued*)

Table 6. (*continued*)

Input Modality	Hyperparameters	MAE Mean ± SD	RMSE Mean ± SD	CC Mean ± SD
Random Forest	n_estimators = 500, min_samples_leaf = 2	1.94 ± 0.64	2.62 ± 1.29	0.51 ± 0.28

5 Discussion

This work explored whether TUG completion time can be estimated from vertical GRF signals recorded during two-minute walk in people with PD and healthy controls. Overall, the results suggest that steady-walking GRF contains substantial information related to functional mobility. Both the raw GRF timeseries signal and GRF summary features-based Perceiver models achieved high predictive accuracy, and the combined GRF configurations (Raw timeseries signals + summary features) produced the best average performance. The Perceiver-based models also outperformed conventional feature-based regressors trained on the same feature-set, which supports the value of learning directly from long raw signals and fusing them with interpretable gait descriptors within a single architecture.

Figure 4 provides a quantitative view of these results, showing that the predictions from all Perceiver configurations cluster closely around the reference line, indicating strong agreement with the measured TUG times for most participants. The largest deviations occur at the extremes of the score distribution, where the slowest participant is consistently underpredicted. Compared with the unimodal models, the Multimodal Data configuration (Raw timeseries signals and summary features) shows prediction slightly closer to the reference line, consistent with the performance metrics reported in Table 2.

The comparison between unimodal and multimodal inputs provides insight into multimodal learning in this context. The raw GRF timeseries signal and GRF summary features models explained most of the variability in TUG time, and combining these two GRF representations produced only a modest improvement but consistent reduction in MAE and RMSE. Although the improvement was modest, it may still be practically relevant, as the multimodal model provided a more reliable estimate of TUG time than either modality alone. This suggests that TUG-related mobility information can be captured from structured walking recordings. However, further work is needed to determine its utility for continuous monitoring in real-world settings. In contrast, adding age, sex, height and weight did not provide consistent benefit and slightly reduced performance. This matches the weak performance of the demographics model and suggests that, once GRF inputs are incorporated, basic demographics add little extra information. These findings should not be interpreted as evidence that demographics are unimportant for mobility in general, but rather that in this dataset they contribute little beyond what is already captured by GRF-based gait dynamics. This is consistent with multimodal learning theory, where fusion is most useful when modalities provide complementary information rather than redundant signals [34, 35].

Subgroup analyses showed higher accuracy in controls than in participants with PD. Prediction error increased error in older age groups, consistent with higher variability in TUG performance in these subgroups. In participants with PD, the model also showed reasonable performance near the clinically relevant 11.5 s cutoff, although some near-threshold cases were placed on the wrong side of the threshold. Therefore, small prediction errors near the cutoff may lead to incorrect fall-risk classification in PD, and predictions in this range should be interpreted carefully.

The Perceiver architecture is well suited for long GRF sequences and for combining multiple modalities in a single model. However, its fusion behavior can influence the contribution of low-dimensional inputs when a high-dimensional modality is much more informative. The model compresses the inputs into a fixed-size bottleneck using cross-attention and refines this representation with latent self-attention blocks [16]. When modalities differ strongly in dimensionality and predictive strength, training can prioritize the modality that reduces the loss fastest. This can lead to modality dominance (optimization imbalance), where gradients are driven mainly by the informative modality unless specific architectural or training strategies are used [36]. In our setting, GRF inputs likely dominate learning, so demographics may be down weighted and contribute little to the final prediction.

Computational efficiency should also be considered when interpreting these results, Although the dataset size was moderate, the multimodal and timeseries-based models included long GRF sequences, which substantially increased computational cost. Therefore, training required approximately 50 h.

Model behavior at the extremes of the TUG distribution also reflects the dataset composition. The cohort mainly includes people with mild-to-moderate PD and healthy controls, and very long TUG times are rare. As a result, severe cases are under-represented during training, prediction errors tend to increase for these rare targets. This corresponds to imbalanced regression, where extreme target values are scarce and models trained with standard losses become calibrated to the dense middle of the distribution [37]. In addition, the analyzed recordings capture level-ground walking and do not include key TUG components such as sit-to-stand, turning, or stand-to-sit phases. The model should therefore be viewed as learning a GRF-based proxy for TUG as a global mobility marker rather than a full surrogate for all TUG phases. Although the model achieved sub-second MAE which is below reported MDC ranges in PD [11], this indicates potential feasibility for longitudinal monitoring. However, the clinical impact of prediction error depends on where the true TUG value lies, as errors near commonly used cut-offs may change risk categorization. For this reason, predictions for individuals with very poor mobility and predictions near the decision threshold should be interpreted with caution.

Several methodological points also affect how these results should be interpreted. MAE and RMSE were selected as primary evaluation metrics because they express prediction error directly in seconds, making them more interpretable for TUG estimation. In contrast, explained-variance metrics such as R^2 are dimensionless and do not reflect the absolute magnitude of error on the original scale. Both the Perceiver models and the conventional regressors were evaluated without systematic hyperparameters optimization. Therefore, the observed performance differences should be interpreted with these methodological considerations in mind. Although both single-task and dual-task gait recordings were included, they were not analyzed separately because both recording conditions were not available for all subjects. Therefore, the reported performance reflects overall model accuracy across available recordings and does not permit a direct comparison between single-task and dual-task conditions. Finally, because the PhysioNet dataset aggregates recordings from multiple studies, cross-cohort validation (e.g., train on one or two cohorts and test on the third) would provide a stronger test of generalizability.

Overall, these findings support steady-walking vertical GRF as a practical tool for functional mobility in this dataset, while highlighting the need for stronger validation and robustness testing before clinical use.

6 Conclusion

This study evaluated a Perceiver-based multimodal framework to estimate TUG time from in-shoe vertical GRF recordings collected during straight, steady walking in people with PD and healthy controls from a publicly available dataset. Models trained on raw GRF timeseries and GRF-derived features achieved sub-second error, and combining both representations within a single architecture outperformed conventional feature-based regressors and prior studies. In this cohort, basic demographic variables showed limited predictive value and did not consistently improve performance when added to GRF inputs. Subgroup analyses indicated higher accuracy in controls than in PD, and errors increased with age.

Future work should prioritize external validation on independent cohorts with broader disease stages to assess generalizations and clinical robustness. Performance should also be reported stratified by TUG severity bands, age, and PD or control status to identify whether accuracy degrades for slow walkers or differs across clinical groups. In addition, model performance should be evaluated separately for single-task and dual-task gait recordings to determine whether cognitive-motor interference influences TUG prediction in PD. A more systematic hyperparameter tuning strategy should be adopted to improve the rigor and reproducibility of the experiments. If non-gait modalities are intended to contribute reliably, modality fusion should be designed explicitly (e.g., modality-specific encoders, conditional fusion, or training strategies that mitigate modality dominance). Finally, longitudinal data and uncertainty-aware prediction could support patient-specific monitoring by indicating low-confidence estimates, particularly for severe cases that are under-represented during training. In addition to TUG estimation, future work should evaluate the model for fall prediction and its potential use as a biomarker for rehabilitation and treatment outcomes.

References

1. Haagsma, J.A., Olij, B.F., Majdan, M., et al.: Falls in older aged adults in 22 European countries: incidence, mortality and burden of disease from 1990 to 2017. Inj. Prev. **26**, i67–i74 (2020). https://doi.org/10.1136/injuryprev-2019-043347
2. Nocera, J.R., Stegemöller, E.L., Malaty, I.A., et al.: Using the timed up & go test in a clinical setting to predict falling in Parkinson's disease. Arch. Phys. Med. Rehabil. **94**, 1300–1305 (2013). https://doi.org/10.1016/j.apmr.2013.02.020

3. World Health Organization: Step Safely: Strategies for Preventing and Managing Falls Across the Life-Course. https://www.who.int/publications/i/item/978924002191-4. Accessed 07 Feb 2024
4. Haddad, Y.K., Miller, G.F., Kakara, R., et al.: Healthcare spending for non-fatal falls among older adults, USA. Inj. Prev. **30**, 272–276 (2024). https://doi.org/10.1136/ip-2023-045023
5. National Council of Aging, Get the Facts on Falls Prevention, https://www.ncoa.org/article/get-the-facts-on-falls-prevention/. Accessed 10 Dec 2025
6. Almada, M., Brochado, P., Portela, D., et al.: Prevalence of fall and associated factors among community-dwelling European older adults: a cross-sectional study. J. Frailty Aging, **10**, 10–16 (2021). https://doi.org/10.14283/jfa.2020.44
7. Mathias, S., Nayak, U.S., Isaacs, B.: Balance in elderly patients: the "get-up and go" test. Arch. Phys. Med. Rehabil. **67**, 387–389 (1986)
8. Podsiadlo, D., Richardson, S.: The timed "Up & Go": a test of basic functional mobility for frail elderly persons. J. Am. Geriatr. Soc. **39**, 142–148 (1991). https://doi.org/10.1111/j.1532-5415.1991.tb01616.x
9. Shumway-Cook, A., Brauer, S., Woollacott, M.: Predicting the probability for falls in community-dwelling older adults using the timed up & go test. Phys. Ther. **80**, 896–903 (2000). https://doi.org/10.1093/ptj/80.9.896
10. Barry, E., Galvin, R., Keogh, C., et al.: Is the timed up and go test a useful predictor of risk of falls in community dwelling older adults: a systematic review and meta- analysis. BMC Geriatr. **14**, 14 (2014). https://doi.org/10.1186/1471-2318-14-14
11. Keus, S.H.J., Munneke, M., Graziano, M., et al.: European Physiotherapy Guideline for Parkinson's Disease. KNGF/ParkinsonNet, The Netherlands (2014)
12. Kristoffersson, A., Lindén, M.: A systematic review of wearable sensors for monitoring physical activity. Sensors **22**, 573 (2022). https://doi.org/10.3390/s22020573
13. Faiem, N., Asuroglu, T., Acici, K., et al.: Assessment of Parkinson's disease severity using gait data: a deep learning-based multimodal approach. In: Säreströniemi, M., et al (eds.) Digital Health and Wireless Solutions, pp. 29–48. Springer, Cham (2024). https://doi.org/10.1007/978-3-031-59091-7_3
14. Aşuroğlu, T., Oğul, H.: A deep learning approach for parkinson's disease severity assessment. Health Technol. **12**, 943–953 (2022). https://doi.org/10.1007/s12553-022-00698-z
15. Aşuroğlu, T., Açıcı, K., Berke Erdaş, Ç., et al.: Parkinson's disease monitoring from gait analysis via foot-worn sensors. Biocybern. Biomed. Eng. **38**, 760–772 (2018). https://doi.org/10.1016/j.bbe.2018.06.002
16. Jaegle, A., Gimeno, F., Brock, A., et al.: Perceiver: General Perception with Iterative Attention, http://arxiv.org/abs/2103.03206 (2021)
17. Zampieri, C., Salarian, A., Carlson-Kuhta, P., et al.: The instrumented timed up and go test: potential outcome measure for disease modifying therapies in Parkinson's disease. J. Neurol. Neurosurg. Psychiatry **81**, 171–176 (2010). https://doi.org/10.1136/jnnp.2009.173740
18. Greene, B.R., O'Donovan, A., Romero-Ortuno, R., et al.: Quantitative falls risk assessment using the timed up and go test. IEEE Trans. Biomed. Eng. **57**(12), 2918–2926 (2010). https://doi.org/10.1109/TBME.2010.2083659
19. Palmerini, L., Mellone, S., Rocchi, L., et al.: Dimensionality reduction for the quantitative evaluation of a smartphone-based Timed Up and Go test. In: 2011 Annual International Conference of the IEEE Engineering in Medicine and Biology Society, pp. 7179–7182 (2011). https://doi.org/10.1109/IEMBS.2011.6091814
20. Vervoort, D., Vuillerme, N., Kosse, N., et al.: Multivariate analyses and classification of inertial sensor data to identify aging effects on the timed-up-and-go test. PLoS ONE **11**, e0155984 (2016). https://doi.org/10.1371/journal.pone.0155984

21. Ortega-Bastidas, P., Gómez, B., Aqueveque, P., et al.: Instrumented timed up and go test (iTUG)—more than assessing time to predict falls: a systematic review. Sensors. **23**, 3426 (2023). https://doi.org/10.3390/s23073426
22. Choi, J., Parker, S.M., Knarr, B.A., et al.: Wearable sensor-based prediction model of timed up and go test in older adults. Sensors. **21**, 6831 (2021). https://doi.org/10.3390/s21206831
23. Polvorinos-Fernández, C., Sigcha, L., Borzì, L., et al.: Evaluating motor symptoms in parkinson's disease through wearable sensors: a systematic review of digital biomarkers. Appl. Sci. **14**, 10189 (2024). https://doi.org/10.3390/app142210189
24. Hausdorff, J.M.: Gait in Parkinson's Disease. https://physionet.org/content/gaitpdb/. (2008). https://doi.org/10.13026/C24H3N
25. Hao, T., Yamada, Y., Rogers, J.L., et al.: An automated digital biomarker of mobility. In: 2023 IEEE International Conference on Digital Health (ICDH), pp. 100–108. IEEE, Chicago, IL, USA (2023). https://doi.org/10.1109/ICDH60066.2023.00022
26. Mostafavi, S.M., Soumma, S.B., Peterson, D., et al.: Detection and severity assessment of parkinson's disease through analyzing wearable sensor data using Gramian angular fields and deep convolutional neural networks. Sensors. **25**, 3421 (2025). https://doi.org/10.3390/s25113421
27. Acosta, J.N., Falcone, G.J., Rajpurkar, P., et al.: Multimodal biomedical AI. Nat. Med. **28**, 1773–1784 (2022). https://doi.org/10.1038/s41591-022-01981-2
28. Sar, A., Puri, P.S., Naz, H., et al.: Multi-modal deep learning framework for early detection of Parkinson's disease using neurological and physiological data for high-fidelity diagnosis. Sci. Rep. **15**, 34835 (2025). https://doi.org/10.1038/s41598-025-21407-6
29. Li, A., Lian, J., Vardhanabhuti, V.: Multi-modal machine learning approach for early detection of neurodegenerative diseases leveraging brain MRI and wearable sensor data. PLOS Digit Health. **4**, e0000795 (2025). https://doi.org/10.1371/journal.pdig.0000795
30. Yogev, G., Giladi, N., Peretz, C., et al.: Dual tasking, gait rhythmicity, and Parkinson's disease: which aspects of gait are attention demanding? Eur. J. Neurosci. **22**, 1248–1256 (2005). https://doi.org/10.1111/j.1460-9568.2005.04298.x
31. Hausdorff, J.M., Lowenthal, J., Herman, T., et al.: Rhythmic auditory stimulation modulates gait variability in Parkinson's disease. Eur. J. Neurosci. **26**, 2369–2375 (2007). https://doi.org/10.1111/j.1460-9568.2007.05810.x
32. Frenkel-Toledo, S., Giladi, N., Peretz, C., et al.: Treadmill walking as an external pacemaker to improve gait rhythm and stability in Parkinson's disease. Mov. Disord. **20**, 1109–1114 (2005). https://doi.org/10.1002/mds.20507
33. Campagne, F.: Adapting Perceiver for learning with text modalities (2021). https://github.com/fac2003/perceiver-multi-modality-pytorch
34. Baltrusaitis, T., Ahuja, C., Morency, L.-P.: Multimodal machine learning: a survey and taxonomy. IEEE Trans. Pattern Anal. Mach. Intell. **41**, 423–443 (2019). https://doi.org/10.1109/TPAMI.2018.2798607
35. Li, S., Tang, H.: Multimodal Alignment and Fusion: A Survey, https://arxiv.org/abs/2411.17040 (2024). https://doi.org/10.48550/ARXIV.2411.17040
36. Peng, X., Wei, Y., Deng, A., et al.: Balanced Multimodal Learning via On-the-fly Gradient Modulation. https://arxiv.org/abs/2203.15332 (2022). https://doi.org/10.48550/ARXIV.2203.15332
37. Ribeiro, R.P., Moniz, N.: Imbalanced regression and extreme value prediction. Mach. Learn. **109**, 1803–1835 (2020). https://doi.org/10.1007/s10994-020-05900-9

Latency-Aware Evaluation of Bleeding Monitoring Algorithms for Real-Time Surgical Applications

Prosper Magara[1(✉)], Sudesh Sivarasu[1], Lamees Ras[1], Ahmed Biyabani[2], and Bessie Malila[3]

[1] University of Cape Town, Observatory, Cape Town 7925, South Africa
mgrpro001@myuct.ac.za

[2] Regional ICT Center of Excellence Bldg, Carnegie Mellon University Africa, Kigali Innovation City, Kigali, Rwanda

[3] University of Johannesburg, Auckland Park Kingsway Campus, Auckland Park, Johannesburg, Gauteng, South Africa

Abstract. Intraoperative bleeding is a critical complication in laparoscopic surgery that can obscure the surgical field, prolong procedures, and increase the risk of adverse outcomes. In surgical telementoring and telesurgery, timely recognition of bleeding is especially important, as delays in visual feedback or decision support can compromise surgical precision and patient safety. While deep learning–based methods have demonstrated strong performance for bleeding detection, their suitability for real-time deployment remains constrained by computational latency. This work presents a latency-aware evaluation of classical computer vision and deep learning approaches for intraoperative bleeding segmentation in laparoscopic surgery video. Classical methods based on colour analysis and motion estimation were compared against representative deep learning models, including MobileNetV2-U-Net and DeepLabV3. Segmentation performance was evaluated using the Dice coefficient, intersection over union (IoU), precision, and recall on both a publicly available dataset and an external local dataset. In addition, a browser-based benchmarking testbench was developed to measure processing latency from video acquisition through local inference, excluding network transmission. Results showed that deep learning models achieved higher segmentation accuracy and produced more spatially coherent bleeding masks across datasets. However, under central processing unit (CPU) execution, these models incurred substantial latency, exceeding clinically recommended thresholds for real-time surgical interaction. In contrast, classical computer vision methods achieved real-time performance with low latency but exhibited reduced segmentation accuracy and sensitivity to visual artefacts. These findings highlight a fundamental trade-off between bleeding segmentation fidelity and real-time feasibility in bleeding detection systems.

Keywords: Intraoperative bleeding · Surgical telementoring · Latency-aware evaluation

M. Säreströniemi et al. (Eds.): NCDHWS 2026, CCIS 3010, pp. 51–69, 2026.
https://doi.org/10.1007/978-3-032-28819-6_4

1 Introduction

Intraoperative bleeding is a potentially life-threatening complication during minimally invasive surgery, particularly in laparoscopic procedures where the surgeon's field of view is constrained and depth perception is reduced [1]. Uncontrolled or excessive bleeding can rapidly obscure the surgical scene, prolong operative time, increase the likelihood of conversion to open surgery, and ultimately lead to adverse patient outcomes [2]. Early detection and continuous monitoring of bleeding events are therefore critical for maintaining situational awareness and ensuring surgical safety, especially when the procedure is performed by a novice surgeon. In this context, computer vision–based approaches that can automatically identify and monitor bleeding in real time have attracted increasing interest as tools for intraoperative decision support, with longer-term implications for autonomous and semi-autonomous robotic surgery [3].

Recent advances in artificial intelligence (AI), particularly deep learning, have demonstrated promising results in automated bleeding detection and segmentation on surgical video [4–9]. Convolutional neural networks (CNNs) and modern segmentation architectures have achieved high accuracy, often surpassing traditional rule-based or classical computer vision methods [5]. However, the majority of existing studies emphasise detection and segmentation accuracy in isolation and largely overlook a key requirement for clinical deployment: processing latency [8–13]. In real-time applications such as surgical telementoring and telesurgery, even modest delays in visual feedback or decision support can degrade performance, impair situational awareness, and compromise patient safety [14]. Consequently, accuracy alone is insufficient as an evaluation metric for surgical AI systems intended for real-world use.

In parallel, classical computer vision techniques based on colour analysis and motion estimation remain relevant due to their interpretability, low computational overhead, and suitability for deployment on resource-constrained platforms [15–17]. Approaches operating in perceptually meaningful colour spaces, such as hue–saturation–value (HSV) and Commission Internationale de l'Éclairage L*a*b* (CIELAB), can effectively highlight blood-like regions, while optical flow provides a mechanism for distinguishing active bleeding from static blood-stained tissue by exploiting temporal motion cues [9,18,19]. Although such methods may struggle in visually complex surgical scenes, their favourable latency characteristics make them valuable baselines for real-time systems. Despite this, systematic, latency-aware comparisons between classical computer vision techniques and deep learning models for intraoperative bleeding detection, as well as comparisons among deep learning methods, remain limited.

Motivated by this gap, this work presents a latency-aware evaluation framework for bleeding detection algorithms in surgical video, with a particular focus on applications in surgical telementoring and telesurgery. Rather than proposing a single novel detection algorithm, the emphasis is on evaluating both classical and deep learning approaches under realistic real-time constraints. To support this, we develop a unified benchmarking testbench that enables frame-level processing, incorporates temporal methods such as optical flow, and provides end-to-end latency measurement under controlled and reproducible conditions.

The contributions of this work are threefold. First, we implement and evaluate a set of classical bleeding detection baselines based on colour analysis and motion estimation. Second, we compare these classical methods against representative deep learning models using both segmentation accuracy metrics and detailed latency measurements, highlighting the trade-offs between detection performance and real-time feasibility. Third, we introduce a reusable latency benchmarking testbench for surgical video analytics, providing a foundation for future low-latency telementoring and telesurgical systems where timely visual feedback is essential. Collectively, these contributions offer practical insights into the design and evaluation of real-time surgical AI systems within the broader context of digital health.

1.1 Related Works

Research on automated intraoperative bleeding monitoring in laparoscopic surgery spans a wide range of methodologies, from classical computer vision to deep learning–based models, with varying degrees of real-time capability and clinical focus. In this section, we summarise representative work, situating our study's latency-aware benchmarking within the broader context of bleeding analysis and surgical video analytics.

AI-Based Bleeding Detection and Segmentation. Deep learning has become a dominant approach for bleeding analysis in surgical video due to its ability to learn complex visual representations. Marullo et al. [7] developed a multi-task convolutional neural network that jointly performs semantic segmentation and blood accumulation event detection, achieving a Dice score of 81.9% and classification accuracy of 90.6% at approximately 21 frames per second on a graphics processing unit (GPU), demonstrating the potential for near-real-time performance in laparoscopic video understanding. Similarly, hybrid spatio-temporal frameworks that fuse image segmentation with temporal action localisation have been proposed to improve recognition of active bleeding events, although reported metrics such as F1 scores remain moderate and latency measurements are often not reported [5,20].

Studies using semantic segmentation architectures tailored for biomedical video, such as DeepLabv3 [9] and MobileNetV2-U-Net [21–23], have also been applied to recognise bleeding regions. For example, Tashiro et al. [24] reported a Dice coefficient of 0.53 and an IoU of 0.42 with inference times under 0.12 s per frame, while Sunakawa et al. [25] achieved a Dice score of 0.77 with GPU-based inference in liver haemorrhage video datasets. These segmentation models highlight the trade-off between spatial accuracy and computational cost: deeper contextual models yield stronger localisation performance but incur higher latency and hardware requirements.

Object detection has likewise been used to identify bleeding points or events. Rus et al. [6] leveraged a YOLOv5 detector in a simulated surgical environment, reporting a precision of 0.73 and a recall of 0.96 with per-frame detection times under 1 s, demonstrating the feasibility of region-based approaches for identifying bleeding regions in video streams. Other bleeding detection studies, such as Horita et al. [4], applied YOLOv7 to clinical colectomy videos, achieving AP50 metrics of 0.574 at 30 frames per second (FPS) on GPU hardware, indicating that modern detector backbones can operate near real time on surgical video. Such work underscores the adoption of deep learning detectors for bleeding localisation and event detection in diverse laparoscopic contexts.

In addition to binary detection and segmentation, related research has investigated broader applications of deep learning in surgical video analytics where bleeding is a component. For example, Checcucci et al. [8] developed a multi-task convolutional framework to detect instances of bleeding onset as part of robotic console overlays, achieving event accuracy above 90% in a retrospective evaluation, though latency was not reported. Other frameworks such as BlooDet have recently extended bleeding analysis tasks to include both region and bleeding point localisation within unified models, achieving region IoU around 64.9% and demonstrating the potential for synergistic multi-task learning; however, these frameworks remain primarily benchmarked on offline metrics rather than real-time performance [20].

Classical Computer Vision Approaches. Before the deep learning era, classical computer vision methods were foundational for bleeding and blood region analysis due to their computational efficiency and interpretability. One of the earliest approaches by Jo et al. [16] combined colour segmentation and Otsu thresholding to distinguish blood pixels from background, reporting sensitivity above 86% and specificity near 59% with processing times of approximately 0.37 s per frame. Similarly, pixel colour ratio algorithms based on B/R and G/R thresholds, integrated into OpenCV and Robot Operating System (ROS) pipelines by García-Martínez et al. [18], achieved frame rates around 24 FPS in combined in-vitro and in-vivo evaluation, illustrating the viability of lightweight colour-based bleeding segmentation in real-time scenarios.

Local entropy filters have also been proposed to capture texture disruptions caused by active bleeding. Daneshgar and Rahbar [17] reported classification accuracy exceeding 97% with extremely low per-frame computational cost, suggesting that lightweight filters can serve as rapid detectors when paired with simple segmentation rules. Optical flow–based approaches integrate motion cues to distinguish active bleeding from static blood residues. Richter et al. [3] combined optical flow with convolutional neural network (CNN) refinement in a robotic suction context, demonstrating how temporal information complements classical vision cues for bleeding dynamics.

While classical methods rarely match deep learning models in complex scenes, their low resource requirements and interpretability make them important candidates for latency-critical deployments. Hybrid models combining classical cues with learning components, such as gauze-tracking methods that integrate CNNs with motion analysis, further illustrate how these paradigms can be complementary. However, systematic head-to-head comparisons across classical and deep learning methods within consistent evaluation benchmarks remain sparse.

Real-Time Performance and Latency Considerations. Across both deep learning and classical paradigms, claims of real-time performance are frequently made, yet the reporting of latency metrics is inconsistent. Some studies include per-frame processing times (for example, Tashiro et al. [24] under 120 ms or YOLO detectors at 30 FPS [4]), while others omit any explicit measurement of latency [8–12,20,26]. Statements such as "real-time capability" are often made based on GPU acceleration without quantifying end-to-end processing delay, making it difficult to assess true feasibility under streaming or edge hardware conditions [5,27,28]. Few works evaluate scalability on non-GPU platforms such as central processing units (CPUs) or embedded devices, further limiting assessment of practical deployment potential.

This inconsistency extends to the choice of evaluation metrics. While accuracy, Dice, and IoU are commonly reported, many bleeding detection studies do not include precision and recall, and even fewer integrate latency metrics into the same evaluation framework. This disconnect between performance metrics and real-time feasibility motivates the need for standardised benchmarks that capture both segmentation quality and responsiveness.

Summary and Research Gap. In summary, existing work demonstrates the technical feasibility of intraoperative bleeding detection across both classical and deep learning approaches, with a wide range of reported segmentation and detection metrics. While some methods claim real-time capability, there is a notable absence of systematic evaluation that concurrently considers detection efficacy and processing latency under consistent conditions. Moreover, the integration of bleeding detection into real-time telementoring pipelines has not been thoroughly benchmarked. These limitations motivate the present study, which introduces a unified, latency-aware benchmarking framework and systematically compares classical and deep learning bleeding detection methods in a controlled, real-time context.

2 Methods and Materials

This section describes the experimental framework used to evaluate intraoperative bleeding detection methods under real-time constraints. Classical computer vision approaches and representative deep learning models were compared using a unified pipeline that standardised data input, preprocessing, visualisation, and latency measurement.

2.1 Dataset and Splits

The deep learning models were trained and evaluated using a publicly available dataset proposed by Rabbani et al. [9], consisting of 751 laparoscopic images and corresponding bleeding segmentation annotations. The images were extracted from over 60 h of video recordings obtained during 96 gynaecologic laparoscopic surgeries; Rabbani et al. [9] report that all participants provided written informed consent under institutional approval. Bleeding regions were annotated by junior surgeons under the supervision of senior surgeons.

A total of 751 images were used in this study, partitioned into training ($n = 525$), validation ($n = 112$), and test ($n = 114$) sets using pre-defined split files. Mutual exclusivity across all three splits was verified, with zero overlap confirmed between every pair.

Binary bleeding masks were derived by thresholding the provided grayscale portable network graphics (PNG) annotations at pixel value > 0. Class prevalence analysis revealed a highly imbalanced distribution at the pixel level: 99.8% of training images contained at least one bleeding region, with a mean bleeding pixel ratio of 3.390%. Both the validation and test sets contained bleeding regions in all images (100%), with mean pixel ratios of 2.657% and 3.552%, respectively. The consistent prevalence across splits confirmed representative partitioning despite the severe foreground/background imbalance.

To assess cross-dataset generalisation and enable direct comparison with classical computer vision methods, an external evaluation dataset of 100 annotated laparoscopic images was constructed from locally acquired videos and supplemented with publicly available laparoscopic footage. Ground-truth masks were manually annotated, and this dataset was used exclusively for testing the bleeding segmentation accuracy of the developed algorithms. Deep learning models were evaluated on both the internal test split and the external dataset, whereas classical methods were evaluated only on the locally annotated dataset. The University of Cape Town Human Research Ethics Committee (HREC; Ref: 541/2025) approved the retrospective use and annotation of laparoscopic surgery videos. Where required, additional institutional approvals were obtained prior to data use. All data were anonymised prior to analysis. The datasets, training scripts, application code, and evaluation scripts are available upon request for non-commercial use.

2.2 Preprocessing and Data Augmentation

All images and corresponding masks were resized to 512×512 pixels. Pixel intensities were normalised using ImageNet channel statistics (mean $[0.485, 0.456, 0.406]$, std $[0.229, 0.224, 0.225]$), yielding a normalised input range of approximately $[-2.12, 2.64]$. No augmentation beyond resizing and normalisation was applied at validation or test time.

Augmentation was applied exclusively during training using the Albumentations library, comprising random horizontal flip ($p = 0.5$), random vertical flip ($p = 0.5$), random rotation within $\pm 10^\circ$ ($p = 0.5$), random brightness and contrast jitter (limit ± 0.2, $p = 0.3$), and Gaussian noise injection ($p = 0.2$). Mini-batches of size 4 were used across all splits, with `drop_last=True` applied to the training loader to avoid instability from incomplete final batches, yielding 131 training batches and 28 validation batches per epoch. No fixed random seed was set during training; results may therefore exhibit minor variance across independent runs.

2.3 Classical Computer Vision Bleeding Segmentation Algorithms

Classical computer vision methods were implemented as training-free baselines to evaluate bleeding detection under strict real-time constraints. All methods operated on individual frames or short temporal windows and produced binary bleeding masks that were overlaid on the original video frames for visualization and latency measurement.

The first baseline employed HSV colour thresholding, exploiting the characteristic chromatic properties of blood [29]. Given an RGB image I, a colour space transformation

$$\mathbf{I}_{\text{HSV}} = (H, S, V) \tag{1}$$

was applied. Candidate bleeding pixels were identified by thresholding the hue and saturation channels within predefined red ranges, such that

$$M_{\text{HSV}}(x, y) = \begin{cases} 1, & H(x, y) \in H_{\text{red}} \cap S(x, y) > \tau_s \\ 0, & \text{otherwise} \end{cases} \tag{2}$$

Morphological filtering [30,31] and connected component analysis [32] were used to suppress noise and remove small, isolated regions. To reduce false positives from non-blood reddish structures, a red-dominance constraint was applied in RGB space by retaining only pixels satisfying

$$R(x, y) > \alpha\, G(x, y) \tag{3}$$

where α is a constant ratio.

A second appearance-based method used CIELAB colour thresholding [16], which provides perceptual separation between blood and surrounding tissue. Frames were transformed to CIELAB space

$$\mathbf{I}_{\text{Lab}} = (L, a, b) \tag{4}$$

and candidate bleeding regions were identified by thresholding the red–green opponent channel:

$$M_{\text{Lab}}(x, y) = \begin{cases} 1, & a(x, y) > \tau_a \cap L(x, y) > \tau_b \\ 0, & \text{otherwise} \end{cases} \tag{5}$$

This formulation emphasizes red chromaticity while suppressing bright specular highlights. The resulting mask was refined using morphological operations and area-based filtering.

Third, a hybrid CIELAB + optical flow [20,33] approach with camera motion compensation was implemented. Dense optical flow,

$$\mathbf{F}(x, y) = \big(u(x, y), v(x, y)\big) \tag{6}$$

was computed between consecutive frames. Global camera motion was estimated using the median flow vector $(\tilde{u}_m, \tilde{v}_m)$ and subtracted to obtain compensated motion:

$$\mathbf{F}'(x, y) = \mathbf{F}(x, y) - (\tilde{u}_m, \tilde{v}_m) \tag{7}$$

Motion magnitude was then calculated as

$$M_{\text{flow}}(x, y) = \sqrt{u'(x, y)^2 + v'(x, y)^2} \tag{8}$$

and thresholding was used to identify dynamically flowing regions. The final active bleeding mask was obtained by intersecting appearance and motion cues:

$$M_{\text{active}} = M_{\text{Lab}} \cap M_{\text{flow}} \tag{9}$$

2.4 AI-Based Bleeding Segmentation Models

Two deep learning–based semantic segmentation models were implemented as learned baselines for intraoperative bleeding detection.

U-Net with MobileNetV2. The first model was a U-Net with a MobileNetV2 encoder [34], constructed using the `segmentation-models-pytorch` library (Fig. 1). The encoder was initialised with ImageNet-pretrained weights. The decoder produces a single-channel output without an integrated activation function; raw logits were used throughout training and inference. All BatchNorm layers were frozen at the start of training.

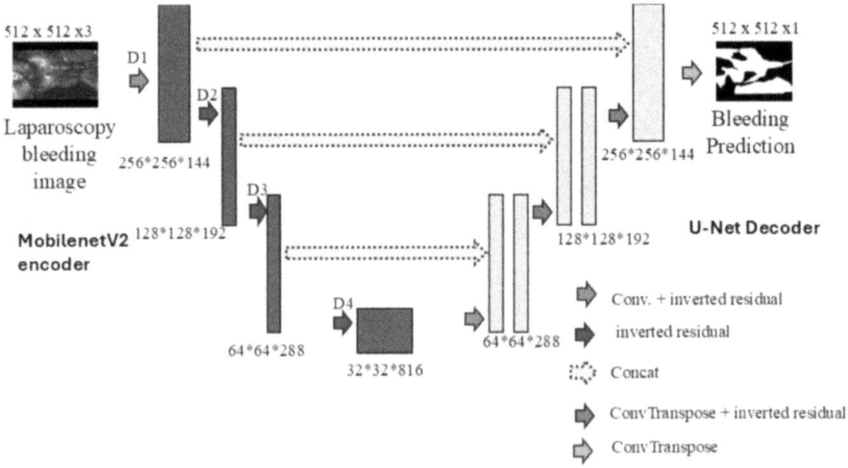

Fig. 1. MobileNetV2-U-Net implementation architecture.

DeepLabV3 with ResNet-50. The second model was a DeepLabV3 architecture with a ResNet-50 backbone (Fig. 2), initialised from weights pretrained for semantic segmentation on the Common Objects in Context (COCO) dataset with Visual Object Classes (VOC) label categories (`DeepLabV3_ResNet50_Weights.COCO_WITH_VOC_LABELS_V1`). The Atrous Spatial Pyramid Pooling (ASPP) module operates with dilation rates of {12, 24, 36} alongside a global average pooling branch, concatenating five 256-channel feature maps (1,280 channels) before projecting to 256 features via a 1×1 convolution with 0.5 dropout. The original classification head was replaced with a 1×1 convolution mapping the 256-dimensional feature space to a single binary output channel. An auxiliary fully convolutional network (FCN) head was retained in the architecture but its output was discarded during both training and inference; only the primary decoder branch was optimised. All BatchNorm layers were frozen throughout training (evaluation mode with gradients disabled) to preserve pretrained running statistics given the small batch size.

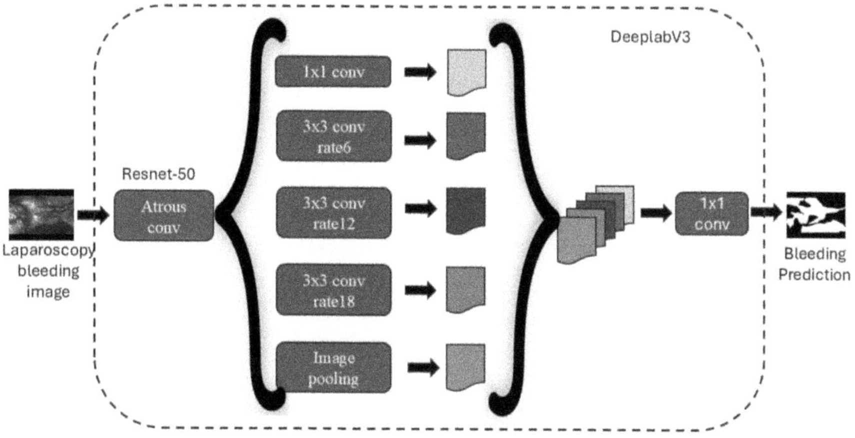

Fig. 2. DeepLabV3 implementation architecture.

2.5 Loss Function and Optimisation

Both models were trained using an identical composite loss combining soft Dice loss and binary cross-entropy with logits, weighted equally:

$$\mathcal{L} = \mathcal{L}_{\text{Dice}} + \mathcal{L}_{\text{BCE}}. \tag{10}$$

The soft Dice loss was computed on sigmoid-activated logits with a smoothing term $\varepsilon = 1 \times 10^{-5}$:

$$\mathcal{L}_{\text{Dice}} = 1 - \frac{2\sum_i p_i t_i + \varepsilon}{\sum_i p_i + \sum_i t_i + \varepsilon}, \tag{11}$$

where $p_i = \sigma(\hat{y}_i)$ is the predicted probability and t_i is the binary ground-truth label at pixel i. The binary cross-entropy term used the standard unweighted formulation.

Both models were optimised using Adam with a fixed learning rate of 1×10^{-4} and default momentum parameters ($\beta_1 = 0.9$, $\beta_2 = 0.999$). No learning-rate scheduling was applied. Training was conducted for 50 epochs on a single NVIDIA T4 GPU.

2.6 Model Selection and Inference Thresholds

At the end of each epoch, soft Dice score was computed on the validation set without thresholding. The checkpoint achieving the highest validation Dice across all 50 epochs was retained for final evaluation. For DeepLabV3, the best checkpoint was saved at epoch 37 with a validation Dice of 0.7683 (training loss decreased from 0.5434 at epoch 1 to 0.2993 at epoch 50). For the U-Net, the best checkpoint was saved at epoch 46 with a validation Dice of 0.7859 (training loss decreased from 0.6578 at epoch 1 to 0.3851 at epoch 50).

For evaluation, sigmoid activation was applied to logits and binary masks were obtained using thresholds selected on the validation set to prioritise sensitivity to sparse bleeding regions: 0.04 for DeepLabV3 and 0.05 for the U-Net.

2.7 Evaluation

The evaluation was designed to assess both segmentation accuracy and processing latency for classical computer vision and deep learning–based intraoperative bleeding detection methods. Deep learning models were first evaluated for segmentation performance using the held-out test split of the dataset proposed by Rabbani et al. [9], providing an internal assessment under conditions consistent with model training. To examine robustness and enable direct comparison with classical computer vision approaches, the same deep learning models were additionally evaluated on an external dataset comprising 100 locally annotated laparoscopic images. This dataset was also used to evaluate the classical computer vision methods, ensuring that all approaches were assessed on identical visual content.

Segmentation performance was quantified using the Dice coefficient, intersection over union (IoU), precision, and recall [35]. Classical computer vision methods were evaluated exclusively on the locally annotated dataset using the same metrics to ensure direct comparability with the deep learning approaches. No additional tuning was performed on the classical methods for individual images, allowing performance differences to reflect inherent methodological characteristics rather than dataset-specific optimisation.

Processing latency was evaluated using a browser-based benchmarking testbench with a Python backend designed to assess real-time feasibility under controlled and repeatable conditions. A prerecorded 3 s laparoscopic video clip with a resolution of 1080×720 was used as the input source to guarantee identical visual content across all latency experiments. Video frames were acquired from a universal serial bus (USB) flash drive connected to the inference computer, processed by the selected bleeding detection method, and rendered in a web browser. Latency was measured on a per-frame basis from frame acquisition through algorithm execution to local browser display, capturing processing and visualisation delays while explicitly excluding network transmission latency.

All latency experiments were manually initiated after selecting the target algorithm and were executed in isolation. Each experiment consisted of three complete iterations of the same video clip at a fixed resolution and target frame rate, ensuring consistent temporal exposure for all methods. For every frame, two synchronised outputs were generated: a raw baseline frame without inference and a processed frame with inference applied. This allowed the computational overhead introduced by each method to be isolated. Inference latency was measured using high-resolution timers, while instantaneous throughput was estimated from inter-frame timing to assess frames-per-second stability and drift during execution. The experiment pipeline for the latency testbench application is shown in Fig. 3.

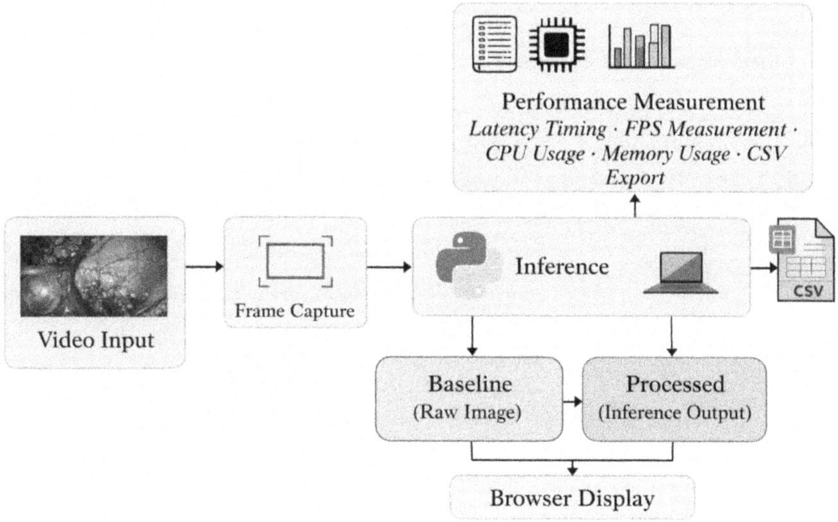

Fig. 3. Experiment pipeline for the latency-testbench application.

System-level resource utilisation was sampled concurrently with inference to contextualise computational performance. CPU utilisation and memory usage were recorded throughout each experiment, and frame-level measurements were aggregated to compute summary statistics, including median (p50) and tail (p95 and p99) inference latencies, the mean and standard deviation of frame rate, and mean CPU and memory usage. Algorithms that could not sustain continuous execution due to excessive computational demand were reported using only the frames successfully processed.

All experiments were conducted on a consumer-grade laptop equipped with an 11th Generation Intel Core i5-1135G7 processor (2.40 GHz), 8 GB of random access memory (RAM), and a 64-bit operating system, with all models executed on the CPU. The browser-based interface was accessed using Google Chrome, reflecting a realistic deployment environment for web-based surgical telementoring and intraoperative decision-support systems.

3 Results and Discussion

This section presents and discusses the segmentation accuracy and latency benchmarking results of the evaluated bleeding detection methods. Results are reported for both the Rabbani dataset (test split) and the local dataset, followed by an analysis of processing latency measured using the browser-based benchmarking testbench. Together, these results highlight the trade-offs between detection performance and real-time feasibility across classical computer vision and deep learning approaches, and they motivate future deployment on GPU-enabled edge devices.

3.1 Segmentation Performance Across Datasets

Quantitative segmentation results are summarised in Table 1 and Table 2, reporting the Dice coefficient, IoU, precision, and recall. Deep learning models were evaluated on both datasets, while classical computer vision methods were evaluated exclusively on the local dataset.

Table 1. Segmentation performance of deep learning models on the Rabbani dataset (test split).

Model	Dice	IoU	Precision	Recall
MobileNetV2-U-Net	0.7170	0.5984	0.7609	0.7912
DeepLabV3	0.7647	0.6264	0.7227	0.8332

Table 2. Segmentation performance of bleeding detection methods on the local dataset.

Method	Model type	Dice	IoU	Precision	Recall
MobileNetV2-U-Net	Deep learning	0.5233	0.3952	0.7542	0.4741
DeepLabV3	Deep learning	0.5818	0.4409	0.7577	0.5354
HSV thresholding	Classical CV	0.4144	0.2987	0.4106	0.5041
CIELAB thresholding	Classical CV	0.3792	0.2643	0.6038	0.3341
CIELAB + optical flow	Classical CV	0.3574	0.2425	0.6176	0.3029

On the Rabbani dataset (test split), both deep learning models achieved strong segmentation performance. MobileNetV2-U-Net attained a Dice score of 0.7170 and an IoU of 0.5984, with a high recall of 0.7912, indicating effective detection of bleeding regions under in-distribution conditions. DeepLabV3 achieved higher overall performance, with a Dice score of 0.7647 and an IoU of 0.6264, alongside a recall of 0.8332, reflecting improved sensitivity to bleeding regions when trained and evaluated within the same domain.

When evaluated on the local dataset, segmentation performance declined for both deep learning models. MobileNetV2-U-Net achieved a Dice score of 0.5233, while DeepLabV3 achieved 0.5818, with IoU values of 0.3952 and 0.4409, respectively. Precision remained relatively high for both models (≥ 0.75), whereas recall decreased compared to the Rabbani dataset. This reduction highlights the impact of domain shift arising from differences in surgical context, acquisition conditions, and visual characteristics between datasets. During latency experiments, DeepLabV3 inference crashed at the tenth frame due to RAM limitations; latency statistics are therefore computed only from the frames successfully processed.

Classical computer vision methods exhibited lower segmentation performance on the local dataset. The HSV-based method achieved a Dice score of 0.4144 with a recall of 0.5041, indicating moderate sensitivity but limited spatial agreement with the ground truth. The CIELAB-based method demonstrated a higher precision of 0.6038 but a lower recall of 0.3341, resulting in a Dice score of 0.3792. The hybrid CIELAB + optical-flow method achieved a Dice score of 0.3574, with improved precision of 0.6176 but reduced recall of 0.3029, reflecting stricter detection of regions exhibiting both blood-like appearance and motion.

3.2 Qualitative Analysis of Segmentation Outputs

Figure 4 presents qualitative segmentation outputs obtained from randomly selected frames processed using the browser-based benchmarking testbench. The HSV-based method frequently missed bleeding regions close to the surgical instrument, where specular highlights and metallic reflections altered the apparent colour distribution. In these regions, the CIELAB-based method produced more consistent detections, indicating improved robustness to illumination changes and tool proximity.

Compared to CIELAB alone, the hybrid CIELAB + optical-flow method generated smaller and more selective segmented regions, emphasising areas associated with active motion. While this reduced detections in static blood-stained tissue, it also resulted in fewer segmented pixels overall, particularly when bleeding motion was subtle.

Both deep learning models produced more solid and spatially coherent segmentation masks compared to classical methods. Bleeding regions were captured with clearer boundaries and greater continuity, even in the presence of surgical instruments and tissue deformation.

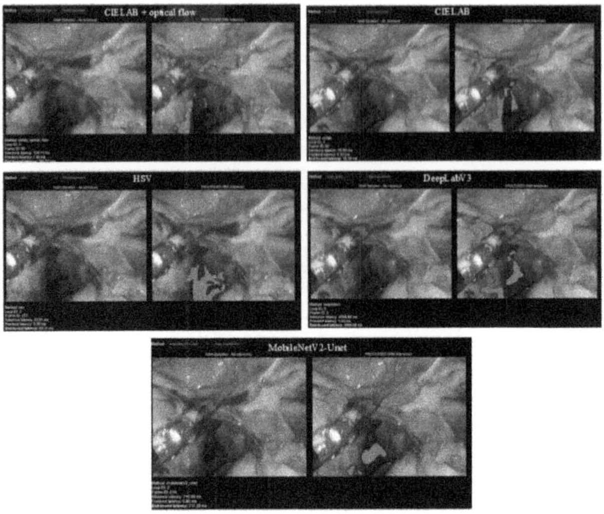

Fig. 4. Qualitative bleeding segmentation results.

3.3 Latency Benchmarking Results

Latency benchmarking results are summarised in Table 3, reporting percentile latency (p50, p95, p99), mean FPS, and system resource utilisation. Latency was measured from video-frame acquisition via a USB source through processing and local browser display.

Purely appearance-based classical methods achieved the lowest latency, with median latencies of 12.73 ms for CIELAB and 16.21 ms for HSV, corresponding to mean frame rates above 25 FPS. The hybrid CIELAB + optical-flow method incurred higher latency, with a median of 109.18 ms and a reduced throughput of 7.59 FPS, reflecting the computational cost of dense motion estimation and camera-motion compensation.

Deep learning models exhibited substantially higher latency under CPU-only execution. MobileNetV2-U-Net achieved a median latency of 679.34 ms, corresponding to 1.42 FPS, while DeepLabV3 demonstrated the highest latency, with a median of 4570.85 ms and 0.22 FPS. These results reflect the computational demands of CNN inference when executed without hardware acceleration in a browser-based pipeline.

Latency requirements for safe and effective telesurgery have been widely discussed in the literature. A recent narrative review by Motiwala et al. [36] reported that telesurgical performance degrades significantly as latency increases, with an ideal end-to-end latency threshold of less than 200 ms required to maintain surgical precision, dexterity, and patient safety. Importantly, this latency budget encompasses not only network transmission delay, but also delays introduced by sensing, computation, rendering, and system-level processing. In this context, the latency measured in the present study represents a component of the overall end-to-end delay in telementoring and telesurgical systems. The reported results therefore provide practical insight into how algorithmic and computational choices contribute to the latency budget that must be satisfied to meet clinically acceptable thresholds.

Table 3. Latency evaluation performed on the latency testbench.

Method	p50 latency (ms)	p95 latency (ms)	p99 latency (ms)	Mean FPS	FPS std	Mean CPU (%)	Mean RAM (%)
HSV	16.21	25.23	28.05	25.25	6.89	24.60	91.89
CIELAB	12.73	20.70	24.07	26.12	7.93	24.23	87.74
CIELAB + optical flow	109.18	155.88	177.89	7.59	1.41	17.59	86.49
MobileNetV2-U-Net	679.34	831.37	1000.43	1.42	0.19	21.16	85.25
DeepLabV3†	4570.85	5618.72	5710.64	0.22	0.03	20.77	95.00

3.4 Implications for Real-Time Deployment and Edge Acceleration

The combined accuracy and latency results indicate that, under CPU-only execution, deep learning–based bleeding detection models are not suitable for real-time deployment in interactive surgical telementoring systems. However, the observed segmentation performance suggests that these models remain strong candidates for real-time use when paired with appropriate hardware acceleration.

GPU-enabled edge devices, such as NVIDIA Jetson-class platforms, offer a promising deployment pathway at an affordable cost [37]. These devices provide dedicated GPU and tensor acceleration while maintaining low power consumption and compact form factors suitable for operating room environments. Lightweight architectures such as MobileNetV2-U-Net are especially well suited to such platforms and may achieve real-time or near-real-time performance when optimised using inference engines such as TensorRT [38]. More computationally intensive models, such as DeepLabV3, may benefit from model pruning, quantisation, or backbone substitution to meet latency constraints [39].

These findings suggest a hybrid design strategy for future bleeding monitoring systems: classical computer vision methods can provide low-latency baseline detection on CPU-only platforms, while deep learning models can be deployed on GPU-enabled edge devices to deliver higher segmentation accuracy without incurring prohibitive delays. The latency-aware benchmarking framework presented in this work provides a practical foundation for evaluating such deployments under realistic system constraints.

4 Conclusion

This study presented a latency-aware evaluation of classical computer vision and deep learning approaches for intraoperative bleeding segmentation in laparoscopic surgery, with particular emphasis on applications in surgical telementoring and telesurgery. By combining segmentation accuracy assessment with a browser-based latency benchmarking framework, the work highlighted the importance of evaluating algorithmic performance within realistic system-level constraints rather than relying on accuracy metrics alone.

Quantitative and qualitative results demonstrated that deep learning models achieved superior segmentation accuracy and produced more spatially coherent bleeding masks across both in-distribution and external datasets. However, when executed under CPU-only conditions, these models incurred substantial processing latency that exceeded clinically acceptable thresholds for real-time surgical interaction. In contrast, classical computer vision methods achieved low latency and real-time throughput, but at the cost of reduced segmentation accuracy and increased sensitivity to illumination changes and tool proximity.

These findings reveal a fundamental trade-off between segmentation fidelity and real-time feasibility in bleeding detection systems. They further emphasise that computational latency constitutes a significant portion of the end-to-end delay budget in web-based surgical platforms. Future work will focus on deploying lightweight deep learning models on GPU-enabled edge devices and integrating model-optimisation strategies to bridge this gap. The latency-aware benchmarking framework introduced in this work provides a practical foundation for evaluating such hybrid and accelerated systems, supporting the development of responsive, scalable, and clinically viable surgical telementoring technologies.

Acknowledgments. This document has been produced with the financial assistance of the European Union (EU) (Grant no. DCI-PANAF/2020/420-028) through the African Research Initiative for Scientific Excellence (ARISE) pilot programme. ARISE is implemented by the African Academy of Sciences (AAS) with support from the European Commission and the African Union Commission (AUC). The statements made and views expressed are solely the responsibility of the authors. This research was also supported by Telkom South Africa via the Telkom Centre of Excellence (CoE) in Broadband Networks at the University of Cape Town, and by the Google PhD Fellowship Program.

Disclosure of Interests. The authors declare no conflicts of interest.

References

1. Qadrie, Z., Maqbool, M., Dar, M.A., Qadir, A.: Navigating challenges and maximizing potential: handling complications and constraints in minimally invasive surgery. Open Health **6**(1), 20250059 (2025). https://doi.org/10.1515/ohe-2025-0059
2. Kaya, A.C., et al.: Intraoperative and postoperative complications of gynecological laparoscopic interventions: incidence and risk factors. Arch. Gynecol. Obstet. **304**(5), 1259–1269 (2021). https://doi.org/10.1007/s00404-021-06192-7
3. Richter, F., et al.: Autonomous robotic suction to clear the surgical field for hemostasis using image-based blood flow detection. IEEE Robot. Autom. Lett. **6**(2), 1383–1390 (2021). https://doi.org/10.1109/LRA.2021.3056057

4. Horita, K., et al.: Real-time detection of active bleeding in laparoscopic colectomy using artificial intelligence. Surg. Endosc. **38**(6), 3461–3469 (2024). https://doi.org/10.1007/s00464-024-10874-z
5. Hua, S., et al.: Automatic bleeding detection in laparoscopic surgery based on a faster region-based convolutional neural network. Ann. Transl. Med. **10**(10), 546 (2022). https://doi.org/10.21037/atm-22-1914
6. Rus, G., et al.: Artificial intelligence-based hazard detection in robotic-assisted single-incision oncologic surgery. Cancers**15**(13) (2023). https://doi.org/10.3390/cancers15133387
7. Marullo, G., Tanzi, L., Ulrich, L., Porpiglia, F., Vezzetti, E.: A multi-task convolutional neural network for semantic segmentation and event detection in laparoscopic surgery. J. Pers. Med.**13**(3) (2023). https://doi.org/10.3390/jpm13030413
8. Checcucci, E. et al.: Development of bleeding artificial intelligence detector (BLAIR) system for robotic radical prostatectomy. J. Clin. Med. **12**(23) (2023). https://doi.org/10.3390/jcm12237355
9. Rabbani, N., Seve, C., Bourdel, N., Bartoli, A.: Video-based computer-aided laparoscopic bleeding management: a space-time memory neural network with positional encoding and adversarial domain adaptation. In: Proceedings of the 5th International Conference on Medical Imaging with Deep Learning (MIDL), pp. 961–974. PMLR (2022). https://proceedings.mlr.press/v172/rabbani22a.html
10. Hong, S., et al.: Amplifying action-context greater: image segmentation-guided intraoperative active bleeding detection. Comput. Methods Biomech. Biomed. Eng. Imaging Vis.**11**(4), 1261–1270 (2023). https://doi.org/10.1080/21681163.2022.2159533
11. Yoon, D., et al.: Automated deep learning model for estimating intraoperative blood loss using gauze images. Sci. Rep. **14**(1), 2597 (2024). https://doi.org/10.1038/s41598-024-52524-3
12. Abaci, H., Soygazi, F.: Blood loss estimation on surgical sponges via machine learning and rate-based pixel counting method. IEEE Access **12**, 196133–196147 (2024). https://doi.org/10.1109/ACCESS.2024.3520245
13. Miao, A.J., et al.: HemoSet: the first blood segmentation dataset for automation of hemostasis management. arXiv:2403.16286 (2024). https://doi.org/10.48550/arXiv.2403.16286
14. Fernandez, C.C., Ruiz, M.G.: Telesurgery and telementoring. Cir. Esp. (Engl. Ed.) **102**, S23–S29 (2024). https://doi.org/10.1016/j.cireng.2024.01.012
15. Rahbar, M.D., Reisner, L., Ying, H., Pandya, A.: An entropy-based approach to detect and localize intraoperative bleeding during minimally invasive surgery. Int. J. Med. Robot. **16**(6), e2166 (2020). https://doi.org/10.1002/rcs.2166
16. Jo, K., et al.: Automatic detection of hemorrhage and surgical instrument in laparoscopic surgery image. In: Proceedings of the 38th Annual International Conference on IEEE EMBC, pp. 1260–1263 (2016). https://doi.org/10.1109/EMBC.2016.7590935
17. Daneshgar Rahbar, M., Ying, H., Pandya, A.: Visual intelligence: prediction of unintentional surgical-tool-induced bleeding during robotic and laparoscopic surgery. Robotics**10**(1) (2021). https://doi.org/10.3390/robotics10010037
18. Garcia-Martinez, A., Vicente-Samper, J.M., Sabater-Navarro, J.M.: Automatic detection of surgical haemorrhage using computer vision. Artif. Intell. Med. **78**, 55–60 (2017). https://doi.org/10.1016/j.artmed.2017.06.002

19. Jiang, J., Lu, Y., Hua, S.: Using spatio-temporal hybrid features for detecting bleeding point in laparoscopic surgery. In: Twelfth International Conference on Graphics and Image Processing (ICGIP 2020), pp. 88–96. SPIE (2021). https://doi.org/10.1117/12.2589338
20. Pei, J. et al.: Synergistic bleeding region and point detection in laparoscopic surgical videos. arXiv:2503.22174 (2025). https://doi.org/10.48550/arXiv.2503.22174
21. Bag, B.C., Maity, H.K., Koley, C.: UNET MOBILENETV2: medical image segmentation using deep neural network (DNN). J. Mech. Cont. Math. Sci. **18**(1), 21–29 (2023). https://doi.org/10.26782/jmcms.2023.01.00002
22. Kanadath, A., Jothi, J.A.A., Urolagin, S.: Histopathology image segmentation using MobileNetV2 based U-net model. In: Proceedings of the International Conference on Intelligent Technologies (CONIT), pp. 1–8 (2021). https://doi.org/10.1109/CONIT51480.2021.9498341
23. Ben Ahmed, I., Ouarda, W., Ben Amar, C.: Hybrid UNET model segmentation for an early breast cancer detection using ultrasound images. TechRxiv (preprint) (2022). https://doi.org/10.36227/techrxiv.19704895.v1
24. Tashiro, Y., et al.: Color-coded laparoscopic liver resection using artificial intelligence: a preliminary study. J. Hepato-Biliary-Pancreat. Sci. **31**(2), 67–68 (2024). https://doi.org/10.1002/jhbp.1388
25. Sunakawa, T., et al.: Deep learning-based automatic bleeding recognition during liver resection in laparoscopic hepatectomy. Surg. Endosc. **38**(12), 7656–7662 (2024). https://doi.org/10.1007/s00464-024-11331-7
26. Li, Y.-J., et al.: A better method for the dynamic, precise estimating of blood/haemoglobin loss based on deep learning of artificial intelligence. Ann. Transl. Med.**8**(19) (2020). https://doi.org/10.21037/atm-20-1806
27. Bamba, Y., et al.: Automated bleeding identification in surgical videos using deep learning. Society of Tokyo Women's Medical University (2022). https://doi.org/10.24488/twmuj.2022005
28. Acharya, D., Guda, R.K.S., Raovenkatajammalamadaka, K.: Enhanced EfficientNet network for classifying laparoscopy videos using transfer learning technique. In: Proceedings of the International Joint Conference on Neural Networks (IJCNN), pp. 1–9 (2022). https://doi.org/10.1109/IJCNN55064.2022.9891989
29. Okamoto, T., Ohnishi, T., Kawahira, H., Dergachyava, O., Jannin, P., Haneishi, H.: Real-time identification of blood regions for hemostasis support in laparoscopic surgery. Signal Image Video Process. **13**(2), 405–412 (2018). https://doi.org/10.1007/s11760-018-1369-7
30. Linghu, S., et al.: Iterative morphological filtering for DEM generation: improving accuracy and robustness in complex terrains. Appl. Sci. **15**(21) (2025). https://doi.org/10.3390/app152111683
31. Morphological filtering. In: The Essential Guide to Image Processing, pp. 293–321. Academic Press (2009). https://doi.org/10.1016/B978-0-12-374457-9.00013-5
32. Preeti, P., Kasi, A., Shetty, M., M., Mamatha, H.R.: Denoising and segmentation of epigraphical estampages by multi scale template matching and connected component analysis. Procedia Comput. Sci. **171**, 1877–1886 (2020). https://doi.org/10.1016/j.procs.2020.04.201
33. Beauchemin, S.S., Barron, J.L.: The computation of optical flow. ACM Comput. Surv. **27**(3), 433–466 (1995). https://doi.org/10.1145/212094.212141
34. Tomar, N.: UNet-with-pretrained-encoder: `U-Net_with_Pretrained_MobileNetV2_as_Encoder.ipynb` (GitHub repository). https://github.com/nikhilroxtomar/Unet-with-Pretrained-Encoder/blob/master/U-Net_with_Pretrained_MobileNetV2_as_Encoder.ipynb. Accessed 29 Jan 2026

35. Kamtam, D.N., et al.: Deep learning approaches to surgical video segmentation and object detection: A scoping review. arXiv:2502.16459 (2025). https://doi.org/10.48550/arXiv.2502.16459
36. Motiwala, Z.Y., et al.: Telesurgery: current status and strategies for latency reduction. J. Robot. Surg. **19**(1), 153–165 (2025). https://doi.org/10.1007/s11701-025-02333-1
37. Kang, P.: Evaluation of GPU-accelerated edge platforms for stochastic simulations: performance and energy efficiency analysis. Mathematics**13**(20) (2025). https://doi.org/10.3390/math13203305
38. Martín, J.J., Flich, J., Hernández, C.: Peformance isolation for inference processes in edge GPU systems. arXiv:2601.07600 (2026). https://doi.org/10.48550/arXiv.2601.07600
39. Lu, H., Alemi, M., Rawassizadeh, R.: The impact of quantization and pruning on deep reinforcement learning models. arXiv:2407.04803 (2024). https://doi.org/10.48550/arXiv.2407.04803

Robust Fatigue Prediction via Hybrid Generative–Ensemble Learning on Wearable Data

Fatemeh Sepehrmanesh(✉), Antti Isosalo, and Erkki Harjula

Centre for Wireless Communications, University of Oulu, Oulu, Finland
{fatemeh.sepehrmanesh,antti.isosalo,erkki.harjula}@oulu.fi

Abstract. Accurate fatigue prediction using wearable sensor data is important for a range of digital health applications, including preventive health management. In real-world settings, however, fatigue datasets are typically small, heterogeneous, and severely imbalanced, which limits the reliability of conventional machine learning and deep learning approaches, especially for detecting less common but more pronounced fatigue conditions. This paper presents a hybrid generative and ensemble learning framework for robust fatigue-level prediction from wearable data. The proposed approach integrates a Conditional Variational Autoencoder (CVAE) with a Light Gradient Boosting Machine (LightGBM) classifier. The CVAE performs class-conditional generative oversampling to synthesize physiologically plausible samples for underrepresented fatigue levels, thereby mitigating data imbalance while preserving fatigue-specific characteristics. The resulting balanced dataset is then used to train a LightGBM classifier, which is well suited for heterogeneous, tabular wearable-sensor features commonly encountered in digital health systems. The framework is evaluated on two benchmark fatigue datasets derived from wearable sensors with different imbalance characteristics using stratified 10-fold cross-validation. Experimental results demonstrate consistent improvements over six baseline models, achieving Macro F1-scores of 0.947 and 0.965, respectively, while substantially reducing misclassification between adjacent fatigue levels. These findings suggest that combining class-aware generative modeling with ensemble-based discriminative learning is an effective strategy for fatigue prediction in imbalanced wearable-sensor datasets.

Keywords: Physiological signal modeling · Class-imbalanced learning · Ensemble decision models · Multiclass prediction

1 Introduction

Fatigue, weariness of exertion, degrades cognitive and motor performance, increases reaction time, and impairs decision-making, thereby elevating the risk of accidents, injuries, and long-term health consequences [1,2]. These risks are especially pronounced in harsh operational settings—such as industrial labor,

M. Säreströniemi et al. (Eds.): NCDHWS 2026, CCIS 3010, pp. 70–93, 2026.
https://doi.org/10.1007/978-3-032-28819-6_5

field operations, surveillance, and outdoor activities in extreme climates—where prolonged physical workload, environmental stressors, and limited access to immediate healthcare amplify the impact of fatigue-related impairment.

Traditional approaches to occupational fatigue assessment primarily rely on self-reported questionnaires or observational evaluations conducted by supervisors [3]. While widely adopted, these methods suffer from subjectivity, limited temporal resolution, and poor reliability in capturing the gradual and cumulative nature of fatigue development [4]. As a result, critical fatigue states can remain undetected until performance degradation or safety incidents occur, limiting the effectiveness of preventive occupational health interventions.

Recent advances in wearable sensor technologies have enabled a shift toward continuous, objective, and data-driven fatigue prediction. Wearable devices equipped with physiological and biomechanical sensors can capture rich information related to muscle activity, movement dynamics, and physical workload, making them particularly suitable for, e.g., long-duration and remote occupational scenarios [5]. Continuous monitoring of cumulative workload and physiological stress aligns closely with the goals of digital health, supporting early intervention, personalized risk assessment, and proactive care pathways [5,6].

Available public fatigue datasets, including those used in this study [7,8] are often limited in size, heterogeneous in sensor modalities, and characterized by pronounced class imbalance, with severe fatigue states occurring less frequently despite their higher safety relevance. These factors degrade the generalization capability of conventional machine learning and deep learning models, which tend to favor majority classes and exhibit poor recall for critical fatigue conditions—an undesirable outcome in health and safety applications.

To address these challenges, this paper proposes a Hybrid Conditional Variational Autoencoder–Light Gradient Boosting Machine (CVAE–LightGBM) framework for robust multiclass fatigue level prediction using wearable sensor data (for CVAE, please refer to [9], and for LightGBM, please refer to [10]). The proposed approach employs class-conditional generative modeling to synthesize physiologically consistent samples for underrepresented fatigue levels, mitigating data imbalance while preserving class-specific characteristics. The augmented dataset is then used to train a LightGBM classifier, which is well suited for heterogeneous, tabular wearable features and capable of modeling complex, nonlinear relationships with modest computational requirements.

The proposed framework is evaluated on two benchmark wearable-based fatigue datasets with distinct sensing configurations, task characteristics, and class imbalance levels using stratified 10-fold cross-validation. The evaluation is designed to systematically assess the effectiveness of integrating class-conditional generative modeling with ensemble-based classification for multiclass fatigue-level prediction under imbalanced data conditions. By focusing on learning architecture, this study examines how class-aware data augmentation combined with gradient-boosted decision trees can support robust fatigue prediction using heterogeneous wearable-derived features in digital health contexts.

This paper makes the following contributions:

- A hybrid CVAE–LightGBM framework for multiclass fatigue prediction from wearable data, combining class-conditional generative modeling with ensemble-based classification.
- A class-aware generative oversampling strategy to mitigate class imbalance by synthesizing physiologically plausible samples for minority fatigue levels.
- A unified evaluation on two heterogeneous wearable fatigue datasets using stratified 10-fold cross-validation, demonstrating consistent improvements over six baseline models.
- Evidence that the proposed approach reduces misclassification between adjacent fatigue levels and improves overall classification performance.

2 Related Work

Recent advances in artificial intelligence (AI) have substantially expanded the role of wearable technologies in digital health, enabling real-time health monitoring, early risk detection, and personalized interventions. In occupational and industrial contexts, AI-enabled wearables are increasingly deployed to monitor physiological responses, detect fatigue and physical strain, analyze posture, and enhance situational awareness in hazardous environments. Occupational healthcare has adopted these systems to improve ergonomics, optimize workflows, and deliver timely safety alerts, thereby reducing injury risks and productivity losses [11]. A growing body of research demonstrates that multimodal sensing approaches consistently outperform single-sensor systems for fatigue detection. Physiological and behavioral signals such as heart rate, electrodermal activity, electromyography (EMG), inertial motion data, and skin temperature capture complementary aspects of physical and mental workload, enabling more robust and context-aware fatigue assessment. Advances in wearable technology have further facilitated non-invasive, continuous, and real-time acquisition of these signals, making fatigue prediction increasingly feasible outside controlled laboratory environments [1,12].

Table 1 summarizes representative studies on wearable-based fatigue detection across occupational and healthcare environments, highlighting sensor configurations, physiological metrics, machine learning techniques, deployment contexts, and classification outcomes.

Liu et al. [13] investigated physical fatigue during repetitive aviation manufacturing tasks over a six-hour protocol. By fusing data from six Shimmer3 inertial measurement units (IMUs), photoplethysmography (PPG), and external force sensors, the study achieved a binary classification accuracy of 94.15% using a polynomial-SVM model. A notable contribution was the demonstration that motion sensors alone can provide high detection accuracy, reducing system complexity and deployment costs.

In construction-oriented research, Gautam and Jebelli [14] introduced a flexible, fractal-based EMG sensor designed to withstand harsh site conditions. EMG signals were transformed into spectrograms and processed using a Vision Transformer (ViT), achieving 87% accuracy for multi-level fatigue classification. This study highlights the potential of combining innovative sensor design with deep learning architectures to improve signal reliability under real-world constraints.

Table 1. Comparison of wearable-based fatigue detection studies.

Ref.	Wearables	Signals/Metrics	Methods	Classes	Acc.
[13]	6 IMUs (hip, spine, arms, shank), PPG ear-clip	IMU(acc/gyro), HR, Borg CR15	LDA, kNN, SVM; PCA; RUS; 10-fold CV	Binary (Low/High)	94.15%
[14]	Flexible EMG sensor	EMG, SNR, Borg RPE	ViT (ImageNet-21K)	Multi (Low/ Med/High)	87.0%
[15]	Empatica E4, Huawei Watch 2, Polar H10	HR, EDA, Temp, Acc; Borg CR10	RF, FFNN; PCA; SG filter	Binary/ Multi	85.48%
[16]	Pulse, eye-blink, IMU	EBR, HRR, motion features	RF, KBIS; 10-fold CV	Binary	100%
[17]	Empatica EmbracePlus	PR, EDA, Temp; Borg	XGBoost, RF, BNN	Multi (3–5 levels)	99.9%
[7]	IMUs (foot, spine, thigh), chest strap	Acc, Gyro, EMG, Lactate; Borg	RF, SVM, ANN, DT, kNN, LR	Multi (4 levels)	98.0%
[8]	OFS elbow brace, IMUs, EMG	EMG, OFS, IMU features, Borg CR10	LightGBM, RF, DT, ET	Multi (Low/ Med/High)	96.2%

Moving beyond laboratory simulations, Rosselli et al. [15] conducted in-the-wild fatigue monitoring across multiple manufacturing companies in alignment with Industry 5.0 principles emphasizing worker well-being. By integrating wearable physiological data with questionnaires and personal attributes, their Random Forest and neural network models achieved 85.48% accuracy, underscoring the importance of ecological validity and long-term deployability.

Several studies have reported very high classification accuracy by combining wearable sensing with advanced machine learning models. Pabolu et al. [16] proposed an Industrial Internet of Things (IIoT)-based knowledge-driven fatigue recognition system incorporating physiological, behavioral, and demographic features, achieving perfect binary classification accuracy under controlled conditions. Albarrán Morillo et al. [17] validated an Industry 4.0 fatigue monitoring solution using a smartwatch-based platform, where XGBoost achieved near-perfect performance for three-level fatigue classification. Pinto-Bernal et al. [7] further demonstrated the feasibility of multi-level fatigue classification during rehabilitation walking tasks using wearable IMUs, achieving over 98% accuracy with a Random Forest model.

Otálora et al. [8] addressed upper-limb fatigue by integrating optical fiber sensors, IMUs, and EMG during repetitive tasks. Their LightGBM-based model achieved 96.2% accuracy for three fatigue levels, while also showing that combinations of non-EMG sensors can provide robust alternatives in industrial settings where EMG reliability is often compromised.

More recent work has explored ensemble and temporal modeling strategies to capture complex fatigue dynamics. Kim et al. [3] proposed the ChronoEnsemble Fatigue Analysis System (CEFAS), integrating multimodal wearable sensing with DeepAR and Temporal Fusion Transformer models, combined via an XGBoost meta-learner. The system demonstrated strong performance in estimating both physical and mental fatigue in smart construction environments, highlighting the benefits of ensemble learning for handling heterogeneous and temporally correlated physiological data.

Conditional Variational Autoencoders (CVAEs) offer significant advantages over traditional oversampling methods such as SMOTE by fundamentally changing the mechanism of synthetic data generation. Whereas SMOTE relies on local linear interpolation between minority samples, CVAEs learn the global data distribution through unsupervised representation learning, enabling the generation of novel and coherent samples that better capture nonlinear feature relationships [18,19]. This capability directly addresses SMOTE's limitations in producing noisy samples in regions of class overlap and its inability to model the complex global structure of minority classes [18]. Unlike interpolation-based methods that ignore information from majority classes, deep generative models such as CVAEs leverage distributional information from all classes to produce minority samples with improved diversity and physiological consistency [18]. CVAEs also offer practical advantages over GANs and diffusion models, including greater training stability and reduced computational cost, while avoiding issues such as mode collapse [20]. Recent extensions further enhance CVAE performance through adversarial training, where discriminators evaluate the realism of generated samples relative to the original dataset [21,22].

3 Materials and Methods

Building upon existing wearable-based fatigue detection studies, this work proposes a conditional variational autoencoder (CVAE) framework (see Sect. 3.2) to enhance classification performance on two publicly available datasets introduced by Pinto-Bernal et al. [7] and Otálora et al. [8]. Both datasets employ multimodal wearable sensors and multi-level fatigue annotations. The proposed approach leverages CVAE-based conditional data generation to synthesize physiologically plausible samples conditioned on fatigue level, enabling more balanced and discriminative training distributions. The effectiveness of the approach is evaluated by integrating the generated samples into existing classification pipelines and benchmarking performance improvements against the original reported results. Using the same CVAE-based framework across both datasets enables a consistent methodological comparison with prior work by Otálora et al. and Pinto-Bernal et al., while demonstrating the generalizability of conditional latent modeling for fatigue detection across different sensing configurations and experimental protocols.

3.1 Datasets Description

This subsection describes the two publicly available datasets used in this study, including their sensing modalities, experimental protocols, labeling strategies, and feature representations.

A) Fourth Fatigue Diagnosis States. The dataset developed by Pinto-Bernal et al. [7] was designed to classify multi-level fatigue states during walking tasks, primarily in rehabilitation contexts. Data were collected from 24 healthy volunteers (14 male, 10 female) with an average age of 21.75 ± 1.16 years. All participants were confirmed to be in a non-fatigued state at baseline using the Multidimensional Fatigue Inventory questionnaire. A multimodal wearable sensor suite was employed to capture physiological and biomechanical data. Four Shimmer3 IMUs recorded acceleration and angular velocity at 128 Hz, with sensors placed on the dominant foot instep and at the L5–S1 spinal segment. Muscle activity was monitored using two Shimmer3 EMG sensors sampling at 512 Hz, positioned on the tibialis anterior, rectus femoris, biceps femoris, and gastrocnemius muscles of the dominant leg. Heart rate data were recorded using a Zephyr HxM BT chest strap at 1 Hz. Fatigue was progressively induced through a structured protocol consisting of treadmill walking interleaved with a high-intensity exercise circuit. The circuit included high knees, jumping jacks, squats, and short runs, repeated across four rounds with increasing duration to induce escalating fatigue levels. After each round, gait and EMG data were recorded during treadmill walking, while blood lactate measurements and Borg CR10 ratings were collected as physiological and perceptual ground truth measures.

B) Upper-Limb Fatigue Dataset. The dataset introduced by Otálora et al. [8] was developed to estimate upper-limb muscle fatigue during repetitive physical tasks using a multimodal wearable sensor setup. Data were collected from 30 healthy volunteers (16 male, 14 female) aged between 18 and 30 years. Participants performed repetitive biceps curl exercises using their dominant arm until reaching physical failure. Load intensity was adjusted by sex, with female participants lifting 2.5 kg and male participants lifting 4.5 kg. The task was terminated when participants reported a Borg CR10 score of 10 or were unable to maintain the required range of motion. Each session began with a one-minute baseline recording in an anatomical position followed by a warm-up phase using lighter weights. Physiological and kinematic signals were collected using three sensing modalities. Surface EMG signals from the biceps brachii were recorded using a Shimmer3 device at 1024 Hz. Elbow joint kinematics were captured using an optical fiber sensor embedded in an elbow brace. In addition, two IMUs placed on the wrist and at the C7 vertebra recorded accelerometer and gyroscope data at 128 Hz to capture movement dynamics and compensatory postural adaptations. A comparative summary of the two datasets, including sensing modalities, fatigue states, and baseline methods, is provided in Table 2.

Table 2. Comparison of reference fatigue datasets and baseline methods

Feature	Fourth fatigue states [7]	Biceps muscle fatigue [8]
Physical Activity	Walking/rehabilitation	Repetitive biceps curls
Fatigue States	4	3
Subjects	24 (14 M, 10 F)	30 (16 M, 14 F)
Sensor Suite	IMUs, EMG, HR	IMUs, OFS, sEMG
Total Features	43	63
Best Model	Random Forest	LightGBM
Ground Truth	Blood lactate + Borg CR10	Borg CR10

Labeling and Fatigue States. Fatigue labeling in both datasets is based on the Borg CR10 scale, a subjective measure of perceived exertion in which lower values indicate minimal fatigue and a score of 10 corresponds to maximal exertion or physical failure. In the dataset by Pinto-Bernal et al. [7], perceived exertion is categorized into four diagnostic states: low (0–3), moderate (4–5), high (6–8), and very high (9–10). These labels are further supported by blood lactate measurements, which provide an objective physiological indicator of metabolic stress and internal workload. The resulting class distribution is imbalanced, with Low Fatigue (32.65%), Moderate Fatigue (26.41%), High Fatigue (25.08%), and Very High Fatigue (15.86%). The fine-grained labeling and multimodal sensor configuration make this dataset particularly suitable for conditional generative modeling approaches.

In contrast, the dataset by Otálora et al. [8] defines three fatigue states, namely Low Fatigue (36.6%), Moderate Fatigue (28.0%), and High Fatigue (35.5%), with subjective Borg CR10 ratings collected at 20-s intervals during repetitive lifting tasks. In this setting, the high-fatigue state primarily corresponds to Borg scores between 7 and 9 and reflects the onset of muscular failure. The dataset exhibits moderate class imbalance and limited subject diversity, which motivates the use of conditional data augmentation techniques.

While both datasets rely on subjective exertion ratings, the walking-based dataset incorporates biochemical validation through lactate measurements, whereas the lifting-based dataset infers fatigue progression through neuromuscular indicators such as EMG spectral shifts and increased kinematic variability. These differences highlight the need for a modeling framework capable of learning class-conditional representations while remaining robust to heterogeneous fatigue definitions.

Wearable Signals and Feature Representation. Both datasets employ engineered feature representations derived from multimodal wearable sensor signals to capture kinematic and physiological changes associated with progressive fatigue. Rather than using raw time-series data, sensor streams are segmented into gait or repetition cycles, from which compact descriptors are extracted to summarize fatigue-relevant dynamics while reducing computational complexity.

The walking-based dataset contains 2,919 samples with 43 features extracted per gait cycle, including IMU-based kinematic descriptors, EMG root-mean-square envelopes, and temporal gait parameters. These features characterize gait stability, temporal variability, and neuromuscular activation patterns. The upper-limb fatigue dataset consists of 1,240 samples with 63 features extracted per repetition cycle, capturing movement dynamics, joint behavior, and fatigue-related spectral changes in muscle activity.

Despite differences in task design and sensing configurations, both datasets share a common abstraction in which wearable-derived features provide structured representations of fatigue progression. This consistency enables the application of a unified conditional generative modeling framework to learn fatigue-aware latent representations across heterogeneous physical activities.

3.2 Conditional Variational Autoencoder for Class Balancing

A central component of the proposed Hybrid CVAE–LightGBM framework is a Conditional Variational Autoencoder (CVAE), employed as a class-aware generative model to address class imbalance. CVAE extends the standard Variational Autoencoder (VAE) by explicitly conditioning both the encoder and decoder on auxiliary information [9], such as class labels or contextual variables [23,24]. By incorporating the condition variable y, the model learns class-specific latent distributions rather than a single shared latent space, enabling structured and discriminative representations. This property makes CVAE particularly suitable for generating realistic synthetic samples for underrepresented fatigue states.

Given an input feature vector $\mathbf{x} \in \mathbb{R}^D$ and its associated class condition $\mathbf{y} \in \{1, \dots, C\}$ (or equivalently a one-hot encoded vector $\mathbf{y} \in \{0,1\}^C$), the conditional data distribution is defined as

$$p_\theta(x \mid y) = \int p_\theta(x \mid z, y)\, p_\theta(z \mid y)\, dz, \tag{1}$$

where $\mathbf{z} \in \mathbb{R}^{d_z}$ denotes a latent variable capturing hidden structure, $p_\theta(x \mid z, y)$ represents the decoder likelihood, and $p_\theta(z \mid y)$ denotes the conditional prior. Conditioning the latent space on y encourages the model to capture intra-class variability while preserving inter-class separation, resulting in more disentangled and interpretable representations [25].

Since the true posterior distribution $p_\theta(z \mid x, y)$ is intractable, an approximate inference model $q_\phi(z \mid x, y)$ is introduced. In practice, this variational posterior is modeled as a multivariate Gaussian with diagonal covariance:

$$q_\phi(z \mid x, y) = \mathcal{N}\big(z; \mu_\phi(x, y), \mathrm{diag}(\sigma_\phi^2(x, y))\big), \tag{2}$$

where $\mu_\phi(x, y)$ and $\sigma_\phi(x, y)$ are the mean and standard deviation vectors predicted by the encoder network. The diagonal covariance assumption implies conditional independence between latent dimensions and enables efficient optimization.

Model training is performed by maximizing the Evidence Lower Bound (ELBO) on the conditional log-likelihood:

$$\log p_\theta(x \mid y) \geq \mathbb{E}_{q_\phi(z \mid x, y)}\left[\log p_\theta(x \mid z, y)\right] - D_{\mathrm{KL}}\big(q_\phi(z \mid x, y) \,\|\, p_\theta(z \mid y)\big), \tag{3}$$

which leads to the following loss function:

$$\mathcal{L}_{\text{cVAE}}(x, y) = \underbrace{\mathbb{E}_{q_\phi(z|x,y)}\left[\log p_\theta(x \mid z, y)\right]}_{\text{Reconstruction Term}} - \underbrace{D_{\text{KL}}(q_\phi(z \mid x, y) \,\|\, p_\theta(z \mid y))}_{\text{KL Divergence}}. \quad (4)$$

Here, the first term encourages accurate reconstruction of the input, and the second term regularizes the latent space by minimizing the Kullback–Leibler (KL) divergence between the approximate posterior and the conditional prior. In practice, the conditional prior is often chosen as a standard Gaussian $p_\theta(z|y) = \mathcal{N}(0, I)$, and the KL divergence term admits a closed-form solution:

$$D_{\text{KL}}(\mathcal{N}(\mu, \sigma^2 I) \,\|\, \mathcal{N}(0, I)) = \tfrac{1}{2}\sum_{i=1}^{d}\left(\sigma_i^2 + \mu_i^2 - 1 - \log \sigma_i^2\right), \quad (5)$$

where μ and $\log \sigma^2$ are outputs of the encoder network.
To enable gradient-based optimization, the reparameterization trick [26] is employed:

$$z = \mu_\phi(x, y) + \sigma_\phi(x, y) \odot \epsilon, \qquad \epsilon \sim \mathcal{N}(0, I), \quad (6)$$

which allows backpropagation through stochastic sampling.

Both the encoder and decoder are typically implemented as neural networks. Their mappings are expressed as:

$$(\mu_\phi, \log \sigma_\phi^2) = f_\phi([x; y]), \qquad \hat{x} = g_\theta([z; y]). \quad (7)$$

The latent variable z thus provides a low-dimensional, condition-aware embedding of the input data.

Once trained, the CVAE is used to generate synthetic feature vectors by sampling from the conditional latent space corresponding to minority fatigue classes and decoding them into the original feature space. This class-conditional oversampling strategy mitigates data imbalance while preserving class-specific feature distributions. In addition, the latent mean $\mu_\phi(x, y)$ serves as an informative representation for downstream classification, enabling seamless integration with gradient-boosted decision tree models.

Overall, the CVAE provides a unified probabilistic framework for conditional generative modeling, structured representation learning, and imbalance-aware data augmentation, making it particularly well suited for wearable-based digital health applications characterized by limited and unevenly distributed labeled data.

3.3 Hybrid CVAE–LightGBM Framework

Figure 1 illustrates the architecture of the proposed Hybrid CVAE–LightGBM framework, which combines a conditional variational autoencoder, a class-aware data balancing module, and a LightGBM classifier, while Algorithm 1 summarizes the associated training and data generation workflow.

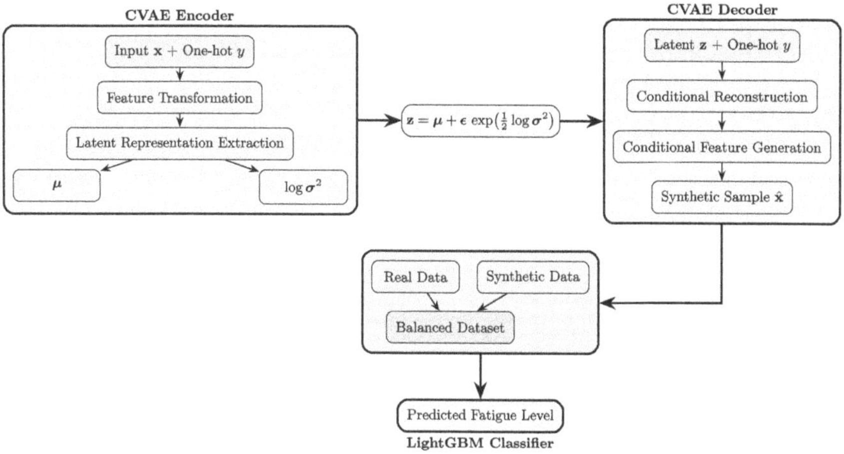

Fig. 1. Hybrid CVAE–LightGBM architecture for fatigue level prediction.

Algorithm 1. Hybrid CVAE–LightGBM (Minimal Version)

Require: Training data $\mathcal{D} = \{(x_i, y_i)\}$, epochs E, batch size B, latent dimension L, number of classes C

Initialize CVAE encoder ϕ, decoder θ, and LightGBM classifier

1. Train Conditional VAE
for epoch $= 1$ to E **do**
  for mini-batch (X, Y) **do**
    $\tilde{Y} \leftarrow$ one-hot(Y)
    $(\mu, \log\sigma^2) \leftarrow \text{Encoder}_\phi([X, \tilde{Y}])$
    $Z \leftarrow \mu + \exp(0.5 \log\sigma^2) \odot \epsilon,\ \epsilon \sim \mathcal{N}(0, I)$
    $\hat{X} \leftarrow \text{Decoder}_\theta([Z, \tilde{Y}])$
    $\mathcal{L} \leftarrow \text{MSE}(X, \hat{X}) + \text{KL}(q_\phi(Z|X, Y) \,\|\, p(Z))$
    Update ϕ, θ using $\nabla\mathcal{L}$
  end for
end for

2. Generate Class-Conditional Synthetic Samples
Compute class counts n_c and target size $n_{\max}$
for each class c **do**
  Sample $Z_{\text{syn}} \sim \mathcal{N}(0, I)$
  Decode: $X_{\text{syn}}^{(c)} \leftarrow \text{Decoder}_\theta([Z_{\text{syn}}, \text{one-hot}(c)])$
end for
Form balanced dataset $\mathcal{D}_{\text{bal}}$

3. Train Classifier
Train LightGBM on $\mathcal{D}_{\text{bal}}$
return trained CVAE and LightGBM

Conditional Encoder. The CVAE encoder receives as input a concatenation of the original feature vector $\mathbf{x} \in \mathbb{R}^D$ and the corresponding class condition $\mathbf{y} \in \{0,1\}^C$, represented using one-hot encoding. Conditioning the encoder on class labels enables the model to learn class-dependent latent representations rather than a single shared latent space. Through successive feature transformation and latent representation extraction stages, the encoder maps the conditional input into the parameters of a variational posterior distribution, namely the latent mean vector $\boldsymbol{\mu}$ and the log-variance vector $\log \boldsymbol{\sigma}^2$.

Latent Space Sampling. A stochastic latent variable $\mathbf{z} \in \mathbb{R}^L$ is sampled from the learned posterior distribution using the reparameterization trick. This mechanism allows efficient gradient-based optimization while preserving the probabilistic nature of the latent space.

Conditional Decoder. The decoder reconstructs feature vectors by conditioning on both the sampled latent representation $\mathbf{z}$ and the class label $\mathbf{y}$. By explicitly incorporating class information during reconstruction, the decoder performs conditional feature generation, producing synthetic samples that are consistent with the statistical characteristics of each fatigue level. The output of the decoder is a reconstructed or synthetic feature vector $\hat{\mathbf{x}} \in \mathbb{R}^D$ in the original feature space.

Class-Conditional Data Balancing. After training, the CVAE is employed as a class-aware generative model to address data imbalance. Synthetic samples are generated for minority fatigue classes by sampling from their corresponding conditional latent distributions. These synthetic samples are merged with the original dataset to form a balanced training set, thereby reducing class bias while preserving intra-class variability.

LightGBM-Based Classification. The balanced dataset is subsequently used to train a Light Gradient Boosting Machine (LightGBM) classifier for fatigue-level prediction. LightGBM is selected due to its strong performance on tabular data, robustness to heterogeneous feature distributions, and ability to capture complex non-linear decision boundaries. By decoupling generative modeling from discriminative learning, the proposed framework leverages the complementary strengths of deep probabilistic representation learning and ensemble-based classification.

Overall, the proposed hybrid architecture enables effective learning from limited and imbalanced wearable-sensor datasets by integrating conditional generative modeling with a high-performance classification backend. This design is particularly well suited for digital health applications, where data scarcity, class imbalance, and reliable decision-making are critical challenges.

3.4 Implementation Details

This subsection describes the practical implementation of the proposed Hybrid CVAE–LightGBM framework, including data preprocessing, CVAE training, synthetic data generation, and classifier configuration. All experiments were implemented in Python, using PyTorch for generative modeling and LightGBM for discriminative classification.

Data Preprocessing and Feature Scaling. For each dataset, the extracted wearable-sensor features were organized into fixed-length feature vectors, and categorical fatigue labels were mapped to integer class indices. To ensure numerical stability and to facilitate effective optimization of the generative model, feature values were normalized using standardization, transforming each feature to zero mean and unit variance based on the training data statistics. To avoid data leakage, preprocessing operations were performed independently within each cross-validation fold. Feature scaling parameters were learned exclusively from the training split and subsequently applied to the corresponding test split. Class labels were converted to one-hot encodings only when used as conditional inputs to the CVAE.

CVAE Training Configuration. The conditional variational autoencoder was trained using only the training portion of each cross-validation fold. The encoder and decoder were implemented as fully connected neural networks, with ReLU activations applied after each hidden layer. The encoder outputs the parameters of the variational posterior distribution, namely the latent mean and log-variance vectors. The CVAE was optimized using the Adam optimizer with a fixed learning rate. The training objective consisted of a reconstruction loss, implemented as mean squared error between the input feature vector and its reconstruction, combined with a Kullback–Leibler (KL) divergence term that regularizes the latent space toward a standard Gaussian prior. Training was performed for a fixed number of epochs, sufficient to ensure convergence without overfitting. The reparameterization trick was employed during training to allow gradient-based optimization through stochastic latent sampling. Class labels were incorporated as conditional information by concatenating one-hot encoded labels with the input features at the encoder and with the latent representation at the decoder.

Synthetic Data Generation and Class Balancing. After training, the CVAE was used as a class-conditional generative model to address class imbalance. For each fatigue class, the number of training samples was compared, and minority classes were augmented until all classes reached the size of the largest class in the training set. Synthetic samples were generated by sampling latent vectors from a standard normal distribution and decoding them together with the corresponding class condition. This process ensures that generated samples follow class-specific feature distributions while preserving intra-class variability. The synthetic samples were then combined with the original training data to form a balanced dataset. Importantly, synthetic data generation was restricted to the training folds only, ensuring that no artificial samples influenced the evaluation on unseen test data.

LightGBM Training Configuration. The balanced training dataset was used to train a Light Gradient Boosting Machine (LightGBM) classifier for fatigue-level prediction. LightGBM was selected due to its strong performance on tabular data, computational efficiency, and robustness to heterogeneous feature distributions commonly observed in wearable-sensor datasets. The classifier was configured using a multiclass objective function, with hyperparameters selected to balance model complexity and generalization performance. The trained model outputs the predicted fatigue level for each test sample, which is then used for quantitative evaluation. By separating generative data augmentation from discriminative classification, the proposed framework allows each component to specialize in its respective task, resulting in a flexible and effective solution for learning from limited and imbalanced digital health datasets.

4 Experimental Setup and Evaluation Protocol

This section describes the experimental setup and evaluation protocol used to assess the proposed Hybrid CVAE–LightGBM framework. All experiments were conducted using a rigorous and reproducible design to ensure fair model comparison and to mitigate biases arising from limited dataset sizes. The overall workflow is illustrated in Fig. 2.

4.1 Experimental Setup

All experiments were performed on a workstation running Python 3.13. PyTorch was used for generative modeling, `scikit-learn` for data preprocessing and evaluation, and LightGBM for gradient-boosting classification, together with standard scientific computing libraries. Both the CVAE and downstream classifiers were trained exclusively on CPU, as dataset sizes are relatively small and training times are modest. To ensure full reproducibility, random seeds were fixed across all components of the experimental pipeline.

The complete experimental workflow—including data preprocessing, CVAE training, synthetic sample generation, oversampling, and classifier training—was executed independently within each fold of a stratified 10-fold cross-validation scheme (Fig. 2). This design guarantees that (i) synthetic samples never appear in the test set, (ii) the CVAE is trained exclusively on the corresponding training split, and (iii) class distributions remain consistent across folds. As a result, the protocol provides an unbiased and robust estimate of generalization performance.

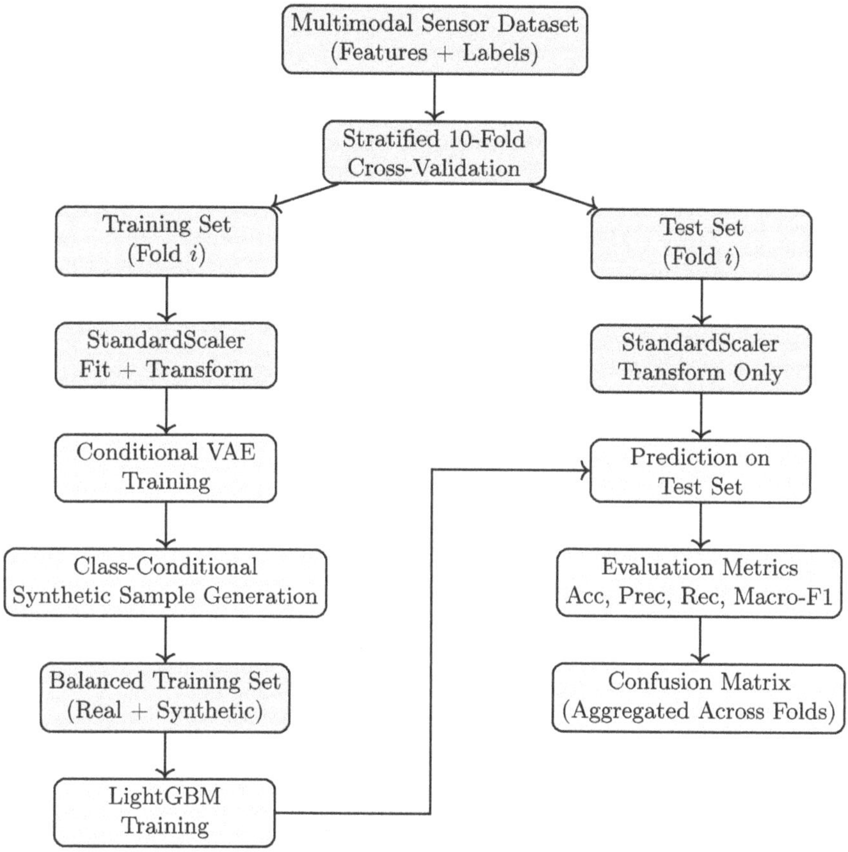

Fig. 2. Experimental workflow for the proposed hybrid CVAE–LightGBM framework using stratified 10-fold cross-validation. The Conditional Variational Autoencoder is trained exclusively on the training subset of each fold to generate class-conditional synthetic samples for mitigating class imbalance, while the test subset remains untouched and is used solely for performance evaluation.

4.2 Datasets and Preprocessing

Experiments were conducted on two wearable-sensor–based fatigue datasets consisting of multivariate tabular features and discrete fatigue-level labels. To facilitate multi-class classification, fatigue labels were mapped to integer class indices and encoded consistently across all experiments. Prior to model training, all feature variables were standardized using z-score normalization. Importantly, normalization parameters (mean and standard deviation) were estimated exclusively from the training portion of each cross-validation fold and subsequently applied to the corresponding test data. This fold-wise preprocessing strategy prevents information leakage and ensures an unbiased evaluation.

4.3 Baseline Models

To contextualize the performance of the proposed Hybrid CVAE–LightGBM framework, several baseline classifiers were evaluated under the same preprocessing pipeline and cross-validation protocol. These included Random Forest (RF) [27], a Multi-Layer Perceptron (MLP) classifier [28], Logistic Regression (LR) [29], Support Vector Machines (SVM) [30], k-Nearest Neighbors (KNN) [31,32], and Decision Trees (DT) [33]. The selected baselines represent widely adopted approaches for tabular physiological and behavioral data, covering linear models, distance-based methods, tree-based classifiers, and neural network-based models. Hyperparameters were selected following the grid-search procedure reported in Otalora et al. [8], who optimized model configurations for the same dataset. Specifically, the Random Forest model used 1400 trees, with the maximum depth of each tree set to 40. The Decision Tree employed the Gini impurity criterion, with the minimum number of samples required to split an internal node set to eight. The Support Vector Machine used a radial basis function (RBF) kernel, with the regularization parameter set to 10 and the gamma value set to 0.01. The K-Nearest Neighbors model used five neighbors, while Logistic Regression was configured with L2 regularization. The Multilayer Perceptron consisted of a single hidden layer with 64 neurons. LightGBM followed the optimized configuration reported in [8], where the number of leaves was set to 181 and the fraction of data used for bagging was set to 0.56. These configurations reflect commonly adopted settings in physiological classification studies and ensure reproducibility.

4.4 Hybrid CVAE–LightGBM Configuration

The proposed Hybrid CVAE–LightGBM framework combines a class-conditional generative oversampling module with a gradient-boosting classifier. The CVAE was trained for 60 epochs using the Adam optimizer with a learning rate of 0.001. A latent dimensionality of 16 was selected to balance representational capacity and regularization. The encoder and decoder followed a symmetric fully connected architecture with hidden layers of sizes 128, 64, and 128 neurons, respectively. This configuration provides sufficient expressive power while mitigating overfitting given the limited dataset size.

Generative oversampling was applied exclusively to the training split within each fold of the stratified cross-validation scheme. Synthetic samples were generated class-conditionally until all fatigue classes reached the size of the majority class, yielding a balanced training distribution without introducing information leakage. For classification, a LightGBM model was trained on the augmented dataset with 181 leaf nodes, a bagging fraction of 0.56, a feature fraction of 0.8, a learning rate of 0.05, and 500 boosting iterations. The multiclass objective function was selected to support fatigue-level prediction. This configuration corresponds to the best-performing setup identified during experimental evaluation.

4.5 Evaluation Metrics

Classification performance was assessed using multiple complementary metrics to account for class imbalance. These included overall accuracy, macro-averaged precision, macro-averaged recall, and macro-averaged F1-score. Macro averaging assigns equal importance to each fatigue class, regardless of class frequency. In addition to scalar metrics, confusion matrices were computed by aggregating predictions across all cross-validation folds. The resulting normalized confusion matrices provide class-wise insight into misclassification patterns and enable qualitative analysis of model behavior across different fatigue levels (Fig. 2).

5 Results

This section presents an evaluation of the proposed Hybrid CVAE–LightGBM framework on two benchmark fatigue datasets. Performance is assessed using stratified 10-fold cross-validation and compared against six baseline classifiers to examine classification accuracy, robustness to class imbalance, and generalization capability. The results provide a comprehensive assessment of the effectiveness of the proposed class-conditional generative oversampling and hybrid classification strategy.

Across both datasets, the proposed Hybrid CVAE–LightGBM framework consistently outperforms all baseline models, demonstrating the effectiveness of integrating class-conditional generative modeling with ensemble-based classification (Table 3 and Fig. 3). On Dataset A, the proposed method achieves a Macro F1-score of 0.947, surpassing strong baseline approaches such as Random Forest (0.922) and the Artificial Neural Network (0.911). This improvement indicates that CVAE-based class-conditional oversampling effectively mitigates class imbalance while enhancing generalization across all fatigue states.

On Dataset B, which represents a more challenging learning scenario due to higher class imbalance and a smaller sample size, the proposed framework achieves near-optimal performance, with an Accuracy of 0.968 and a Macro F1-score of 0.965. These results suggest that the CVAE-generated synthetic samples capture class-specific feature characteristics effectively, enabling the LightGBM classifier to maintain strong discriminative performance even under limited data conditions.

Overall, the results confirm that combining a Conditional Variational Autoencoder with a gradient-boosted decision tree classifier improves multiclass fatigue-level prediction. The proposed hybrid approach alleviates the adverse effects of class imbalance while enhancing the model's ability to capture subtle physiological differences between fatigue levels. These findings support the suitability of the Hybrid CVAE–LightGBM framework for real-world digital health applications, particularly in low-resource or imbalanced data environments.

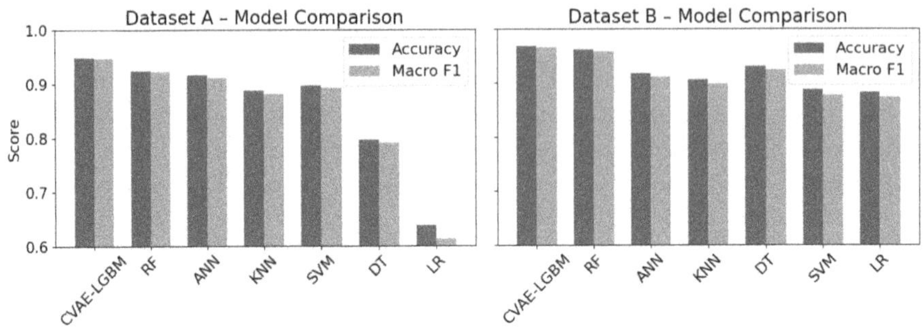

Fig. 3. Visual comparison of baseline models and the proposed Hybrid CVAE–LightGBM across Dataset A and Dataset B.

Table 3. Performance comparison of baseline models and the proposed Hybrid CVAE–LightGBM using stratified 10-fold cross-validation.

Model	Accuracy	Macro Precision	Macro Recall	Macro F1
Dataset A: Fourth Fatigue States Dataset [7]				
CVAE–LGBM	**0.949**	**0.945**	**0.947**	**0.947**
RF	0.924	0.925	0.921	0.922
ANN	0.916	0.913	0.910	0.911
KNN	0.887	0.884	0.880	0.881
SVM	0.896	0.895	0.890	0.892
DT	0.796	0.798	0.789	0.791
LR	0.637	0.618	0.612	0.612
Dataset B: Biceps Muscle Fatigue Dataset [8]				
CVAE–LGBM	**0.968**	**0.966**	**0.966**	**0.965**
RF	0.961	0.958	0.959	0.958
ANN	0.917	0.912	0.910	0.910
KNN	0.906	0.899	0.896	0.897
DT	0.930	0.925	0.925	0.924
SVM	0.887	0.879	0.877	0.877
LR	0.882	0.876	0.872	0.873

5.1 Confusion Matrix Analysis

Figure 4 presents the normalized confusion matrices of the proposed Hybrid CVAE–LightGBM framework for Dataset A and Dataset B. Overall, the model exhibits strong and well-balanced classification performance across all fatigue classes in both datasets, with low confusion between neighboring fatigue levels.

For Dataset A (left), more than 94% of samples in each fatigue class are correctly classified, indicating robust class-wise performance. Misclassifications are primarily limited to adjacent fatigue levels, which is expected given the gradual physiological transitions between fatigue states. Notably, Class 3, corresponding to the most severe fatigue level, is detected with an accuracy of approximately 95%, highlighting the framework's reliability in identifying critical fatigue conditions that are particularly relevant for occupational safety applications.

For Dataset B (right), classification performance is further improved despite higher class imbalance and a smaller sample size. Class 0 is recognized with perfect accuracy (100%), while Classes 1 and 2 achieve classification accuracies of approximately 95%. Off-diagonal error rates remain below 5%, demonstrating the model's ability to distinguish subtle inter-class differences and maintain high discriminative performance under challenging data conditions.

These confusion matrix results provide additional evidence of the effectiveness of the proposed CVAE-based class-conditional oversampling strategy. By generating a balanced and representative training distribution, the framework enhances classifier generalization across all fatigue levels, directly contributing to the strong macro-averaged performance metrics reported in Table 3.

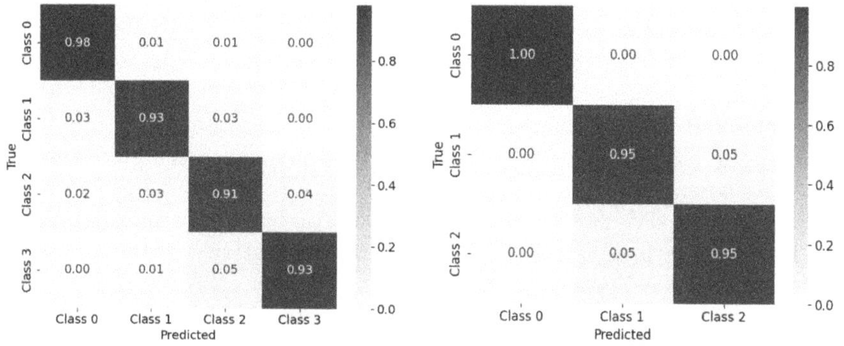

Dataset A — Proposed Method   Dataset B — Proposed Method

Fig. 4. Normalized confusion matrices of the proposed Hybrid CVAE–LightGBM framework. Left: Dataset A (4 classes: no, mild, moderate, severe fatigue). Right: Dataset B (3 classes: no, moderate, severe fatigue). Each matrix shows class-wise prediction accuracy and misclassification rates.

The experimental results demonstrate that the proposed Hybrid CVAE–LightGBM framework consistently achieves strong and balanced performance across datasets with differing sensing configurations, class distributions, and sample sizes. In particular, the improvements observed in macro-averaged metrics and class-wise prediction accuracy indicate that class-conditional generative oversampling plays a critical role in mitigating imbalance-related performance degradation. These findings motivate a deeper discussion of the underlying factors contributing to the observed performance gains, the comparative advantages of CVAE-based oversampling over conventional approaches, and the practical implications of the proposed framework for wearable-based fatigue prediction in real-world occupational and digital health settings.

6 Discussion and Future Work

The experimental results demonstrate that the proposed Hybrid CVAE–LightGBM framework provides a robust and effective solution for multiclass fatigue-level detection under class-imbalanced conditions. By integrating class-conditional generative modeling with an ensemble-based classifier, the framework consistently outperforms conventional machine learning approaches across two heterogeneous wearable-based fatigue datasets, achieving modest but consistent performance improvements.

6.1 Generative Oversampling and Non-linear Physiological Dynamics

A key contribution of this work lies in the use of class-conditional generative modeling to address data imbalance in wearable-derived physiological features. Physiological signals such as heart rate variability, electromyography, and inertial measurements exhibit inherently non-linear and non-stationary behavior due to complex interactions among autonomic regulation, neuromuscular activation, and biomechanical adaptation. These interactions give rise to multiscale patterns that are difficult to approximate under linear modeling assumptions.

Conventional oversampling strategies based on linear interpolation in feature space may therefore struggle to preserve the underlying structure of such data, particularly when class boundaries overlap or when minority classes exhibit distinct fatigue-related dynamics. In contrast, the Conditional Variational Autoencoder learns structured, class-aware latent representations, enabling the synthesis of physiologically consistent samples that better reflect non-linear class-conditional distributions. This capability is reflected in the reduced confusion between adjacent fatigue levels observed in the confusion matrix analysis, which is especially important for reliable fatigue prediction in real-world occupational settings.

6.2 Synergy Between Generative and Discriminative Learning

The proposed framework benefits from the complementary strengths of generative and discriminative models. The CVAE enriches the training distribution by mitigating class imbalance while preserving intra-class variability, whereas the LightGBM classifier effectively exploits these enriched representations to model complex, non-linear decision boundaries. Gradient-boosted decision trees are particularly well suited for heterogeneous, tabular wearable-sensor features, capturing feature interactions that linear models may fail to represent adequately. The consistent performance gains over Random Forests, Support Vector Machines, and neural network baselines indicate that this decoupled yet synergistic design enhances both robustness and generalization.

6.3 Comparison with Previous Studies

The performance of the proposed CVAE–LightGBM framework is significant when compared to both the baseline methodologies established by the creators of these datasets and subsequent evaluative studies. In the walking-task study introduced by Pinto-Bernal et al. [7], a Random Forest model achieved a reported high accuracy; however, this result was strongly influenced by the substantial class imbalance in the dataset, where the critical 'Very High' fatigue state represented only 15.86% of samples, and our reproduction yielded an accuracy of 92%. Our framework addresses this limitation through class-aware generative oversampling, enabling more reliable detection across all four fatigue levels and achieving a balanced Macro F1-score of 0.947. This compares favorably to works such as Bustos et al. [12], who applied the Pinto-Bernal et al. [7] approach to firefighters and reported varying accuracies (69–93%) across categories, and Narteni et al. [34], who used the same dataset for explainable AI and obtained accuracies between 82% and 84% for regional diagnostics. Similarly, for the upper-limb dataset by Otalora et al. [8], which originally achieved 96.2% accuracy using LightGBM, our hybrid approach reached an accuracy of 0.968 and a Macro F1-score of 0.965. By leveraging a Conditional Variational Autoencoder (CVAE) to learn the global data distribution, our model reduces misclassification between adjacent fatigue levels—a challenge noted in the original studies—and demonstrates superior stability compared to non-augmented implementations.

6.4 Occupational Health Scenario

The framework demonstrates consistent performance improvements across two datasets with distinct sensing modalities, task designs, and imbalance characteristics. This robustness of the developed method suggests that the proposed approach can generalize across a range of digital health monitoring scenarios. By addressing class imbalance through class-conditional generative modeling, the proposed approach improves sensitivity also to underrepresented states. Furthermore, the use of wearable-derived tabular features and computationally efficient models supports potential deployment in resource-constrained settings, enabling practical monitoring and decision support for remote or safety-critical occupational environments.

6.5 Limitations and Future Directions

Despite its strengths, the proposed framework has several limitations that warrant further investigation. First, the current approach relies on static, cycle-level feature representations and does not explicitly model temporal fatigue progression. Extending the framework to incorporate sequential generative models or temporal feature learning could improve sensitivity to gradual fatigue development. Second, the CVAE is trained offline, which may limit adaptability in dynamic or long-term monitoring scenarios. In addition, while this study adopts a grid-search procedure for hyper-parameter tuning, more advanced optimization strategies—such as Grey Wolf Optimization or Bayesian optimization—could further enhance model performance in future work. Future research may also explore lightweight updating mechanisms and edge-compatible implementations to support real-time deployment. Finally, integrating uncertainty estimation and explainability techniques would enhance transparency and trust, facilitating adoption in safety-critical and clinical decision-support systems.

7 Conclusion

This paper presented a Hybrid CVAE–LightGBM framework for multiclass fatigue-level prediction from wearable sensor data under class-imbalanced conditions. By combining class-conditional generative modeling with a robust ensemble-based classifier, the proposed approach addresses a persistent challenge in digital health analytics: reliable learning from limited and unevenly distributed physiological data. Experimental evaluation on two heterogeneous wearable-based fatigue datasets demonstrates consistent and meaningful performance improvements over conventional machine learning and neural network baselines. The results confirm that class-aware synthetic data generation using Conditional Variational Autoencoders enhances discriminative learning, particularly for minority fatigue classes that are critical in health and safety monitoring. When coupled with LightGBM—well suited for heterogeneous, tabular wearable features—the framework achieves strong predictive accuracy, improved macro-averaged recall, and reduced confusion between adjacent fatigue states. These properties are especially important for fatigue monitoring applications, where accurate classification directly influence user safety, well-being, and operational decision-making.

Beyond predictive accuracy, the proposed framework provides a flexible methodological basis for wearable-based fatigue analysis. While the present study focuses on offline learning using static feature representations, the hybrid modeling paradigm is amenable to future extensions involving temporally enriched features, adaptive learning strategies, and uncertainty-aware prediction. Such extensions may further improve robustness and interpretability, which are essential considerations for fatigue-aware decision support.

Disclosure of Interests. No conflicts of interest, financial or otherwise, are declared by the authors.

References

1. Adão Martins, N.R., Annaheim, S., Spengler, C.M., Rossi, R.M.: Fatigue monitoring through wearables: a state-of-the-art review. Front. Physiol. **12**, 790292 (2021). https://doi.org/10.3389/fphys.2021.790292
2. Gholami, M., Napier, C., Patiño, A.G., Cuthbert, T.J., Menon, C.: Fatigue monitoring in running using flexible textile wearable sensors. Sensors **20**, 5573 (2020). https://doi.org/10.3390/s20195573

3. Kim, B., et al.: Internet of things and ensemble learning-based mental and physical fatigue monitoring for smart construction sites. J. Big Data **11**, 115 (2024). https://doi.org/10.1186/s40537-024-00978-7
4. Yang, L., et al.: Towards smart work clothing for automatic risk assessment of physical workload. IEEE Access **6**, 40059–72 (2018). https://doi.org/10.1109/ACCESS.2018.2855719
5. Matijevich, E.S., Volgyesi, P., Zelik, K.E.: A promising wearable solution for the practical and accurate monitoring of low back loading in manual material handling. Sensors **21**, 340 (2021). https://doi.org/10.3390/s21020340
6. Vo, D.K., Trinh, K.T.L.: Advances in wearable biosensors for healthcare: current trends, applications, and future perspectives. Biosensors **14**, 560 (2024). https://doi.org/10.3390/bios14110560
7. Pinto-Bernal, M.J., Cifuentes, C.A., Perdomo, O., Rincón-Roncancio, M., Múnera, M.: A data-driven approach to physical fatigue management using wearable sensors to classify four diagnostic fatigue states. Sensors **21**, 6401 (2021). https://doi.org/10.3390/s21196401
8. Otálora, S., Segatto, M.E., Monteiro, M.E., Múnera, M., Díaz, C.A., Cifuentes, C.A.: Data-driven approach for upper limb fatigue estimation based on wearable sensors. Sensors **23**, 9291 (2023). https://doi.org/10.3390/s23229291
9. Sohn, K., Lee, H., Yan, X.: Learning structured output representation using deep conditional generative models. In: Proceedings of the 29th International Conference on Neural Information Processing Systems, pp. 3483–3491 (2015). https://doi.org/10.5555/2969442.2969628
10. Ke, G., et al.: LightGBM: a highly efficient gradient boosting decision tree. Neural Inf. Process. Syst. (2017). https://doi.org/10.5555/3294996.3295074
11. Melders, L., Smigins, R., Birkavs, A.: Recent advances in vehicle driver health monitoring systems. Sensors **25**, 1812 (2025). https://doi.org/10.3390/s25061812
12. Bustos, D., et al.: Exploring the applicability of physiological monitoring to manage physical fatigue in firefighters. Sensors **23**, 5127 (2023). https://doi.org/10.3390/s23115127
13. Liu, G., Dobbins, C., D'Souza, M., Phuong, N.: A machine learning approach for detecting fatigue during repetitive physical tasks. Pers. Ubiquit. Comput. **27**, 2103–20 (2023). https://doi.org/10.1007/s00779-023-01718-z
14. Gautam, Y., Jebelli, H.: Design of flexible polyimide-based serpentine EMG sensor for AI-enabled fatigue detection in construction. Sens. Bio-Sens. Res. **46**, 100713 (2024). https://doi.org/10.1016/j.sbsr.2024.100713
15. Rosselli, M., et al.: Workers fatigue monitoring for well-being improvement in manufacturing. IFAC-PapersOnLine **58**, 61–6 (2024). https://doi.org/10.1016/j.ifacol.2024.09.092
16. Pabolu, V.K.R., Shrivastava, D., Kulkarni, M.S.: Intelligent system for assembly-line worker's fatigue recognition and facilitation. Comput. Ind. Eng. **198**, 110726 (2024). https://doi.org/10.1016/j.cie.2024.110726
17. Morillo, C.A., Demichela, M., Jawla, D., Kelleher, J.: Wearable technology and machine learning for assessing physical fatigue in Industry 4.0. Hum. Factors Wearable Technol. **141**, 28–36 (2024). https://doi.org/10.54941/ahfe1005052
18. Zare, A., et al. Uncertainty-Aware Generative Oversampling Using an Entropy-Guided Conditional Variational Autoencoder (2025). arXiv preprint arXiv:2509.25334. https://doi.org/10.48550/arXiv.2509.25334
19. Chen, B., Zhang, L., Liu, T., Li, H., He, C.: Lightweight network with variable asymmetric rebalancing strategy for small and imbalanced fault diagnosis. Machines **10**, 879 (2022). https://doi.org/10.3390/machines10100879

20. Di Salvo, F., Nguyen, H.H.M., Ledig, C.: Embedding-based federated data sharing via differentially private conditional VAEs. In: International Conference on Medical Image Computing and Computer-Assisted Intervention, pp. 138–147. Springer, Heidelberg (2025). https://doi.org/10.48550/arXiv.2507.02671
21. Sabeel, U., Heydari, S.S., Elgazzar, K., El-Khatib, K.: CVAE-AN: atypical attack flow detection using incremental adversarial learning. In: IEEE Global Communications Conference (GLOBECOM), pp. 1–6. IEEE. (2021). https://doi.org/10.1109/GLOBECOM46510.2021.9685699
22. Wang, C., Xu, D., Li, Z., Niyato, D.: Effective intrusion detection in highly imbalanced IoT networks with lightweight S2CGAN-IDS. IEEE Internet Things J. **11**, 15140–51 (2023). https://doi.org/10.1109/JIOT.2023.3342638
23. Xu, X., Tsang, I., Liu, C.: Improving generalization via attribute selection on out-of-the-box data. Neural Comput. **32**, 485–514 (2020). https://doi.org/10.1162/neco_a_01256
24. Ramchandran, S., Tikhonov, G., Lönnroth, O., Tiikkainen, P., Lähdesmäki, H.: Learning conditional variational autoencoders with missing covariates. Pattern Recogn. **147**, 110113 (2024). https://doi.org/10.1016/j.patcog.2023.110113
25. Lavda, F., Kalousis, A.: Semi-supervised variational autoencoders for out-of-distribution generation. Entropy **25**, 1659 (2023). https://doi.org/10.3390/e25121659
26. Kingma, D.P., Rezende, D.J., Mohamed, S., Welling, M.: Semi-supervised learning with deep generative models. In: Proceedings of the 28th International Conference on Neural Information Processing Systems, pp. 3581–3589 (2014). https://doi.org/10.5555/2969033.2969226
27. Breiman, L.: Random forests. Machine learning **45**, 5–32 (2001). https://doi.org/10.1023/a:1010933404324
28. Murtagh, F.: Multilayer perceptrons for classification and regression. Neurocomputing **2**, 183–97 (1991). https://doi.org/10.1016/0925-2312(91)90023-5
29. Hosmer, D.W., Jr., Lemeshow, S., Sturdivant, R.X.: Applied Logistic Regression. John Wiley & Sons, Hoboken (2013). https://doi.org/10.1002/9781118548387
30. Vapnik, V.N.: The support vector method. In: Gerstner, W., Germond, A., Hasler, M., Nicoud, J.-D. (eds.) ICANN 1997. LNCS, vol. 1327, pp. 261–271. Springer, Heidelberg (1997). https://doi.org/10.1007/BFb0020166
31. Kramer, O.: K-nearest neighbors. In: Dimensionality Reduction with Unsupervised Nearest Neighbors, pp. 13–23. Springer, Heidelberg (2013). https://doi.org/10.1007/978-3-642-38652-7
32. Cunningham, P., Delany, S.J.: K-nearest neighbour classifiers: (with Python examples) (2020). arXiv preprint arXiv:2004.04523. https://doi.org/10.1145/3459665
33. Breiman, L., Friedman, J., Olshen, R.A., Stone, C.J.: Classification and Regression Trees. Chapman and Hall/CRC, Boca Raton (2017). https://doi.org/10.1201/9781315139470
34. Narteni, S., Orani, V., Cambiaso, E., Rucco, M., Mongelli, M.: On the intersection of explainable and reliable AI for physical fatigue prediction. IEEE Access **10**, 76243–60 (2022). https://doi.org/10.1109/ACCESS.2022.3191907

Early Detection of Emerging SARS-CoV-2 Variants via Contrastive Siamese BiLSTM Embeddings and Temporal Outlier Persistence

Adnane Touiyate[1(✉)], Chaïmaâ Kissi[2], and Tarik Boujiha[1]

[1] Engineering Science Laboratory, National School of Applied Sciences, Ibn Tofail University, Kenitra, Morocco
{adnane.touiyate,tarik.boujiha}@uit.ac.ma

[2] Advanced Systems Engineering Laboratory, National School of Applied Sciences, Ibn Tofail University, Kenitra, Morocco
chaimaa.kissi@uit.ac.ma

Abstract. Early detection of emerging viral variants remains a key challenge in genomic surveillance, particularly before formal lineage designation or widespread prevalence. Most existing approaches rely on phylogenetic reconstruction or supervised classification and are therefore retrospective and label-dependent.

We propose an unsupervised, alignment-free early-warning framework that models SARS-CoV-2 variant emergence as temporally persistent anomaly detection in a learned genomic embedding space. Fixed-length genomic windows are encoded using a contrastive Siamese Bidirectional Long Short-Term Memory (BiLSTM), and candidate anomalies are identified using a distribution-aware Mahalanobis distance and validated through temporal persistence across consecutive time windows.

Applied to longitudinal SARS-CoV-2 data, the framework identifies approximately 5% of sequences (100 out of 2,000) as statistically significant anomalies based on a 95th percentile Mahalanobis threshold, with persistent temporal patterns observed across consecutive months. Post-hoc attention analysis highlights localized model focus in biologically relevant Spike regions, supporting the plausibility of detected signals. The method serves as an interpretable screening layer that complements existing genomic surveillance pipelines.

Keywords: SARS-CoV-2 · Genomic surveillance · Anomaly detection · Contrastive learning · Siamese networks · BiLSTM · Attention mechanism

1 Introduction

The rapid and continuous evolution of the SARS-CoV-2 genome underscores the importance of genomic surveillance frameworks capable of identifying emerging variants at a very early stage, when public-health response and monitoring efforts are most effective. As the volume and diversity of viral sequences

M. Säreströniemi et al. (Eds.): NCDHWS 2026, CCIS 3010, pp. 94–112, 2026.
https://doi.org/10.1007/978-3-032-28819-6_6

steadily increase, surveillance methodologies must not only scale efficiently but also remain resilient to practical challenges such as label noise, inconsistent lineage definitions across geographic regions, and irregular temporal sampling [11,18]. In this setting, the early identification of unusual or atypical genomic patterns often provides greater value than retrospective variant classification performed after widespread circulation has already occurred.

Most existing genomic surveillance approaches rely on phylogenetic reconstruction or supervised classification strategies [10,12]. Although these methods are valuable for downstream and retrospective analyses, they typically depend on predefined mutation signatures or sufficiently dense temporal data to reliably capture early divergence events [3,12]. Furthermore, supervised models are intrinsically limited by the scope of previously observed variant classes, which restricts their ability to detect genuinely novel genomic configurations that do not conform to known categories [3,13].

An alternative formulation treats early variant detection as an anomaly detection problem. Under this perspective, the majority of sequenced genomes define a reference distribution representing dominant evolutionary dynamics, while emerging variants manifest as distributional anomalies relative to this background [2,10,15]. This paradigm enables detection without relying on mutation labels, lineage names, or epidemiological outcomes. However, most existing anomaly detection approaches implicitly assume temporal independence among samples, overlooking the persistent recurrence of anomalous patterns over time as a critical indicator of true variant emergence [15].

Recent advances in deep representation learning have shown promise for biological sequence analysis, particularly through self-supervised and contrastive learning strategies [5,8]. Siamese neural networks trained with contrastive objectives can learn similarity-preserving embeddings of biological sequences in an unsupervised setting and have been successfully applied to viral genome modeling and subtyping [4]. Bidirectional Long Short-Term Memory (BiLSTM) networks are well suited for genomic data due to their ability to capture long-range contextual dependencies, while attention mechanisms enhance post-hoc interpretability by highlighting sequence regions that contribute most strongly to learned representations [9]. Prior work has demonstrated that alignment-free Siamese BiLSTM architectures can generate informative genomic embeddings with minimal prior knowledge, without requiring mutation prediction or lineage classification [16].

In this paper, we propose an unsupervised and explicitly time-aware framework that reformulates early variant emergence as a problem of temporally persistent anomalies in a learned genomic embedding space. Unlike conventional approaches based on phylogenetic reconstruction or supervised classification, the proposed method is agnostic to lineage assignment, mutation patterns, and sequence alignment.

Robustness to isolated noise and sequencing artifacts is achieved by explicitly incorporating temporal persistence as a validation criterion for candidate anomalies. Interpretability is addressed through post-hoc attention analysis, enabling biological plausibility assessment without claiming mutation-level causality. The proposed system is designed to function as an early-warning screening component that complements, rather than replaces, downstream phylogenetic and epidemiological analyses.

1.1 Related Work and Positioning

Early detection of emerging SARS-CoV-2 variants has been investigated through multiple methodological paradigms, including phylogenetic reconstruction, feature-based anomaly detection, and unsupervised embedding or clustering approaches. While effective for retrospective analysis of the above approaches for the detection of SARS-CoV-2 variants, their ability to be used for *early-warning surveillance* remains limited, especially when the genetic difference is small and precedes the establishment of a new lineage.

The conceptual comparison of the above approaches, as presented in the literature, is given in Table 1.

Table 1. Comparison of representative existing approaches for early detection of emerging SARS-CoV-2 variants.

Approach	Method Type	Sup.	Align.	Temporal	Early-Warning
Phylogenetic reconstruction [12]	Tree-based evolutionary analysis	No	Yes	Implicit	No
Feature-based anomaly detection [15]	Engineered features + distance metrics	No	Often	No	Limited
Embedding-based clustering [3,10]	Unsupervised embedding + clustering	No	No	No	Partial
Deep anomaly learning (DeepAutoCoV) [13]	Deep autoencoder-based anomaly detection	No	No	Indirect	Partial

As summarized in Table 1, most existing approaches do not explicitly integrate temporal persistence as a decision criterion, and typically rely on retrospective confirmation of variant emergence.

This study is guided by the following research question:

> *Can an unsupervised contrastive Siamese BiLSTM framework, trained on fixed-length Spike-derived genomic windows, identify temporally persistent outlier patterns in SARS-CoV-2 sequences that may serve as early signals of emerging variant divergence, while remaining alignment-free, label-independent, and biologically interpretable?*

2 Materials and Methods

This section describes the proposed unsupervised and time-aware framework for early detection of emerging SARS-CoV-2 variants. The methodology is designed as an alignment-free genomic anomaly detection pipeline that integrates representation learning, distribution-aware outlier scoring, and temporal persistence validation. While the framework is virus-agnostic and the Siamese encoder is trained using genomic sequences from multiple viral families to encourage generalizable representation learning, anomaly detection and temporal analysis are performed exclusively on SARS-CoV-2 as a clinically relevant case study. An overview of the end-to-end pipeline is shown in Fig. 1, and the anomaly detection and temporal validation logic is illustrated in Fig. 2.

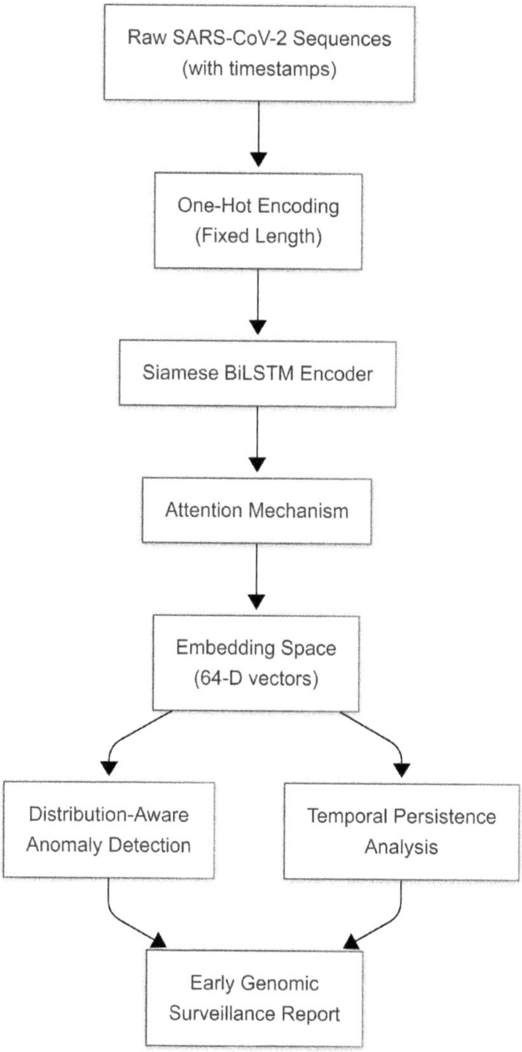

Fig. 1. High-level overview of the proposed unsupervised framework for early detection of emerging SARS-CoV-2 variants.

2.1 Dataset Construction and Scope

Genomic sequences were collected from the NCBI GenBank repository, a widely used public database for viral genomic surveillance [18]. The dataset includes six viral pathogens: SARS-CoV-2, Influenza A, Dengue, Zika, Lassa, and Nipah viruses. Sequences were retained only if they exhibited valid nucleotide composition after cleaning and were associated with collection timestamps to enable longitudinal analysis. A summary of the dataset is provided in Table 2.

After quality control and preprocessing, a total of 3,878 sequences were retained across all viruses. For further investigation as case studies, 2000 SARS-CoV-2 sequences were extracted for the detection of outliers and examination of the temporal persistence. The temporal granularity was limited to the monthly level based on available collection date metadata. This approach fosters the notion of early-warning surveillance, considering signals that persist through time rather than being one-off anomalies, consistent with calls for scalable and resilient genomic surveillance [11].

Table 2. Summary of the SARS-CoV-2 dataset used in this study.

Property	Value
Data source	NCBI GenBank
Total cleaned sequences (all viruses)	3,878
SARS-CoV-2 sequences (case study)	2,000
Fixed-length window size	3,000 bp
Encoding	One-hot (A,C,G,T,N)
Embedding dimension	64
Time span (SARS-CoV-2)	Aug 2022–Oct 2025
Temporal granularity	Monthly

2.2 Fixed-Length Windowing and Input Encoding

To maintain architectural and computational coherence, all sequences were normalized to 3,000 bp in length. If the read sequence was longer than the target length, it was trimmed; if shorter, it was padded with ambiguous bases (N), which act as a neutral symbol under one-hot encoding.

Fixed-length windowing mitigates the need for multiple sequence alignment and enables scalable deep learning on genomic sequences [1]. In the current implementation, sequences were not explicitly cropped using gene coordinates during preprocessing. Instead, the model processes fixed-length nucleotide windows extracted from consistently ordered GenBank records. For SARS-CoV-2, these windows tend to overlap Spike-associated sequence regions due to the consistent genome organization and preprocessing strategy employed in dataset construction, rather than anything intrinsic; however, attention is over sequence positions within a fixed window, not gene labels (Sect. 2.5). This results in a method that does not depend on annotation completeness but can still be used for post-hoc biological interpretation.

Each nucleotide sequence was encoded using a one-hot representation over the alphabet $\{A, C, G, T, N\}$, producing input tensors of shape (3000×5). One-hot encoding preserves positional information and avoids handcrafted features, making it suitable for unsupervised representation learning [5,8].

The choice of a 3,000 bp window represents a trade-off between capturing sufficient genomic context and maintaining computational tractability. While smaller windows may better localize mutations, larger windows provide a more stable representation of sequence context for contrastive learning. Importantly, the method does not assume exact alignment with gene boundaries and is designed to remain robust to variations in genomic segmentation.

Importantly, the framework does not assume that the fixed-length window precisely matches Spike gene boundaries; interpretability analyses are performed strictly post-hoc and do not influence model training or anomaly detection.

2.3 Contrastive Pair Construction

To train the Siamese architecture, contrastive learning was employed using pairs of sequences. Positive and negative pairs were generated using weak supervision based on relative sequence similarity, without requiring lineage labels, mutation annotations, or predefined variant classes. Pair labels are used solely to shape the geometry of the embedding space and do not represent biological ground-truth classes.

In practice, sequence similarity for pair construction is approximated using simple heuristic measures derived from nucleotide composition and positional similarity, allowing weak supervision without reliance on lineage annotations. This design ensures that the learned embedding space is shaped by relative sequence similarity rather than predefined biological labels.

Contrastive learning has been shown to be effective for learning similarity-preserving representations under limited supervision, including biological sequence modeling [6–8]. This formulation is particularly suitable for early-stage variant detection where reliable labels may be unavailable or delayed.

2.4 Siamese BiLSTM Encoder

The representation learning backbone consists of a Siamese neural network composed of two identical branches with shared parameters. Each branch processes a one-hot encoded sequence and outputs a fixed-dimensional latent representation.

Each branch is implemented using a Bidirectional Long Short-Term Memory (BiLSTM) network, which captures long-range contextual dependencies in both forward ($5'$–$3'$) and reverse ($3'$–$5'$) directions. BiLSTM architectures are well suited for genomic sequence modeling due to their ability to model sequential dependencies without requiring explicit alignment [4,5]. The encoder design follows an alignment-free Siamese representation learning strategy previously validated in our prior work [16].

2.5 Attention Mechanism and Embedding Formation

The BiLSTM hidden representations are passed through an attention mechanism that computes a weighted aggregation over sequence positions. Attention weights quantify the relative contribution of individual positions within the fixed-length window to the final embedding.

Attention is not used to supervise training or impose biological priors. Instead, it is analyzed post-hoc as an interpretability aid, following recent recommendations for cautious attention-based interpretation in biological sequence models [9]. Biological interpretation is performed by mapping regions of elevated attention (sequence position indices) to known functional domains of the SARS-CoV-2 Spike protein in downstream analysis. Attention is therefore used for interpretability rather than mutation calling, gene prediction, or lineage assignment.

The attention-weighted representations are globally pooled to produce compact 64-dimensional embeddings for each sequence. Compact embedding representations are particularly important for scalable genomic surveillance pipelines operating under computational and resource constraints [14].

2.6 Contrastive Training Objective

The Siamese network is trained using a contrastive loss function that encourages embeddings of similar sequence pairs to be close in Euclidean space while enforcing separation between dissimilar pairs:

$$L = (1 - y) \cdot D^2 + y \cdot \max(0, m - D)^2, \tag{1}$$

where D denotes the Euclidean distance between paired embeddings, $y \in \{0, 1\}$ is the pair label, and m is a margin hyperparameter. Contrastive objectives of this form are widely used in metric learning and representation learning [6,8].

2.7 Training Configuration and Optimization

The Siamese network was trained on contrastive pairs encoded as tensors of shape (3000×5). Each Siamese branch shares a common encoder mapping sequences to a 64-dimensional embedding space, and the distance between paired embeddings is computed using the Euclidean (L2) metric.

Optimization was performed using Adam with an initial learning rate of 1×10^{-4} and contrastive loss margin $m = 1.0$. Training was run for up to 15 epochs using a small batch size of 2 due to the high-dimensional sequential input. To prevent overfitting and stabilize convergence, early stopping was applied using validation loss with a patience of 5 epochs and restoration of best weights. In addition, ReduceLROnPlateau was used to halve the learning rate when validation loss plateaued for 3 consecutive epochs. Since the study focuses on representation learning and anomaly detection rather than computational benchmarking, hardware-specific performance metrics are not reported.

From a computational perspective, the model scales approximately linearly with sequence length and dataset size, and benefits from compact embedding representations for efficient downstream anomaly detection.

2.8 Distribution-Aware Anomaly Detection

After training, embeddings are extracted for SARS-CoV-2 sequences only. Anomaly detection is performed by modeling the reference embedding distribution using its empirical mean and covariance, and computing the Mahalanobis distance for each embedding.

Mahalanobis distance provides a distribution-aware measure of deviation in high-dimensional spaces and is commonly used for anomaly detection in biological and genomic settings [2,15]. Sequences exceeding a percentile-based threshold of the Mahalanobis distance distribution are flagged as anomalous candidates. The percentile-based threshold is intentionally conservative and is not intended to produce a definitive variant assignment, but rather to flag candidate deviations for subsequent temporal validation.

2.9 Temporal Persistence Analysis

To mitigate sensitivity to isolated noise and sequencing artifacts, anomaly detection is coupled with temporal analysis. SARS-CoV-2 embeddings are grouped by collection month, and the persistence of anomalous signals is examined across consecutive temporal windows.

An emerging variant signal is defined as an anomalous pattern that persists across multiple consecutive months rather than appearing sporadically. This temporal persistence criterion is motivated by two key considerations: First, sustained persistence reflects long-term evolutionary divergence rather than transient fluctuations; second, it mitigates well-known limitations of point anomaly detection in high-dimensional biological data [10,12]. Accordingly, the framework explicitly rejects isolated singleton outliers and prioritizes long-lasting signals, in keeping with biological expectations that viral diversification will be gradual, followed by population-level growth.

2.10 Attention-Based Interpretation and Reporting

For the temporally persistent anomaly sequences, we examine attention weight distributions to see which parts of the sequence play a role in embedding deviation. The analyses presented here provide biological plausibility but do not suggest any causal impact of the mutations.

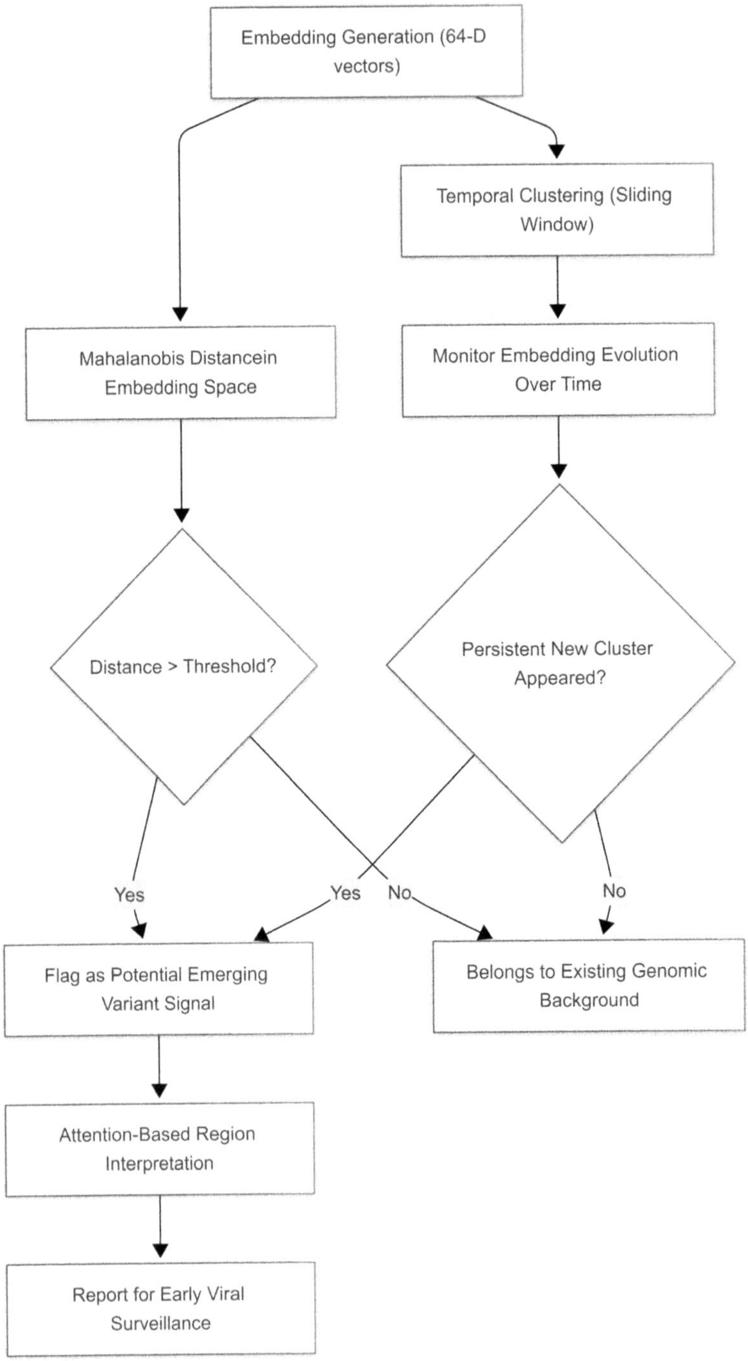

Fig. 2. Anomaly detection and temporal validation logic.

Overall, the proposed framework is intended as an AI-assisted early-warning screening tool that complements existing phylogenetic and epidemiological pipelines rather than replacing them, consistent with modern genomic surveillance guidance [11,18].

Attention weights are not used as explanatory evidence of causal mutations but are analyzed solely to assess whether the model focus aligns with biologically plausible regions.

3 Results

This section presents the experimental results obtained using the proposed unsupervised framework for early detection of emerging SARS-CoV-2 variants. The evaluation focuses on four complementary aspects: (i) the structure of the learned embedding space, (ii) statistical detection of anomalous sequences, (iii) temporal persistence of detected anomalies, and (iv) biological interpretability through attention analysis. All results are reported without the use of lineage labels or supervised variant annotations.

3.1 Embedding Space Structure and Anomaly Separation

We begin by examining the structure of the learned 64-dimensional embedding space in order to evaluate whether the Siamese BiLSTM encoder captures meaningful genomic representations. Figure 3 presents a two-dimensional PCA projection of the embeddings, in which the majority of SARS-CoV-2 sequences form a dense and compact manifold, while detected outliers are located in lower-density peripheral regions of the space.

This clear spatial separation between typical and atypical sequences indicates that the model learns a structured and informative representation of Spike-derived genomic diversity, rather than collapsing inputs into an undifferentiated embedding cloud. It should be emphasized that PCA is used here solely for visualization purposes; all anomaly detection decisions are performed in the original high-dimensional embedding space.

Taken together, these observations suggest that the learned embeddings preserve biologically relevant variation among sequences, enabling downstream statistical analysis without dependence on explicit variant labels or supervised classification.

3.2 Statistical Detection of Anomalous Sequences

In order to measure the degree of deviation from the learned genomic background, the Mahalanobis distance is calculated for each of the embeddings relative to the learned distribution of the normal SARS-CoV-2 genome. The distribution of the distance is shown in Fig. 4, where the threshold is also indicated.

The anomaly threshold is set as the 95th percentile of the distance distribution, which is equal to ($D = 5.09$). This is the upper tail of the historical

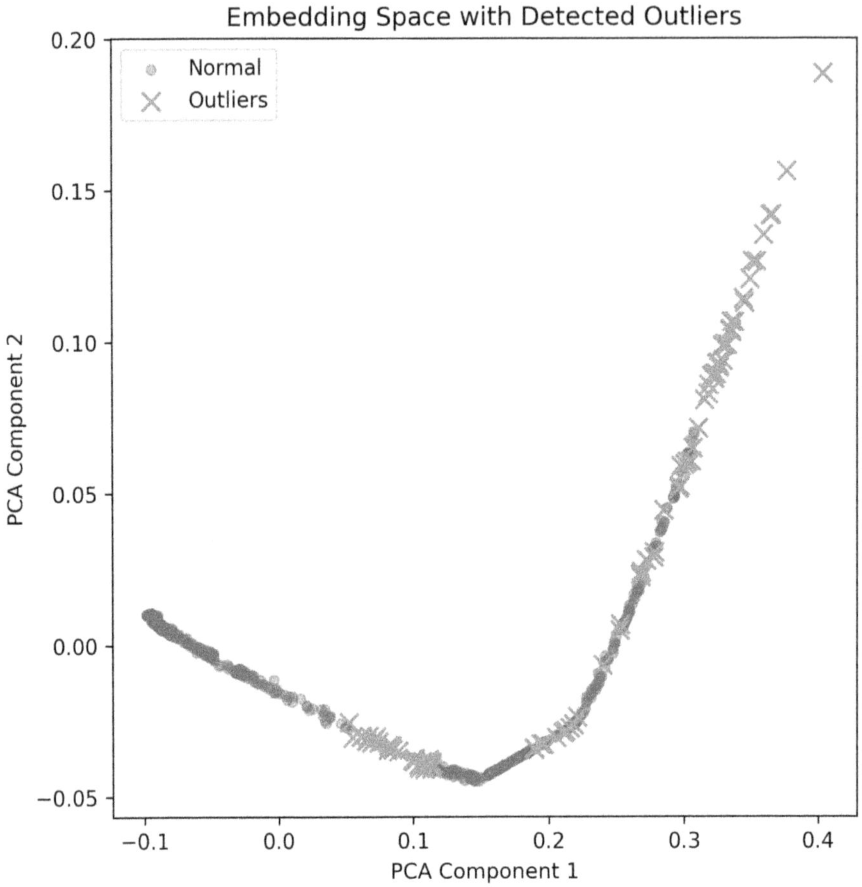

Fig. 3. PCA projection of 64-dimensional Spike sequence embeddings. Normal SARS-CoV-2 sequences form a compact manifold, while detected outliers occupy low-density peripheral regions.

embedding space. This is a data-driven choice that is particularly important for early warning surveillance. Under this choice, 100 out of 2,000 sequences are identified as anomalous candidates. This percentile-based threshold provides a conservative operating point that prioritizes specificity, thereby reducing the likelihood of false positives in early-warning settings.

The majority of the sequences are concentrated in the low distance regime, while a few are located in the higher distance regime. This results in a long-tailed distribution. The sequences that are above the threshold are identified as statistically significant deviations from the learned background. This approach avoids heuristic cutoffs or clustering-dependent decisions and provides a principled, distribution-aware mechanism for anomaly detection.

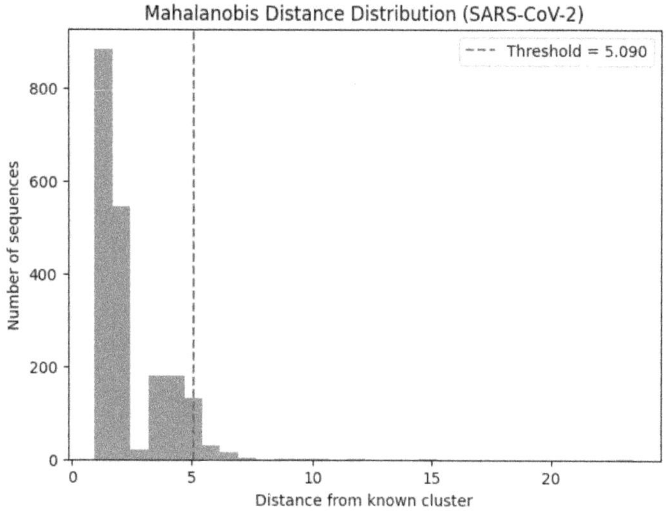

Fig. 4. Distribution of Mahalanobis distances from the reference SARS-CoV-2 embedding distribution. The dashed line indicates the anomaly detection threshold used to flag outlier sequences.

The presence of a pronounced tail in the distance distribution supports the interpretation that the detected anomalies reflect genuine departures from historical SARS-CoV-2 genomic patterns rather than random noise or minor fluctuations.

3.3 Temporal Emergence of Anomalous Sequences

While the detection of anomalous sequences is crucial for monitoring variants, determining whether identified anomalies exist over time is also equally important. In Fig. 5, we plot the temporal emergence of the detected anomalous SARS-CoV-2 sequences.

Anomalous sequences are essentially not present, or they occur at a very low rate during the initial observation period (as depicted in the figure). Then the number of abnormal sequences grows with time. This temporal pattern of anomalous sequences is strong evidence that the type of anomalies identified may not be attributed to chance errors in sequencing.

On the contrary, the temporal emergence of anomalous sequences is consistent with the gradual emergence of a new subgroup of the viral genome. Importantly, isolated or short-lived anomalies are not considered sufficient evidence of variant emergence under this framework.

By explicitly incorporating temporal continuity as a validation criterion, the proposed framework filters out transient artifacts and prioritizes anomalies that exhibit sustained deviation over consecutive time periods.

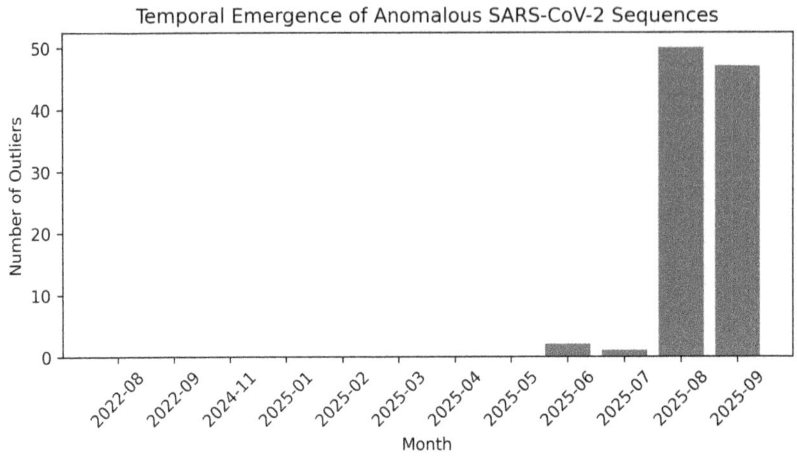

Fig. 5. Temporal emergence of anomalous SARS-CoV-2 sequences aggregated by month.

3.4 Attention-Based Interpretation of Emerging Variants

To assess whether the detected anomalies are associated with structured differences in model focus, we analyze the attention weights produced by the Siamese BiLSTM encoder. Figure 6 compares the mean attention profiles of anomalous and normal sequences across the full 3,000 bp Spike window.

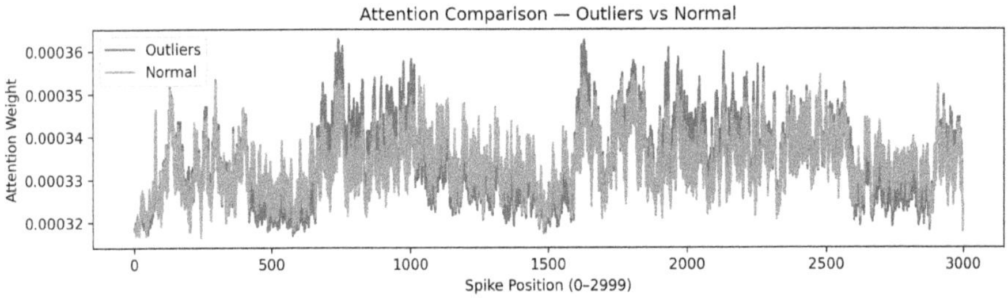

Fig. 6. Comparison of mean attention profiles between anomalous and normal SARS-CoV-2 Spike sequences across the full 3,000 bp window.

Although both groups share a broadly similar baseline structure, anomalous sequences consistently exhibit elevated and locally differentiated attention in specific regions. These differences are not uniformly distributed along the Spike sequence, suggesting that the model emphasizes particular genomic segments when encoding anomalous inputs.

To further examine this effect, Fig. 7 presents a focused view of the HR1/HR2 region. In this region, anomalous sequences display systematically higher and more variable attention compared to normal sequences. The HR1 and HR2 domains are known to play a central role in membrane fusion and viral entry, making them biologically plausible loci for divergence.

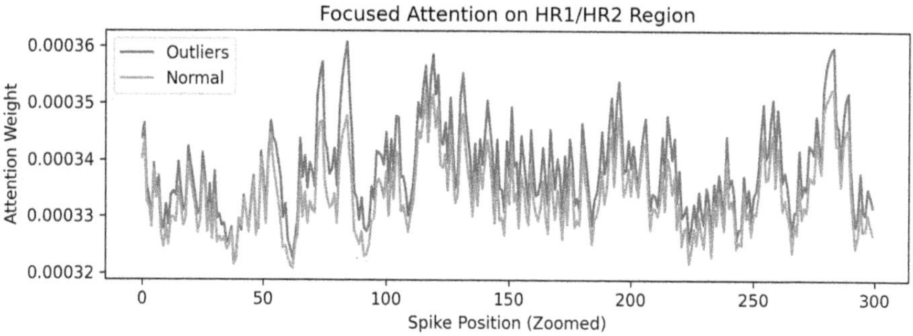

Fig. 7. Zoomed attention comparison over the HR1/HR2 region of the Spike protein.

It is important to stress that attention weights are interpreted here as indicators of model focus rather than as direct evidence of causal mutations. Attention analysis is used strictly as a post-hoc interpretability tool to assess biological plausibility and does not imply mutation-level or mechanistic conclusions.

4 Discussion

This section discusses the implications of the proposed framework for existing genomic surveillance approaches and highlights its methodological contributions.

Table 3 highlights the key design choices of the proposed framework, emphasizing its explicit focus on temporal persistence and its suitability for early-warning genomic surveillance.

Table 3. Positioning of the proposed framework relative to existing approaches.

Criterion	Proposed Framework
Supervision required	No
Sequence alignment required	No
Explicit temporal persistence modeling	Yes
Designed for early-warning screening	Yes
Interpretability support	Attention-based (post-hoc)
Variant labels required	No

4.1 Interpretation of Results and Methodological Implications

The constant and rapid evolution of the SARS-CoV-2 virus poses a major challenge to existing genomic surveillance infrastructures. Conventional phylogenetic reconstruction and lineage assignment are time-consuming processes that require sufficient genetic divergence between sequences, curated reference data, and expert interpretation. As a result, the early stages of newly emerging variants often remain undetected until they reach substantial prevalence in the population.

In this context, this unsupervised anomaly-detection framework provides a complementary approach for identifying atypical genomic patterns without relying on prior variant knowledge. The applicability of unsupervised anomaly detection to SARS-CoV-2 genomic data has been demonstrated in previous studies, including feature-based anomaly detection approaches [15] and deep anomaly learning systems such as DeepAutoCoV [13]. However, most existing methods rely on static anomaly scores or clustering outputs and lack explicit mechanisms for distinguishing persistent evolutionary signals from transient noise.

The proposed framework extends conventional unsupervised anomaly detection methods by directly learning representations from Spike-derived nucleotide sequences using a contrastive Siamese BiLSTM architecture. As shown in Fig. 3, the learned embedding space is structured such that anomalous sequences occupy low-density peripheral regions, while historically dominant SARS-CoV-2 sequences form a compact and well-organized manifold.

Initial candidate anomalies are identified using a statistically grounded Mahalanobis distance criterion. While distance-based detection alone may be sensitive to transient noise, this limitation is addressed by incorporating temporal persistence as a validation criterion. As illustrated in Fig. 5, anomalous sequences persist across consecutive months rather than appearing as isolated sequencing artifacts. Similar behavior has been reported in retrospective studies, where genomic anomalies were observed prior to formal lineage designation [12].

Biological plausibility of the detected signals is further supported through attention-based interpretation. The analysis reveals consistent differences between anomalous and normal sequences, with elevated attention concentrated in the HR1 and HR2 regions of the Spike protein (Fig. 7). These domains play a central role in membrane fusion and viral entry. Importantly, attention weights are interpreted as indicators of model focus rather than evidence of causal mutations, serving as a post-hoc validation tool rather than a mechanistic explanation.

4.2 Key Findings and Current Limitations

The experimental results show that the proposed framework: (i) can learn structured and discriminative genomic embeddings in an unsupervised and alignment-free manner; (ii) can effectively discover a concise set of statistically significant genomic anomalies; (iii) can corroborate detected anomalies via explicit temporal persistence; (iv) can provide interpretable indicators to highlight biologically important parts of the Spike protein.

The current limitations of our framework should be acknowledged. The proposed framework does not perform lineage, mutation, or clinical impact prediction. As such, genomic sequences detected as anomalous require validation via phylogenetic analysis, epidemiological context, and expert analysis. The above limitation is consistent with the proposed framework's intended role as an early warning screening tool rather than a diagnostic or classification tool. Accordingly, the framework is intended to support early situational awareness and prioritization rather than to replace downstream phylogenetic or epidemiological analyses.

In addition, the current study is limited by the relatively small dataset size and the absence of quantitative benchmarking against baseline methods. Future work will focus on large-scale evaluation, including quantitative evaluation and retrospective validation against known variant emergence timelines.

4.3 Future Work and Perspectives

There are a few possible directions for future work to enhance the proposed approach. Expanding beyond, one possible direction for future work would be to test our framework in larger and more diverse genomic data sets (e.g., multi-country samples, aggregate surveillance data). These extensions make it applicable to a wider variety of evolutionary processes and noise properties in real surveillance systems.

Unsupervised anomaly detection has increasingly been recognized as a valuable strategy for early-warning genomic surveillance, particularly in scenarios where labeled data are scarce or unavailable [17]. In this regard, future research might explore the incorporation of other types of contextual information (e.g., geographic or time metadata) in order to make available richer situational awareness and therefore enable more informed downstream analysis.

Although this study focuses on SARS-CoV-2 as a representative case study, the proposed time-aware anomaly detection framework is not virus-specific. The same methodology can be readily adapted to other rapidly evolving viral pathogens, including influenza, respiratory syncytial virus, and other zoonotic viruses. As such, the framework has the potential to serve as a general AI-assisted screening tool for genomic surveillance and early warning in future epidemic and pandemic preparedness efforts.

5 Conclusion

The current work presents a novel, time-sensitive, and unsupervised method for the early discovery of newly emerging SARS-CoV-2 variants. The method is designed as an AI-assisted genomic screening tool. Unlike existing approaches that focus on phylogenetic analysis, lineage prediction, and classification, the current method formulates early SARS-CoV-2 variant discovery as a time-sensitive anomaly detection problem. The framework employs contrastive representation learning through a Siamese BiLSTM architecture with attention to learn structured and biologically meaningful genomic representations without requiring sequence alignment or mutation calling. The identified variants are then validated on the basis of their persistence over time. This explicit incorporation of temporal persistence constitutes the central methodological contribution of the proposed framework. This distinction sets the proposed framework apart from existing embedding- or clustering-based approaches, which typically treat samples as temporally independent.

The findings indicate that the approach consistently identifies a small number of statistically-significant outliers that appear across multiple months and act cohesively in embedding space. A post-hoc attention analysis also provides biological plausibility for the detected signals, as attended regions in the Spike protein include loci involved in viral entry and fusion, specifically at the S1/S2 cleavage site and in the HR1/HR2 region. Crucially, the framework is not designed to predict specific mutations nor lineage assignments. Instead, it provides an interpretable early-warning signal that can be used for further phylogenetic, epidemiological, and clinical investigation.

The proposed framework should be considered a screening program for SARS-CoV-2 to support genomic surveillance, in combination with other genomic and epidemiological surveillance approaches. The main contribution of this work is situational awareness, an early warning sign for persistent genomic divergence that precedes formal classification and broad dissemination. This makes it most suitable for surveillance, which is forecasting-oriented.

Although in this work SARS-CoV-2 has been described as a clinical case study, the proposed method is conceptually general. The applicability toward alignment-free representation learning, distribution-aware anomaly detection, and temporal persistence validation allows this work to serve as an easy-to-use scheme for other emerging viral pathogens (in addition to SARS-CoV-2), which are expected in future epidemic preparedness.

Acknowledgements. The authors acknowledge Ibn Tofail University and the National School of Applied Sciences for providing the academic environment and resources that supported this research.

Disclosure of Interests. The authors declare that they have no competing interests.

References

1. Alser, M., et al.: Technology dictates algorithms: recent developments in read alignment. Genome Biol. **22**(1), 249 (2021). https://doi.org/10.1186/s13059-021-02443-7
2. Chandola, V., Banerjee, A., Kumar, V.: Anomaly detection: a survey. ACM Comput. Surv. **41**(3), 1–58 (2009)
3. Chandra, R., Bansal, C., Kang, M.: Unsupervised machine learning framework for discriminating major variants of concern during covid-19. arXiv (2022)
4. Chen, T., Sun, Y.: Siamdna: self-supervised siamese networks for viral subtyping. Cell Syst. **13**(2), 134–145 (2022)
5. Eraslan, G., Avsec, Z., Gagneur, J., Theis, F.J.: Deep learning: new computational modelling techniques for genomics. Nat. Rev. Genet. **20**, 389–403 (2019)

6. Hadsell, R., Chopra, S., LeCun, Y.: Dimensionality reduction by learning an invariant mapping. In: Proceedings of the IEEE Conference on Computer Vision and Pattern Recognition, vol. 2, pp. 1735–1742 (2006)
7. Le, T., Patel, N., Kim, J.: Contrastive learning for unsupervised protein sequence classification. Bioinformatics **39**(1), btac782 (2023). https://doi.org/10.1093/bioinformatics/btac782
8. Li, Y., Zhang, J., Sun, L.: Contrastive representation learning for viral genome clustering. Bioinformatics **39**(6), btad456 (2023). https://doi.org/10.1093/bioinformatics/btad456
9. Nguyen, E., Kumar, R., Wang, L.: Interpretable attention maps for pathogen surveillance. Nat. Comput. Sci. **3**(1), 23–31 (2023)
10. Nicora, G., Salemi, M., Marini, S., Bellazzi, R.: Predicting emerging SARS-CoV-2 variants of concern through a one-class dynamic anomaly detection algorithm. BMJ Health Care Inform. **29**(1), e100643 (2022)
11. Pronyk, P.M., de Alwis, R., Rockett, R.J., Basile, K.: Advancing pathogen genomics in resource-limited settings. Cell Genomics **3**(Supplement 1), 100443 (2023). https://doi.org/10.1016/j.xgen.2023.100443
12. Ramazzotti, D., Maspero, D., Angaroni, F., Spinelli, S.: Early detection and improved genomic surveillance of sars-cov-2 variants from deep sequencing data. iScience **25**, 104487 (2022)
13. Rancati, S., Nicora, G., Prosperi, M., Bellazzi, R., Marini, S., Salemi, M.: Forecasting dominance of sars-cov-2 lineages by anomaly detection using deepautocov. Briefings Bioinform. **25**(6), bbae535 (2024). https://doi.org/10.1093/bib/bbae535
14. Rao, R., Tan, A., Qian, L.: Lightweight architectures for genomic deep learning. Proc. Natl. Acad. Sci. **121**(3), e2309487120 (2024). https://doi.org/10.1073/pnas.2309487120
15. Ren, H., Li, Y., Huang, T.: Anomaly detection models for sars-cov-2 surveillance based on genome k-mers. Microorganisms **11**(11), 2773 (2023)
16. Touiyate, A., Boujiha, T., Kissi, C., Moumen, I.: Alignment-free DNA sequence clustering using deep siamese bilstm and attention mechanisms. In: 2025 12th International Conference on Wireless Networks and Mobile Communications (WINCOM), pp. 1–6 (2025). https://doi.org/10.1109/WINCOM65874.2025.11313377
17. Trezza, A.: Unsupervised learning in precision medicine: unlocking the potential of anomaly detection. Appl. Sci. **14**(20) (2024)
18. World Health Organization: Genomic surveillance in low-resource settings (2023). https://www.who.int/publications/i/item/9789240063459

Explainable Video-Based Facial Expression Analysis for Quantifying Temporal Emotion Dynamics: A Methodological Framework Toward ADHD Research

Sameera Gamage(✉)

University of Oulu, P.O. Box 123, 90014 Oulu, Northern Ostrobothnia, Finland
sameera.gamage@oulu.fi

Abstract. Facial feature analysis is commonly used to study emotional responses in affective computing and mental health research. Automated facial expression recognition allows emotions to be analyzed from video data. Since facial expression patterns have been reported in the literature to differ in conditions like ADHD, it is important to use transparent and interpretable methods. This paper presents an explainable, video-based macro facial expression recognition (FER) pipeline designed as a methodological foundation for future ADHD-oriented research. The proposed approach integrates standardized visual stimuli, a fine-tuned Vision Transformer (ViT) model for basic emotion classification, temporal analysis of emotion dynamics (including emotion duration, switching behavior, and confidence trajectories), and post-hoc explainability using LIME. The feasibility of the pipeline is demonstrated using participant video recordings collected under controlled conditions. To evaluate methodological sensitivity, participants are grouped using a non-clinical attribute (male versus female), serving solely as a methodological comparison. The results indicate that the proposed pipeline can classify facial expressions, extract interpretable temporal emotion features, and generate visual explanations of model predictions. This work does not aim to perform clinical diagnoses or to interpret gender-based emotional differences. This paper does not include participants with ADHD and does not draw any ADHD-related conclusions. Instead, it presents a reproducible methodological baseline that can be used in future clinical studies involving diagnosed ADHD populations, subject to ethical approval. Such a pipeline can support future digital health research by providing reproducible, interpretable measures of emotional response dynamics from video data.

Keywords: facial expression recognition · explainable AI · emotion dynamics · Vision Transformer · method validation

1 Introduction

Facial expressions play an important role in communication and emotion regulation. Automated facial expression recognition from video data enables contin-

M. Säreströniemi et al. (Eds.): NCDHWS 2026, CCIS 3010, pp. 113–130, 2026.
https://doi.org/10.1007/978-3-032-28819-6_7

uous analysis of emotional responses over time. In mental health research, such methods must be transparent, interpretable, and ethically designed, especially when applied to conditions such as Attention-Deficit/Hyperactivity Disorder (ADHD), where emotion processing and social interaction can be affected. While many existing facial expression recognition studies focus on single-frame accuracy, fewer works analyze how emotional responses evolve over time. Temporal emotion dynamics may provide richer information about emotional regulation patterns, which are relevant in mental health research.

Facial expressions are a key component of non-verbal communication, and difficulties in recognizing or responding to emotional cues have been reported in individuals with ADHD. Recent advances in computer vision make it possible to analyze facial expressions automatically from video recordings, creating new opportunities to study emotional responses under controlled conditions. However, the use of such techniques in mental health research requires transparent and interpretable models, as well as carefully designed and ethically sound methodologies.

In this paper, we present an explainable video-based FER pipeline designed as a methodological reference for future ADHD-oriented research. The proposed framework integrates standardized visual stimuli, a fine-tuned Vision Transformer (ViT) model for basic emotion classification, temporal analysis of emotion dynamics, and post-hoc explainability using LIME. The focus of this research is not clinical diagnosis but rather the validation of technical feasibility, interpretability, and reproducibility. To demonstrate methodological sensitivity, participant recordings are analyzed using a non-clinical grouping variable that serves solely as a validation step. This work establishes a transparent and ethically sound framework that can be extended to future clinically approved studies involving diagnosed ADHD populations. Importantly, this paper does not test ADHD-related hypotheses and does not use any ADHD-labeled data. The ADHD context is included only to explain the need for interpretability and careful methodology in future clinical studies.

1.1 Research Question

How can an explainable, video-based facial expression recognition pipeline be used to quantify and interpret emotional response dynamics to standardized visual stimuli in a way that supports future ADHD-oriented research?

1.2 Objectives

To address the research question, this study aims to design an explainable video-based facial expression recognition pipeline for analyzing macro facial expressions over time. A Vision Transformer model is fine-tuned for basic emotion classification, and temporal features such as emotion duration, switching rate, and confidence trajectories are extracted. Post hoc explainability using LIME is integrated to support transparent interpretation of model predictions. The feasibility and interpretability of the proposed pipeline are demonstrated using participant recordings collected under standardized visual stimuli. The overall objective is to establish a reproducible and ethically sound methodological foundation for future ADHD-oriented research.

1.3 Contributions

This paper presents a methodological contribution and does not propose a new model architecture. The main contribution is combining several components into one explainable pipeline to analyze temporal emotion dynamics from video data. Specifically, the contributions are:

1. An end-to-end video-based facial expression recognition pipeline that includes emotion classification, temporal feature extraction, and explainability.
2. The use of interpretable temporal features such as emotion duration, switching rate, and confidence trajectories to analyze how emotions change over time.
3. The use of LIME to explain model predictions at the frame level.
4. A reproducible and ethically designed framework that can be used in future ADHD-related research.

Most existing work focuses mainly on classification accuracy. In contrast, this study focuses on interpretability, temporal analysis, and a clear and reproducible methodology.

2 Related Work

Facial Expression Recognition (FER) is a well-established research area in computer vision that focuses on the automatic analysis of human affective states from visual data. Early FER methods relied on handcrafted facial features, while more recent deep learning approaches learn discriminative representations directly from data, leading to improved emotion recognition performance [6]. Convolutional Neural Networks (CNNs) and Vision Transformer (ViT)-based architectures have demonstrated strong accuracy and robustness across multiple emotion classes and datasets [7,8]. As FER systems are increasingly applied in sensitive domains such as healthcare, model interpretability has become an important requirement. Explainable Artificial Intelligence (XAI) techniques, including Grad-CAM, are commonly used to highlight salient facial regions contributing to classification decisions, supporting transparency and trust [14]. Reviews on digital phenotyping further emphasize the importance of interpretable affective computing systems in mental health research [15].

In parallel, research in psychology and neuroscience has examined facial emotion processing in individuals with Attention-Deficit/Hyperactivity Disorder (ADHD). Evidence suggests that children and adolescents with ADHD often show reduced accuracy in facial emotion recognition compared to typically developing peers [4]. Studies using dynamic facial stimuli and eye-tracking methods report reduced attention to key facial regions, such as the eyes, and difficulties in recognizing emotions such as anger and disgust [3]. A systematic review confirms that these challenges are observed across both static and dynamic tasks while also highlighting heterogeneity related to age, comorbidity, and experimental design [2].

Despite these advances, most existing studies focus on recognition accuracy or behavioral outcomes and provide limited analysis of how facial emotional responses evolve over time. In addition, few works integrate video-based temporal emotion analysis with explainable AI in an end-to-end framework suitable for future clinical research. This paper addresses this gap by proposing an interpretable, video-based facial expression recognition pipeline that extracts temporal emotion dynamics from facial responses to standardized visual stimuli. The framework is designed as a reproducible methodological foundation for future ethically approved ADHD research rather than as a diagnostic tool.

3 Methodology

This research adopts a methodological empirical (constructive) research [9,10] approach with a method-oriented design to validate an explainable facial expression recognition pipeline. It also focuses on validating the designed pipeline for future use. The research demonstrates the feasibility of capturing and explaining macro facial expression dynamics from visual stimuli and does not make clinical or diagnostic claims.

3.1 Proposed Facial Emotion Analysis Pipeline

The proposed method consists of three main stages: (1) fine-tuning a Vision Transformer (ViT) model for facial expression recognition, (2) preparation of stimulus videos and collection of facial response data, and (3) frame extraction, emotion prediction, and temporal emotion dynamics analysis. The Vision Transformer architecture was selected due to its ability to capture global facial patterns, which is beneficial for modeling holistic facial expressions in video data. All implementation scripts were developed in Python and are publicly available for reproducibility[1]. The overall workflow is illustrated in Fig. 1. The framework is presented as a methodological foundation and does not imply a clinical diagnosis.

3.2 Facial Expression Model and Training

In this research, emotions were recognized using a predefined set of basic facial expressions commonly used in facial expression recognition research. The emotion labels were taken from standard FER datasets and should be interpreted as computational outputs rather than as actual human emotions. A Vision Transformer (ViT) architecture was selected for its ability to capture global facial

[1] Code and materials are available at https://github.com/Sameera-G/Facial_Expressions_Detection_in_ADHD_Diagnosis.

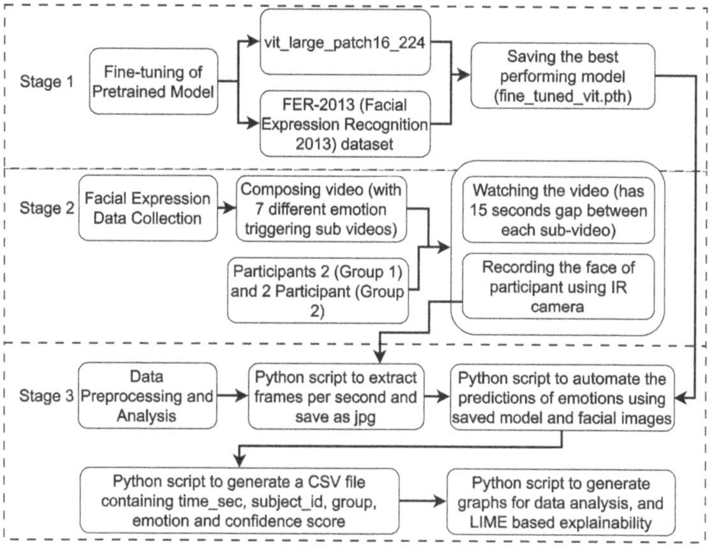

Fig. 1. Overview of the proposed pipeline.

patterns. The pre-trained `vit_large_patch16_224` model from the `timm` library was fine-tuned to classify seven basic macro facial expressions: *angry, disgust, fear, happy, sad, surprise, and neutral.* Model training was performed using the FER-2013 dataset, with images resized to 224×224 pixels and standard data augmentation applied to improve generalization. Although FER-2013 is widely used for benchmarking, it is not a clinically validated dataset and is used here solely to establish technical feasibility. The final classification layer was adapted to target the emotion categories. Training was conducted for 10 epochs using the AdamW optimizer with a learning rate of 7×10^{-5}, a weight decay of 1×10^{-11}, and categorical cross-entropy loss. A very small weight decay value was used to avoid excessive regularization, as the goal was to preserve expressive facial features rather than enforce strong parameter sparsity. The model checkpoint with the highest validation accuracy was used for all experiments.

3.3 Stimulus Design and Data Collection

A single composed stimulus video was created and shown to all participants. The stimulus consisted of seven short emotion-eliciting clips intended to predominantly trigger happy, sad, disgust, fear, angry, surprise, and neutral emotional responses. To reduce carry-over effects between emotional segments, each clip was separated by a 15-s neutral interval. After the final clip, an additional 15-second black screen was appended to the stimulus video.

The total duration of the composed stimulus video was 15 min and 30 s. All participants viewed the same stimulus video under controlled conditions, and their facial responses were recorded continuously while watching the video. After data collection, participant recordings were processed by extracting one frame per second across the full duration of the recording. This resulted in a total of 2,115 facial images extracted from all participant recordings combined, which were used for frame-level emotion prediction and temporal emotion analysis. The grouping variable, male versus female, is used only as a methodological sensitivity check and does not represent a biological, psychological, or clinical comparison.

Participant Scope. This study uses a very small sample (4 participants) because the goal is not population-level analysis. The goal is to validate the technical pipeline end-to-end (video → frames → predictions → temporal features → explainability) under controlled conditions. For this reason, the results should be interpreted as a feasibility demonstration, not as generalizable evidence. This small sample size is intentionally chosen for pipeline validation and does not aim to support statistical generalization or hypothesis testing.

3.4 Stimulus-to-Emotion Mapping

The stimulus video contains seven short sub-clips. Each sub-clip was selected to predominantly elicit one target emotion and was separated by a neutral interval to reduce carry-over effects. Table 1 summarizes the stimulus structure used in the study. A neutral interval of 15 s was placed between consecutive emotion clips to reduce carry-over effects and to support clearer separation between stimulus segments during analysis. Film and short-video clips are commonly used as standardized emotion-elicitation stimuli in affective computing and psychology research [11–13].

The table summarizes the conceptual structure of the stimulus video; all segments were combined into a single continuous video with a total duration of 15 min and 30 s.

These labels describe the intended dominant emotion of the stimulus segment. We do not assume that participants will show the same emotion continuously during the segment, which is why we analyze temporal emotion dynamics rather than only clip-level outcomes. For this reason, the analysis focuses on temporal emotion dynamics rather than assuming a fixed emotional response throughout each stimulus segment.

3.5 Frame Extraction, Analysis, and Explainability

Recorded videos were processed by extracting one frame per second, which was sufficient to capture macro facial expressions while reducing temporal redundancy and computational overhead. Each frame was passed through the fine-tuned ViT model to obtain an emotion label and the corresponding confidence score. Predictions were stored in a structured CSV file containing `time_sec`, `subject_id`, `group`, `emotion`, and confidence values. Based on frame-level predictions, temporal emotion features were computed, including emotion occurrence frequency, dominant emotion duration, emotion switching rate, and confidence trajectories. These features were analyzed at both individual and group

Table 1. Structure of the composed stimulus video shown to participants.

Segment	Intended emotion	Description
Clip 1	Happy	Emotion-eliciting video segment
Gap 1	Neutral	15 s neutral interval
Clip 2	Sad	Emotion-eliciting video segment
Gap 2	Neutral	15 s neutral interval
Clip 3	Disgust	Emotion-eliciting video segment
Gap 3	Neutral	15 s neutral interval
Clip 4	Fear	Emotion-eliciting video segment
Gap 4	Neutral	15 s neutral interval
Clip 5	Angry	Emotion-eliciting video segment
Gap 5	Neutral	15 s neutral interval
Clip 6	Surprise	Emotion-eliciting video segment
Gap 6	Neutral	15 s neutral interval
Clip 7	Neutral	Neutral emotion segment
End	Neutral	15 s black screen

levels to examine emotional response dynamics. To support interpretability, the Local Interpretable Model-agnostic Explanations (LIME) method was applied to selected frames, highlighting facial regions that contributed most to the predicted emotions. LIME was selected over gradient-based methods because it provides model-agnostic and localized explanations that support interpretation of individual frame-level predictions in video data.

3.6 Frame Preprocessing

During model training on the FER-2013 dataset, standard data augmentation and spatial cropping were applied to improve generalization. In particular, random resized cropping, horizontal flipping, and rotation were used during training to help the model learn robust facial expression features under spatial and appearance variations. For participant video analysis, a simpler preprocessing strategy was used. Recorded videos were first processed by extracting one frame per second. Each extracted frame was then resized to 224×224 pixels and normalized using the same settings as in training. No explicit face detection or face cropping was applied during inference. Instead, the full video frame was used as model input.

This design choice keeps the inference pipeline simple and reproducible and avoids introducing additional errors from automatic face detection. Face detection and cropping are not always reliable, especially under changes in lighting, pose, and image quality, and they can affect the overall system performance [17,18]. In addition, previous studies show that preprocessing steps can influence recognition accuracy in different ways depending on the dataset and conditions

[16,19]. Because our recordings were collected in a controlled environment with a stable frontal view and a plain background, the face remains the main region in the frame. For this reason, using the full frame is sufficient for demonstrating the proposed methodological pipeline without adding extra preprocessing steps.

In addition, the Vision Transformer model can capture global spatial features, which allows it to focus on relevant facial regions even when the full frame is used as input. We also visually inspected a sample of frames and confirmed that the face is centered with minimal background variation. The pipeline is also designed with future real-world use in mind, such as mobile or remote monitoring applications. In such scenarios, users may not maintain consistent face alignment, and recording conditions may vary. Studies in real-world facial expression recognition show that face detection can fail or produce inaccurate bounding boxes under unconstrained conditions, which can lead to the loss of important facial features [19]. Using the full frame helps reduce this risk and makes the system more robust to variations in user behavior and recording conditions.

In less controlled environments, the absence of face detection may reduce accuracy. Therefore, future work will include face detection and cropping and evaluate their impact on model performance using larger and more diverse datasets.

3.7 Frame Sampling

Frames were extracted from each participant video at a rate of one frame per second. This sampling rate was chosen to balance between capturing meaningful facial expression information and reducing unnecessary redundancy.

Facial expressions that reflect emotional reactions (macro-expressions) usually last longer than a fraction of a second and are visible across multiple frames. In contrast, very brief micro-expressions, which occur for only a tiny fraction of a second, require high frame rates to detect reliably. Because our focus is on overall emotional responses over longer stimulus segments rather than on subtle, fleeting changes, sampling one frame per second is appropriate for extracting stable temporal emotion patterns. This strategy reduces computational cost and simplifies the analysis while preserving the temporal dynamics of interest for our method.

3.8 Temporal Emotion Feature Computation

For each participant recording, facial emotion predictions are obtained at regular time intervals of one second. Let e_t denote the predicted emotion label at time step t, and let c_t denote the corresponding model confidence score, where $t = 1, \ldots, T$ and T is the total number of extracted frames. Emotion occurrence describes how frequently each emotion appears during the recording. It is computed by counting the number of time steps for which the predicted label equals a given emotion e.

Emotion duration captures how long an emotion persists over time. It is defined as the length of consecutive time intervals during which the same emotion label is predicted. For example, if the predicted emotion remains unchanged for six consecutive time steps, the duration of that emotion segment is six seconds.

Emotion switching rate measures how frequently the predicted emotion changes from one time step to the next. Research on emotion dynamics emphasizes that emotions are time-varying and can change in both intensity and form over short periods (e.g., second-by-second), which motivates the use of measures that capture how often emotional states shift across time [20]. Emotion switching rate, denoted as S, measures how frequently the predicted emotion changes from one time step to the next. It is defined as,

$$S = \frac{1}{T-1} \sum_{t=2}^{T} I(e_t \neq e_{t-1}), \tag{1}$$

where $I(\cdot)$ is an indicator function that equals 1 when the emotion label changes and 0 otherwise. This measure provides a simple and interpretable summary of how dynamically emotional states change over time. A higher switching rate indicates greater moment-to-moment variability in the predicted emotional state.

Confidence trajectory is defined as the sequence of confidence values $\{c_t\}_{t=1}^{T}$ across time. This concept is commonly used in time-series analysis to study how model confidence evolves and to understand prediction stability over time [20]. This trajectory provides information about the stability or uncertainty of model predictions throughout the stimulus duration.

3.9 Dataset Scope and Domain Shift

The ViT model was fine-tuned using FER-2013, which consists of posed facial expressions collected under different recording conditions than our participant videos. FER-2013 is not a clinical dataset and is not matched to ADHD populations. It is used here only to establish technical feasibility.

Because participant recordings were collected using different camera setups and lighting conditions, prediction noise and accuracy differences may occur due to domain shift. For this reason, the purpose of the participant analysis is to demonstrate the pipeline and temporal feature extraction rather than to claim strong emotion recognition validity in real-world settings. To reduce noise caused by domain shift, we include confidence scores in the output and avoid interpreting frames with low confidence. We also plan two simple stabilization steps that do not change the model, such as a short sliding-window majority vote to smooth brief changes and confidence-based filtering, where low-confidence frames are marked as uncertain and excluded from duration calculations.

We do not compare with baseline CNN or temporal models in this study, as the focus is on demonstrating the feasibility of the proposed pipeline. Future work will include benchmarking against baseline FER models and temporal deep learning approaches to better understand performance under domain shift.

3.10 Ethical Considerations

All participants provided informed consent prior to participation. Data were anonymized, and recordings were deleted after analysis unless explicit permission was granted. This research does not involve clinical diagnosis or intervention and is intended solely as a methodological feasibility study. Future clinical evaluation will require separate ethical approval.

4 Results

This section presents results that address the research question by evaluating whether the proposed explainable FER pipeline can extract and interpret temporal emotion dynamics from video data. The focus is on methodological feasibility, interpretability, and reproducibility rather than clinical conclusions. The results are reported in two parts. First, the performance of the fine-tuned Vision Transformer (ViT) model is summarized using standard classification metrics. Second, the pipeline is applied to participant recordings to demonstrate how temporal emotion dynamics can be extracted and interpreted. The results are intended to validate methodological feasibility rather than to support clinical evaluation.

4.1 Model Evaluation Setup

Model performance was evaluated using standard classification metrics on the FER-2013 benchmark. The reported values represent overall model behavior on a held-out evaluation set and are used only to confirm that the fine-tuned model is functioning as expected before applying it to participant recordings.

Since the main goal of this paper is methodological validation of a temporal analysis pipeline, we do not claim that these metrics guarantee clinical-level emotion recognition performance. Future work should evaluate performance on datasets closer to the target recording conditions and with human-verified labels.

4.2 Performance of the Fine-Tuned Vision Transformer Model

The performance of the fine-tuned ViT model was evaluated on the FER-2013 dataset using standard classification metrics, including accuracy, sensitivity (recall), specificity, F1-score, and area under the receiver operating characteristic curve (AUROC). The overall performance is summarized in Table 2. These metrics are reported to confirm functional model behavior and are not the primary contribution of this work.

We do not include a direct comparison with state-of-the-art (SOTA) FER models, as the main goal of this work is not to improve classification accuracy but to demonstrate a complete and explainable temporal analysis pipeline. The reported metrics are included solely to demonstrate that the model achieves satisfactory performance on a standard benchmark. Future work will include

Table 2. Overall Performance Metrics of the Fine-Tuned ViT Model

Sensitivity	Specificity	Accuracy	F1 Score	AUROC
0.6503	0.9436	0.6683	0.6650	0.9165

comparisons with baseline CNN and transformer-based FER models under the same experimental settings.

The FER-2013 dataset was used exclusively for model training and evaluation, while the collected participant video recordings were used only for downstream emotion inference and temporal analysis. Finally, the model shows stable performance across emotion classes, with higher recognition accuracy for visually distinctive emotions such as *happy* and *surprise*, and relatively lower performance for visually similar emotions such as *sad* and *fear*. These trends are consistent with previous facial expression recognition studies. To support interpretability, a representative LIME explanation is shown in Fig. 2. The explanation highlights facial regions such as the eyes and mouth, indicating that the model focuses on semantically meaningful facial features rather than background artifacts. We generated LIME explanations for multiple frames with different predicted emotions. In general, the explanations highlight facial regions around the eyes, eyebrows, and mouth, which are expected areas for macro-expression cues. Due to space limitations, we present one representative example.

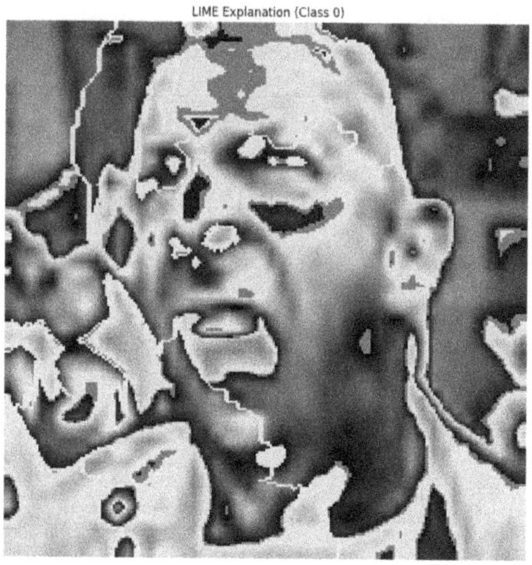

Fig. 2. LIME explanation highlighting facial regions contributing to an example emotion prediction.

The Vision Transformer model was fine-tuned using the FER-2013 dataset, which provides a diverse set of facial expressions captured under varied conditions. This training enables the model to learn general facial expression features that can be transferred to new video data. The participant recordings differ from FER-2013 in terms of camera setup, lighting, and recording context, which may introduce a domain shift. For this reason, the participant analysis is intended to demonstrate the feasibility of applying the trained model to controlled video recordings rather than to establish absolute recognition accuracy. The focus of the subsequent analysis is on relative temporal emotion patterns rather than frame-level classification performance.

4.3 Illustrative Analysis of Emotion Response Dynamics

Following model validation, the pipeline was applied to participant recordings to demonstrate how temporal emotion dynamics can be extracted from video data. No statistical significance testing is reported, as the analysis is intended to illustrate methodological sensitivity rather than population-level inference. Because the participant count is small, we report only descriptive results and visualization. We use these results to show that the pipeline runs reliably and produces interpretable temporal features. We avoid any population-level claims.

4.4 Validation and Repeatability Checks

To reduce the risk that the observed findings are driven by randomness in the analysis pipeline, we conducted two simple checks. First, we re-ran the complete analysis using the same extracted frames and verified that the predicted labels and computed temporal features remained identical. Second, we compared the model behavior during neutral gaps and emotion-eliciting clips. As expected, the neutral gaps showed predominantly neutral predictions and lower label switching compared to the emotion clips. These checks suggest that the pipeline captures meaningful temporal changes across the stimulus timeline, even within this small feasibility setting.

4.5 Emotion Occurrence Patterns

Figure 3 presents the frequency of predicted emotions across participant recordings, grouped by male and female participants. The results illustrate variability in facial expression responses to the same standardized visual stimuli, while overall emotion distributions remain comparable across groups.

Average prediction confidence values were generally similar between groups across emotions and are therefore not shown separately.

4.6 Emotion Duration and Switching Behavior

Temporal analysis further reveals differences in emotion persistence and transition behavior. Figure 4 shows (a) the distribution of emotion durations using a logarithmic scale and (b) the emotion switching rate, indicating how frequently

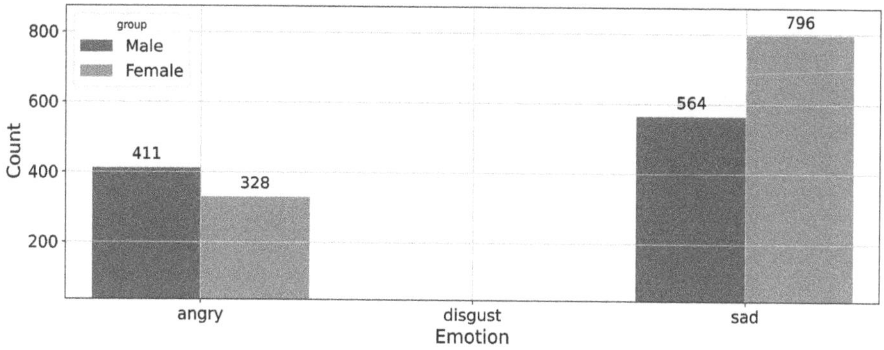

Fig. 3. Emotion occurrence count by group (male vs. female). Only the most frequently occurring emotions are shown for clarity.

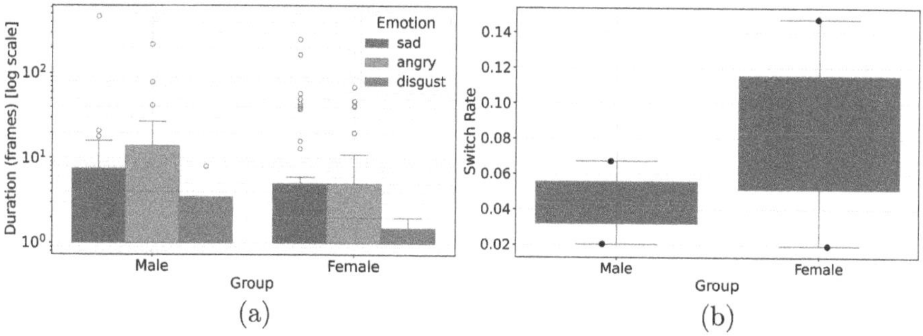

Fig. 4. (a) Emotion duration distribution (log-scale due to skewed duration values). (b) Emotion switching rate by group.

emotional states change over time. Together, these features demonstrate the ability of the proposed pipeline to capture structured temporal characteristics of emotional responses beyond frame-level classification.

These results demonstrate that the proposed explainable facial expression recognition pipeline can reliably extract, quantify, and visualize temporal emotion dynamics from video data. This suggests that the proposed temporal features are sensitive to changes in emotional responses over time. It also indicates that the pipeline can capture meaningful patterns in facial expression dynamics, even in a small and controlled dataset. This ability to capture between-group variability supports the method as a foundation for future ethically approved clinical studies. These analyses illustrate the sensitivity of the proposed temporal features rather than implying population-level differences. Temporal confidence trajectories over the full stimulus duration can be reproduced using the publicly available analysis scripts provided in the project repository.

In addition to emotion duration and switching behavior, the stability of model predictions over time was examined using confidence trajectories. For each participant, the model's prediction confidence was recorded at one-second intervals across the full stimulus duration. This analysis shows how confident the model is at different time points and allows for the observation of periods where predictions remain stable, as well as periods where confidence changes during the recording. Figure 5 presents the temporal confidence trajectories for all participants across the stimulus presentation.

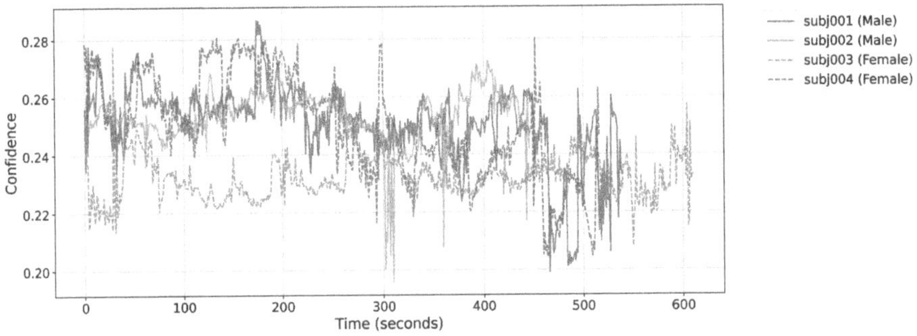

Fig. 5. Time-series of model prediction confidence per participant across the full stimulus duration, showing how confidence changes over time.

5 Discussion

This research addressed the research question by examining how an explainable, video-based facial expression recognition pipeline can be used to quantify and interpret emotional response dynamics elicited by standardized visual stimuli. The results show that this is feasible within a transparent and reproducible methodological framework, supporting the aim of future ADHD-oriented research. All stated objectives were achieved. The proposed pipeline successfully captured macro facial expressions from video data, applied a fine-tuned Vision Transformer model for emotion classification, extracted temporal emotion features, and integrated LIME to support interpretable model outputs. The model showed stable performance on a standard dataset and acceptable generalization to controlled participant recordings, which is sufficient for methodological validation but not intended for clinical use. Such interpretable temporal emotion features may be particularly valuable for digital health applications that require transparent monitoring of affective responses over time.

The extracted temporal features, including emotion occurrence, dominant emotion duration, emotion switching rate, and confidence trajectories, provide a structured way to describe how emotional responses evolve over time. The use of a non-clinical grouping variable demonstrated methodological sensitivity, indicating that the pipeline can capture variability without implying biological or diagnostic meaning. From an ADHD research perspective, these results suggest that the proposed approach can support future ethically approved studies by providing interpretable and reproducible measures of emotional response dynamics. While no clinical conclusions are drawn, this work establishes a methodological foundation aligned with the research objectives and is suitable for extension to clinically diagnosed populations.

5.1 Positioning Toward Future ADHD Research

ADHD is heterogeneous, and emotion-related differences can be influenced by age, comorbidities, medication status, and task design. For this reason, this paper does not attempt to infer ADHD traits from facial expressions. Instead, it proposes a transparent pipeline that can measure temporal emotion dynamics in a reproducible way.

With ethically approved data from diagnosed cohorts and clinically validated protocols, the same temporal features could support future ADHD-oriented analysis. In this paper, the participant grouping is used only as a non-clinical sensitivity check and should not be interpreted as evidence for any mental health conclusions. In summary, ADHD is considered only as a future application area. The current results are not interpreted as ADHD traits or ADHD-specific emotion patterns. Any ADHD-related interpretation would require ethically approved data from diagnosed participants and a clinically validated study design.

5.2 How to Use This Pipeline in a Future ADHD Study

This pipeline is intended to be used as a technical measurement tool in a future ADHD study. In a clinically approved setup, the same stimulus design and temporal features can be applied to a diagnosed ADHD cohort and a matched control cohort. The main outputs would include emotion occurrence, emotion duration, emotion switching rate, and confidence trajectories, supported by explainability methods. Clinical interpretation should be performed only with appropriate ground truth labels, relevant clinical metadata (such as age, medication status, and comorbidities), and an ethically approved protocol. In this paper, we focus only on demonstrating that the proposed method functions end-to-end and produces interpretable and reproducible outputs.

5.3 Limitations

Several limitations should be noted. First, the number of participants is small and intended for methodological validation rather than statistical generalization, so the results are not representative of broader populations. This limitation is intentional and aligns with the methodological focus of the study. Second, emotion labels are based on automated model predictions rather than human annotated ground truth, and uncertainty remains, especially for visually similar emotions. Third, frames were extracted at one frame per second, focusing on macro facial expressions and not capturing brief micro expressions. In addition, the visual stimuli were not formally validated, and the analysis relies solely on facial expression data. In addition, no statistical significance testing is performed due to the small sample size. Future studies with larger datasets will include statistical analysis to validate the observed temporal patterns. Future work will explore simple temporal smoothing strategies, such as sliding-window majority voting, to reduce short-term prediction fluctuations caused by blinking or minor head movements. In this study, all temporal features were computed directly from frame-level predictions without additional stabilization. These limitations are acceptable, as the primary goal of this research was to establish a transparent and reproducible methodological baseline.

6 Conclusion

This paper presented an explainable, video-based facial expression recognition pipeline as a methodological framework for analyzing macro facial expression dynamics in response to visual stimuli. The framework integrates a fine-tuned Vision Transformer, temporal emotion dynamics analysis, and explainable AI to provide a transparent and interpretable approach to facial expression analysis. The results demonstrate that the pipeline can reliably classify basic facial expressions, extract temporal features such as emotion duration, switching rate, occurrence, and confidence trajectories, and generate meaningful visual explanations of model predictions. The male–female grouping is used only for methodological demonstration and shows that the extracted features capture measurable variability without clinical labels.

This work does not aim to perform clinical diagnosis or mental health classification. Instead, it establishes a methodological foundation for future research. With appropriate ethical approval, larger participant cohorts, and clinically validated datasets, the proposed framework can be extended to study emotion response dynamics in conditions such as Attention-Deficit/Hyperactivity Disorder (ADHD). Future work will focus on expanding the dataset, incorporating clinically validated stimuli, and integrating additional modalities such as EEG to provide complementary physiological context. These extensions aim to support the development of robust, explainable, and ethically responsible tools for mental health research and digital health applications.

Acknowledgments. The initial dataset used in this research was obtained from a publicly available Kaggle repository. This research is supported by FAST (Finnish Software Engineering Doctoral Research Network), funded by the Finnish Ministry of Education and Culture, and conducted as part of the doctoral program at the University of Oulu in close collaboration with academic and industrial partners.

Disclosure of Interests. The author has no competing interests to declare that are relevant to the content of this article.

References

1. Papa, G., et al.: Emotion processing difficulties in attention-deficit/hyperactivity disorder: a Bayesian meta-analysis of emotion recognition and processing. Eur. Child Adolescent Psychiatry (2025). https://doi.org/10.1007/s00787-025-02647-3
2. Olaya-Galindo, M.D., Vargas-Cifuentes, O.A., Vélez Van-Meerbeke, A., Talero-Gutiérrez, C.: Establishing the relationship between attention deficit hyperactivity disorder and emotional facial expression recognition deficit: A systematic review. J. Atten. Disord. **27**(11), 1181–1195 (2023). https://doi.org/10.1177/10870547231154901
3. Bozkurt, A., Yıldırım Demirdöğen, E., Kolak Çelik, M., Akıncı, M.A.: An assessment of dynamic facial emotion recognition and theory of mind in children with ADHD: An eye-tracking study. PLoS ONE **19**(2), e0298468 (2024). https://doi.org/10.1371/journal.pone.0298468
4. Economides, A., Laouris, Y., Conson, M., Esposito, A.: Facial emotion recognition skills and measures in children and adolescents with attention deficit hyperactivity disorder (ADHD). In: Esposito, A., Faundez-Zanuy, M., Morabito, F.C., Pasero, E. (eds.) Progresses in Artificial Intelligence and Neural Systems. SIST, vol. 184, pp. 435–475. Springer, Singapore (2021). https://doi.org/10.1007/978-981-15-5093-5_39
5. Li, S., Deng, W.: Deep facial expression recognition: a survey. IEEE Trans. Affect. Comput. **14**(2), 1195–1215 (2023). https://doi.org/10.1109/TAFFC.2021.3114365
6. Kus, I., Kocak, C., Keles, A.: A systematic review of vision transformer and explainable artificial intelligence advances in multimodal facial expression recognition. Intell. Syst. Appl. **29**, 200615 (2026). https://doi.org/10.1016/j.iswa.2025.200615
7. Muralidharan, M., Alagarsamy, K., Ramyasree, K.: Enhanced facial emotion recognition using vision transformer models. J. Electr. Eng. Technol. (2024). https://doi.org/10.1007/s42835-024-02118-w
8. Tian, Y., Zhu, J., Yao, H., Chen, D.: Facial expression recognition based on vision transformer with hybrid local attention. Appl. Sci. **14**(15), 6471 (2024). https://doi.org/10.3390/app14156471
9. Crnkovic, G.D.: Constructive research and info-computational knowledge generation. In: Magnani, L., Carnielli, W., Pizzi, C. (eds.) Model-Based Reasoning in Science and Technology. Studies in Computational Intelligence, vol. 314, pp. 359–389. Springer, Heidelberg (2010). https://doi.org/10.1007/978-3-642-15223-8_20
10. Beyer, D., Winter, S.: Artifact evaluations for stronger research results. In: Proceedings of the 33rd ACM International Conference on the Foundations of Software Engineering (FSE 2025), pp. 1234–1237. Association for Computing Machinery (2025). https://doi.org/10.1145/3696630.3728623
11. Gross, J.J., Levenson, R.W.: Emotion elicitation using films. Cogn. Emot. **9**(1), 87–108 (1995). https://doi.org/10.1080/02699939508408966
12. Li, K., Shen, X., Chen, Z., He, L., Liu, Z.: Effectiveness of emotion eliciting of video clips: a self-report study. In: Meng, H., Lei, T., Li, M., Li, K., Xiong, N., Wang, L. (eds.) ICNC-FSKD 2020. LNDECT, vol. 88, pp. 523–542. Springer, Cham (2021). https://doi.org/10.1007/978-3-030-70665-4_59
13. Koelstra, S., et al.: DEAP: a database for emotion analysis using physiological signals. IEEE Trans. Affect. Comput. **3**(1), 18–31 (2012). https://doi.org/10.1109/T-AFFC.2011.15
14. Selvaraju, R.R., Cogswell, M., Das, A., Vedantam, R., Parikh, D., Batra, D.: Grad-CAM: visual explanations from deep networks via gradient-based localization. In:

Proceedings of the IEEE International Conference on Computer Vision (ICCV), pp. 618–626. IEEE (2017). https://doi.org/10.1109/ICCV.2017.74
15. Bufano, P., Laurino, M., Said, S., Tognetti, A., Menicucci, D.: Digital phenotyping for monitoring mental disorders: systematic review. J. Med. Internet Res. **25**, e46778 (2023). https://doi.org/10.2196/46778
16. Rehman, A., Mujahid, M., Elyassih, A., AlGhofaily, B., Bahaj, S.A.O.: Comprehensive review and analysis on facial emotion recognition: performance insights into deep and traditional learning with current updates and challenges. Comput. Mater. Continua **82**(1), 41–72 (2025). https://doi.org/10.32604/cmc.2024.058036
17. Haq, M.U., Sethi, M.A.J., Ahmad, S., Ahmad, N., Anwar, M.S., Kutlimuratov, A.: A comprehensive review of face detection/recognition algorithms and competitive datasets to optimize machine vision. Comput. Mater. Continua **84**(1), 1–24 (2025). https://doi.org/10.32604/cmc.2025.063341
18. Mohana, M., Subashini, P.: Facial expression recognition using machine learning and deep learning techniques: a systematic review. SN Comput. Sci. **5**(4), 432 (2024). https://doi.org/10.1007/s42979-024-02792-7
19. Soekarta, R., Ku-Mahamud, K.R.: Recent facial image preprocessing techniques: a review. Eng. Proc. **84**(1), 39 (2025). https://doi.org/10.3390/engproc2025084039
20. Kuppens, P., Verduyn, P.: Emotion dynamics: patterns and change over time. Curr. Opin. Psychol. **17**, 22–26 (2017). https://doi.org/10.1016/j.copsyc.2017.06.004

A Modern Hopfield Network Approach for Alzheimer's and Dementia Classification Using EEG Signals

Bhargava Bhamidipati[1](✉), Sarthak Acharya[2], and Rajkumar Saini[1]

[1] Luleå University of Technology, 97187 Luleå, Sweden
bhargavabhamidipati@gmail.com, rajkumar.saini@Ltu.se
[2] M3S Research Group, SEIS Unit, ITEE, University of Oulu, Oulu, Finland
sarthak.acharya@oulu.fi

Abstract. More than two-thirds of dementia cases are attributed to Alzheimer's disease (AD), while the remaining cases include frontotemporal dementia (FTD), vascular dementia, and other related disorders. Electroencephalography (EEG) is among the most cost-effective methods for supporting the diagnosis of these conditions and can serve as a valuable source of information for AI-assisted diagnostic systems. This paper focuses on the classification of EEG data from patients with FTD, Alzheimer's disease, and healthy controls. Our study focused on two key issues in this setting. First, the reliable differentiation between FTD and AD. Secondly, EEG data are noisy, difficult to Pre-process, and often limited in their ability to capture long-range relationships. Modern Hopfield networks offer a promising direction because they are effective in pattern storage and retrieval and are closely related to attention mechanisms. In this work, four neural network architectures integrated with modern Hopfield networks are investigated on a publicly available dataset. A standardized workflow was adopted so that all models were trained and evaluated under identical conditions. The models were assessed using 5-fold stratified cross-validation together with hold-out evaluation. The best-performing model achieved 96% accuracy in the present experimental setting. Overall, the results show that the more expressive Hopfield-based architectures improve performance within the proposed model family and suggest that modern Hopfield networks are a promising component for EEG-based dementia classification.

Keywords: Electroencephalography (EEG) · Modern Hopfield Networks · Dementia Classification

1 Introduction

Dementia is characterized by a progressive decline in cognitive and emotional functioning, which can significantly interfere with daily activities [1]. Alzheimer's disease (AD) and frontotemporal dementia (FTD) are among the leading causes

M. Särestöniemi et al. (Eds.): NCDHWS 2026, CCIS 3010, pp. 131–144, 2026.
https://doi.org/10.1007/978-3-032-28819-6_8

of dementia [1]. However, distinguishing between AD and FTD remains clinically challenging, highlighting the need for more reliable diagnostic approaches [1].

With advancements in electroencephalography (EEG) sensor technology, EEG has emerged as a reliable and non-invasive diagnostic tool for neurological disorders such as AD and FTD [1–11]. EEG captures the brain's electrical activity and enables the identification of abnormal neural patterns that may indicate neurodegenerative diseases [12]. A variety of signal processing and analytical techniques can be applied to EEG data to study these patterns and facilitate accurate disease classification [12].

In recent years, numerous studies have explored the use of machine learning and deep learning techniques for the identification of neurodegenerative diseases. Mlinarič et al. [2] employed a stacked ensemble learning approach on a publicly available dataset using a leave-one-subject-out (LOSO) validation strategy. Their stacked model successfully differentiated AD and FTD from healthy controls (HC), achieving ROC–AUC values of 81.80% and 71.37%, respectively. Additionally, they reported an accuracy of 85% when distinguishing between AD and FTD using a single base classifier.

Mehran et al. [3] applied statistical feature selection methods, including the Mann–Whitney U-test and t-test, to identify the most discriminative features. They evaluated four machine learning algorithms and found that support vector machines performed best. Using 10-fold cross-validation, their approach achieved 87.8% accuracy for AD versus FTD classification and 93.5% accuracy for dementia versus healthy controls.

Quoc et al. [4] generated EEG topographic maps across different frequency bands and applied deep learning techniques for disease classification. Their method achieved accuracy rates of 83.0%, 85.5%, and 87.3% for AD/FTD, AD/HC, and FTD/HC classification tasks, respectively. Jacob et al. [5] proposed a novel convolutional neural network (CNN) architecture that incorporates dynamic mode decomposition and segments eyes-open EEG signals into shorter temporal windows. A 3D CNN was then used to learn spatiotemporal–spectral features. Their approach outperformed traditional spectral machine learning methods and FFT-based CNNs in AD classification. Moreover, they observed that excluding the delta band improved contrast for AD detection.

Khan et al. [6] proposed a lightweight and explainable EEG-based deep learning framework using temporal convolutional network–long short-term memory (TCN–LSTM) architectures. Their method employed a modified relative band-power feature set across six frequency bands and integrated SHAP values for model interpretability. The proposed framework achieved 99.7% accuracy in binary classification and 80.34% in multiclass classification.

Chen et al. [7] introduced a dual-branch feature fusion network that combines convolutional neural networks and vision transformers to capture both local texture features and global semantic patterns from EEG signals for Alzheimer's disease diagnosis. Their approach also incorporated spatial and channel attention mechanisms to identify abnormal EEG patterns. To improve diagnostic reliability, EEG prediction consistency analysis was combined with Mini-Mental

State Examination (MMSE) scores, yielding a multiclass classification accuracy of 80.23%.

Wang et al. [8] extracted topological features from network graphs constructed using disease characteristics and scalp EEG data. Both machine learning and deep learning models were subsequently applied for AD classification, achieving an accuracy of 97.8%.

Despite these advances, reliably distinguishing between AD and FTD remains one of the primary challenges in EEG-based analysis. EEG signals also exhibit inherent limitations in capturing long-range or global relationships and in providing robust associative recall under noisy or limited data conditions. Modern Hopfield networks present a promising solution to these challenges. They excel at pattern storage and retrieval and are mathematically linked to attention mechanisms, enabling them to model global dependencies that may be overlooked by conventional CNN and LSTM architectures. Furthermore, modern Hopfield networks can be seamlessly integrated as layers within deep learning models, introducing memory-like computation and enhancing feature representation, robustness, and interpretability in EEG-based clinical applications.

Motivated by these considerations, this study investigates four deep learning architectures integrated with modern Hopfield layers. The architectures follow a unified design philosophy, with incremental modifications introduced across models. Accordingly, the main objective of this paper is to perform a controlled comparison within the Hopfield-based model family, examining how architectural choices such as depth, normalization, residual connections, and Hopfield layer formulation influence EEG-based neurodegenerative disease classification. To provide broader context, the performance of the proposed models is also discussed in relation to previously reported classical machine learning and deep learning studies from the literature.

2 Methodology

All experiments follow the standardized workflow shown in Fig. 1. First, the raw data are preprocessed to remove artifacts and improve signal quality. A consistent set of features is then extracted from the preprocessed data and used as standardized input for all four model architectures proposed in Subsect. 2.3. These features are subsequently used for model training and evaluation, and the resulting performance metrics are finally summarized in tabular form. Within this workflow, two classification tasks are performed: multiclass classification and binary classification.

2.1 Dataset

The experiments were conducted on the publicly available EEG dataset introduced by Miltiadous et al. in A Dataset of Scalp EEG Recordings of Alzheimer's Disease, Frontotemporal Dementia and Healthy Subjects from Routine EEG [12]. This is the only dataset used in the present study, and therefore its characteristics

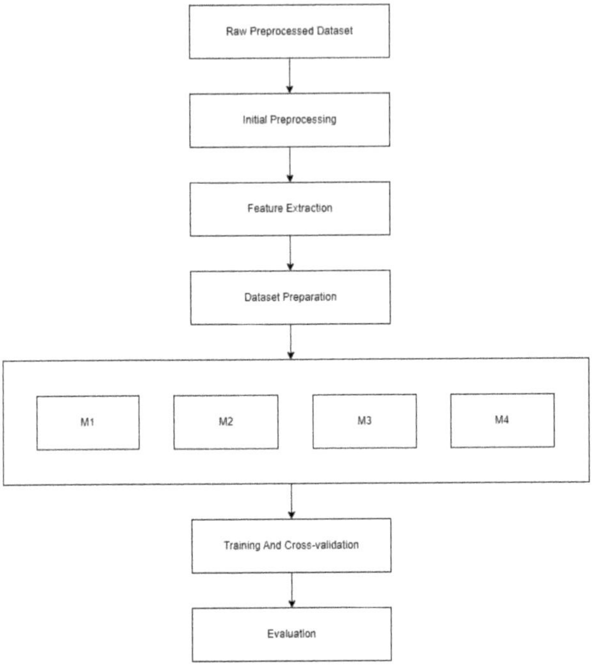

Fig. 1. High-level methodological workflow diagram

define both the training and evaluation setting. The data were collected in Greece from routine clinical EEG examinations and later organized in BIDS format at the University of Ioannina. The cohort comprises 88 subjects: 36 patients with Alzheimer's disease (AD), 23 patients with frontotemporal dementia (FTD), and 29 healthy controls (HC). At a high level, the dataset represents an older adult clinical population, with mean ages of 66.4 ± 7.9 years for AD, 63.6 ± 8.2 years for FTD, and 67.9 ± 5.4 years for HC. Mean MMSE scores were 17.75 for AD, 22.17 for FTD, and 30 for HC, indicating more severe cognitive impairment in the AD group than in the FTD group, while controls were cognitively intact. The median reported disease duration was 25 months (IQR 24–28.5) for the patient groups.

EEG was recorded during an eyes-closed resting-state condition using 19 scalp electrodes placed according to the international 10–20 system, with two reference electrodes and a sampling rate of 500 Hz. Recording duration was not identical across subjects: each EEG lasted approximately 13.5 min in the AD group (range 5.1–21.3 min), 12.0 min in the FTD group (range 7.9–16.9 min), and 13.8 min in the HC group (range 12.5–16.5 min). In total, the dataset contains 485.5 min of AD recordings, 276.5 min of FTD recordings, and 402 min of HC recordings. The dataset includes both raw and preprocessed EEG recordings.

2.2 Preprocessing

The preprocessed dataset was used for all experiments. Preprocessing was performed in multiple steps for each subject. First, the EEG signals were re-referenced to the average of the A1 and A2 electrodes. The data were then band-pass filtered between 0.5 Hz and 45 Hz to remove low-frequency noise and high-frequency artifacts outside the EEG frequency range.

To improve signal quality, artifact subspace reconstruction (ASR) was applied. Following ASR, the EEG data were decomposed into independent components using independent component analysis (ICA). Major artifacts, such as eye blinks and muscle activity, were identified and removed using ICLabel. The cleaned signals were subsequently reconstructed through back-projection.

Baseline correction and signal smoothing were then applied to further reduce residual noise. The cleaned EEG data were segmented into 5-second epochs with 50% overlap. From these epochs, frequency-domain, time-domain, complexity-based, and statistical features were extracted.

All extracted features were organized into a tabular format, with subject IDs and corresponding labels (AD, FTD, or HC) assigned to each epoch. To reduce overfitting, features exhibiting a correlation coefficient greater than 0.90 were removed. The resulting dataset was used as an input for the experiments.

2.3 Proposed Model Architectures

The four proposed models share a common architectural framework consisting of a feedforward feature extraction block, an associative memory layer based on modern Hopfield networks, and a linear output head. All four model architectures are shown in Fig. 2. The models differ in terms of depth, normalization strategies, regularization techniques, and post-associative processing. These variations are introduced to systematically investigate the impact of each component on the classification of neurodegenerative diseases. SELU activation function was used in M1 and M2 to support self-normalization in shallow architectures. GELU activations combined with layer normalization were used in M3 to improve training stability. Residual connections are introduced to preserve associative memory outputs and mitigate gradient degradation. The post-associative transformation block is included to enhance representational capacity while maintaining stable optimization.

Let (B) denote the batch size and (in_dim) the input dimensionality. M1 is a shallow feedforward neural network integrated with a modern Hopfield network layer, as shown in Fig. 2a. The model accepts an input tensor of shape ([B, in_dim]), which is first passed through a linear transformation that projects the input from the original feature space into a hidden feature space of dimensionality (hidden). A SELU activation function is applied to introduce nonlinearity and promote self-normalizing behavior. The resulting output has the shape ([B, hidden]).

To prepare the hidden representations for the associative memory layer, the tensor is reshaped to ([B, 1, hidden]) by adding a singleton dimension. The

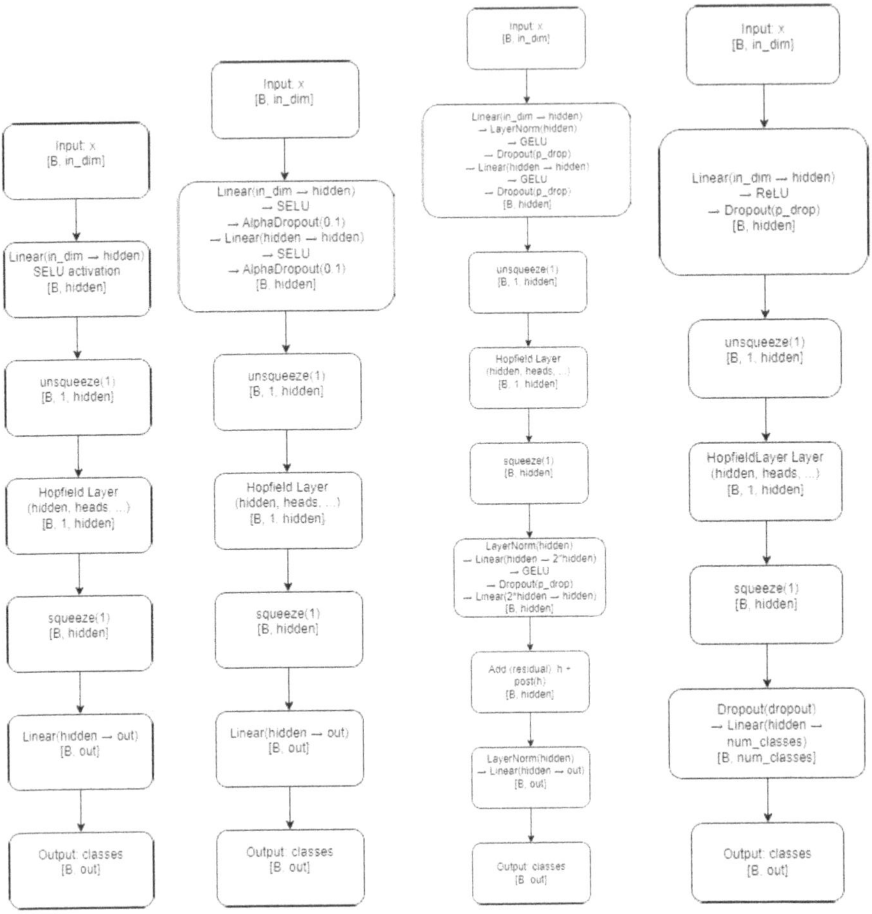

(a) M1 (b) M2 (c) M3 (d) M4

Fig. 2. Architecture diagrams of Models M1–M4.

Hopfield layer operates as a content-addressable memory mechanism, enhancing the representation by modeling global dependencies within the hidden space. The output of the Hopfield layer retains the same shape ([B, 1, hidden]). The singleton dimension is subsequently reduced, restoring the tensor shape to ([B, hidden]). Finally, a linear output layer maps the hidden features to the output space of dimension ([B, out]), corresponding to the class logits.

M2 extends M1 by incorporating deeper embedding layers and additional regularization prior to the associative memory retrieval, aiming to produce more expressive and stable hidden representations as shown in Fig. 2b. The input tensor of shape ([B, in_dim]) is processed through a stack of two fully connected layers. The first layer projects the input into the hidden feature space and is followed by a SELU activation function. AlphaDropout with a dropout rate of

0.1 is applied to improve generalization. The second linear layer maintains the same dimensionality and is also followed by AlphaDropout with the same rate. The output of this embedding stack has the shape ([B, hidden]). The associative memory pipeline follows the same procedure as in M1, producing final outputs of shape ([B, out]).

M3 further extends M1 and M2 by introducing residual connections, replacing the SELU activation with GELU, and adding a post-associative transformation block to enhance training stability and representational capacity. A detailed architecture diagram of M3 is present in the Fig. 2c. Similar to M2, the input vector is passed through two stacked fully connected layers. However, in this model, layer normalization is applied before the activation function in each layer to stabilize feature-wise activations. The GELU activation function is used, followed by dropout with probability (p_drop). The output of this embedding block has the shape ([B, hidden]).

The resulting representation is then processed through the same associative memory pipeline as in the previous models, yielding a tensor of shape ([B, hidden]). This output is subsequently passed through a post-associative transformation block. This block begins with layer normalization, followed by a linear expansion from (hidden) to (2 * hidden), GELU activation, dropout with rate (p_drop), and a linear projection back to (hidden). The output of this block, denoted as (h), is combined with the output of the associative memory pipeline through a residual connection. The resulting vector is then normalized using layer normalization and passed through a final linear layer to produce the class logits.

M4 is proposed to study the HopfieldLayer introduced by Ramsauer et al. [13] in modern Hopfield networks, as shown in Fig. 2d. This model closely resembles M1 but incorporates additional normalization and regularization techniques. The input vector is passed through a linear transformation followed by a ReLU activation function and dropout regularization with rate (p_drop). The regularized representation is reshaped to ([B, 1, hidden]) and then processed by the HopfieldLayer. After applying a squeeze operation, the resulting tensor of shape ([B, hidden]) is fed into a lightweight output head consisting of dropout followed by a linear projection from the hidden dimension to the number of output classes (out).

2.4 Training and Testing

To ensure a fair comparison among models, identical training and evaluation conditions were applied to all four models. The input data were selected according to the task type: for binary classification, the dataset included only the relevant class pairs, whereas for multiclass classification, all three classes were retained. All non-numerical features and columns unrelated to the target variable were removed.

For each task, all four models were trained using 5-fold stratified cross-validation. Within each fold, the data were normalized, class imbalance was addressed using weighted loss functions, and early stopping was employed to reduce overfitting. Performance metrics were computed for each fold and subsequently aggregated to obtain cross-validated results. In addition, a separate stratified 20% hold-out split was used for a final evaluation stage. Since this split also served for early stopping and checkpoint selection during final model training, it does not represent a strictly untouched test set; rather, it provides an additional hold-out evaluation of model performance. The same evaluation protocol was consistently applied to both multiclass and pairwise binary classification tasks, ensuring uniformity across all experimental settings.

All proposed models were optimized using the AdamW optimizer with a learning rate of 0.001, a weight decay coefficient of 0.0001, and a mini-batch size of 512. To address class imbalance, the optimization objective was defined as class-weighted cross-entropy loss, with class weights assigned inversely proportional to class frequencies in the training set. Training was performed for up to 60 epochs, with early stopping based on validation loss (patience = 8) to reduce overfitting. During inference, class labels were assigned according to the standard argmax rule applied to the output logits, and model performance was assessed using accuracy, sensitivity, precision, and F1-score. These hyperparameters were selected as part of a stable empirical training configuration and evaluated consistently within the 5-fold stratified cross-validation framework.

3 Results and Analysis

The classification of neurodegenerative diseases was conducted using four proposed neural network architectures integrated with modern Hopfield layers. Model performance was evaluated for both multiclass and binary classification tasks using cross-validation and stratified hold-out test sets. The evaluation metrics included accuracy, precision, recall, and F1-score. The results for all tasks are presented in Tables 1, 2, 3, 4 and 5.

3.1 Binary Classification Results

For the binary classification task, M1 achieved cross-validated accuracies ranging from 88% to 94%, with the lowest performance observed when distinguishing between AD and FTD. The hold-out test results followed a similar trend. Additionally, the evaluation metrics indicate that M1 struggled to effectively separate the AD and FTD classes.

M2 demonstrated improved performance over M1, achieving cross-validated accuracies between 91.6% and 95.6%, with comparable results on the hold-out test set. Consistent improvements were also observed across the other evaluation metrics, suggesting enhanced class separability resulting from deeper embedding layers and the incorporation of regularization techniques.

Among all four models, M3 achieved the highest performance in the binary classification task, with cross-validated accuracies exceeding 96% and hold-out test accuracies ranging from 96% to 98%. The corresponding precision, recall, and F1-score further confirm a high degree of class separation.

M4, which employs a single-step Hopfield layer, achieved cross-validated accuracies between 94.7% and 97.2%, and hold-out test accuracies ranging from 94% to 96%. Its performance lies between that of M2 and M3, indicating that multi-step Hopfield updates and additional architectural components contribute positively to classification performance.

Table 1. Cross-validated accuracy (mean ± std) for binary and multiclass classification tasks

Model	AD vs FTD	FTD vs HC	AD vs HC	AD vs FTD vs HC
M1	0.889 ± 0.012	0.940 ± 0.006	0.928 ± 0.007	0.889 ± 0.006
M2	0.916 ± 0.005	0.956 ± 0.004	0.955 ± 0.004	0.924 ± 0.006
M3	0.965 ± 0.006	0.980 ± 0.002	0.974 ± 0.007	0.966 ± 0.005
M4	0.947 ± 0.008	0.972 ± 0.005	0.959 ± 0.005	0.941 ± 0.004

Table 2. Hold-out test accuracies for binary and multiclass classification tasks

Model	AD vs FTD	FTD vs HC	AD vs HC	AD vs FTD vs HC
M1	0.88	0.93	0.94	0.88
M2	0.90	0.96	0.95	0.92
M3	0.96	0.98	0.97	0.96
M4	0.94	0.96	0.96	0.93

3.2 Multiclass Classification Results

For the multiclass classification task, the cross-validated accuracies of M1 to M4 were 88%, 92%, 96%, and 94%, respectively. Precision, recall, and F1-score analyses reveal that M1 encountered difficulties in accurately classifying the FTD class. In contrast, M2 and M3 exhibited substantial improvements, particularly in handling inter-class variability. A similar performance trend was observed on the hold-out test set, with accuracies of 88%, 92%, 96%, and 93% for M1 to M4, respectively. The multiclass setting is more challenging because the model must simultaneously distinguish disease-specific EEG patterns across AD, FTD, and HC. The results show that M3 maintained the strongest balance across all classes, indicating better representation learning and more stable class separation than the other variants.

Table 3. Hold-out test precision for binary and multiclass classification tasks

Model	AD vs FTD	FTD vs HC	AD vs HC	AD vs FTD vs HC
M1	0.93/0.80	0.95/0.90	0.95/0.93	0.90/0.89/0.83
M2	0.95/0.83	0.98/0.94	0.95/0.95	0.94/0.95/0.85
M3	0.98/0.93	0.98/0.97	0.97/0.97	0.97/0.97/0.94
M4	0.97/0.89	0.97/0.95	0.97/0.96	0.94/0.93/0.91

Table 4. Hold-out test recall for binary and multiclass classification tasks

Model	AD vs FTD	FTD vs HC	AD vs HC	AD vs FTD vs HC
M1	0.88/0.89	0.93/0.93	0.94/0.94	0.84/0.92/0.88
M2	0.89/0.92	0.95/0.97	0.96/0.93	0.89/0.94/0.94
M3	0.96/0.96	0.98/0.97	0.97/0.97	0.95/0.97/0.97
M4	0.94/0.95	0.97/0.95	0.96/0.96	0.92/0.95/0.92

3.3 Analysis

The results shown in Tables 1, 2, 3, 4 and 5 for M1 indicate that a shallow architecture integrated with modern Hopfield layers can perform neurodegenerative disease classification but remains limited in effectively distinguishing between AD and FTD. The introduction of deeper embedding layers and regularization strategies in M2 led to noticeable improvements in classification performance, underscoring the importance of robust feature representation learning. M3 significantly outperformed the other architectures across both binary and multiclass classification tasks. This performance gain can be attributed to the use of normalization, deeper nonlinear projections, and residual connections surrounding the Hopfield layer. M4, which integrates a Hopfield layer within a minimal architectural framework, outperformed M1 and M2 despite its simplicity. However, further architectural refinement is necessary to fully exploit its classification potential. While these findings establish the relative strengths of the proposed Hopfield-based variants, it is also important to position the results with respect to prior EEG-based dementia classification studies.

3.4 Comparison to Prior Work

The Subsects. 3.1, 3.2 and 3.3 provide a controlled comparison among four Hopfield-based architectures trained under the same preprocessing and evaluation pipeline. To place these findings in a broader context, the performance of the proposed models can be qualitatively compared with prior EEG-based studies on Alzheimer's disease and frontotemporal dementia classification discussed in Sect. 1. Earlier research has reported competitive results using both classical machine learning and non-Hopfield deep learning approaches, including stacked ensemble learning, support vector machines, convolutional neural network-based

Table 5. Hold-out test F1-scores for binary and multiclass classification tasks.

Model	AD vs FTD	FTD vs HC	AD vs HC	AD vs FTD vs HC
M1	0.90/0.84	0.94/0.92	0.95/0.94	0.87/0.90/0.85
M2	0.92/0.87	0.96/0.95	0.95/0.94	0.92/0.95/0.89
M3	0.97/0.94	0.98/0.97	0.97/0.97	0.96/0.97/0.95
M4	0.95/0.92	0.97/0.95	0.97/0.96	0.93/0.94/0.92

models, temporal convolutional network and long short-term memory frameworks, and convolutional neural network and vision transformer fusion models. Reported results in the literature include 85% accuracy for Alzheimer's disease versus frontotemporal dementia classification in a stacked ensemble setting [2], 87.8% accuracy for the same task using classical machine learning with feature selection [3], 83.0% to 87.3% accuracies across EEG topographic map-based deep learning tasks [4], 80.34% multiclass accuracy in a temporal convolutional network and long short-term memory framework [6], 80.23% multiclass accuracy in a convolutional neural network and vision transformer fusion approach [7] and 97.8% accuracy in a graph-based Alzheimer's disease classification study [8]. In comparison, the best-performing model in the present work achieved 96% accuracy in the current experimental setting, suggesting that Hopfield-based architectures are competitive with previously reported EEG classification approaches.

At the same time, this comparison should be interpreted with caution because the studies differ in dataset composition, number of subjects, preprocessing pipelines, feature extraction procedures, class definitions, and validation strategies. In particular, some prior work relies on leave-one-subject-out validation, whereas others use k-fold cross-validation in task-specific binary classification settings, which limits the direct comparability of reported accuracies. Furthermore, non-Hopfield baselines were not retrained under the identical experimental setting in the present work. For this reason, the current study does not claim definitive superiority over classical machine learning methods or other deep learning model families. Rather, the main conclusion supported by the present experiments is that, within a standardized and controlled pipeline, the more expressive Hopfield-based variants, especially M3, consistently outperform simpler Hopfield-based alternatives. These findings indicate that modern Hopfield layers are a promising architectural component for EEG-based dementia classification, while also showing that their effectiveness depends strongly on the surrounding network design.

4 Discussion

Differentiating between frontotemporal dementia (FTD) and Alzheimer's disease (AD) remains a significant challenge. In addition, EEG data are limited and difficult to acquire, and preprocessing remains particularly challenging. EEG signals contain substantial noise, making it difficult to completely filter out artifacts, and capturing long-range temporal dependencies further complicates the analysis.

The experiments in this paper investigate integrating modern Hopfield networks into deep learning architectures. Modern Hopfield networks are highly effective at storing and retrieving patterns and inherently incorporate attention mechanisms. Integrating such networks could help learn complex associative patterns that may be less effectively captured by conventional machine learning algorithms or by existing deep learning architectures such as LSTMs and CNNs.

This paper proposes four deep learning model architectures integrated with modern Hopfield networks and follows a data-driven, standardized approach to classify neurodegenerative diseases. A thorough evaluation of all four models is presented for both binary and multiclass classification tasks. The results demonstrate that M3 outperforms the other models, likely due to its deep embedding layers, use of regularization techniques, and residual connections. M4 shares a similar backbone structure with the other models; however, it incorporates a HopfieldLayer rather than a Hopfield module. Its performance falls between that of M2 and M3. Notably, the results suggest that, even with a relatively shallow architecture, M4 achieved better performance than simpler architectures without Hopfield-layer integration [14].

We employed 5-fold cross-validation at the sample level due to the limited amount of available data. While this strategy enabled consistent evaluation across all experiments, it may result in samples from the same subject appearing in both the training and testing folds, leading to optimistic performance estimates. For this reason, the reported results should be interpreted cautiously, and subject-wise validation should be examined in future work. In addition, the study is constrained by a relatively small dataset and class imbalance across subjects. The present experiments also do not investigate the interpretability of Hopfield networks through analysis of the stored patterns. Moreover, the evaluation does not include classical machine learning baselines or non-Hopfield deep learning baselines trained under the same preprocessing and testing pipeline. Consequently, the findings primarily establish the relative behavior of the four proposed Hopfield-based architectures rather than a definitive advantage over other model families. Although the quantitative comparison with prior studies indicates that the proposed approach is competitive, a fully controlled benchmark against conventional baselines remains an important direction for future research.

5 Conclusion

This paper suggests that integrating modern Hopfield networks into deep learning models can enhance class separability and representation learning, both of which are important for EEG-based pattern analysis. The results indicate that M3 is the most effective among the four proposed Hopfield-based architectures under the present experimental setting. While the findings are promising, further validation across larger and more diverse clinical datasets is necessary. Future work should investigate subject-specific validation, include controlled comparisons with classical machine learning and non-Hopfield deep learning baselines, and further explore the interpretability of modern Hopfield networks to improve transparency and support deployment in real clinical workflows. Furthermore, neural architecture search may provide a systematic way to identify more effective Hopfield-based configurations and to refine the design of future EEG-based models for neurodegenerative disease classification.

Acknowledgments. This work was supported by the University of Oulu and the Research Council of Finland, Profi6 336449.

References

1. Miltiadous, A., et al.: Alzheimer's disease and frontotemporal dementia: a robust classification method of EEG signals and a comparison of validation methods. Diagnostics **11**(8), 1437 (2021)
2. Mlinarič, T., Van Den Kerchove, A., Barinaga, Z.I., Van Hulle, M.M.: EEG-based classification of Alzheimer's disease and frontotemporal dementia using functional connectivity. Sci. Rep. (2026)
3. Rostamikia, M., Sarbaz, Y., Makouei, S.: EEG-based classification of Alzheimer's disease and frontotemporal dementia: a comprehensive analysis of discriminative features. Cogn. Neurodyn. **18**(6), 3447–3462 (2024)
4. Sercek, I., et al.: A new quantum-inspired pattern based on Goldner-Harary graph for automated Alzheimer's disease detection. Cogn. Neurodyn. **19**(1), 71 (2025)
5. Kang, J., Kang, H., Seo, J.-H.: CNN-based framework for Alzheimer's disease detection from EEG via dynamic mode decomposition. Front. Neuroinform. **19**, 1706099 (2025)
6. Khan, W., et al.: An explainable and efficient deep learning framework for EEG-based diagnosis of Alzheimer's disease and frontotemporal dementia. Front. Med. **12**, 1590201 (2025)
7. Chen, Y., Wang, H., Zhang, D., Zhang, L., Tao, L.: Multi-feature fusion learning for Alzheimer's disease prediction using EEG signals in resting state. Front. Neurosci. **17**, 1272834 (2023)
8. Wang, Z., Song, J., Wang, Y., Liu, W.: Alzheimer's disease classification detection based on brain electrical signal graph structure. In: 2023 3rd International Conference on Frontiers of Electronics, Information and Computation Technologies (ICFEICT), pp. 294–300. IEEE (2023)
9. Saini, R., et al.: Evaluating the generalizability of EEG-based ai models in Alzheimer's and dementia diagnosis. medRxiv, pp. 2025–09 (2025)
10. Saini, R., et al.: An EEG analysis framework for brain disorder classification using convolved connectivity features. In: 2024 9th International Conference on Frontiers of Signal Processing (ICFSP), pp. 158–162. IEEE (2024)
11. Rajasekhar, D.: Unveiling diagnostic significance: investigating EEG biomarkers for enhanced dementia diagnosis (2023)
12. Miltiadous, A., et al.: A dataset of scalp EEG recordings of Alzheimer's disease, frontotemporal dementia and healthy subjects from routine EEG. Data **8**(6), 95 (2023)

13. Ramsauer, H., et al.: Hopfield networks is all you need. arXiv preprint arXiv:2008.02217 (2020)
14. Bhamidipati, B.: EEG-based classification of neurodegenerative diseases using modern hopfield networks (2025)

Synthetic Data–Guided Feature Selection for Robust Activity Recognition in Older Adults

Shuhao Que[1(✉)], Dieuwke van Dartel[1,2], Ilse Heeringa[1], Han Hegeman[1,2], Miriam Vollenbroek-Hutten[1,3], and Ying Wang[1]

[1] University of Twente, Drienerlolaan 5, 7522 NB Enschede, The Netherlands
s.que@utwente.nl
[2] Ziekenhuis Groep Twente, Zilvermeeuw 1, 7609 PP Almelo, The Netherlands
[3] Medisch Spectrum Twente, Koningstraat 1, 7512 KZ Enschede, The Netherlands

Abstract. Physical activity during hip fracture rehabilitation is essential for mitigating long-term functional decline in geriatric patients. However, it is rarely quantified in clinical practice. Existing continuous monitoring systems with commercially available wearable activity trackers are typically developed in middle-aged adults and therefore perform unreliably in older adults with slower and more variable gait patterns. This study aimed to develop a robust human activity recognition (HAR) system to improve continuous physical activity recognition in the context of hip fracture rehabilitation. 24 healthy older adults aged $\geq$ 80 years were included as an age-matched feasibility cohort. Participants performed activities of daily living under simulated free-living conditions for 75 min while wearing two accelerometers positioned on the lower back and anterior upper thigh. To address and enhance model robustness to inter-person variability, a novel synthetic data generation scheme was proposed to capture common gait characteristics across individuals. Our real data and synthetic data have been published along with this work. Leveraging this synthetic dataset, a feature selection pipeline was subsequently applied to identify a compact set of six discriminative features for classifying walking, standing, sitting, lying down, and postural transfers. Model robustness was evaluated using leave-one-subject-out cross-validation. The synthetic data demonstrated potential to improve generalization across participants. The resulting feature intervention model (FIM), aided by synthetic data guidance, achieved reliable activity recognition with mean F1-scores of 0.896 $\pm$ 0.100 for walking, 0.927 $\pm$ 0.039 for standing, 0.997 $\pm$ 0.004 for sitting, 0.937 $\pm$ 0.202 for lying down, and 0.816 $\pm$ 0.120 for postural transfers. Compared with a control condition model without synthetic data, the FIM significantly improved the postural transfer detection, i.e., an activity class of high clinical relevance that is often overlooked in existing HAR literature. In conclusion, these preliminary results demonstrate the feasibility of robust activity recognition in older adults. Further validation in hip fracture patient populations is required to assess the clinical utility of the proposed monitoring system.

M. Säreströniemi et al. (Eds.): NCDHWS 2026, CCIS 3010, pp. 145–171, 2026.
https://doi.org/10.1007/978-3-032-28819-6_9

Keywords: Synthetic data · DBA · Activity detection · Hip fracture · Machine learning

1 Introduction

Hip fractures pose a growing burden on healthcare systems due to population ageing [38]. Although surgical treatment is often successful, more than half of patients fail to regain prefracture mobility within one year [10,65], resulting in reduced independence in activities of daily living (ADL) [48] and long-term declines in health-related quality of life (HRQoL) [29]. Increasing physical activity during rehabilitation is one of the few modifiable strategies shown to improve mobility and ADL independence [67], and to reduce secondary fracture risk by preventing sarcopenia and balance impairments [62]. Despite this clinical importance, physical activity is rarely quantified in routine care [61]. Wearable activity trackers have therefore been introduced in postoperative hip fracture rehabilitation [51], yet their accuracy remains uncertain, as they perform poorly for low-intensity movements such as slow or shuffling gait, which are prevalent in geriatric patients [27,44].

Recent validation work reinforces these concerns. In our previous study [64], a commercial human-activity-recognition (HAR) algorithm [2] substantially underestimated walking time in hip-fracture patients aged 82 $\pm$ 6 years, frequently misclassifying walking as standing. Such errors arise because most HAR algorithms are calibrated on middle-aged adults, whereas older adults present slower gait and altered movement amplitudes [6]. As a result, HAR models developed in younger populations often fail to capture ambulation behavior in geriatric users [22].

Accurate monitoring also requires recognizing the functional milestones that determine clinical discharge readiness, including sitting, standing, lying down, walking, and transfers (sit-to-stand, stand-to-sit, sit-to-lie, lie-to-sit) [41]. Yet most HAR studies involving older adults overlook transfers [20]. The only system addressing all milestones, developed by Allen et al. [1], was not evaluated in free-living conditions (FLC), where individual habits and environmental unpredictability introduce substantial intra-activity variation [60].

Collecting data under FLC introduces its own challenges. Because participants perform activities at self-selected frequency and duration, sensor data become highly imbalanced [14]. Imbalances can limit the representation of diverse gait patterns and reduce robustness to inter-person variability—one of the major determinants of generalization failure in HAR [21]. This indicates the following methodological gap: HAR development for geriatric monitoring must account simultaneously for free-living variability and inter-subject gait differences.

To address these gaps, we developed a new HAR algorithm for detecting hospital-discharge-relevant activities in the context of geriatric hip fracture rehabilitation. Specifically, we developed the HAR system on an age-appropriate cohort of healthy older adults aged $\geq$ 80 years, whose gait characteristics better reflect the target clinical population [33]. Our study design captured intra-activity variation by collecting wearable-sensor data under simulated FLC rather than scripted laboratory tasks. To improve robustness to inter-person gait variability and reduce overfitting to idiosyncratic patterns under realistic free-living class imbalance, we proposed a novel synthetic data generation scheme, which captured common movement characteristics across individuals. Rather than explicitly rebalancing activity classes, class-specific synthetic data were generated to enrich the representation of shared gait patterns within each activity, thereby increasing the effective diversity of underrepresented classes and mitigating class-imbalance-induced overfitting in the feature selection process. The synthetic data generation scheme was developed to support more reliable physical activity monitoring during hip fracture rehabilitation in the future.

2 Methods

2.1 Data Collection

This prospective observational study was conducted at the eHealth House (eHH) of the TechMed Simulation Centre, University of Twente (Enschede, The Netherlands). The dataset is publicly available (DOI: 10.5281/zenodo.18222937). The eHH is a controlled environment designed to simulate free-living conditions (FLC) and includes a living room, kitchen, bedroom, and bathroom. All experimental sessions were recorded using five fixed cameras installed throughout the eHH. Participants were eligible if they were aged 80 years or older and physically able to participate independently. Individuals with cognitive impairments or mobility disorders that impeded task performance were excluded. According to Dutch law, and based on a ruling from the Medical Research Ethics Committee (MREC) Arnhem–Nijmegen, the study was exempt from the Medical Research Involving Human Subjects Act. Ethical approval was granted by the Ethics Committee of the Natural Sciences and Engineering Sciences of the University of Twente. All participants provided written informed consent prior to participation.

Each participant visited the eHH once for a 75-minute session. During the visit, participants performed a set of activities of daily living (ADL) at their own pace and in their preferred order. These tasks reflected functional discharge criteria for geriatric hip fracture patients and included: (1) walking inside the eHH (between the living room, kitchen, bedroom, and front door), (2) visiting the toilet once, (3) getting in and out of bed once (sit-to-lie, lying, and lie-to-sit), (4) preparing a meal (walking to the kitchen, cutting food, and returning to the living room), and (5) preparing a drink (walking to the kitchen, pouring a drink, and returning to the living room).

Participants' movements and postures were recorded using two wearable devices: the MOX activity monitor (Maastricht Instruments, The Netherlands) and the APDM activity tracker (Hankamp Rehab BV, The Netherlands). The MOX is a waterproof device containing a single triaxial accelerometer and was attached to the upper thigh, approximately 10 cm above the knee, using a medical plaster. Data were recorded at 25 Hz. This placement was selected based on evidence that upper-leg accelerations exhibit low inter-person variability, facilitating better generalization in HAR [36]. The APDM comprises a triaxial accelerometer, gyroscope, and magnetometer, and was worn on the lower back using a strap. Data were recorded at 128 Hz. This location provides robust measurements of sedentary behaviors with low sensitivity to postural differences [68], and captures representative whole-body motion due to its proximity to the body's center of mass. The combination of thigh and lower-back sensors (Fig. 1) was considered necessary to reliably distinguish all static and dynamic activities, as a single sensor location was insufficient.

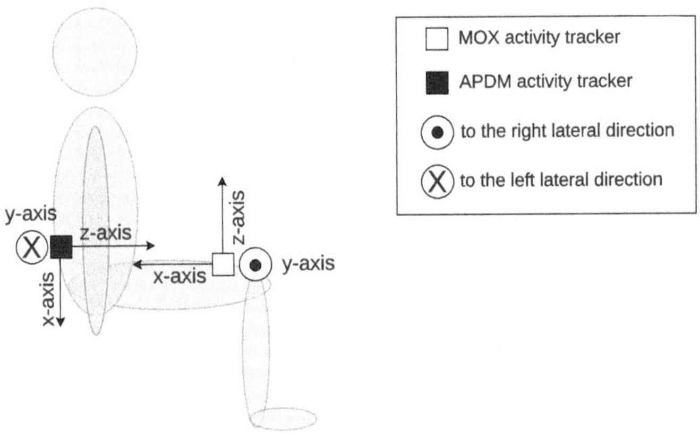

Fig. 1. Schematic of activity trackers' placements on the upper thigh and lower back.

To obtain gold-standard labels, two independent reviewers annotated the video recordings into the following activity classes: walking, standing, sitting, lying (supine, left lateral recumbent, right lateral recumbent), and transfers (stand-to-sit, sit-to-stand, sit-to-lie, and lie-to-sit). Disagreements were resolved by a third reviewer. The activity annotations were synchronized with the sensor recordings by aligning the timestamps of the first annotated sit-to-stand transfer observed in the videos with the corresponding acceleration signals.

After synchronization, all subsequent analyses were performed using accelerometer data only. The gyroscope and magnetometer signals were excluded, as previous studies showed that accelerometers alone outperform multimodal sensor combinations for comparable HAR tasks, with no significant performance gains from sensor fusion [58,59]. All data processing was conducted in MATLAB (R2022a, MathWorks Inc., Natick, MA, USA).

2.2 Models

To improve robustness to inter-person variability and reduce overfitting to idiosyncratic patterns due to class imbalance, we constructed a class-specific synthetic dataset (see Sect. 2.4) representing common gait patterns across individuals. Using this dataset, an HAR model incorporating synthetic data was proposed and compared against a control condition model trained solely on real data.

The synthetic data-guided model, termed the feature intervention model (FIM) (left flow chart in Fig. 2), examined whether synthetic data could better guide the identification of generalizable features than the real data. Specifically, for the FIM model, feature selection was performed solely on the complete synthetic dataset while excluding the real data. This design choice was motivated by the hypothesis that the synthetic data suppresses individual-specific variability, thereby encouraging the feature selection process to capture fundamental, subject-invariant activity characteristics rather than incidental or participant-specific patterns, even in the presence of class imbalance. Combining features selected from both real and synthetic data was intentionally avoided, since features identified from real data may encode subject-specific or dataset-specific biases, which could dilute the intended regularization effect of the synthetic data and compromise robustness to inter-person variability. After feature selection on synthetic data, the selected features were extracted from the real data. Model training and evaluation were subsequently conducted on the real data using leave-one-subject-out cross-validation. The control condition model (CCM) (right flow chart in Fig. 2) followed the standard activity recognition chain (ARC) using only real data. Feature selection was performed on 25% of the real data, after which the selected features were used to train and evaluate the model on the remaining 75% using leave-one-subject-out cross-validation.

Both HAR models followed the standard activity recognition chain (ARC) [14], comprising preprocessing, feature extraction, feature selection, model training, and model evaluation. Each component is described in detail in the following sections.

2.3 Preprocessing

Random high-frequency noise was suppressed by smoothing all physical-activity signals using a Savitzky–Golay filter [55]. This filter was preferred over a moving average due to its superior ability to preserve peak shape and amplitude during smoothing [56]. The filter was configured with a frame length of 0.12 s and a second-order polynomial. The selected frame length was previously shown to be suitable for smoothing gait signals in older adults [11], while a polynomial order of 2 was sufficient to capture local movement characteristics in accelerometer data [40].

After filtering, signals were segmented into non-overlapping 2-s windows. Non-overlapping windows were chosen because overlapping windows increase computational cost without improving generalization performance in HAR systems [21]. A window length of 2 s was selected as it has been shown to yield low classification error rates across a wide range of physical activities [7], and is particularly suitable for older adults [11]. Windows containing mixed activity annotations were excluded to avoid classification ambiguity [5].

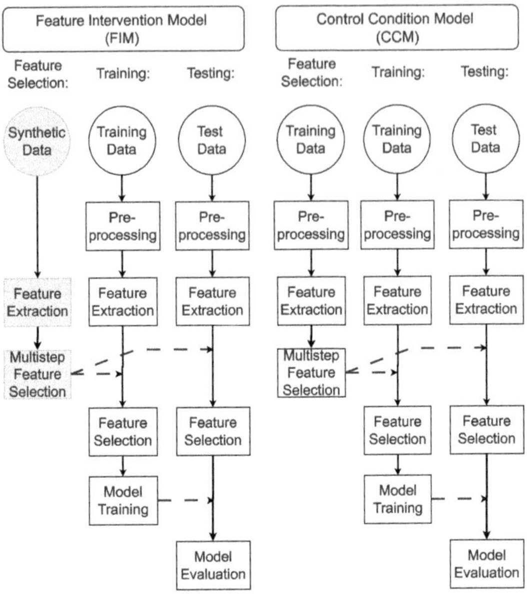

Fig. 2. General workflow of two proposed human activity recognition models. The process blocks involving the direct usage of synthetic data or derived features are colored in green. (Color figure online)

2.4 Synthetic Data Generation

Synthetic data were generated by extracting generalized gait representations that capture common characteristics across individuals while minimizing participant-specific biases. The synthetic dataset is publicly available (DOI: 10.5281/zenodo.18230770). First, raw acceleration signals were visually inspected for anomalies. For walking, large baseline drifts along the APDM z-axis were observed in a small number of participants. As no kinematically plausible explanation could be identified, these drifts were removed using a noncausal fourth-order high-pass filter with a cut-off frequency of 0.5 Hz.

Second, generalized activity representations were generated using dynamic time warping barycentre averaging (DBA) [50]. DBA is a DTW-based averaging technique that aligns time series with varying temporal dynamics by nonlinear stretching or compression, while enforcing alignment of the first and last samples [45]. After alignment, the barycentre of the aligned signals is computed, yielding a representative time series that captures common temporal patterns despite inter-individual variability [49]. Synthetic windows were generated for walking, standing, sitting, supine lying, left and right lateral recumbent lying, sit-to-stand, stand-to-sit, sit-to-lie, and lie-to-sit transfers. To ensure a fair comparison, the number of 2-s windows per activity was matched between the real and synthetic datasets, preserving identical class imbalance conditions.

A summary of the custom DBA protocol is shown in Fig. 3. The protocol consisted of four steps. First, for each activity, data availability was assessed. If at least 100 windows were available, one window per participant (i.e., 24 windows from 24 participants) was randomly sampled per DBA iteration. Otherwise, a subset-based sampling strategy was adopted: windows were randomly sampled from 20% of the participants (6 windows per iteration), a proportion chosen empirically, to increase combinatorial diversity, as 134,596 unique combinations exist when selecting 6 participants from 24.

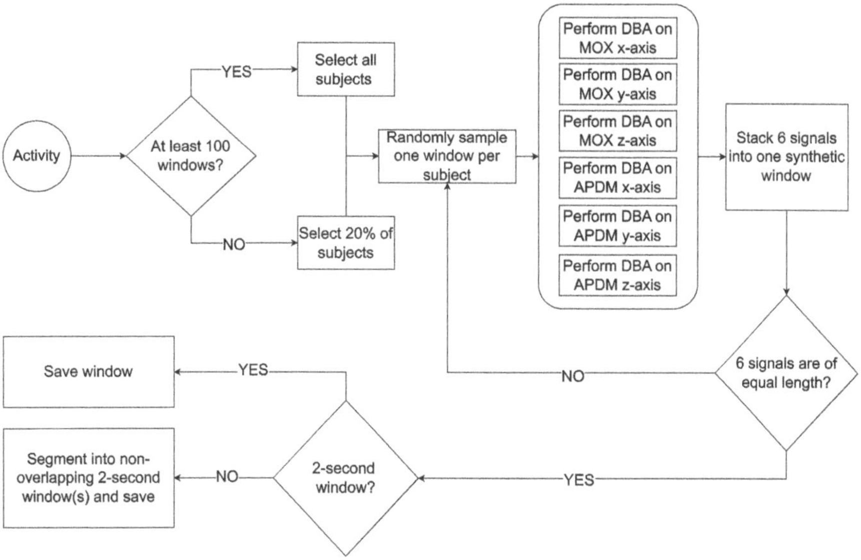

Fig. 3. General protocol for the generation of synthetic data using dynamic time warping barycentre averaging (DBA), on both MOX and APDM sensory data.

Second, one window was randomly sampled per selected participant. Each window comprised synchronized MOX and APDM signals along the x-, y-, and z-axes. Window length was activity-dependent to reduce DTW boundary artifacts. For walking, 4-s windows were used to exploit periodicity, after which the central 2 s were retained. Transfers were processed from start to end due to their variable duration, while static activities were processed using fixed 2-s windows without concern for boundary effects.

Third, DBA was applied separately to each axis of both sensors, resulting in six signals per synthetic window. For transfers, temporal consistency across the six signals was verified, as DTW can yield outputs of unequal length. If inconsistencies were detected, the sampling process was repeated.

Finally, post-processing was applied to obtain 2-s windows. For walking, the first and last seconds of the 4-s window were discarded. Transfer signals longer than 2 s were segmented into non-overlapping 2-s windows. No post-processing was required for static activities, as their windows were already of fixed length.

2.5 Feature Extraction

Handcrafted features were used instead of deep learning–based automated feature extraction for two reasons. First, deep learning methods require large datasets to achieve robust generalization [42], which was not feasible in this study. Second, a primary target of this work was the detection of transfer activities, which occur infrequently in HAR datasets and are therefore poorly suited to data-hungry deep learning approaches [52].

The candidate feature set was selected based on prior HAR literature. Although both time- and frequency-domain features are commonly employed [26], only time-domain features were considered in this study. Frequency-domain features incur higher computational cost without consistent evidence of superior discriminative performance [36]. Moreover, they are primarily effective for quasi-periodic movements with distinct frequency content [1]. Since most activities in this study were static or aperiodic, frequency-domain features were expected to contribute limited additional information and were therefore excluded.

To further reduce multicollinearity, redundant time-domain features were preemptively removed based on domain knowledge. For example, pairs of features such as mean and median, or variance, standard deviation, and mean absolute deviation, were expected to encode largely overlapping information. This pruning resulted in a total of 62 candidate features (Table 1). Such pre-selection of features is recommended to improve the reliability of subsequent feature selection algorithms [66] and to reduce instability in feature optimization procedures [54].

2.6 Multistep Feature Selection

To improve the generalizability of the HAR models, a feature selection (FS) pipeline was developed to identify a minimal and robust subset of features from the initial candidate set. The pipeline, applied identically to real and synthetic data, is summarized in Fig. 4. It addresses two key challenges in FS.

First, no single FS algorithm is universally optimal, as performance strongly depends on the application and data characteristics [12,57]. To mitigate this limitation, a heterogeneous feature selection ensemble (HFSE) was employed [12]. By combining multiple FS algorithms with complementary selection heuristics, HFSEs have been shown to produce more generalizable feature sets than individual algorithms [24,57]. Second, FS results are often sensitive to small variations in the data [66]. To improve robustness, FS stability was imposed as a secondary criterion. Following [37], the FS procedure was repeated 10 times on activity-stratified subsamples with approximately 78% overlap. The resulting feature sets were aggregated by vote counting: a feature was retained if it was selected in at least 5 out of 10 repetitions. This threshold is commonly used to eliminate features selected by chance [15].

Table 1. Overview of the time domain features before selection. Each feature was computed for both the MOX and APDM signals across a window of size N. Except for the axial correlations and signal vector magnitude, all features were computed along each acceleration axis $a \in \{x, y, z\}$. This resulted in a total of 62 features.

Feature and interpretation	Formula	References
The **mean** provides postural information.	$\mu_a = \frac{1}{N} \sum_{i=1}^{N} a_i$	[11,36]
The **standard deviation** provides information about the intensity of a physical activity.	$\sigma_a = \sqrt{\frac{\sum_{i=1}^{N} (a_i - \mu_a)^2}{N-1}}$	[17,36]
The **root mean square** is identical to the standard deviation for signals with a mean of zero.	$\mathrm{RMS}(a) = \sqrt{\frac{1}{N} \sum_{i=1}^{N} a_i^2}$	[17,36]
Axial correlations distinguish unidirectional vs. multidirectional translations (e.g., walking vs. stair climbing).	$\frac{\mathrm{cov}(x,y)}{\sigma_x \sigma_y}, \quad \frac{\mathrm{cov}(x,z)}{\sigma_x \sigma_z}, \quad \frac{\mathrm{cov}(y,z)}{\sigma_y \sigma_z}$	[4,17]
The **minimum** describes the lowest value measured along a single sensing axis.	$\min(a_1, a_2, \ldots, a_N)$	[36,47]
The **maximum** describes the highest value measured along a single sensing axis.	$\max(a_1, a_2, \ldots, a_N)$	[18,36]
The **interquartile range** separates sedentary behaviours from physical activities.	$Q_3 - Q_1$	[17,36]
The **skewness** describes the distribution asymmetry of movement accelerations.	$\frac{\sum_{i=1}^{N} (a_i - \mu_a)^3}{(N-1)\, \sigma_a^3}$	[17,25]
The **kurtosis** describes the likelihood of extreme values in a movement signal.	$\frac{\sum_{i=1}^{N} (a_i - \mu_a)^4}{(N-1)\, \sigma_a^4}$	[17,19]
The **mean-crossing rate** captures how often accelerations change sign relative to the mean.	$\frac{1}{2} \sum_{i=2}^{N} \Big\lvert \mathrm{sgn}(a_i - \mu_a) - \mathrm{sgn}(a_{i-1} - \mu_a) \Big\rvert$	[4,17]
The **signal vector magnitude** distinguishes sedentary from active behaviours. All accelerations were high-pass filtered (noncausal, 4th-order, 0.5 Hz cutoff) beforehand.	$\frac{1}{N} \sum_{i=1}^{N} \sqrt{x_i^2 + y_i^2 + z_i^2}$	[26,36]

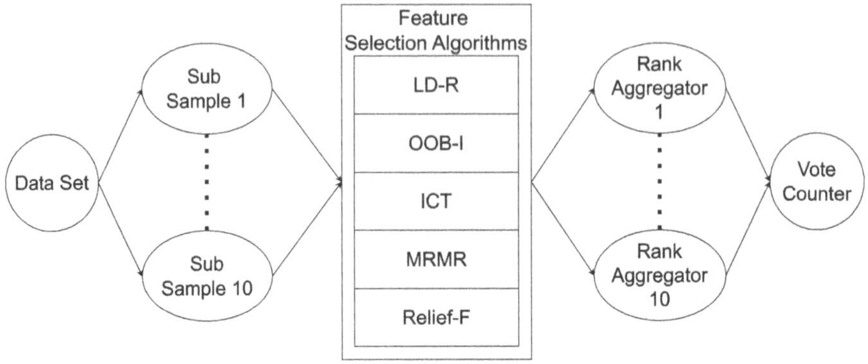

Fig. 4. Overview of the multistep feature selection (FS) pipeline. The pipeline was applied to the real data to build the control condition model, and it was applied to the synthetic data to build the complete data intervention model and the feature intervention model. Five FS algorithms were selected in this work, including Relief-F [63], maximum relevance minimum redundancy (MRMR) [23], interaction-curvature tests embedded into a decision tree (ICT) [43], out-of-bag feature importance by permutation embedded into a random forest (OOB-I) [13], and regularization embedded into a linear discriminant (LD-R) [31].

The HFSE design consisted of two steps: (1) selecting the constituent FS algorithms, and (2) aggregating their ranking outputs.

For the first step, five FS algorithms were included: Relief-F [63], maximum relevance minimum redundancy (MRMR) [23], interaction–curvature tests embedded in a decision tree [43], out-of-bag permutation importance from a random forest (OOB-I) [13], and regularized linear discriminant analysis (LD-R) [31]. Algorithm selection was guided by two criteria: diversity of selection heuristics and algorithmic stability [12]. Diversity ensured that the strengths of one algorithm compensated for the limitations of another (Table 2). For example, Relief-F captures feature interactions but does not address redundancy, whereas MRMR explicitly penalizes redundant features but ignores interactions.

Feature selection should identify features that reflect true activity characteristics rather than artifacts of a particular data split. We therefore assessed algorithm stability by examining how consistently each feature selection method selected the same features across repeated subsamples of the data. Algorithm stability was quantified using the Tanimoto similarity T. Each FS algorithm was applied to 10 activity-stratified subsamples of the synthetic data, producing 10 ranking lists. Following standard practice [12,37], the top 10 features from each ranking were used to form feature subsets, and T was computed for all 45 unique subset pairs (i.e., the number of unique unordered pairs that can be formed from 10 subjects):

$$T(s, s') = 1 - \frac{|s| + |s'| - 2\, s \cap s'|}{|s| + |s'| - |s \cap s'|} \tag{1}$$

Table 2. Overview of the feature selection algorithms used in the heterogeneous feature selection ensemble, with their properties highlighted. NA indicates not applicable.

Algorithm	Type	Relationship	Feature redundancy	Classifier type
Relief-F	Filter	Multivariate	Not accounted for	NA
MRMR	Filter	Univariate	Accounted for	NA
ICT	Embedded	Multivariate	NA	Nonlinear & greedy
OOB importance	Embedded	Univariate	NA	Nonlinear & non-greedy
Regularisation	Embedded	Univariate	NA	Linear

MRMR: maximum relevance minimum redundancy, ICT: interaction-curvature tests, OOB: out-of-bag.
Embedded into a decision tree classifier,
Embedded into a random forest classifier,
Embedded into a linear discriminant classifier.

where s and s' denote two feature subsets, $|\cdot|$ their cardinality, and $s \cap s'$ their intersection. $T = 0$ indicates no overlap and $T = 1$ identical subsets. The stability of an FS algorithm was defined as the average T across all subset pairs.

For the second step, robust rank aggregation (RRA) [39] was used to combine the feature rankings. Each feature received five ranks, i.e., one from each FS algorithm, ranging from 1 to m, where m is the total number of features. Ranks were normalized to $r_i \in (0, 1]$, yielding $\boldsymbol{r} = (r_1, \ldots, r_5)$, which was reordered such that $r_{(1)} \leq \cdots \leq r_{(5)}$.

RRA evaluates the probability of observing a rank that is $r_{(k)}$ or smaller under the null hypothesis that all ranks are independently drawn from a uniform distribution $\mathcal{U}(0, 1)$. This probability is given by the binomial distribution

$$\beta_{(k)} := \sum_{\ell=k}^{5} \binom{5}{\ell} r_{(k)}^{\ell} \left(1 - r_{(k)}\right)^{(5-\ell)} \tag{2}$$

$$p(\boldsymbol{r}) = \min\left(1, 5 \cdot \underset{k \in \{1,2,3,4,5\}}{\arg\min}\ \beta_{(k)}(\boldsymbol{r})\right) \tag{3}$$

which includes a Bonferroni correction. Features with p-values < 0.05 were identified as consistently informative across FS algorithms.

2.7 Model Training

For the CCM and FIM, the same classification algorithm and hyperparameters were used to ensure fair comparisons. The k-nearest neighbors (KNN) classifier was selected because it has consistently demonstrated strong performance across HAR studies [36], typically requires fewer features and shorter window lengths to achieve high accuracy [7], and remains robust across different sensor placements [36].

Hyperparameter tuning was not performed due to severe class imbalance and limited data availability for minority classes, which made partitioning the data into reliable tuning sets infeasible. Instead, hyperparameters were selected based on established findings in the literature. Prior studies indicate that values of k in the range $[3, 10]$ yield comparable performance across diverse HAR tasks, with minimal sensitivity to the exact choice [36]. Based on these findings, $k = 5$ was selected. Smaller values of k were avoided due to increased overfitting risk [35], while excessively large values reduce KNN's sensitivity to local structure [36]. An odd value was preferred to prevent ties in majority voting [59]. The Euclidean distance metric was used, as it has been shown to perform optimally in extensive KNN evaluations for HAR [36]. Because KNN is sensitive to feature scale, all features were Z-standardized prior to classification to ensure equal contribution across feature dimensions [32].

All models were trained to recognize five activity classes: walking, standing, sitting, lying, and transfers. Supine, left, and right lateral recumbent positions were merged into a single lying class, as they are functionally equivalent and difficult to distinguish reliably under free-living conditions due to sensor orientation variability. Due to limited samples for individual transfer types (sit-to-stand, stand-to-sit, sit-to-lie, and lie-to-sit), these were also merged into a single transfer class.

2.8 Evaluation

Model performance was quantified using the F1-score, defined as:

$$\begin{aligned}\text{F1-score} &= 2 \cdot \frac{\text{precision} \cdot \text{recall}}{\text{precision} + \text{recall}} \\ \text{precision} &= \frac{\text{true positives}}{\text{true positives} + \text{false positives}} \\ \text{recall} &= \frac{\text{true positives}}{\text{true positives} + \text{false negatives}}\end{aligned} \tag{4}$$

Differences in participant-level F1-scores across models were evaluated using the Friedman test with Wilcoxon signed-rank post-hoc comparisons (Bonferroni-corrected).

3 Results

3.1 Dataset

An overview of the dataset is provided in Table 3. A total of 24 participants were included in the study (11 males, 13 females). The cohort had a median age of 82 years (interquartile range: 81–85 years). Data collection under simulated free-living conditions resulted in pronounced imbalance at multiple levels. First, substantial class imbalance was observed, with transfers constituting the minority class (1.4%) and sitting the majority class (73.5%). Second, participation imbalance was present across activities; for example, only five and two participants contributed data for left and right lateral recumbent positions, respectively. Third, the number of observations per participant varied considerably within activities. For right lateral recumbent lying, one participant contributed only 6 windows, whereas another contributed 305 windows.

Table 3. Overview of the number of 2-s windows for all physical activities. # denotes the number of windows per activity, % the proportion of windows relative to the total dataset, and N the number of participants contributing to each activity. 23*: the sit-to-lie transfer of one participant was missing as the activity could not be verified with the video recordings due to a faulty camera orientation.

Physical activity	Available windows		N	Windows per participant	
	#	%		Mean	Min - Max
Walking	2,244	8.0	24	90.5	58 - 139
Standing	3,258	11.6	24	133	36 - 234
Sitting	20,677	73.5	24	967	322 - 1,487
Supine	929	3.3	21	19	5 - 171
Left lateral recumbent	300	1.1	5	24	15 - 206
Right lateral recumbent	311	1.1	2	155.5	6 - 305
Sit-to-stand transfer	178	0.6	24	8	2 - 10
Stand-to-sit transfer	163	0.6	24	7	3 - 11
Sit-to-lie transfer	35	0.1	23*	1	1 - 3
Lie-to-sit transfer	41	0.1	24	1.5	1 - 4

3.2 Feature Selection

All five individual FS algorithms demonstrated sufficient stability to contribute to the HFSE, with Tanimoto similarity scores ranging from 0.648 to 1.0, indicating good to excellent stability [12]. The HFSE outcomes across 10 subsamples of the real and synthetic datasets are shown in Fig. 5.

For the real data, three features were stably selected across all subsamples: mean accelerations from the upper thigh (Mean-X UT, Mean-Z UT) and the minimum acceleration from the lower back (Min-X LB). For the synthetic data, six features were stably selected: mean accelerations (Mean-X UT, Mean-Z UT, Mean-X LB), minimum acceleration (Min-X UT), and root mean square accelerations (RMS-X UT, RMS-X LB). Among these, only the two upper-thigh mean acceleration features overlapped with those selected from the real data.

Class-conditional value distributions of the selected features for the real and synthetic datasets are shown in Fig. 6. In both datasets, the selected features displayed distinct value ranges across activity classes, with mean acceleration features separating static postures and Min-X UT and RMS-X UT differentiating standing from walking. Feature separability appeared stronger in the synthetic dataset, consistent with lower within-class variability. Visual comparison with the representative DBA traces (Fig. 7) did not suggest systematic discrepancies between the real and synthetic distributions, indicating preservation of the principal activity-related signal characteristics.

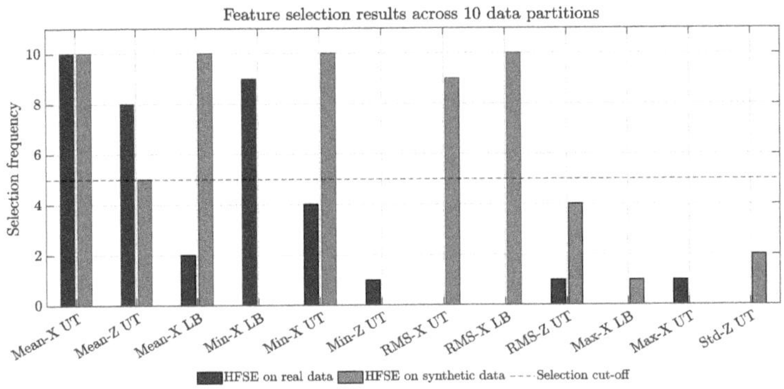

Fig. 5. Overview of feature selection results using the heterogeneous feature selection ensemble (HFSE) across the 10 subsamples of the real and synthetic data. X and Z denote the acceleration axes. UT, LB, and RMS are abbreviations for upper thigh, lower back, and root-mean-square, respectively.

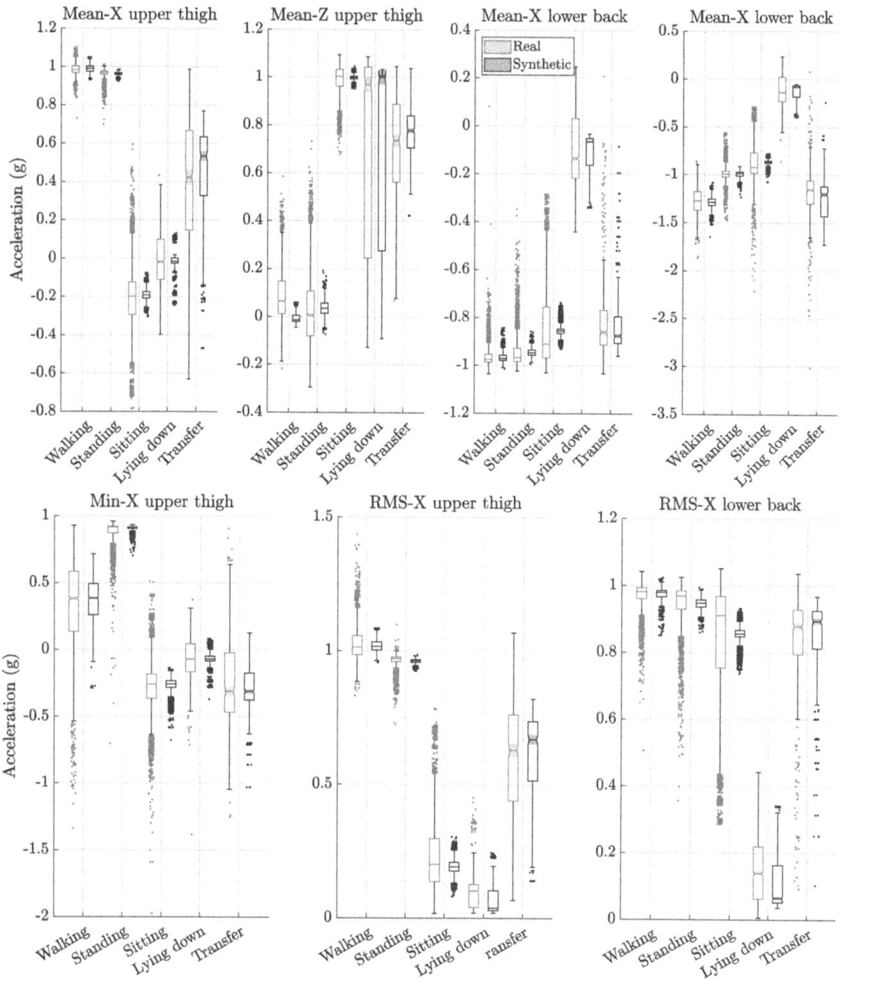

Fig. 6. Class-conditional value distributions of the features selected in accordance with the heterogeneous feature selection ensemble pipeline across the complete real and synthetic datasets. X and Z denote the acceleration axes. RMS is the abbreviation for root-mean-square.

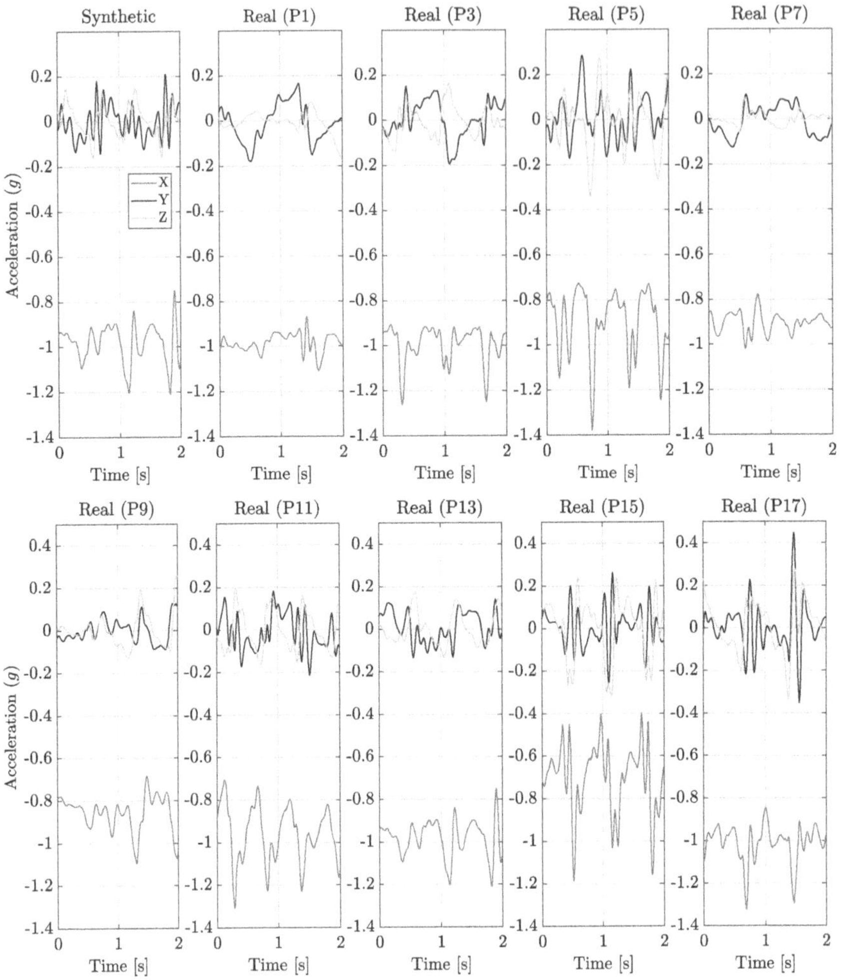

Fig. 7. Example tri-axial physical activity signals during walking from synthetic and real datasets. Data from all 24 participants were used to generate the synthetic signals. 9 participants (i.e., P1, P3, P5, P7, P9, P11, P13, P15, and P17) were randomly sampled to provide a general impression of the real signals.

3.3 Model Evaluation

Control Condition Model. The classification performance of the CCM estimated through leave-one-subject-out cross-validation is shown in Table 4. Overall, the CCM yielded a mean precision of 0.932±0.045, a mean recall of 0.885±0.064, and a mean F1-score of 0.896±0.075 across all 24 participants. Upon examining the recognition rates of the individual activities, inter-person variability in classification performance appeared to be large for recognition of walking (F1-score range: 0.107–1.0), lying down (F1-score range: 0.154–1.0), and transfers (F1-score range: 0.176–0.929).

Table 4. Performance of control condition model evaluated with leave-one-subject-out cross-validation.

Physical activity	Precision		Recall		F1-score	
	Mean ± SD	Range	Mean ± SD	Range	Mean ± SD	Range
Walk	0.894±0.072	0.744-1.0	0.861±0.197	0.058-1.0	0.861±0.172	0.107-1.0
Stand	0.914±0.070	0.708-1.0	0.912±0.086	0.654-1.0	0.911±0.066	0.680-1.0
Sit	0.994±0.006	0.977-1.0	0.999±0.002	0.993-1.0	0.997±0.003	0.987-1.0
Lie down	0.986±0.037	0.833-1.0	0.956±0.187	0.083-1.0	0.955±0.172	0.154-1.0
Transfer	0.871±0.187	0.100-1.0	0.698±0.130	0.438-0.867	0.755±0.159	0.176-0.929

Table 5. Performance of the feature intervention model evaluated with leave-one-subject-out cross-validation.

Physical activity	Precision		Recall		F1-score	
	Mean ± SD	Range	Mean ± SD	Range	Mean ± SD	Range
Walk	0.922±0.037	0.855-1.0	0,889±0.138	0.288-1.0	0.896±0.100	0.448-0.966
Stand	0.924±0.051	0.768-1.0	0.932±0.051	0.769-1.0	0.927±0.039	0.833-0.975
Sit	0.994±0.008	0.961-1.0	0.999±0.001	0.996-1.0	0.997±0.004	0.980-1.0
Lie down	0.929±0.205	0-1.0	0.948±0.204	0-1.0	0.937±0.202	0-1.0
Transfer	0.909±0.136	0.417-1.0	0.758±0.151	0.500-1.0	0.816±0.120	0.500-1.0

Feature Intervention Model. The classification performance of the FIM estimated through leave-one-subject-out cross-validation is shown in Table 5. Overall, the FIM yielded a mean precision of 0.936±0.055, a mean recall of 0.905±0.066, and a mean F1-score of 0.915±0.064 across all 24 participants. Upon examining the recognition rates of the individual activities, inter-person variability in classification performance appeared to be large for recognition of lying down (F1-score range: 0–1.0), and moderately large for walking (F1-score range: 0.448–0.966) and transfers (F1-score range: 0.500–1.0).

Performance Comparison. On average, the FIM achieved the highest overall F1-score and the lowest inter-participant variability (0.915 ± 0.064), outperforming the CCM (0.896 ± 0.075). Pairwise comparisons demonstrated a statistically significant difference between models (Friedman test, p-value < 0.05), with post-hoc Wilcoxon signed-rank tests indicating that the FIM significantly outperformed the CCM (p-value < 0.05).

In comparison with the CCM, the FIM provided consistent participant-level improvements, particularly for transfers. The FIM increased the transfer F1-score for 18 of 24 participants, maintained identical performance for one participant, and reduced performance for five. Notably, the per-participant transfer F1-score range increased from 0.176–0.929 under the CCM to 0.500–1.0 under the FIM, indicating a statistically significant upward shift in the lower bound (p-value < 0.05).

Failure Cases of the Best Classification Model. The best classification model, FIM, still produced relatively poor F1-scores (<0.5) for lying down and walking in two participants. Specifically, all 12 cases of lying down were misclassified as sitting for participant 18, and 33 out of 48 cases of walking were misclassified as standing for participant 1. Through analyzing the gait patterns, it was observed that most participants, including the best classified participant, exhibited Mean-X LB values between –0.1 and 0.1 g. This acceleration range entailed that the vertical axis of the upper body was oriented (nearly) parallel to the bed's surface while lying down. By comparison, for participant 18, the Mean-X LB values were more deviant with fluctuations around –0.4 g, which were in the vicinity of the Mean-X LB range observed during sitting. As for participant 1, based on Min-X UT, the walking accelerations exhibited considerably smaller amplitudes than those of most participants, and the difference is especially noticeable compared to the best classified participant. As shown in Fig. 6, the Min-X UT was found to separate most cases of walking and standing from each other. However, the low amplitudes of participant 1 caused the Min-X UT values during walking to fall within the Min-X UT value range observed during standing.

4 Discussions

Despite the absence of hip fracture patients in our study cohort, the contributions of this work are valuable regardless. Contrary to commercially available activity trackers, we developed our HAR algorithm in a demographic age group (age ≥ 80) that is representative of the hip fracture patient population. Beyond demonstrating that continuous physical activity monitoring in older adults can be achieved under simulated free-living conditions and across all clinically relevant functional milestones (walking, standing, sitting, lying, and transfers), this study introduced a structured strategy to manage inter-individual variability using synthetic gait representations. The synthetic data supported the multi-step FS pipeline in identifying features that generalized better across different individuals. By using the proposed feature set selected from the synthetic data to train a classifier on the real data, i.e., the FIM, the classification performance and robustness to inter-person variability improved slightly with statistical significance compared to the baseline model CCM. Such improvements were most noticeable in the classifications of transfers.

4.1 Real vs. Synthetic Data

The differences between the real and synthetic data are worth examining to infer how they complement each other in the development of the FIM. We previously observed that the synthetic data exhibited a lower intra-activity variation than the real data. It is postulated that this was due to a reduced inter-person variability, since DBA produced generalized gait patterns based on the common characteristics across different individuals. This reduction in individual gait deviations can be interpreted as a form of noise suppression, which facilitates the identification of stable and representative activity patterns. This interpretation is consistent with Bai et al. [6], who reported that reduced variability in HAR data improves the stability of pattern recognition in machine learning.

For the final feature set used in the FIM, only the features selected from the synthetic dataset were retained. Although two upper-thigh mean acceleration features (Mean-X UT and Mean-Z UT) overlapped between the real and synthetic selections, one feature selected exclusively from the real data (Min-X LB) was deliberately excluded. Because the synthetic data effectively suppresses individual-specific variability, feature selection performed on the synthetic dataset is more likely to capture fundamental, subject-invariant activity characteristics rather than incidental patterns driven by sampling noise or subject-specific gait traits in the real dataset. Moreover, consistently stronger feature stability and class separability were observed in the synthetic data, while visual inspection of class-conditional distributions and representative DBA traces confirmed that the principal activity-related signal structure was preserved without systematic distortion. Therefore, prioritizing synthetic data-selected features supports improved robustness and generalizability of the FIM, particularly for deployment in heterogeneous clinical populations. Nevertheless, as future work, it is worth investigating the impact of combining features selected from both the real and synthetic data.

4.2 Synthetic Data-Selected Feature Analysis

The FIM was able to classify most physical activities correctly using solely six features selected from the synthetic data with the multistep FS method. The features included Mean-X UT, Mean-Z UT, Mean-X LB, Min-X UT, RMS-X UT, and RMS-X LB. As shown in Fig. 6, we observed that the mean accelerations primarily supported the discrimination between standing, sitting, and lying down. These findings are in line with previous HAR studies, which characterized body postures using the mean. For example, Capela et al. [16] tested three different FS algorithms and found that mean accelerations were consistently selected to distinguish between sitting, standing, and lying down, in able-bodied older adults (74 ± 6.3 years). Similarly, Pannurat et al. [47] found that mean accelerations of the waist were ranked among the six most important features for classification of walking, standing, sitting, and lying down in healthy adults (average age of 67.5 years). Bijnens et al. [11] demonstrated the feasibility of using mean accelerations of the upper thigh to distinguish between standing, sitting, and lying down in healthy older adults between the ages of 60–88 years. Hence, our findings underscore and affirm the importance of the mean acceleration values in distinguishing between static activities whose differences are primarily defined by posture. To distinguish between standing and walking, which are similar in posture, Min-X UT and RMS-X UT appeared to provide discriminative information. Despite the widespread use of the minimum [36] and RMS [9,17] in HAR, their exact discriminative properties are ill-defined in the literature. Nevertheless, it is known that the RMS is sensitive to signal variability and that the minimum is sensitive to signal amplitudes. Both of these properties are distinctive for static and dynamic activities, which could explain their ability to discriminate between standing and walking.

The contribution of the aforementioned features in relation to the recognition of transfers remains challenging to explain. The primary challenge resides in the fact that transfers always occur in between two other activities, which causes their feature values to overlap. In the feature selection study by Capela et al. [16], no generalizable features for the characterization of transfers could be identified. However, others found that accelerations of the chest, waist, and upper thigh effectively captured the range of motion of transfers, and thereby enhanced recognition rates [5]. We extracted features from two similar locations: the lower back and upper thigh. We demonstrated that the six features extracted from these locations could collectively recognize transfers accurately with an F1-score of 0.816 ± 0.120. Hence, since the most crucial features could not be pinpointed from a univariate standpoint, it is postulated that interactions between these features underpinned the success of the good transfer recognition rate.

4.3 Two Failure Cases

Although our FIM model generally performed well on most participants, some pronounced misclassification errors were found for participants 18 and 1. First, the FIM model misclassified all instances of lying down as sitting for participant 18. Among participants for whom lying down was mostly correctly classified, the Mean-X LB values primarily varied between -0.1 and 0.1 g. By contrast, the Mean-X LB values of participant 18 were near -0.4 g, which may also be observed during a backward leaning sitting posture. This could potentially explain why instances of lying down were misclassified as sitting for participant 18. There are several external factors that may also have caused this deviating feature value, such as physiological differences between participants, which altered the sensor orientation or displacement during the execution of ADL tasks. Clinical practitioners may need to be particularly mindful of the latter, as displacements are more likely to occur during long-term monitoring in FLC [5], which may harm the HAR algorithm's ability to accurately recognize physical activities [8]. Second, the FIM model misclassified most instances of walking as standing for participant 1. The misclassifications were postulated to be due to the fact that participant 1 showcased noticeably smaller acceleration amplitudes during walking, which decreased the discriminative properties of Min-X UT to distinguish it from standing. This may explain why walking was often mistaken for standing in participant 1.

4.4 Failure Cases' Implication on Real-World Patients

These two failure cases indicate that our HAR algorithm recognizes ambulation behaviors less accurately in individuals whose walking accelerations exhibit lower amplitudes, e.g., due to slower or shuffling gait. Such a limitation presents a potential challenge when applying our proposed HAR algorithm to the hip fracture patient population. Because these forms of ambulation may be more prominent among geriatric hip fracture patients, considering that more than half of them do not regain their prefracture mobility level within the first postoperative year [10,65]. In addition, following hip fracture surgery, increased double support time, increased single support asymmetry, decreased cadence, and increased step length may be observed among such patients [28]. These factors highlight the need to consider the unique gait characteristics of hip fracture patients.

Apart from deviating ambulation patterns, transfers may also carry different characteristics in hip fracture patients. Compared to healthy older adults (69.4 ± 10.9 years), patients recovering from a hip fracture (76.4 ± 7.1 years) rely significantly more on force compensations from the contralateral side of the fractured hip to perform sit-to-stand transfers [34]. Besides force asymmetry in the lower extremities, transfer durations are generally prolonged for hip fracture patients. The cohort examined in our study showcased an average sit-to-stand transfer duration of 2.16 s. This is comparable to other studies examining healthy older adults, in which an average sit-to-stand transfer duration of 2.41–2.90 s was reported [3,30,46,53]. However, for rehabilitating hip fracture patients, the average transfer duration was previously estimated at approximately 5.35 s [3]. Similar deviations in movement symmetry, timing, and motor control are also commonly observed in other neurological and musculoskeletal populations, such as stroke survivors and patients with Parkinson's disease, suggesting that these generalization challenges may extend beyond hip fracture patients. In conclusion, the deviating transfer movements and prolonged transfer durations highlight the potential generalization problems that may be encountered when using our HAR algorithm in the real-world patient population.

4.5 Future Work

Based on the aforementioned limitations and in line with a systematic review on HAR for health research [60], it is imperative to further develop our HAR algorithm in a diverse participant pool, especially including real-world hip fracture patients, as well as patients that survived a stroke or have Parkinson's, to improve the algorithm's population-level impact. In addition, future work should also explore more expressive synthetic generation schemes beyond DBA. While DBA effectively captures average gait characteristics and suppresses inter-individual variability, it smooths temporal dynamics and may insufficiently represent atypical or pathological patterns such as slow, shuffling, or asymmetric gait in patients with neurological or musculoskeletal conditions. Deep generative models and hybrid artificial intelligence approaches that embed biomechanical or physiological constraints could generate more diverse yet physiologically plausible motion patterns, enabling targeted augmentation of underrepresented behaviors and further improving robustness and generalizability of our HAR algorithm in heterogeneous clinical populations.

5 Conclusion

This study focused on developing a continuous physical activity monitoring system that leverages a novel synthetic data generation scheme to aid in the multi-step feature selection process, thereby enhancing HAR performance and generalizability across individuals. The cohort consisted of healthy older adults aged ≥ 80 years, providing an age-matched first step toward future deployment in hip fracture rehabilitation. The investigated activities comprised walking, standing, sitting, lying down, and postural transfers. First, intra-activity variation was addressed by collecting sensor data under simulated free-living conditions. Second, robustness to inter-person variability was supported by generating a synthetic data set that represented common gait characteristics across individuals. We found that feature selection based on synthetic data improved downstream classification on real data, with the most notable gains observed in the recognition of transfers. The resulting monitoring system demonstrated good predictive performance using only six features, selected based on synthetic data and derived from two accelerometers placed on the upper thigh and lower back. While these preliminary results are encouraging, further validation in real-world patient populations remains essential to determine the clinical utility of the proposed monitoring system.

References

1. Allen, F.R., Ambikairajah, E., Lovell, N.H., Celler, B.G.: Classification of a known sequence of motions and postures from accelerometry data using adapted Gaussian mixture models. Physiol. Meas. **27**(10), 935–951 (2006). https://doi.org/10.1088/0967-3334/27/10/001
2. Annegarn, J., et al.: Objective physical activity assessment in patients with chronic organ failure: a validation study of a new single-unit activity monitor. Arch. Phys. Med. Rehabil. **92**(11) (2011). https://doi.org/10.1016/j.apmr.2011.06.021
3. Arcelus, A., Herry, C.L., Goubran, R.A., Knoefel, F., Sveistrup, H., Bilodeau, M.: Determination of sit-to-stand transfer duration using bed and floor pressure sequences. IEEE Trans. Biomed. Eng. **56**(10), 2485–2492 (2009). https://doi.org/10.1109/TBME.2009.2026733, conference Name: IEEE Transactions on Biomedical Engineering
4. Arif, M., Kattan, A.: Physical activities monitoring using wearable acceleration sensors attached to the body. PLoS ONE **10**(7), e0130851 (2015). https://doi.org/10.1371/journal.pone.0130851
5. Atallah, L., Lo, B., King, R., Yang, G.Z.: Sensor positioning for activity recognition using wearable accelerometers. IEEE Trans. Biomed. Circuits Syst. **5**(4), 320–329 (2011)
6. Bai, C., Wanigatunga, A.A., Saldana, S., Casanova, R., Manini, T.M., Mardini, M.T.: Are machine learning models on wrist accelerometry robust against differences in physical performance among older adults? Sensors (Basel, Switzerland) **22**(8), 3061 (2022). https://doi.org/10.3390/s22083061
7. Banos, O., Galvez, J.M., Damas, M., Pomares, H., Rojas, I.: Window size impact in human activity recognition. Sensors **14**(4), 6474–6499 (2014)

8. Banos, O., Toth, M.A., Damas, M., Pomares, H., Rojas, I.: Dealing with the effects of sensor displacement in wearable activity recognition. Sensors (Basel, Switzerland) **14**(6), 9995–10023 (2014). https://doi.org/10.3390/s140609995
9. Bennasar, M., Price, B.A., Gooch, D., Bandara, A.K., Nuseibeh, B.: Significant features for human activity recognition using tri-axial accelerometers. Sensors **22**(19), 7482 (2022). https://doi.org/10.3390/s22197482, number: 19 Publisher: Multidisciplinary Digital Publishing Institute
10. Bertram, M., Norman, R., Kemp, L., Vos, T.: Review of the long-term disability associated with hip fractures. Inj. Prev. **17**(6), 365–370 (2011). https://doi.org/10.1136/ip.2010.029579
11. Bijnens, W., Aarts, J., Stevens, A., Ummels, D., Meijer, K.: Optimization and validation of an adjustable activity classification algorithm for assessment of physical behavior in elderly. Sensors **19**(24), 5344 (2019)
12. Bolón-Canedo, V., Alonso-Betanzos, A.: Ensembles for feature selection: a review and future trends. Information Fusion **52**, 1–12 (2019). https://doi.org/10.1016/j.inffus.2018.11.008
13. Breiman, L.: Random forests. Mach. Learn. **45**(1), 5–32 (2001). https://doi.org/10.1023/A:1010933404324
14. Bulling, A., Blanke, U., Schiele, B.: A tutorial on human activity recognition using body-worn inertial sensors. ACM Comput. Surv. (CSUR) **46**(3), 1–33 (2014)
15. Bunea, F., She, Y., Ombao, H., Gongvatana, A., Devlin, K., Cohen, R.: Penalized least squares regression methods and applications to neuroimaging. Neuroimage **55**(4), 1519–1527 (2011). https://doi.org/10.1016/j.neuroimage.2010.12.028
16. Capela, N.A., Lemaire, E.D., Baddour, N.: Feature selection for wearable smartphone-based human activity recognition with able bodied, elderly, and stroke patients. PLoS ONE **10**(4), e0124414 (2015). https://doi.org/10.1371/journal.pone.0124414
17. Chen, J., Sun, Y., Sun, S.: Improving human activity recognition performance by data fusion and feature engineering. Sensors (Basel, Switzerland) **21**(3), 692 (2021). https://doi.org/10.3390/s21030692
18. Chernbumroong, S., Cang, S., Atkins, A., Yu, H.: Elderly activities recognition and classification for applications in assisted living. Expert Syst. Appl. **40**(5), 1662–1674 (2013). https://doi.org/10.1016/j.eswa.2012.09.004
19. Cleland, I., et al.: Optimal placement of accelerometers for the detection of everyday activities. Sensors **13**(7), 9183–9200 (2013). https://doi.org/10.3390/s130709183
20. Davoudi, A., et al.: The effect of sensor placement and number on physical activity recognition and energy expenditure estimation in older adults: validation study. JMIR Mhealth Uhealth **9**(5), e23681 (2021). https://doi.org/10.2196/23681
21. Dehghani, A., Sarbishei, O., Glatard, T., Shihab, E.: A quantitative comparison of overlapping and non-overlapping sliding windows for human activity recognition using inertial sensors. Sensors **19**(22), 5026 (2019)
22. Del Rosario, M.B., Wang, K., Wang, J., Liu, Y., Brodie, M., Delbaere, K., Lovell, N.H., Lord, S.R., Redmond, S.J.: A comparison of activity classification in younger and older cohorts using a smartphone. Physiol. Meas. **35**(11), 2269–2286 (2014). https://doi.org/10.1088/0967-3334/35/11/2269
23. Ding, C., Peng, H.: Minimum redundancy feature selection from microarray gene expression data. J. Bioinform. Comput. Biol. (2011). https://doi.org/10.1142/S0219720005001004, publisher: Imperial College Press

24. Drotár, P., Gazda, M., Vokorokos, L.: Ensemble feature selection using election methods and ranker clustering. Inf. Sci. **480**, 365–380 (2019). https://doi.org/10.1016/j.ins.2018.12.033
25. Erdaş, Ç.B., Atasoy, I., Açıcı, K., Oğul, H.: Integrating features for accelerometer-based activity recognition. Procedia Comput. Sci. **98**, 522–527 (2016). https://doi.org/10.1016/j.procs.2016.09.070
26. Figo, D., Diniz, P.C., Ferreira, D.R., Cardoso, J.M.P.: Preprocessing techniques for context recognition from accelerometer data. Pers. Ubiquit. Comput. **14**(7), 645–662 (2010). https://doi.org/10.1007/s00779-010-0293-9
27. Fleig, L., et al.: Sedentary behavior and physical activity patterns in older adults after hip fracture: a call to action. J. Aging Phys. Act. **24**(1), 79–84 (2016). https://doi.org/10.1123/japa.2015-0013
28. Gausden, E.B., et al.: Gait analysis after intertrochanteric hip fracture: does shortening result in gait impairment? J. Orthop. Trauma **32**(11), 554–558 (2018). https://doi.org/10.1097/BOT.0000000000001283
29. Gjertsen, J.E., Baste, V., Fevang, J.M., Furnes, O., Engesæter, L.B.: Quality of life following hip fractures: results from the norwegian hip fracture register. BMC Musculoskelet. Disord. **17**(1), 1–8 (2016). https://doi.org/10.1186/s12891-016-1111-y
30. Goffredo, M., Schmid, M., Conforto, S., Carli, M., Neri, A., D'Alessio, T.: Markerless human motion analysis in gauss-laguerre transform domain: an application to sit-to-stand in young and elderly people. IEEE Trans. Inf. Technol. Biomed. **13**(2), 207–216 (2009). https://doi.org/10.1109/TITB.2008.2007960, conference Name: IEEE Transactions on Information Technology in Biomedicine
31. Guo, Y., Hastie, T., Tibshirani, R.: Regularized linear discriminant analysis and its application in microarrays. Biostatistics **8**(1), 86–100 (2007). https://doi.org/10.1093/biostatistics/kxj035
32. Gupta, P., Dallas, T.: Feature selection and activity recognition system using a single triaxial accelerometer. IEEE Trans. Biomed. Eng. **61**(6), 1780–1786 (2014). https://doi.org/10.1109/TBME.2014.2307069
33. Haleem, S., Lutchman, L., Mayahi, R., Grice, J., Parker, M.: Mortality following hip fracture: trends and geographical variations over the last 40 years. Injury **39**(10), 1157–1163 (2008). https://doi.org/10.1016/j.injury.2008.03.022
34. Houck, J., Kneiss, J., Bukata, S.V., Puzas, J.E.: Analysis of vertical ground reaction force variables during a Sit to Stand task in participants recovering from a hip fracture. Clin. Biomech. **26**(5), 470–476 (2011). https://doi.org/10.1016/j.clinbiomech.2010.12.004
35. James, G., Witten, D., Hastie, T., Tibshirani, R.: An Introduction to Statistical Learning, vol. 112, chap. 10, pp. 373–413. Springer, Cham (2013). https://link.springer.com/content/pdf/10.1007%2F978-1-4614-7138-7.pdf
36. Janidarmian, M., Roshan Fekr, A., Radecka, K., Zilic, Z.: A comprehensive analysis on wearable acceleration sensors in human activity recognition. Sensors **17**(3), 529 (2017)
37. Kalousis, A., Prados, J., Hilario, M.: Stability of feature selection algorithms: a study on high-dimensional spaces. Knowl. Inf. Syst. **12**(1), 95–116 (2007). https://doi.org/10.1007/s10115-006-0040-8
38. Kannus, P., Parkkari, J., Sievänen, H., Heinonen, A., Vuori, I., Järvinen, M.: Epidemiology of hip fractures. Bone **18**(1), S57–S63 (1996). https://doi.org/10.1016/8756-3282(95)00381-9
39. Kolde, R., Laur, S., Adler, P., Vilo, J.: Robust rank aggregation for gene list integration and meta-analysis. Bioinformatics **28**(4), 573–580 (2012). https://doi.org/10.1093/bioinformatics/btr709

40. Lee, H., Lee, H., Whang, M.: An enhanced method to estimate heart rate from seismocardiography via ensemble averaging of body movements at six degrees of freedom. Sensors **18**(1), 238 (2018)
41. Lee, K.J., Um, S.H., Kim, Y.H.: Postoperative Rehabilitation after hip fracture: a literature review. Hip Pelvis **32**(3), 125–131 (2020). https://doi.org/10.5371/hp.2020.32.3.125
42. Logacjov, A., Bach, K., Kongsvold, A., Bårdstu, H.B., Mork, P.J.: HARTH: a human activity recognition dataset for machine learning. Sensors **21**(23), 7853 (2021). https://doi.org/10.3390/s21237853
43. Loh, W.Y.: Regression trees with unbiased variable selection and interaction detection. Stat. Sin. **12**, 361–386 (2002)
44. Matthews, C.E., Ainsworth, B.E., Thompson, R.W., Bassett, D.R.: Sources of variance in daily physical activity levels as measured by an accelerometer. Med. Sci. Sports Exerc. **34**(8), 1376–1381 (2002). https://doi.org/10.1097/00005768-200208000-00021
45. Müller, M.: Information Retrieval for Music and Motion. Springer, Berlin, Heidelberg (2007). https://doi.org/10.1007/978-3-540-74048-3
46. Najafi, B., Aminian, K., Loew, F., Blanc, Y., Robert, P.: Measurement of stand-sit and sit-stand transitions using a miniature gyroscope and its application in fall risk evaluation in the elderly. IEEE Trans. Biomed. Eng. **49**(8), 843–851 (2002). https://doi.org/10.1109/TBME.2002.800763, conference Name: IEEE Transactions on Biomedical Engineering
47. Pannurat, N., Thiemjarus, S., Nantajeewarawat, E., Anantavrasilp, I.: Analysis of optimal sensor positions for activity classification and application on a different data collection scenario. Sensors **17**(4), 774 (2017). https://doi.org/10.3390/s17040774
48. Pasco, J.A., Sanders, K.M., Hoekstra, F.M., Henry, M.J., Nicholson, G.C., Kotowicz, M.A.: The human cost of fracture. Osteoporos. Int. **16**(12), 2046–2052 (2005). https://doi.org/10.1007/s00198-005-1997-y
49. Petitjean, F., Gançarski, P.: Summarizing a set of time series by averaging: from steiner sequence to compact multiple alignment. Theoret. Comput. Sci. **414**(1), 76–91 (2012)
50. Petitjean, F., Ketterlin, A., Gançarski, P.: A global averaging method for dynamic time warping, with applications to clustering. Pattern Recogn. **44**(3), 678–693 (2011)
51. Resnick, B., Galik, E., Boltz, M., Hawkes, W., Shardell, M., Orwig, D., Magaziner, J.: Physical activity in the post-hip-fracture period. J. Aging Phys. Act. **19**(4), 373 (2011). https://doi.org/10.1123/japa.19.4.373, publisher: NIH Public Access
52. Reyes-Ortiz, J.L., Oneto, L., Samà, A., Parra, X., Anguita, D.: Transition-aware human activity recognition using smartphones. Neurocomputing **171**, 754–767 (2016)
53. Salarian, A., Russmann, H., Vingerhoets, F.J.G., Burkhard, P.R., Aminian, K.: Ambulatory monitoring of physical activities in patients with Parkinson's disease. IEEE Trans. Biomed. Eng. **54**(12), 2296–2299 (2007). https://doi.org/10.1109/TBME.2007.896591, conference Name: IEEE Transactions on Biomedical Engineering
54. Salarian, A., Russmann, H., Vingerhoets, F.J.G., Burkhard, P.R., Aminian, K.: Ambulatory monitoring of physical activities in patients with Parkinson's disease. IEEE Trans. Biomed. Eng. **54**(12), 2296–2299 (2007). https://doi.org/10.1109/TBME.2007.896591, conference Name: IEEE Transactionson Biomedical Engineering

55. Savitzky, A., Golay, M.J.: Smoothing and differentiation of data by simplified least squares procedures. Anal. Chem. **36**(8), 1627–1639 (1964)
56. Schafer, R.W.: On the frequency-domain properties of savitzky-golay filters. In: 2011 Digital Signal Processing and Signal Processing Education Meeting (DSP/SPE), pp. 54–59. IEEE (2011)
57. Seijo-Pardo, B., Bolón-Canedo, V., Alonso-Betanzos, A.: Testing different ensemble configurations for feature selection. Neural Process. Lett. **46**(3), 857–880 (2017). https://doi.org/10.1007/s11063-017-9619-1
58. Shoaib, M., Bosch, S., Incel, O.D., Scholten, H., Havinga, P.J.: Fusion of smartphone motion sensors for physical activity recognition. Sensors **14**(6), 10146–10176 (2014)
59. Shoaib, M., Bosch, S., Incel, O.D., Scholten, H., Havinga, P.J.: Complex human activity recognition using smartphone and wrist-worn motion sensors. Sensors **16**(4), 426 (2016)
60. Straczkiewicz, M., James, P., Onnela, J.P.: A systematic review of smartphone-based human activity recognition methods for health research. NPJ Digit. Med. **4**(1), 1–15 (2021). https://doi.org/10.1038/s41746-021-00514-4
61. Talkowski, J.B., Lenze, E.J., Munin, M.C., Harrison, C., Brach, J.S.: Patient participation and physical activity during rehabilitation and future functional outcomes in patients after hip fracture. Arch. Phys. Med. Rehabil. **90**(4), 618–622 (2009). https://doi.org/10.1016/j.apmr.2008.10.024
62. Taylor, D.: Physical activity is medicine for older adults. Postgrad. Med. J. **90**(1059), 26–32 (2014). https://doi.org/10.1136/postgradmedj-2012-131366
63. Urbanowicz, R.J., Meeker, M., La Cava, W., Olson, R.S., Moore, J.H.: Relief-based feature selection: introduction and review. J. Biomed. Inform. **85**, 189–203 (2018). https://doi.org/10.1016/j.jbi.2018.07.014
64. van Dartel, D., Hegeman, J.H., Vollenbroek-Hutten, M.M.R.: Feasibility and usability of wearable devices for ambulatory monitoring of the rehabilitation process of older patients after hip fracture surgery. In: Proceedings of the 18th International Conference on Wireless Networks and Mobile Systems - WINSYS. pp. 59–66. INSTICC, SciTePress (2021). https://doi.org/10.5220/0010522500590066
65. Vochteloo, A.J., et al.: More than half of hip fracture patients do not regain mobility in the first postoperative year: mobility and hip fracture. Geriatr. Gerontol. Int. **13**(2), 334–341 (2013). https://doi.org/10.1111/j.1447-0594.2012.00904.x
66. Wallisch, C., Dunkler, D., Rauch, G., de Bin, R., Heinze, G.: Selection of variables for multivariable models: opportunities and limitations in quantifying model stability by resampling. Stat. Med. **40**(2), 369–381 (2021). https://doi.org/10.1002/sim.8779
67. Willems, E., Visschedijk, J., van Balen, R., Achterberg, W.: Physical activity, physical function and fear of falling after hip fracture. Orthop. Res. Physiotherapy **3**(1), 1–6 (2017). https://doi.org/10.24966/ORP-2052/100031
68. Yang, C.C., Hsu, Y.L.: A review of accelerometry-based wearable motion detectors for physical activity monitoring. Sensors **10**(8), 7772–7788 (2010)

Establishing an AI Competence Center in a Public Healthcare Organization: A Multidisciplinary Learning Pathway

Timo Alalääkkölä[1](✉), Aappo Keränen[1], Jaana Kokko[1], Niko Korhonen[1], Roni Huhta[3], Joonas Haataja[1], Tenho Moilanen[1], Miika T. Nieminen[1,2], Mikko Reinikka[1], Jarmo Reponen[2], and Heikki Mikkonen[1]

[1] Wellbeing Services County of North Ostrobothnia, Kajaanintie 50, 90220 Oulu, Finland
timo.alalaakkola@pohde.fi

[2] Research Unit of Health Sciences and Technology, University of Oulu, Oulu, Finland

[3] ESKO Systems Ltd, Oulu, Finland

Abstract. The rapid evolution of Artificial Intelligence (AI) requires public healthcare organizations to balance innovation with strict regulatory compliance. This paper describes the establishment of an AI competence center at the Wellbeing Services County of North Ostrobothnia (Pohde) and at Oulu University Hospital (OYS). The AI competence center was designed to bridge the gap between wellbeing services county organization's needs and technological capabilities through a multidisciplinary structure involving the University of Oulu and industry partners. In addition to establishment activities, we present the AI competence center's "learning pathway," a four-phase methodology consisting of service delivery domain level scouting, market alignment, feasibility ranking, and hackathon-based validation. The results indicate that a centralized, cross-functional competence center accelerates the identification and operationalization of high-value AI solutions.

Keywords: AI competence center · healthcare · public-private innovation

1 Introduction

The integration of Artificial Intelligence (AI) into public healthcare offers significant potential for improving operational efficiency and patient workflows [1]. However, the implementation of AI in public healthcare sector is often fragmented and hindered by limited resources and complex regulatory frameworks, such as the Medical Device Regulation (MDR) and data privacy laws (GDPR) [2]. In the Wellbeing Services County of North Ostrobothnia (Pohde), which operates Oulu University Hospital (OYS) alongside other health, social and rescue services, the need to coordinate diverse AI development initiatives has led to the establishment of a centralized AI competence center. While Pohde has previously gained experience in AI development [1, 3–5] and orchestrating public-private innovation collaboration [6], these efforts have been operated as isolated projects without organization level coordination.

M. Särestöniemi et al. (Eds.): NCDHWS 2026, CCIS 3010, pp. 172–176, 2026.
https://doi.org/10.1007/978-3-032-28819-6_10

The objective of our AI competence center was not only to implement technology, but to create a sustainable structure that aligns diverse stakeholders including service delivery domains representation, legal services, IT administration, and external partners like the University of Oulu and in-house hospital information system provider Esko Systems. The structural formation of the AI competence center notes established digital transformation models in healthcare [7] and addresses field-specific opportunities and challenges identified in the public health sector AI application utilization [8, 9]. This paper outlines the structural formation of the AI competence center and the systematic "learning pathway" adopted to identify and prioritize AI initiatives.

2 Materials and Methods

2.1 Structure of the Competence Center

From the organizational perspective, the AI competence center of Pohde is a virtual organization and a denominator for joint AI development related activities which take place in the form of a regularly meeting working group. Officially established on November 27th 2025, the AI competence center is structured to have representation of each service delivery domain (family and social services, elderly care services, disability services, health and medical services, hospital services and emergency care, fire and rescue services) and support functions across the wellbeing services county organization. In total, the competence center has 35 members.

The governance model consists of two primary layers: I) The core group has representatives from research and development unit, IT management unit, information services, each service delivery domain and Esko Systems; II) Supporting experts are providing critical guidance on legal services, information security, data protection and MDR compliance, alongside external technology providers and academic research support from the University of Oulu. The close collaboration with experienced AI researchers enables knowledge based development.

2.2 The Learning Pathway

The AI competence center has monthly meetings on premise at the development center OYS TestLab, which is the innovation laboratory of Pohde enabling also public-private innovation collaboration [6]. In the first meeting of the AI competence center, the targets and the working model of the group were defined and the participants got familiar with each other. To operationalize the center, a four-phase methodology was developed to scout and validate potential AI application development needs. The learning pathway phases are as follows (see Fig. 1.):

I) Digital leap scouting: In the first meeting, each participant got a task to scout and define the "digital technology leap" within their own service delivery domain, identifying specific clinical or administrative challenges solvable by AI.

II) Market alignment: To ensure that internal ideas matched external capabilities, in the second meeting the topic was market alignment. The group collaborated with one of the leading industry partners (CGI) to gain insight into the current state of AI development in the market and especially in healthcare.

III) Feasibility ranking with prioritization matrix: In the third meeting the findings from the digital leap scouting phase were mapped together onto an "Impact vs. Feasibility" matrix. This allowed the group to rank initiatives based on their potential benefit to the Pohde operations versus the technical and regulatory complexity of implementation.

IV) Validation through initial development (Hackathon): The process culminated in a hackathon event organized in collaboration with an industry partner (Microsoft). The top three ideas/challenges identified in the scouting and ranking phases were presented to development teams to solve. This worked as a rapid validation of technical viability and provided a starting point for actual production-ready solution development.

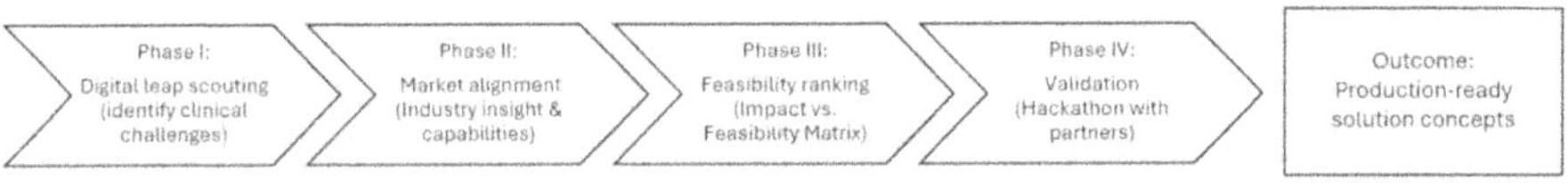

Fig. 1. The four-phase learning pathway for identifying and validating AI solution needs and concepts

3 Results

The establishment of the Pohde AI competence center has thus far successfully transformed isolated development ideas into a managed portfolio of AI initiatives. The "digital leap" scouting process revealed a diverse range of needs across different service delivery domains and support functions. By utilizing the impact vs. feasibility matrix, the competence center group was able to filter these needs, prioritizing those with high clinical, social or productivity impact and realistic implementation pathways. The AI solution development typically requires external funding. With the coordinated working model and prioritized needs, the resources can be focused on high quality and impactful project applications.

The inclusion of diverse professions in the ranking process ensured that regulatory bottlenecks were identified early. The Hackathon provided tangible proof-of-concept for the top three selected challenges, demonstrating that external partnerships (Microsoft, CGI) could be leveraged to accelerate problem-solving when the problem definition has been carried out in a mature way.

4 Discussion

Establishing an AI competence center in a public healthcare setting requires moving beyond a purely technical focus. Our experience at Pohde highlights the importance of a "Triple Helix" collaboration model [10], integrating the public sector (Pohde), academia (University of Oulu), and private industry representatives (Esko Systems, Microsoft, CGI).

The structure of the Pohde AI competence center allows agile operational work while ensuring that regulatory compliance (MDR, legal) is ensured. The organization-wide engagement of personnel is relevant in the need identification and innovative solution planning phases as well as in the solution implementation. A structured "learning pathway" from scouting to hackathons offers a replicable model for other wellbeing services counties aiming to systematize their AI development. Future work will focus on ensuring the development resources and the full-scale deployment of the solutions validated during the hackathon phase.

Acknowledgments. We would like to thank Finnish Innovation Fund SITRA for co-funding AI DocLog project (grant number 495601), which started the Pohde AI core team activity eventually leading to establishment of Pohde AI competence center.

Disclosure of Interests. The authors have no competing interests that are relevant to the content of this article.

References

1. Jansson, M., et al.: Artificial intelligence-enhanced care pathway planning and scheduling system: content validity assessment of required functionalities. BMC Health Serv. Res. **22**, 1513 (2022)
2. International Association of Privacy Professionals (IAPP): Organizational Digital Governance Report 2024. IAPP. https://iapp.org/resources/article/organizational-digital-governance-report/. Accessed 39 Jan 2026
3. Isosalo, A.: Medical image analysis and computing in breast cancer evaluation using mammography data. Doctoral dissertation. (University of Oulu) (2024)
4. Kokko, J., et al.: Co-development is crucial for implementing large language models for social and health care. In: Proceedings of the 29th Finnish National Conference on Telemedicine and eHealth (2024)
5. Reinikka, M., et al.: AI-assisted drafting of patient records: challenges, opportunities, and quality considerations. In: Proceedings of the eHealth2025 International Conference, Finnish Society of Telemedicine and eHealth, Helsinki/Stockholm, Finland, Sep. 17–18 (2025)
6. Alalääkkölä, T., Torvinen, H., Hurmelinna-Laukkanen, P., Mainela, T.: From value creation to value capture practices in healthcare innovation collaborations. Innovation **27**(1), 21–42 (2023)
7. Kraus, S., Jones, P., Kailer, N., Weinmann, A., Chaparro-Banegas, N., Roig-Tierno, N.: Digital Transformation: An Overview of the Current State of the Art of Research. Sage Open, **11**(3). (2021)
8. Wirtz, B.W., Weyerer, J.C., Geyer, C.: Artificial intelligence and the public sector—applications and challenges. Int. J. Public Adm. **42**(7), 596–615 (2019)
9. Berkhout, W.E.M., van Wijngaarden, J.J., Workum, J.D., et al.: Operationalization of artificial intelligence applications in the intensive care unit: a systematic review. JAMA Netw. Open **8**(7), e2522866 (2025)
10. Etzkowitz, H., Leydesdorff, L.: The dynamics of innovation: from national systems and "mode 2" to a triple helix of university–industry–government relations. Res. Policy **29**(2), 109–123 (2000)

Extending Customer Journey Modelling Language for Complex Healthcare: A Design Science Research Approach in Kidney Cancer Care

Essi Miettinen[1], Anu Vehkamäki[1], and Märt Vesinurm[1,2](✉)

[1] Department of Industrial Engineering and Management, Aalto University School of Science, Espoo, Finland
mart.vesinurm@aalto.fi

[2] Faculty of Medicine, Department of Public Health, University of Helsinki, Helsinki, Finland

Abstract. Complex healthcare services operate in inherently fragmented multi-provider environments where decision-making relies on both clinical data and shared information. This creates challenges for coordinating care across independent providers while maintaining continuity. While designing well-functioning patient processes is essential for quality care, a universally accepted modelling method that adequately supports patient engagement is yet to be established. Existing methods often prioritize institutional workflows over the patient's actual experience. This study addresses this gap by applying a Design Science Research (DSR) approach to extend the Customer Journey Modelling Language (CJML) using the kidney cancer care process as a case example. Data were collected through collaborative workshops with healthcare professionals and a patient interview to map the distinct requirements of patient journeys and pathways which were then modelled using CJML. Through iterative modelling and expert validation, specific limitations in the current CJML framework were identified regarding its ability to represent complex process logics. To resolve these, this paper proposes and validates specific extensions to CJML, namely improved notations for sub-processes, modules, decision points, non-linear timelines, angled connectors, looping, data objects, repeat actions, and discussion points. This study contributes modelling artefacts that enhance the capability of CJML to visualize complex patient journeys, supporting both operational efficiency and patient-centred care.

Keywords: Customer Journey Modelling Language (CJML) · Design Science Research · patient journey · process modelling · kidney cancer care

1 Introduction

As life expectancies increase and the human population grows, healthcare systems face increasing pressure to deliver complex, high-quality care at scale [1]. Increasing demand for resources is evident especially in chronic diseases with multimorbidity on the rise [2]. Patients with complex diagnostics account for a large part of healthcare system resource

M. Säreströniemi et al. (Eds.): NCDHWS 2026, CCIS 3010, pp. 177–192, 2026.
https://doi.org/10.1007/978-3-032-28819-6_11

use, while the quality of care does not consistently meet expectations and intentions [3, 4]. This creates an urgent challenge: healthcare providers must optimize processes to ensure efficiency without compromising patient outcomes.

Addressing the widespread impact of chronic diseases has become a central priority for healthcare organizations, policymakers and governments. One way healthcare providers can support these goals is by encouraging patients to take a more active role in managing their own illness (i.e. by making use of value co-creation) [5, 6]. However, meaningful patient involvement requires transparent and well-coordinated care pathways, which remain difficult to achieve in healthcare systems characterized by fragmented responsibilities and multiple detached service producers [7]. This fragmentation often leads to a lack of shared understanding of patient care processes and their planning [8]. Consequently, the modelling and clear representation of care pathways become critical enablers for improving both patient engagement and operational efficiency. Yet, achieving such clarity is far from simple. The underlying challenge is the complexity of care systems, which shapes daily patient care [7, 9]. Patient pathways themselves are inherently complex concepts operating within equally complex healthcare systems [7, 8].

Process modelling plays a foundational role by clarifying how care is structured, delivered and supported through information. This understanding is also essential for making effective use of health data systems such as electronic health records (EHR). For instance, EHRs can help identify patients at risk due to missed follow-ups [10], or improve clinical practice and continuity of care [11]. However, having access to data but no process model to compare it against makes it impossible to study where the reality deviates from what is expected [12]. Therefore, process models not only guide care planning but also enable the purposeful application of data within systems like EHRs. While process modelling offers methods to evaluate costs, resource consumption and bottlenecks [13], applications in healthcare require careful consideration of the unique challenges and complexities inherent in healthcare processes [7]. Notably, a standardised methodological approach for patient-centred healthcare service modelling is still lacking [14, 15].

This study builds on the Customer Journey Modelling Language (CJML) for mapping complex patient pathways [16–20]. CJML is a formalised visual language designed to model service delivery specifically to represent the perspective of the end-user. CJML emphasizes the sequence of interactions or "touchpoints" between the patient and various service providers. Uniquely, the language offers two complementary views: a customer journey diagram (later referred to as journey diagram) for capturing an individual's specific experience, and a journey network diagram (later referred to as network diagram) for representing the network of service touchpoints and inter-provider handovers experienced by the patient [21]. This dual perspective makes it particularly suitable for healthcare [17]. CJML can be a helpful tool for service providers and researchers in service design, operations management, and information systems design.

There is no single representation method that satisfies all needs in complex patient pathways and health systems. This paper focuses on kidney cancer as an illustrative example of a complex care process. In this study, the CJML notation is further developed to enhance its use in patient journey modelling. This study has three main aims. First, to deepen the understanding of how the care of long-term illnesses is organised by identifying the key characteristics relevant to modelling. Second, to assess whether these characteristics can be effectively represented as a patient journey aligned with healthcare system requirements. Third, to evaluate how CJML can be further improved to support this representation.

The study is guided by the following research question:

RQ: How can CJML be developed to better support patient journey modelling in complex healthcare settings?

By addressing this question, this paper contributes to the development of a shared, interpretable modelling method suitable for diverse stakeholders beyond healthcare professionals, including business analysts and IT specialists [15].

2 Methods

This study followed a design science research (DSR) process [22, 23]. An iterative process was adopted to develop and evaluate artefacts through workshops and expert feedback.

2.1 Empirical Setting

This study was conducted in Finland, where the healthcare system is well-performing yet faces structural fragmentation with financing and service provision divided among wellbeing counties, national insurance, employers, and private actors [24]. This results in a variety of care access and differing care pathways depending on the patient's entry point into the system. Within this landscape, the Helsinki University Hospital (HUS). HUS plays a central role as the country's largest healthcare producer. The study focuses on HUS's Comprehensive Cancer Center, Finland's largest cancer treatment unit, which provides extensive specialised services including radiation therapy, drug therapy, and palliative care.

2.2 Research Process

This study followed the design science research (DSR) methodology [22] as illustrated in Fig. 1. DSR was selected as it supports the rigorous creation of artefacts, in this case, extensions to the CJML notation, to address specific problems in unique contexts [22]. The process consisted of five distinct phases, where demonstration and evaluation were combined into a single iterative cycle to maximize expert feedback.

(1) **Problem identification and motivation.** The process began by establishing a practical understanding of complex patient processes. Data were collected through interviews with healthcare professionals (HCPs) specializing in kidney cancer (n = 3), a patient (n = 1) and a literature review on existing CJML modelling techniques. This aligned with the core principle in DSR: the research must produce an "artefact created to address a problem" [23].

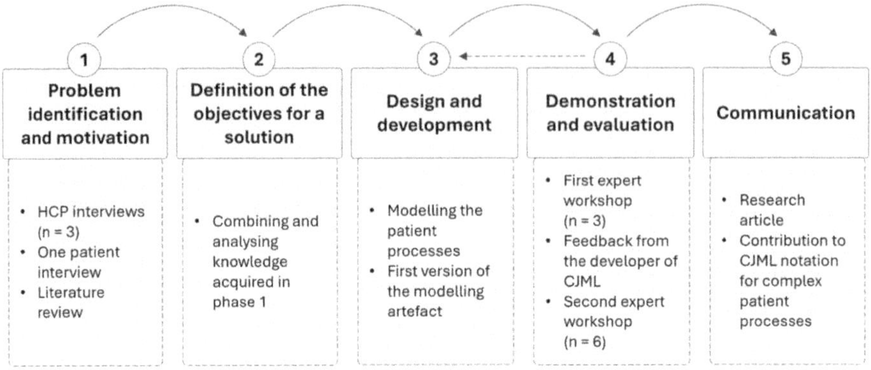

Fig. 1. Research process, methods and outputs.

(2) **Defining objectives for a solution.** Based on the problem identification, we defined the objectives for the new modelling artefact [22]. New insights from the interviews were integrated with existing modelling methodologies to establish a scientific foundation. Specifically, we used the interview data to map the typical kidney cancer care pathway, identifying where CJML currently failed to capture complexity.
(3) **Design and development.** This phase focused on creating the artefact itself [22]. Using the workshops and modelling guidelines, we developed specific CJML extensions. By applying these extensions to the real-world kidney cancer case, we were able to test the strengths and weaknesses of the language in a practical setting.
(4) **Demonstration and evaluation.** As shown by the feedback loop in Fig. 1, demonstration and evaluation were performed iteratively. This phase included two expert workshops (n = 3; n = 6). Between these sessions, the original developer of CJML provided specific feedback, which was incorporated into the second workshop. Following Hevner et al. [23], the artefacts were evaluated against specific criteria including accuracy, completeness, fit with the organization, and usability. The goal was to receive actionable proposals that combine both theoretical and practical contributions to further develop the artefacts.
(5) **Communication.** This paper serves as the final phase, documenting the research process, the problem, and the resulting artefacts [22]. As noted in [23], DSR must be presented effectively to both technology-oriented and management-oriented audiences. The proposed extensions to CJML presented in the Results s5ction constitute the primary contribution of this process.

2.3 Data Collection

Data collection was conducted primarily during the problem identification (phase 1) and demonstration and evaluation (phase 4) stages. During the problem identification phase, four semi-structured interviews were organized as detailed in Table 1. The participants included one oncologist, two oncology nurses, and one patient diagnosed with kidney cancer. The HCPs were chosen and recruited by the HUS for their expertise in kidney cancer treatment. The patient had been treated for kidney cancer for several years, thus having experience of several stages of treatment from a patient's perspective.

The interviews took place between April and May 2023, with each session lasting between 60 and 90 min. All HCP participants were recruited from the HUS Comprehensive Cancer Center. Prior to the interviews, all participants were provided with a summary of the research to ensure informed participation. Two researchers attended every session; one author facilitated the interviews while the other was responsible for taking field notes. All interviews were audio-recorded for verification and analysis.

Table 1. Backgrounds of the participating HCPs and the patient.

Role	Experience	Length
Oncologist	In oncology for 1 year, 3 months	1 h 30min
Oncology Nurse	In oncology for 11 years	1 h 30 min
Oncology Nurse	Long career in oncology – exact years remained unknown	1 h 6 min
Patient	Chronic kidney cancer of 6 years	1 h 12 min

Following the initial development of the artefacts, the validation process involved two sequential expert workshops. The approach was iterative: the model and proposed improvements were refined between sessions, with feedback from the first workshop directly informing the development of the second.

Participating experts evaluated the artefacts using a structured framework (Table 2) consisting of six dimensions: accuracy, clarity, user benefit, reliability, need, and completeness. The evaluation dimensions were derived from the work by Hevner et al. [23]. In addition to scoring, participants were encouraged to provide qualitative feedback on specific notation elements.

Table 2. Evaluation framework

Dimension	Guiding questions
Accuracy	Does the proposed extension enable more precise or correct representation of processes?
Clarity	Does the proposed extension enhance the visual clarity and comprehensibility of CJML models?
User benefit	Does the proposed extension improve the user experience? Does it add practical value for real-world use? How well does this align with the modelling needs of healthcare?
Reliability	Will the proposed extension behave predictably and consistently across cases?
Need	Does the proposed extension respond to a common need? Is it easy and intuitive for modelers and stakeholders to adopt and use?
Completeness	Does the proposed extension help model relevant aspects that are currently missing in CJML?

Participants were selected based on their specialized knowledge of healthcare operations and modelling methodologies.

Workshop 1: The first workshop served as a pilot evaluation, focusing on the model's applicability in real-world organizational settings. Participants (n = 3) were chosen for their research experience in patient journeys, integrated care, and multimorbidity management (Table 3).

Validation Interval: Between the two workshops, the original developer of CJML provided written feedback on the models and development proposals. This step primarily served to validate terminology and ensure the proposed visual notations aligned with the core logic of the language.

Workshop 2: The second workshop recruited experts (n = 6) with direct experience in CJML and digital health research. This panel included members of the research team responsible for developing CJML, as well as experts with hands-on experience applying the language to clinical pathways. Their collective background provided a comprehensive base for critically validating the technical robustness of the proposed extensions.

Table 3. Backgrounds of expert evaluators in workshops 1 and 2.

Participant	Experience	Length
Workshop 1		
1	One year of research experience in patient journey efficiency and care continuity	1 h 40min
2	2 years of research experience in integrated care	
3	4 years of research experience in the management of complex patient journeys, with knowledge in modelling languages	
Workshop 2		
1	Less than a year of experience in modelling customer journeys	1 h 49 min
2	2 years of research experience in journey modelling, including using CJML	
3	1,5 years of research experience in longitudinal studies on patient pathways	
4	Multiple years of experience in digital health research, most recently from visual modelling of patient pathways	
5	2 years of relevant research experience, most recently form modelling pathways using CJML	
6	15 years of research experience from human-computer interaction to service innovation and modelling of patient pathways. Currently overseeing the development of CJML	

2.4 Data Analysis

Insights from the workshops with experts were mapped immediately after each session. All workshops were recorded for analysis verification. The material gathered during the discussions was first consolidated into a digital timeline using Microsoft PowerPoint, ensuring a coherent sequence of events and insights. This preliminary representation, intentionally not modelled using any formal language, was reviewed by the research group and then fact-checked against the recordings before being transformed into a process model.

Following the first iteration of the pathway model, key points and essential elements of the patient journey were identified. Consequently, the pathway was rebuilt in Microsoft PowerPoint using the official visual notation. It was subsequently evaluated, refined, and approved within the research group.

2.5 Ethical Considerations

The research herein has received ethical approval from the Aalto University Research Ethics Committee (Decision D/662/03.04/2022) and research permit (13/2023) from Helsinki University Hospital.

3 Results

3.1 Identifying the Kidney Cancer Journey

The HCP interviews and the patient interview identified the core structural elements typical of kidney cancer cases treated at the Helsinki University Hospital (HUS) Comprehensive Cancer Center. The patient journey was categorized into five distinct phases: detection, diagnosis, treatment, post-treatment survivorship, and end-of-life care. Figure 2 exemplifies the application of CJML to model the detection phase specifically as a network diagram ("swimlane diagram") [21]. Transitions between these phases emerged as critical focal points; the analysis highlighted that these interfaces are often where knowledge sharing and communication between the patient and care providers are most vulnerable to disruptions.

The workshops further revealed that the influence of different care roles evolves significantly across the patient journey. During the initial detection phase, the interface between primary care and the patient is decisive for the progression to diagnosis. As the patient moves into the treatment phase, the influence shifts primarily to the Kidney Cancer Specialist team. However, this specialized support often diminishes as the patient completes oncology treatment and transitions into long-term survivorship, leaving a potential gap in guidance.

Finally, the highly fragmented, multi-producer nature of the care ecosystem was evident. The process model generated in the workshops mapped a minimum of 10 distinct care providers throughout all five distinct care phases, suggesting that the actual operational network involved in a patient's full care trajectory is likely even more extensive.

In Fig. 2, the first phase, "detection," is presented. Kidney cancer detection typically begins in primary healthcare, where a general practitioner ("public side"), an occupational doctor or a private doctor are alternative entry points into the care process for the patient. The receiving HCP depends on the availability of resources and personal preferences of the patient. At the end of the detection phase, the patient is referred to specialised care. The referral process has minor differences depending on the HCP-type the patient sought care from in the beginning. Touchpoints, highlighted in blue, illustrate a communication point and the initiator, for example the sender of certain information – this is standard in CJML. Touchpoints T2 ("Goes to the doctor's office…"), T6 ("Receives information…"), and T7 ("Receives a referral") are non-standard CJML elements and have been compressed for illustrative purposes. In standard CJML, only a single flow can exist between touchpoints, not parallel arrows as shown here.

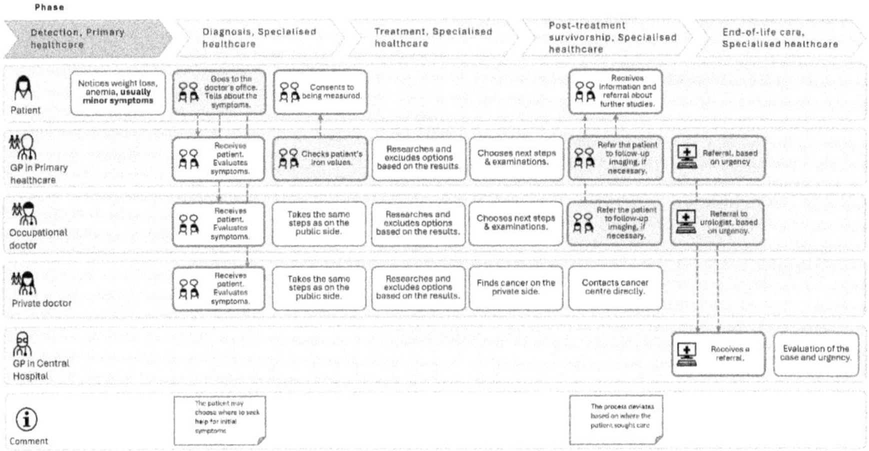

Fig. 2. CJML model of the detection phase of kidney cancer care.

3.2 Developing the CJML Artefacts

While CJML is designed to be a user-friendly and easily interpretable language, its inherent simplicity requires adaptations when applied to complex healthcare processes. The study identified several specific areas where the notation required further development to accurately model the intricacies of the kidney cancer care pathway (Table 4).

Table 4. The artefacts developed in the study as extensions of the CJML

Artefact	Notation	Added value
Sub-processes	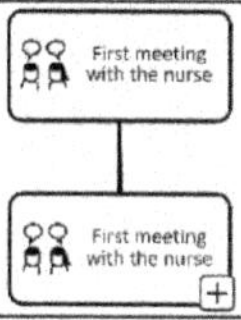	Enables detailed breakdown of complex touchpoints while maintaining a clear overview. For example, a meeting with a nurse can be further elaborated into distinct steps when appropriate.
Modules	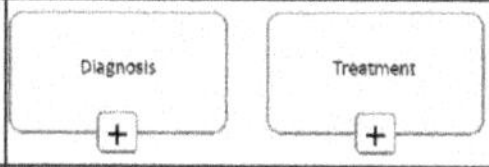	Similar to phases but allowing for collapsing. Encourages structured and reusable modelling.
Decision point	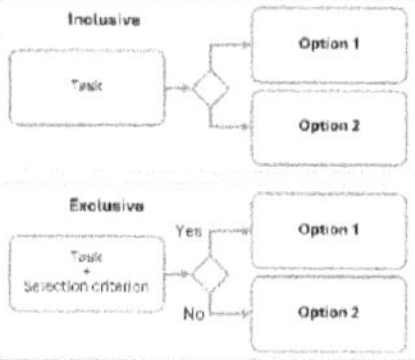	Enables clear visualisation of decision points and branching paths in a network diagram. An inclusive notation is used when all options are valid, whereas an exclusive notation is applied when a specific selection criterion determines which path to follow.
Temporary, non-linear timeline	N/A	Allows for simplified process models for alternative care pathways. For example, flows could be directed "backwards" (right-to-left).
Angled connectors		Enables clear and accurate depiction of the process flow, even in complex cases for message flow (dashed) and sequence flow (solid).
Looping mechanism	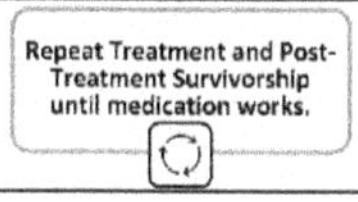	Supports representation of iterative actions and repeated behaviours within a process.
Data object	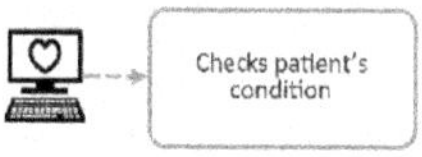	Provides a way to visualise and track uploaded and retrieved data within process steps. Distinct from a communication channel and rather representing databases.
Repeat action	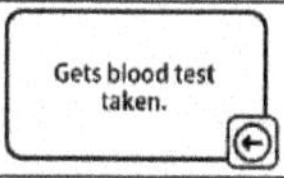	Facilitates repeat of standardised processes by referencing external process logic.
Discussion point	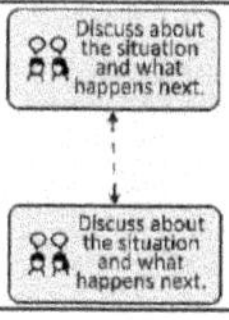	Two-sided arrow enables a visual representation of a shared touchpoint to capture the collaborative nature in patient-centred care.

Sub-processes and Modularity. The inclusion of sub-processes allows for the decomposition of complex patient pathways into manageable, discrete set of touchpoints. Cancer care involves distinct sequences, such as treatment planning, administration, surveillance, and follow-up, which are effectively modelled as separate modules. This modularity allows different stakeholders to focus on the process segments most relevant to their role. Sub-processes should not be conflated with phases, as CJML uses phases to define the overarching progression of a care journey, whereas sub-processes capture the operational breakdown of activities within those phases.

Decision Points. Current guidelines for CJML network diagrams lack a formal mechanism for decision logic, supporting it only in journey diagrams. Integrating decision points into network diagrams is essential for planning aggregate patient flows. Furthermore, the proposed extension distinguishes between inclusive decisions (where multiple valid pathways may be taken simultaneously) and exclusive decisions (where a specific criterion forces a single path). This improvement enables the clear visualisation of branching logic within the planned network.

Temporary, Non-linear Timeline. To reduce repetition and improve clarity, some flows were directed temporally "backwards" (right-to-left). While process models typically follow a strict left-to-right progression, rigid adherence to this rule can lead to cluttered diagrams in complex repetitive care scenarios. Supporting temporary, non-linear timelines simplifies the representation without sacrificing the logical order of care. Some possible early examples have been previously published [9].

Angled Connectors. In complex diagrams, message flows often overlap, obscuring the visualisation. We introduced angled connectors to clarify the directionality of sequence (solid) and message (dashed) flows. Additionally, these connectors visually emphasize temporal latency, for example, illustrating that a physical letter does not arrive at the exact moment it is sent. The official CJML visual notation document has examples of angled connectors being used for non-synchronous touchpoints, such as sending physical letters, where the sending and receiving time is different [21].

Looping Mechanism. A formal looping mechanism was introduced to handle phases where the process structurally repeats until a specific condition is met, such as iterating through medication options during treatment. This mechanism significantly reduces visual repetition in the model.

Data Object. To emphasize points requiring specific evidence or information exchange, a Data Object element was introduced. This element represents a knowledge repository or information system. The retrieval or upload of data is visualised by referencing this object, with distinct icons available to denote different underlying systems (e.g., EHR, patient portal).

Repeat Action. This element refers to a specific activity that has been defined previously and is stored externally as a separate CJML diagram. It functions as a specialized subtype of a sub-process. The key distinction is that while a standard sub-process can be modified for the specific context of the parent diagram, a repeat action functions as a fixed reference to an unmodifiable, standardized sequence of touchpoints.

Discussion Point. The final extension addresses the visualisation of shared decision-making. In standard CJML, interactions are touchpoints that can have one of two types; (1) a communication point where the patient (or customer) interacts with a service provider notated with a circle, and (2) an action where an event occurs or an activity is undertaken within the patient (or customer) journey [18]. However, in patient-centric, co-created care models, collaborative decision-making is a distinct event. To capture this importance, a dedicated Discussion Point visual element, distinctive from a communication point, was proposed to explicitly mark moments of joint deliberation between the patient and a service provider.

3.3 Expert Validation of Artefacts

The simultaneous demonstration and evaluation phases provided critical feedback on the proposed CJML extensions. Experts assessed the artefacts' ability to accurately represent both the planned organizational workflows and the complex realities of the kidney cancer patient journey against the defined evaluation criteria. The validation results can be categorized based on the maturity and reception of the proposals.

First, the **high-maturity extensions**: sub-processes, modules and decision points. These two extensions emerged as the most mature and ready for continued development. Sub-processes were consistently identified across both workshops as the highest priority improvement, meeting the majority of the evaluation criteria for clarity and user benefit. By the conclusion of the second workshop, half of the experts (3 out of 6) considered the sub-process notation ready for immediate implementation. Relatedly, experts noted that modules should be structured as reusable building blocks within sub-processes and not confused with existing CJML process phases.

Second, **extensions requiring refinement**: looping mechanism, data objects, and interactions. The proposals addressed recognized critical gaps in CJML but require further iteration before adoption. The looping mechanism was acknowledged as a promising solution to a common modelling need, but experts concluded the current visual representation requires refinement to ensure immediate clarity for diverse users. The data object was evaluated as highly beneficial for addressing the gap in representing information flows. However, experts emphasized that its referencing mechanism must be unambiguously defined to prevent confusion. A concrete proposal emerging from the workshops suggested placing information systems (like EHRs) in separate swimlanes and using consistent iconography to reference data objects. This approach would minimize cluttered sequence flows while maintaining high visibility of data interactions. Repeat action was noted as promising but requires that processes be presented as modules. The visualization needs further refinement to avoid user confusion. The visualization of discussion points was praised as clear and providing a more realistic representation of collaborative interactions. However, experts noted that defining clear usage guidelines for this common need is challenging and necessitates further research and testing.

Third, **contentious proposals**: timeline and flow adjustments. Proposals involving the alteration of standard temporal flows faced significant resistance. In Workshop 1, experts strongly advised against breaking the linear timeline, even temporarily. They argued that while the complexity of care is real, it should be managed through alternative simplification strategies (like sub-processes) rather than disrupting the fundamental left-to-right flow logic of the diagrams. Regarding angled connectors and non-linear timelines, the original developer of CJML confirmed that while these practices are technically permitted, they currently lack clear definitions within existing guidelines, highlighting a need for formal standardization.

4 Discussion

In this study we have outlined how CJML could be further developed to better support patient journey modelling in complex healthcare environments. Our findings confirm that while CJML is inherently user-centric, its standard notation previously lacked the technical granularity necessary to capture the intricacies of complex clinical pathways. This study demonstrates that by introducing new notation, such as modularity through sub-processes and specific interaction elements such as discussion points, CJML can better bridge the gap between the rigid patient pathways and more fluid patient journeys. The expert validation highlights that these extensions allow the model to retain its empathetic, patient-facing focus while improving the structural rigor required for operational care planning.

The introduction of sub-processes, modules, and decision points aligns CJML with established conventions found in mature process modelling languages, such as Business Process Model and Notation (BPMN) [25]. While these structural elements are staples in systems engineering for managing complexity [26, 27], their absence in CJML's formal guidelines [16] previously forced users to adopt ad-hoc workarounds. Notably, decision points are inherent to any clinical pathway planning; our analysis suggests that modellers were likely already using decision logic implicitly within CJML diagrams, despite the lack of official syntax. The high expert prioritization of sub-processes also confirms that stakeholders were actively seeking a sanctioned method to manage the complexity of reality through modularity, bringing CJML to a level of maturity comparable to other standard modelling languages without losing its specific user-centric focus [15, 28].

A significant theoretical contribution of this study is the distinction between a standard touchpoint and the newly proposed discussion point. Process modelling languages generally lack syntax for 'bargaining' or 'negotiation' inherent to many healthcare processes [29]. Traditional service modelling often portrays the patient journey as a linear sequence of transactional events, where a service is delivered to a passive recipient [30]. However, modern healthcare paradigms posit that value is not delivered but co-created through the active collaboration of the patient and provider [6]. Our findings suggest that standard CJML touchpoints failed to adequately capture these moments of bi-directional exchange, effectively rendering the work of the patient invisible. The expert validation confirmed that the discussion point provides a more realistic representation of interaction, specifically capturing the collaborative nature inherent in patient-centred care.

Despite CJML being a younger modelling language, its flexibility allowed for successful adaptation to modelling needs. However, shortcomings emerged in more advanced use cases. In these instances, the user-friendliness that benefits novice users [20] began to work against effective modelling. While ease of use can promote broader adoption, overly open-ended guidelines may lead to variation in modelling quality and interpretation. These challenges highlight the tension between user-friendly, flexible design and the need for formal structure when aiming for scalable or automated modelling applications. Addressing this tension has direct practical implications for the hospital environment. For healthcare management, the introduction of formal decision logic and sub-processes transforms these diagrams from simple illustrations into diagnostic tools capable of identifying operational bottlenecks. By mapping the precise logical flow of care, management can better pinpoint resource constraints using methods such as process mining [31–35]. For IT and system developers, the new data object explicitly visualizes when and where data is retrieved or uploaded to the EHR, enabling developers to build IT systems that align with the actual workflow of clinicians rather than theoretical assumptions. Finally, these validated, clearer models serve as powerful communication tools. By accurately depicting the journey, providers can offer patients a transparent roadmap of their care, reducing the anxiety caused by uncertainty and empowering them to navigate their treatment with confidence, resulting in improved health outcomes [36].

The primary strength of this study is the application DSR. By employing an iterative cycle of development, demonstration, and evaluation, the study ensured that the proposed CJML extensions were not merely theoretical but were practically validated by domain experts facing real-world clinical and modelling challenges. Furthermore, the collaboration with HUS Comprehensive Cancer Center provided access to highly specialized knowledge, ensuring that the resulting artefacts reflect the actual complexity of tertiary care rather than a simplified abstraction. However, this study also has several limitations. First, the data collection was based on a limited sample of healthcare professionals ($n = 3$), one patient, and modelling experts ($n = 3$ and $n = 6$), which limits the generalisability of the evaluation results. Second, the HUS Cancer Center primarily treats stage IV kidney cancer patients. Consequently, the interviewees possessed detailed knowledge of late-stage, complex care pathways but lacked equivalent insight into earlier stages of the disease, potentially skewing the case model. Finally, the developed modelling artefacts, while effective for this specific use case, require further validation to determine their applicability.

In conclusion, this study demonstrates that while the CJML offers a strong foundation for patient-centric design, it requires specific structural enhancements to effectively model the complexity of modern healthcare systems. By developing and validating extensions, we have shown that it is possible to bridge the gap between the operational requirements and patient-centricity. These artefacts help move CJML from a purely descriptive visualization tool into a functional instrument for care planning, capable of identifying bottlenecks, mapping data flows, and formalizing the critical role of value co-creation. Ultimately, this study contributes to the broader field of health informatics and healthcare operations management by offering a validated approach to modelling that respects both the systemic logic of medical treatment and the human reality of the patient experience. In this paper, we set out to find how CJML could be developed to better support patient journey modelling in complex healthcare settings. Nine artefacts for expanding CJML were developed using an iterative DSR process. Future research should validate these CJML extensions across diverse chronic conditions and complex customer journeys also beyond the healthcare domain. This would establish their generalisability, given their potential applicability to non-healthcare service contexts.

Acknowledgments. The authors would like to thank all the informants and acknowledge the contributions of the Pathway project members, especially Ragnhild Halvorsrud for her support. This work was funded by the Research Council of Norway under the Pathway project (no. 316342).

Disclosure of Interests. The authors have no competing interests.

References

1. World Health Organization: World report on Ageing and Health. World Health Organization, Luxemburg (2015)
2. Hajat, C., Stein, E.: The global burden of multiple chronic conditions: a narrative review. Prev. Med. Rep. **12**, 284–293 (2018). https://doi.org/10.1016/j.pmedr.2018.10.008
3. OECD, European Union: Health at a Glance: Europe 2022: State of Health in the EU Cycle. OECD Publishing (2022)
4. Busse, R., Klazinga, N., Panteli, D., Quentin, W.: Improving Healthcare Quality in Europe: Characteristics. OECD, Effectiveness and Implementation of Different Strategies (2019)
5. Danaher, T.S., Danaher, P.J., Sweeney, J.C., McColl-Kennedy, J.R.: Dynamic customer value cocreation in healthcare. J. Serv. Res. **27**, 177–193 (2024). https://doi.org/10.1177/10946705231161758
6. Peng, Y., Wu, T., Chen, Z., Deng, Z.: Value cocreation in health care: systematic review. J. Med. Internet Res. **24**, e33061 (2022). https://doi.org/10.2196/33061
7. Vesinurm, M.: Managing Complex Patient Journeys: A Healthcare Operations Management Perspective. PunaMusta Oy, Helsinki (2025)
8. Seys, D., et al.: Care pathways are complex interventions in complex systems: new European Pathway Association framework. Int. J. Care Coord. **22**, 5–9 (2019). https://doi.org/10.1177/2053434519839195
9. Halvorsrud, R., Lillegaard, A.L., Røhne, M., Jensen, A.M.: Managing complex patient journeys in health care. In: Pfannstiel, M.A., Rasche, C. (eds.) Service Design and Service Thinking in Healthcare and Hospital Management: Theory, Concepts. Practice. Springer International Publishing, Cham (2019)
10. Murphy, D.R., et al.: Electronic health record-based triggers to detect potential delays in cancer diagnosis. BMJ Qual. Saf. **23**, 8–16 (2014). https://doi.org/10.1136/bmjqs-2013-001874
11. Reis, Z.S.N., Maia, T.A., Marcolino, M.S., Becerra-Posada, F., Novillo-Ortiz, D., Ribeiro, A.L.P.: Is there evidence of cost benefits of electronic medical records, standards, or interoperability in hospital information systems? Overview of systematic reviews. JMIR Med. Inform. **5**, e7400 (2017). https://doi.org/10.2196/medinform.7400
12. Vesinurm, M., Sylgren, I., Bengts, A., Torkki, P., Lillrank, P.: Concept analysis of patient journey disruptions: the obstacle of integrated care. J. Integr. Care **32**, 37–58 (2024). https://doi.org/10.1108/JICA-08-2023-0060
13. Aspland, E., Gartner, D., Harper, P.: Clinical pathway modelling: a literature review. Health Syst. **10**, 1–23 (2021). https://doi.org/10.1080/20476965.2019.1652547
14. Cassidy, S., Solvang, Ø.S., Lintvedt, O.K., Solvoll, T., Granja, C.: Assessing Methods to Model Patient-Centric Care Pathways across Multiple Healthcare Systems
15. Bogale, B., Vesinurm, M., Lillrank, P., Celius, E.G., Halvorsrud, R.: Visual modeling languages in patient pathways: scoping review. Interact. J. Med. Res. **13**, e55865 (2024). https://doi.org/10.2196/55865
16. Halvorsrud, R., Kvale, K., Følstad, A.: Improving service quality through customer journey analysis. J. Serv. Theory Pract. **26**, 840–867 (2016). https://doi.org/10.1108/JSTP-05-2015-0111
17. Larsen, A.G., Halvorsrud, R., Berg, R.E., Vesinurm, M.: Dual-perspective modeling of patient pathways: a case study on kidney cancer. In: Säreströniemi, M., et al. (eds.) Digital Health and Wireless Solutions, pp. 51–68. Springer, Cham (2024)

18. Halvorsrud, R., Sanchez, O.R., Boletsis, C., Skjuve, M.: Involving users in the development of a modeling language for customer journeys. Softw. Syst. Model. **22**, 1589–1618 (2023). https://doi.org/10.1007/s10270-023-01081-w
19. Halvorsrud, R., Lee, E., Haugstveit, I.M., Følstad, A.: Components of a visual language for service design. Presented at the ServDes. 2014 Service Future, Proceedings of the fourth Service Design and Service Innovation Conference , Lancaster University, United Kingdom (2014)
20. Halvorsrud, R., Haugstveit, I.M., Pultier, A.: Evaluation of a modelling language for customer journeys. In: 2016 IEEE Symposium on Visual Languages and Human-Centric Computing (VL/HCC), pp. 40–48 (2016)
21. SINTEF Digital: CJML – Customer Journey Modelling Language, https://cjml.no/cjml/
22. Peffers, K., Tuunanen, T., Rothenberger, M.A., Chatterjee, S.: A design science research methodology for information systems research. J. Manag. Inf. Syst. **24**, 45–77 (2007). https://doi.org/10.2753/MIS0742-1222240302
23. Hevner, A.R., March, S.T., Park, J., Ram, S.: Design science in information systems research. MIS Q. **28**, 75–105 (2004). https://doi.org/10.2307/25148625
24. Karanikolos, M., Tynkkynen, L.-K., Keskimäki, I.: Finland: Health System Summary, 2024. European Observatory on Health Systems and Policies, WHO Regional Office for Europe, Copenhagen (2024)
25. Jordan, D., Evdemon, J.: Business Process Model And Notation (BPMN) Version 2.0. (2011)
26. Bartels, E.A., Meijboom, B.R., Nahar-van Venrooij, L.M.W., De Vries, E.: How service modularity can provide the flexibility to support person-centered care and shared decision-making. BMC Health Serv. Res. **21**, 1245 (2021). https://doi.org/10.1186/s12913-021-07267-6
27. Silander, K.: From borders to interfaces: Modularizing specialized outpatient services. (2019)
28. Følstad, A., Kvale, K.: Customer journeys: a systematic literature review. J. Serv. Theory Pract. **28**, 196–227 (2018). https://doi.org/10.1108/JSTP-11-2014-0261
29. Lillrank, P.: The logics of healthcare: the professional's guide to health systems science. Taylor & Francis, Boca Raton, Florida (2018)
30. Vargo, S.L., Lusch, R.F.: Evolving to a new dominant logic for marketing. J. Mark. **68**, 1–17 (2004). https://doi.org/10.1509/jmkg.68.1.1.24036
31. Rebuge, Á., Ferreira, D.R.: Business process analysis in healthcare environments: a methodology based on process mining. Inf. Syst. **37**, 99–116 (2012). https://doi.org/10.1016/j.is.2011.01.003
32. Gatta, R., et al.: Clinical guidelines: a crossroad of many research areas. challenges and opportunities in process mining for healthcare. In: Di Francescomarino, C., Dijkman, R., Zdun, U. (eds.) Business Process Management Workshops. pp. 545–556. Springer, Cham (2019)
33. Batista, E., Solanas, A.: Process mining in healthcare: a systematic review. In: 2018 9th International Conference on Information, Intelligence, Systems and Applications (IISA), pp. 1–6 (2018)
34. Yang, W., Su, Q.: Process mining for clinical pathway: literature review and future directions. In: 2014 11th International Conference on Service Systems and Service Management (ICSSSM), pp. 1–5 (2014)
35. Aversano, L., Iammarino, M., Madau, A., Pirlo, G., Semeraro, G.: Process mining applications in healthcare: a systematic literature review. PeerJ Comput. Sci. **11**, e2613 (2025). https://doi.org/10.7717/peerj-cs.2613
36. Liu, P.L., Zhang, L., Ma, X., Zhao, X.: Communication matters: the role of patient-centered communication in improving old adults' health competence and health outcomes. Health Commun. **39**, 363–375 (2024). https://doi.org/10.1080/10410236.2023.2166209

Focus is Not just on the Eyes – Constructing Dynamic Areas of Interest for Eye-Tracking

Jaakko Kauramäki[1,2](✉) and Kerttu Huttunen[2]

[1] University of Helsinki, 00014 Helsinki, Finland
jaakko.kauramaki@helsinki.fi
[2] University of Oulu, 90014 Oulu, Finland

Abstract. The use of video stimuli in eye-tracking experiments has become increasingly common. However, for such dynamic stimuli, traditionally manually defined fixed areas of interest (AOIs) are limited and require substantial effort to create. This work presents an automated dynamic AOI pipeline for front-facing facial video stimuli, suitable for tasks such as emotion recognition and language related research, including speechreading. We leveraged the openly available machine learning-based facial landmark toolkit OpenFace and extended its landmark points to define a richer collection of AOIs across the facial region. Particular attention was given to accurately isolating the eyebrow areas by systematically separating the eye and eyebrow AOIs. Results from an eye-tracking dataset demonstrate that automatically generated, large, dynamic AOIs covering the face perform effectively, revealing task dependent individual gaze behavior patterns in children.

Keywords: Dynamic area of interest · AOI · video stimuli · speechreading · lipreading

1 Introduction

1.1 Background on Human Looking Behaviour and Eye-Tracking

People direct their gaze toward areas of the visual field that attract their attention, as well as toward facial regions that provide information relevant to their goals [1]. In free viewing situations, a large proportion of glances, especially initial ones, are directed to the eyes because of their importance for emotional and social cues (see [2], for a review). However, during speechreading of silent speech [3] and during the perception of audiovisual speech [4], particularly in background noise [5, 6], gaze increasingly or predominantly shifts toward the mouth. Viewers tend to focus on the eyes when observing still photographs, whereas their attention typically moves to the mouth when watching a person speak. Despite these general patterns, gaze allocation varies depending on the specific behaviour being observed [7]. Moreover, visual speech information is distributed across the entire face, not only the mouth. Speech is also rarely produced with a completely neutral facial expression, meaning that emotional expressions and visual speech cues frequently co-occur and interact.

M. Särestöniemi et al. (Eds.): NCDHWS 2026, CCIS 3010, pp. 193–205, 2026.
https://doi.org/10.1007/978-3-032-28819-6_12

Visual prosody refers to facial expressions that accompany speech. For example, increases in vocal amplitude or rising intonation may be accompanied by raised eyebrows [8]. Such visual information remains present in originally audiovisual video material even when the audio track is removed for silent-speech experiments. The upper part of the face [1], including the eyebrows [9], has been shown to provide important cues for intonation patterns, even when speech is silent.

Human gaze behaviour can be examined to reveal what a person finds interesting on another person's face or in the surrounding environment. According to the *Eye-Mind Hypothesis* [10], gaze patterns can be used to infer cognitive processes, that is, what a person is mentally processing while looking at something. Gaze behaviour has been studied using human observers who classify where participants direct their gaze [11]. However, such observer-based methods are time consuming and require careful experimental design to avoid distracting or otherwise influencing participants.

Since the early 1990s, advances in eye-tracking technology have provided powerful tools for obtaining objective information about what people look at and how they allocate their visual attention.

When studying eye movement behaviour, most researchers are interested in the number of fixations, i.e. the time points where the eyes are fixed on a certain target, and saccades, the eye movements from one fixation point to another [12, 13]. Dwell time is the total time gaze stays within a certain area predefined by the researchers. The basic output values the eye-tracking devices provide are the x and y eye gaze coordinates on the visual field, from sample to sample, possibly mapped to screen coordinates if the stimulus presentation is computer-driven, and from these data the saccades and fixations can be quantified as the higher-level features [12]. Additional measures to quantify e.g. pupil diameter, blinks, and moments of smooth pursuit can be used to further obtain new features.

1.2 Static and Dynamic Areas of Interest in Researching Facial Expressions and Speechreading

The earliest attempts to illustrate where participants looked on the human face were technically very modest [see, e.g., [1]]. Over the years, concept of Areas of Interest (AOIs), also called Regions of Interest (ROIs), was formed. With AOI it is possible to determine whether gaze is directed at a predefined region around the target point. It helps to pool the complicated gaze behavior to more easily understandable form. In addition to AOIs, heat maps and scan paths have also been frequently utilized in eye-tracking analyses [for a review, see [12]] but, compared to heat maps, AOIs can provide more refined information about, for example, speechreading.

In studies examining the perception of facial expressions and speech, the coverage of different facial regions, as well as the number, size, and shape of AOIs, has varied considerably across studies. For example, some studies have defined one or two AOIs for the eyes and one for the mouth, whereas others have used a single AOI only for the mouth. When studying infants, young children, or individuals with conditions such as autism spectrum, researchers have often employed robust (i.e., large) AOIs [14–16].

Vehlen and colleagues [17] recommend using larger AOIs when gaze data are less accurate (i.e., noisier) and, when accuracy is sufficient, opting for smaller AOIs to reduce misclassifications. Regarding smaller AOIs, one specific example concerns the eyebrows: they have typically been included within AOIs representing the eyes [e.g., 6, 7, 18]. In other cases, eyebrows have been excluded from AOIs covering the eyes or forehead, without being examined as independent regions [e.g., 19, 20]. Given the importance of the eye region and the role of the eyebrows in interpreting facial expressions, such variation in AOI construction may lead to differences in research findings.

The nature of the stimuli, whether still or dynamic, may also influence results. For example, in a study by Schurgin and colleagues [21], which examined how 51 young adults directed their gaze when viewing still photographs of facial expressions, slightly more than one third of dwell time was allocated to the eyes. The nose attracted even more attention (approximately 38%), whereas the eyebrows and forehead together accounted for less than 2% of dwell time. However, although the AOIs differed in size, this did not correspond to differences in the number of fixations allocated to each AOI.

There is considerable variation not only in the number and size of AOIs but also in how they are spatially defined in relation to one another. Some studies include small or large gaps between AOIs that are not of analytical interest [e.g., 22], whereas in rarer cases AOIs are positioned seamlessly side by side. For example, in the study by Viktorsson and colleagues [23], a single horizontally bounded AOI encompassed half of the forehead, the eyebrow, the eye, and even most of the cheek.

Visual acuity is highest when eye movements direct information to the fovea, a small pit located near the center of the retina. Efficient allocation of visual attention may therefore require parafoveal strategies that rely on peripheral vision (processing information just outside the region of sharpest focus) to avoid frequent shifts between the mouth and other facial regions. Despite the general tendency to look at the mouth during speech perception [24], there is substantial interindividual variability in gaze patterns when watching someone speak. These patterns appear highly stable: some individuals consistently prefer to fixate on the eyes, whereas others predominantly fixate on the mouth [25].

Research indicates that fixating on the mouth is particularly beneficial when speechreading is used to support the perception of audiovisual speech in noisy conditions [24]. Nevertheless, some individuals tend to fixate on the nose or the eyes instead [3, 6]. This raises an interesting question about the range of gaze behaviours that may facilitate speechreading. As Lansing and McConkie [1] suggested, peripheral vision may assist in perceiving coarse movements and even broader segmental aspects of speech. When fixating on the nose, the visual parafovea still encompasses the mouth [7]. However, peripheral vision alone is insufficient for detecting rapid movements or fine-grained distinctions between articulated speech segments. It is therefore reasonable to assume that the size and shape of AOIs influence whether fixations on the nose or cheeks can be shown to support speechreading. Peripheral vision may also provide information about emotional expressions, which can help maintain attention and aid in interpreting the spoken message.

In summary, AOIs constructed for children and for populations with developing or atypical gaze patterns must be defined robustly. However, in studies examining facial expressions and visual speech, particularly when these cues co-occur, smaller AOIs are necessary if the aim is to analyse visual prosody or the contribution of peripheral vision to visual processing.

For research on emotion recognition and speechreading, video stimuli are essential rather than static images. With dynamic facial stimuli, static AOIs are limited because facial features change slightly during video playback. Evidence suggests that, for reproducible research, relatively large dynamic AOIs can be generated automatically without manual intervention [26].

When studying speechreading, it is important to include the mandible (lower jaw) within the dynamic mouth AOI, as jaw lowering is a key component of articulating open vowels such as [ɑ] and [æ]. Consequently, the choices made when constructing AOIs can influence how researchers interpret the relationship between speechreading accuracy and gaze allocation during visual speech perception. If AOIs are fixed or too small, valuable information may be lost or misrepresented. This is especially critical when studying speechreading and emotional expressions simultaneously, as dynamic AOIs of appropriate size and coverage around moving facial regions are essential.

1.3 Present Goals

The aim of the present study was to implement dynamic AOIs suitable for video-based stimuli and high-quality gaze tracking. We quantified AOIs frame by frame from the original stimulus videos using an automated labeling algorithm. This process relied on facial landmarks extracted with OpenFace [27] for each video. Using these landmarks, we were able to efficiently define seven AOIs, described later in the Materials and Methods section. Our AOI construction was inspired by earlier Voronoi tessellation based approaches [17, 26], but here we specifically aimed to create more detailed AOIs for the eyebrows rather than relying solely on eye-based regions. Furthermore, another motivation for opting for a novel implementation was to obtain AOIs for dynamic video-based rather than simpler still image-based stimuli.

MATLAB (MathWorks Inc., Natick, USA) provides a widely used scientific computing environment for analyzing data from various eye-tracking systems, and the same OpenFace based landmark detection and AOI generation algorithm can be implemented on other platforms as well.

2 Materials and Methods

2.1 Analysis Pipeline

The first step in our dynamic AOI pipeline (Fig. 1A) involved extracting facial landmarks from the stimulus videos by running OpenFace [27] and using the resulting per stimulus comma-separated values (CSV) file as input for our MATLAB script. OpenFace can be run on a standard office laptop, and processing the stimulus video files used in this study, each under 20 s in duration, took only a few minutes per file.

Dynamic AOI definition under MATLAB. Because OpenFace landmarks focus on facial features, no points are provided above the eyebrows. To address this, we extrapolated a forehead centroid by taking 75% of the line length between points 27 and 33, starting at point 27 and extending upward (Fig. 1C). Face width was defined as the distance between points 0 and 16, and additional geometric features were computed to support AOI construction (Fig. 1C). The initial radius for the central AOI was set to 33% of the facial width, which provided a suitable compromise for our stimulus set. As the first step, circular AOIs for the left eye, right eye, and mouth were created as MATLAB *polyshape* objects, as were all subsequent AOIs. A triangular nose AOI was then defined using selected mid points of OpenFace landmarks as its vertices (see Fig. 1C).

Eyebrow AOIs were constructed using MATLAB's *polybuffer* function by sliding a circle along predefined control points, with a fixed pixel radius of 30. This radius was appropriate for our full HD (1920 × 1080) input videos, which were normalised so that faces appeared at comparable sizes across stimuli. The radius is parameterised and can be adjusted for future datasets with different face proportions or video resolutions.

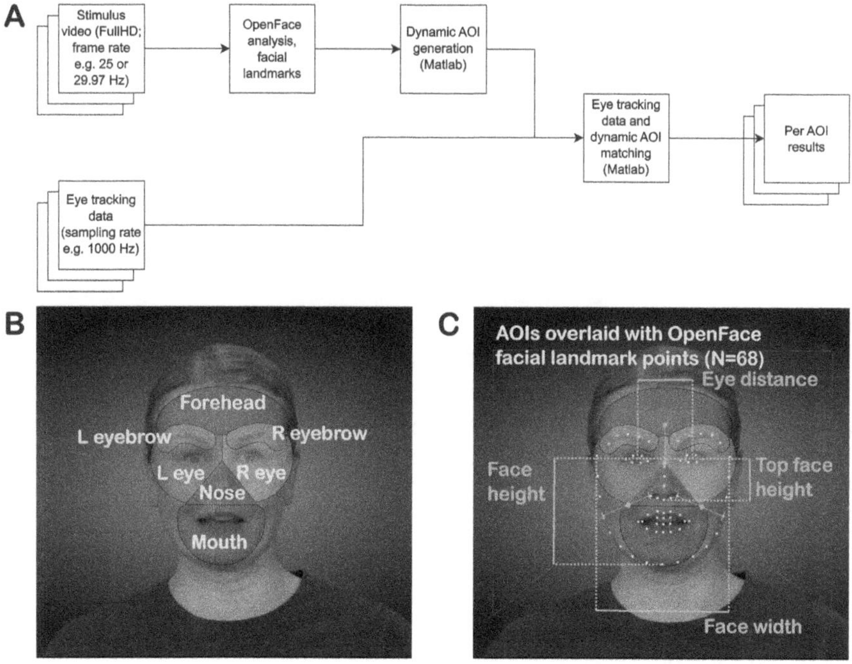

Fig. 1. A) Flow chart of the analysis pipeline. B) Dynamic AOIs shown in different colours, quantified for each frame. C) AOIs overlaid with OpenFace landmark points, which served as the basis for AOI calculations. Additional temporary features and derived landmark points were computed to support AOI construction.

The forehead AOI was defined as an oval shape, with its horizontal radius set to half of the face width and its vertical radius to 90% of the upper face height (Fig. 1C). This oval was rotated according to the face angle, calculated as the angle between the eyes relative to the horizontal axis. In our stimulus material, a human talking head video used for speechreading, we observed some issues with this AOI, as synchronized changes in forehead height occurred during articulation (see the example video on the project GitHub).

All final and temporary AOIs, represented as *polyshape* objects in MATLAB, were then intersected as needed to produce the desired AOI layout. For some stimuli (e.g., angry expressions with a forward tilted head), we observed overlap between the eyebrow and eye AOIs. To address this, we used the OpenFace eye landmarks to generate additional "helper" eye AOIs that carved out overlapping regions, preserving a more ecologically valid eye area and slightly reducing the size of the eyebrow AOIs (Fig. 2).

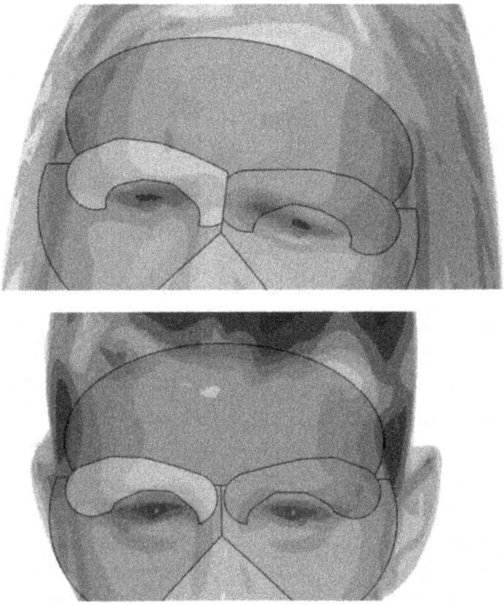

Fig. 2. Examples of cases in which the dynamic eye AOIs and eyebrow AOIs partially overlapped due to the close proximity of the eyes and eyebrows. In these instances, the safety buffers around the eyes carved out portions of the eyebrow AOIs, resulting in distinct shapes. The illustrations derived from video frames have been modified to protect the identity of the child actors.

The resulting AOIs represented a good balance between objective, automated generation and practical usability. The algorithm performed best with frontal facial images, such as those shown in Fig. 1, although some noticeable warping occurred when the face was tilted or rotated. These issues were mitigated effectively through the use of the robust landmark detection OpenFace provides and the incorporation of head rotation parameters. Additional pixel-based AOI quantification steps could have been replaced with measures derived directly from landmark distances and facial geometry, but because the current approach produced sufficiently accurate results for our purposes, we did not implement these further optimizations.

2.2 Experimental Stimulus Selection

We applied the algorithm to data from four different eye-tracking experiment stimuli used in the multidisciplinary and multiprofessional research project *Gaze on lips?*[1]. The Regional Medical Ethical Board of the Northern Ostrobothnia Hospital District, Finland, approved the study protocol. The project has been described and prospectively registered in the Clinical Trials Register of the U.S. National Library of Medicine (identifier NCT05854719[2]). Adults appearing in the still photographs and videos used as stimulus materials provided written consent for their participation and granted permission for the public presentation and publication of the unmasked materials.

The experiments were conducted with typically developing children and children with hearing loss. Participant demographics for the speechreading and emotion discrimination tasks are not presented here, as the focus of this paper is on the use of the experimental stimuli. In three of the four experiments, we used video stimuli depicting (1) a person producing words and sentences (with audio removed during editing), (2) a person expressing an emotion, or (3) both. Examples of these stimuli are shown in Fig. 1 and Fig. 2 and more are available in the project's GitHub repository[3].

2.3 Application to Eye-Tracking Experiment

To evaluate the applicability of the dynamic AOIs and to assess the stability of within participant looking profiles, we applied the algorithm to real world eye-tracking data from a small set of participants. Eye-tracking was conducted using the EyeLink 1000 system (SR Research Ltd., Ottawa, Ontario, Canada), which recorded right eye gaze at 1000 Hz. The data were imported into MATLAB using the *edfImport*[4] libraries, and the per frame dynamic AOIs were used to segment the experimental timeline into the corresponding AOI categories.

We did not compute fixation or saccade metrics for specific AOIs; instead, we relied solely on per sample assignment of gaze points to AOIs. As a result, the current data are not directly comparable to measures such as fixation duration. Rather, they approximate total dwell time within each AOI, a metric shown to be informative for emotional stimuli [28]. More extensive eye-tracking analyses will be reported in the future.

3 Results

3.1 Example Run on Selected Participants

As expected, the distribution of gaze samples differed across experiments according to task demands and instructions. Experiment 1 involved speechreading only, and therefore all participants showed a high proportion of gaze samples within the mouth AOI (leftmost column in Fig. 3 and Fig. 4). Experiment 2 combined speechreading and emotion discrimination tasks, whereas Experiments 3 and 4 focused solely on emotion discrimination, using either still images (Exp. 3) or short video clips (Exp. 4) as stimuli.

[1] https://www.oulu.fi/en/projects/gaze-lips.
[2] https://clinicaltrials.gov/study/NCT05854719.
[3] https://github.com/jkauramaki/dynamic_aoi
[4] https://github.com/alexander-pastukhov/edfImport.

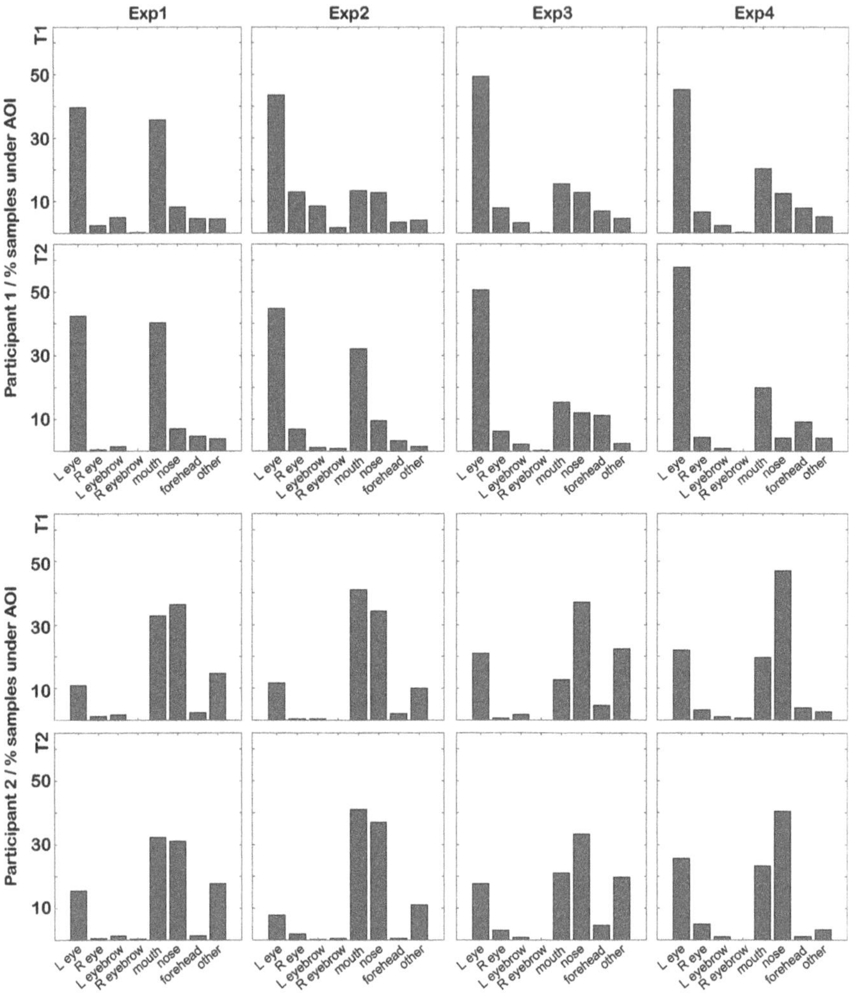

Fig. 3. Example data from two participants (P1, P2) illustrating participant-specific gaze distributions, each showing clear similarity between the two data collection points (T1 and T2). Experiment 1 was a speechreading task, which explains the high proportion of gaze samples falling under the mouth AOI.

To further evaluate our eyebrow specific AOIs, we expanded the subset to ten participants, four of whom were included in the data shown in Fig. 3 and Fig. 4. For this analysis, we contrasted selected stimuli depicting angry versus neutral expressions (Fig. 5). The results demonstrate the usefulness of the eyebrow-specific AOIs across different stimulus types: angry expressions consistently elicited a higher proportion of gaze samples within the eyebrow AOIs, particularly in Experiment 3, where participants viewed still images of emotional expressions.

Experiment 1 is not included in Fig. 5, as it focused solely on speechreading skills and, based on preliminary data inspection, showed no meaningful differences in gaze

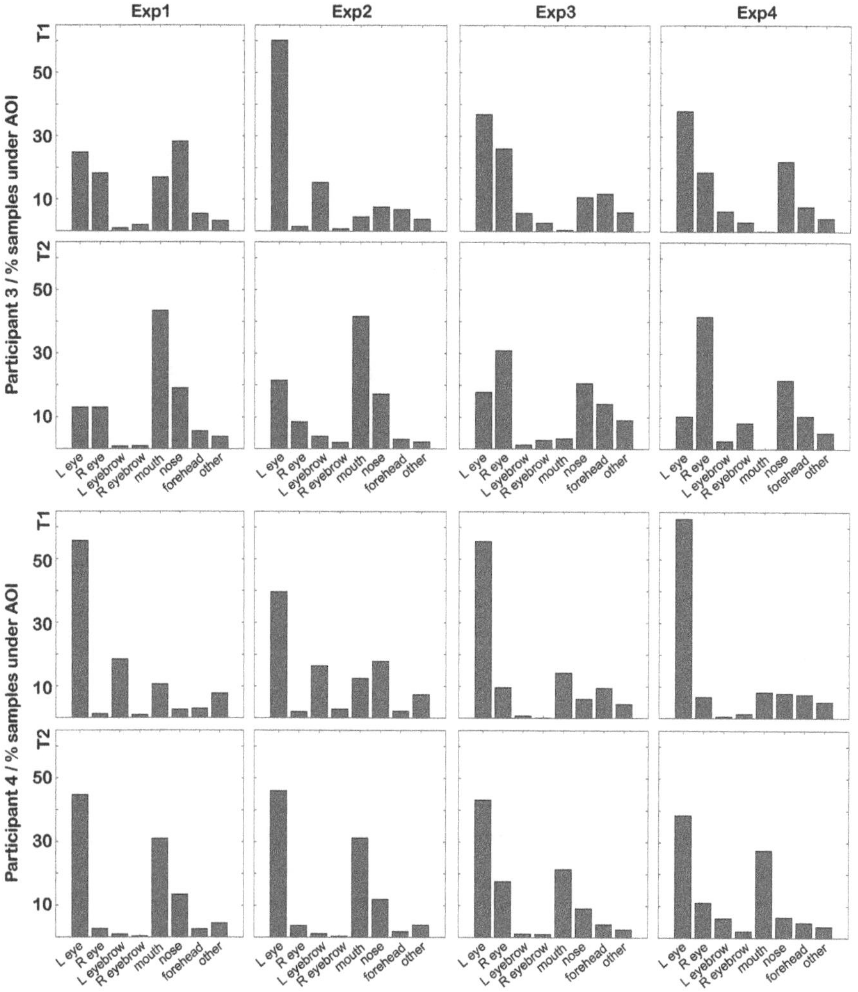

Fig. 4. Additional example data from participants P3 and P4. As in Fig. 3, the plots show within-subject similarity, although the two data collection points (T1 and T2) differ more noticeably here. For example, both participants focus more on the mouth AOI during the speechreading based Experiment 1, with this effect being more pronounced at T2 (showing more than a two-fold increase compared to T1). Interestingly, both participants also show more than 15% of their gaze samples directed toward the left facing eyebrow in Experiment 2, but only at the first time point (T1).

patterns across stimuli. All stimuli in Experiment 1 featured a neutral facial expression, with consistent intonation and voice amplitude, so additional information from eyebrow movements was not expected to contribute to speechreading performance [see 8].

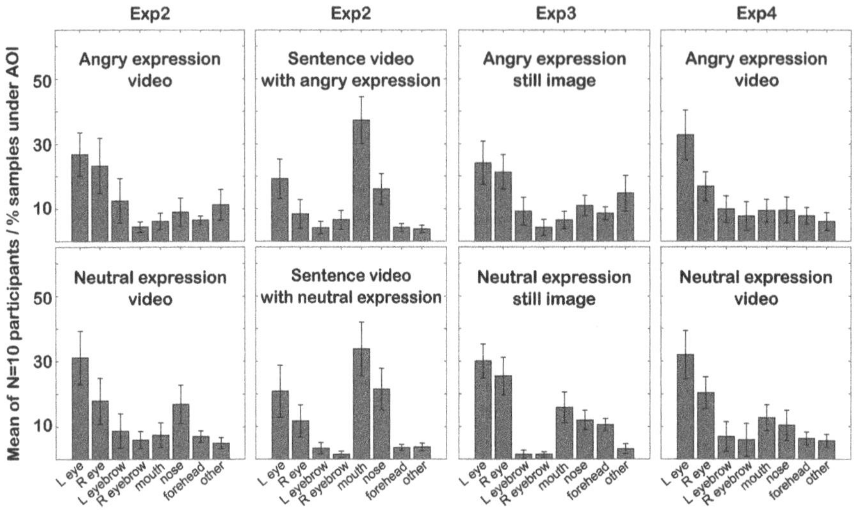

Fig. 5. Representative stimuli used to compare gaze distributions between angry expressions (top row) and neutral expressions (bottom row). Each graph displays the mean ± standard error of the mean (SEM) for N = 10 participants, averaged across two data collection points.

4 Discussion

We presented an automated dynamic area of interest pipeline for front view facial video stimuli. The pipeline is openly available for anyone to test, use, and further develop. AOI generation is fully automated and requires specifying only a few parameters, yet it already performs well for many appropriately edited video stimuli. Importantly, our approach extends previous work by incorporating eyebrow-specific AOIs, which are often merged into broader eye or upper face regions. Based on our preliminary data, eyebrow AOIs appear to be a valuable addition for analysing emotional stimuli and language-related tasks such as speechreading.

4.1 Limitations of the Study

Our implementation was tested using well-edited stimulus videos featuring a single face at a time, recorded from a viewing angle that was easy to interpret and with relatively consistent facial landmark configurations. More dynamic videos, such as those capturing children's expressive movements in front of the camera (not shown here), introduced challenges, as the frame-by-frame AOIs occasionally changed in shape and extent. However, these distortions may be less problematic if OpenFace reliably detects the landmark points, since the AOI boundaries remain within the facial region. Our relatively small selection of stimuli (57 video clips and 12 still images) is one limitation of the study overall. Additional testing with a wider range of viewing angles would be beneficial. At minimum, when applied to new stimulus videos AOIs should be overlaid onto them, as demonstrated in the example script, at project GitHub page3, to verify whether any observed distortions are meaningful.

4.2 Future Steps

In future research, we shall examine how typically hearing children and children with hearing loss allocate their gaze to the dynamic AOIs we constructed, and whether individual or group level differences emerge in gaze behaviour. We also aim to investigate the relationships among speechreading accuracy, facial expression discrimination, and gaze use in children. Such information may support speech and language therapists in guiding children during speechreading training. More broadly, understanding the patterns and dynamics of gaze use contributes to a deeper understanding of the mechanisms underlying face identification and the interpretation of facial expressions.

5 Conclusions

Our approach for creating dynamic AOIs was considered suitable and adequate for the analysis of static photographs of facial expressions as well as dynamic video stimuli comprising facial expressions, speechreading sequences, or both.

Acknowledgments. We warmly thank the individuals who appeared in the photographs and videos used as stimuli, the children who participated in the test sessions and their parents, and the researchers involved in planning the experiment and collecting the eye-tracking data. Partial financial support was provided by the Eudaimonia Institute of the University of Oulu, Finland.

Disclosure of Interests. The authors have no competing interests to declare that are relevant to the content of this article.

References

1. Lansing, C.R., McConkie, G.W.: Attention to facial regions in segmental and prosodic visual speech perception tasks. J. Speech Lang. Hear. Res. **42**, 526–539 (1999). https://doi.org/10.1044/jslhr.4203.526
2. Birmingham, E., Kingstone, A.: Human social attention. Ann. N. Y. Acad. Sci. **1156**, 118–140 (2009). https://doi.org/10.1111/j.1749-6632.2009.04468.x
3. Lansing, C.R., McConkie, G.W.: Word identification and eye fixation locations in visual and visual-plus-auditory presentations of spoken sentences. Percept. Psychophys. **65**, 536–552 (2003). https://doi.org/10.3758/BF03194581
4. Lusk, L.G., Mitchel, A.D.: Differential gaze patterns on eyes and mouth during audiovisual speech segmentation. Front. Psychol. **7** (2016). https://doi.org/10.3389/fpsyg.2016.00052
5. Mitchel, A.D., Lusk, L.G., Wellington, I., Mook, A.T.: Segmenting speech by mouth: the role of oral prosodic cues for visual speech segmentation. Lang. Speech **66**, 819–832 (2023). https://doi.org/10.1177/00238309221137607
6. Vatikiotis-Bateson, E., Eigsti, I.-M., Yano, S., Munhall, K.G.: Eye movement of perceivers during audiovisual speech perception. Percept. Psychophys. **60**, 926–940 (1998). https://doi.org/10.3758/BF03211929
7. Võ, M.L.-H., Smith, T.J., Mital, P.K., Henderson, J.M.: Do the eyes really have it? Dynamic allocation of attention when viewing moving faces. J. Vis. **12**, 3 (2012). https://doi.org/10.1167/12.13.3

8. Munhall, K.G., Jones, J.A., Callan, D.E., Kuratate, T., Vatikiotis-Bateson, E.: Visual prosody and speech intelligibility: head movement improves auditory speech perception. Psychol. Sci. **15**, 133–137 (2004). https://doi.org/10.1111/j.0963-7214.2004.01502010.x
9. Srinivasan, R.J., Massaro, D.W.: Perceiving prosody from the face and voice: distinguishing statements from echoic questions in English. Lang. Speech **46**, 1–22 (2003). https://doi.org/10.1177/00238309030460010201
10. Just, M.A., Carpenter, P.A.: A theory of reading: From eye fixations to comprehension. Psychol. Rev. **87**, 329–354 (1980). https://doi.org/10.1037/0033-295X.87.4.329
11. Suri, K.N., Whedon, M., Lewis, M.: Perception of audio-visual synchrony in infants at elevated likelihood of developing autism spectrum disorder. Eur. J. Pediatr. **182**, 2105–2117 (2023). https://doi.org/10.1007/s00431-023-04871-y
12. Mahanama, B., et al.: Eye Movement and pupil measures: a review. Front. Comput. Sci. **3** (2022). https://doi.org/10.3389/fcomp.2021.733531
13. Carter, B.T., Luke, S.G.: Best practices in eye tracking research. Int. J. Psychophysiol. **155**, 49–62 (2020). https://doi.org/10.1016/j.ijpsycho.2020.05.010
14. Berdasco-Muñoz, E., Nazzi, T., Yeung, H.H.: Visual scanning of a talking face in preterm and full-term infants. Dev. Psychol. **55**, 1353–1361 (2019). https://doi.org/10.1037/dev0000737
15. Zamuner, T.S., Rabideau, T., Mcdonald, M., Yeung, H.H.: Developmental change in children's speech processing of auditory and visual cues: an eyetracking study. J. Child Lang. **50**, 27–51 (2023). https://doi.org/10.1017/S0305000921000684
16. Liu, Q., et al.: Audio-visual speech synchrony impacts gaze patterns in autism. J. Autism Dev. Disord. (2025). https://doi.org/10.1007/s10803-025-06998-3
17. Vehlen, A., Standard, W., Domes, G.: How to choose the size of facial areas of interest in interactive eye tracking. PLoS ONE **17**, e0263594 (2022). https://doi.org/10.1371/journal.pone.0263594
18. Yang, J., et al.: Exploring the relationship between children's facial emotion processing characteristics and speech communication ability using deep learning on eye tracking and speech performance measures. Comput. Speech Lang. **76**, 101389 (2022). https://doi.org/10.1016/j.csl.2022.101389
19. Rigoulot, S., Pell, M.D.: Emotion in the voice influences the way we scan emotional faces. Speech Commun. **65**, 36–49 (2014). https://doi.org/10.1016/j.specom.2014.05.006
20. Watanabe, K., Matsuda, T., Nishioka, T., Namatame, M.: Eye gaze during observation of static faces in deaf people. PLoS ONE **6**, e16919 (2011). https://doi.org/10.1371/journal.pone.0016919
21. Schurgin, M.W., Nelson, J., Iida, S., Ohira, H., Chiao, J.Y., Franconeri, S.L.: Eye movements during emotion recognition in faces. J. Vis. **14**, 14 (2014). https://doi.org/10.1167/14.13.14
22. Wang, J., et al.: An eye-tracking study on audiovisual speech perception strategies adopted by normal-hearing and deaf adults under different language familiarities. J. Speech Lang. Hear. Res. **63**, 2245–2254 (2020). https://doi.org/10.1044/2020_JSLHR-19-00223
23. Viktorsson, C., Valtakari, N.V., Falck-Ytter, T., Hooge, I.T.C., Rudling, M., Hessels, R.S.: Stable eye versus mouth preference in a live speech-processing task. Sci. Rep. **13**, 12878 (2023). https://doi.org/10.1038/s41598-023-40017-8
24. Yi, A., Wong, W., Eizenman, M.: Gaze patterns and audiovisual speech enhancement. J. Speech Lang. Hear. Res. **56**, 471–480 (2013). https://doi.org/10.1044/1092-4388(2012/10-0288)
25. Mehoudar, E., Arizpe, J., Baker, C.I., Yovel, G.: Faces in the eye of the beholder: unique and stable eye scanning patterns of individual observers. J. Vis. **14**, 6 (2014). https://doi.org/10.1167/14.7.6
26. Hessels, R.S., Kemner, C., van den Boomen, C., Hooge, I.T.C.: The area-of-interest problem in eyetracking research: a noise-robust solution for face and sparse stimuli. Behav. Res. Methods **48**, 1694–1712 (2016). https://doi.org/10.3758/s13428-015-0676-y

27. Baltrusaitis, T., Zadeh, A., Lim, Y.C., Morency, L.-P.: OpenFace 2.0: facial behavior analysis toolkit. In: 2018 13th IEEE International Conference on Automatic Face & Gesture Recognition (FG 2018), pp. 59–66 (2018). https://doi.org/10.1109/FG.2018.00019
28. Hunter, L., Roland, L., Ferozpuri, A.: Emotional expression processing and depressive symptomatology: eye-tracking reveals differential importance of lower and middle facial areas of interest. Depress. Res. Treat. **2020**, 1049851 (2020). https://doi.org/10.1155/2020/1049851

Breath-Hold Effect on the Prefrontal Cortex Hemodynamics When Measured by fNIRS at Source–Detector Distances of 3 and 5 cm

Sadegh Moradi[1(✉)], Hany Ferdinando[2], Davood Simyar[2], and Teemu Myllylä[2]

[1] Advanced Electronics Centre, University of Oulu, Oulu, Finland
sadegh.moradi@oulu.fi
[2] Research Unit of Health Science and Technology, University of Oulu, Oulu, Finland

Abstract. Functional near-infrared spectroscopy (fNIRS) is a non-invasive optical technique that measures changes in oxygenated and deoxygenated hemoglobin within the cortical surface of the brain. To ensure sufficient cortical sensitivity, researchers commonly use a 3 cm source–detector separation, which is widely regarded as the standard distance. However, additional or unique information that could potentially be obtained at longer separations has not been extensively researched. In this study, we investigated cerebral oxyhemoglobin response of breath hold when measured at 3 and 5 cm source–detector distances using a highly sensitive low-cost photo detector. The results show that the oxyhemoglobin recovery rate at 5 cm is higher than 3 cm.

Keywords: Near-infrared spectroscopy · brain · cerebral hemodynamics · photodetector

1 Introduction

In functional near-infrared spectroscopy (fNIRS) brain monitoring, source–detector (S–D) separation is one of the most important parameters controlling the probing depth and sensitivity to brain tissue. Because light transport in biological tissue is dominated by multiple scattering, photons do not travel in straight lines. Instead, they follow diffuse paths whose spatial distribution depends strongly on the distance between the light source and the detector. When NIR light illuminates the scalp, photons start to absorb and scatter in the tissue randomly to different directions wavelength dependent. The region of highest sensitivity between a source and a detector forms a characteristic banana-shaped volume, extending from the source into the tissue and back to the detector. As the source–detector distance increases, the maximum sensitivity region moves deeper into the head, and the probability of photons reaching the cortex increases [1].

Conversely, small S–D separations below 1.5 cm primarily measures superficial tissues such as the scalp and skull. As a commonly used rule of thumb in adult human heads is the mean penetration depth is approximately one-third to one-half of the source–detector separation [2]. Therefore, at 30–40 mm separation, a significant sensitivity to

M. Säreströniemi et al. (Eds.): NCDHWS 2026, CCIS 3010, pp. 206–211, 2026.
https://doi.org/10.1007/978-3-032-28819-6_13

cortical gray matter is expected. However, this relationship is not linear and depends on tissue optical properties, wavelength, and head anatomy, in particular, skin and skull thickness that vary between individuals, but it provides a useful practical guideline [1].

Increasing the S–D separation allows deeper penetration, but it also introduces important trade-offs. Light intensity decreases exponentially with distance due to absorption and scattering, resulting in fewer photons detection and lower signal-to-noise ratio (SNR). As a result, there is an optimal range of S–D distances that balances depth sensitivity and measurement reliability.

S-D of 3 cm remains the preferred S-D among fNIRS device manufacturers and researchers for several reasons:

1. **Photon loss and signal-to-noise ratio (SNR):** Beyond 3 cm, the amount of photons that reach the detector decreases significantly, making detection technically challenging and lowering SNR. Achieving adequate performance at larger S-D distances typically requires highly sensitive detectors such as avalanche photodiodes or photomultipliers, which increase cost and size of the receiver reducing suitability for wearable systems.
2. **Sufficient cortical sensitivity:** An S-D distance of around 3 cm has been shown to provide reliable and physiologically meaningful information about cortical hemodynamics.
3. **Power considerations:** Larger S-D distances require higher source intensity to compensate for photon loss, leading to increased electrical power consumption which is in battery powered wearable applications unsuitable.

These constraints raise an important question: What additional information can be gained by measuring at even longer S-D distances? Only few studies have attempted to address this. Guerouah et al. investigated breath hold (BH) responses using hyperspectral NIRS at S-D distances up to 4 cm and identified the 700–900 nm range as optimal for detecting BH related cerebral changes. Changes in cytochrome c oxidase redox state (rCCO) associated with BH were detected at a 4 cm source–detector separation without the use of short-separation regression. Incorporation of the 1 cm channel within a two-layer regression model revealed both cerebral hemodynamic and rCCO responses at a 3 cm separation. The main aim of this study was to determine an optimal wavelength range for cerebral hemodynamics studies [3]. Re et al. examined resting-state brain oscillations using 20 Hz time-domain NIRS with measurements extending to 5 cm. This study is performed using highly sensitive photomultiplier detector and two 828 and 689 nm laser sources [4]. This study suggested using longer S-D distances to get less fraction of scalp-contained photons and avoid skin effect suppression analysis.

In the present study, we demonstrate the BH response at S-D of 5 cm and compare these measurements to the conventional 3 cm standard. The primary objective of this research was to demonstrate that by utilizing the most recent sensor technologies, it is feasible to develop an affordable and low-power NIRS device suitable for wearable applications. For this, we used a low-cost silicon photodiode (developed by Elfys) capable of detecting very low-intensity light levels to enable use of S-D distance even up to 5 cm.

We selected 5 cm distance to be compared with 3 cm because, in most of participants, 5 cm was the maximum separation at which an acceptable SNR and cardiac-band signal were observed.

2 Materials and Methods

SM322, manufactured by Elfys [5], is a surface mount silicone photodiode designed for a spectral range of 400–1100 nm. This photodiode presents high sensitivity and quantum efficiency at this NIR window. In Table 1 a quick comparison of SM322 and S5971 (also a highly sensitive photodiode from Hamamatsu [6]) is shown.

Table 1. Comparison of SM322 and S5971 properties for three selected wavelengths

Properties	Elfys SM322	S5971
Sensitive area size	3.22 mm^2	1.1 mm^2
Dark current @ VR = 0.1v	80 pA	8 pA
Capacitance @ 1v bias	30 pF	9 pF
Sensitivity at 690 nm (A/W)	0.53	0.47
Sensitivity at 830 nm (A/W)	0.65	0.6
Sensitivity at 980 nm (A/W)	0.71	0.52
Calculated QE at 690 nm [7]	95.24%	84.46%
Calculated QE at 830 nm	97.1	89.63
Calculated QE at 980 nm	89.83	65.8

The in-house–designed fNIRS test device having one light source and two detectors (SM322 and S5971) measures cerebral hemodynamic activity in the forehead region (Fig. 1). It consists of two main components: a sensor module with one LED light source having four wavelengths and two detectors positioned on the forehead; and a battery-powered main unit responsible for data acquisition and signal preprocessing. The main unit has an analog-to-digital converter (ADC) operating at a sampling rate of 250 Hz with 16-bit resolution.

For preliminary studies, five adult male participants were recruited. Every subject was performed two BH cycles (normal breathing 88 s and 32 s BH) in sitting position while being measured simultaneously by two detectors positioned at 3 cm and 5 cm (Fig. 1).

3 Results

The recorded NIRS signals were first filtered using a band-pass filter of 0.1–5 Hz, then applied to concentration calculation equations to extract HbO response to BH, presented in Fig. 2.

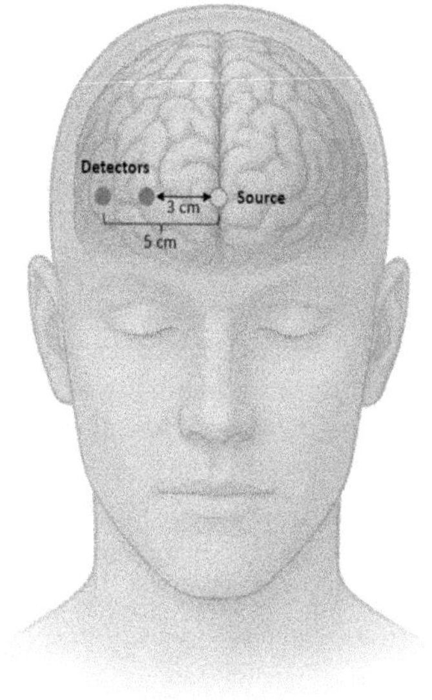

Fig. 1. The measurement was done from right hemisphere; Light source was placed in the middle of forehead and detectors were placed 3 and 5 cm distances from the source.

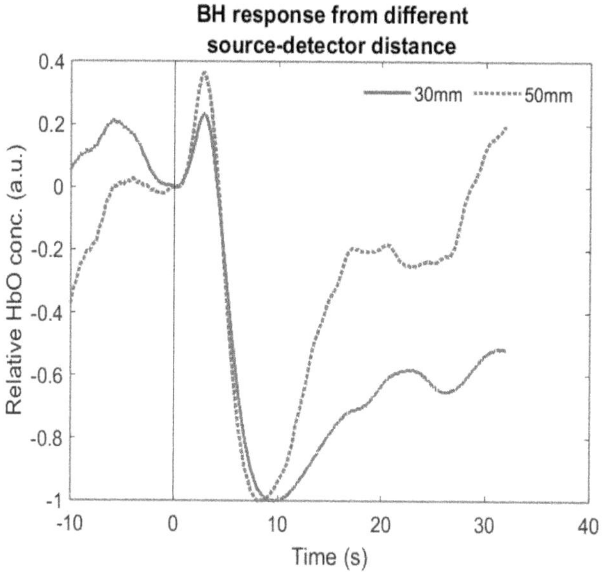

Fig. 2. An example of HbO BH response at S-D distances of 30 mm and 50 mm. As can be observed, HbO effect differs at 5 cm compared to 3 cm distance. In particular, the recovery of the HbO level after the BH seems faster at longer distance.

4 Discussions and Conclusions

In this study we demonstrated that it is possible to realise a wearable low power consumption NIRS device when using latest photo detector technology to reach high sensitivity capable of detecting photons at 5 cm S-D distances when measured from forehead.

Our preliminary study on BH effects comparison at 3 cm vs. 5 cm indicates that HbO trend at 5 cm presents different timing properties in response to BH task (see Fig. 2). In other words, HbO has higher recovery rate in deeper brain tissue (at 5 cm S-D distance). This may be related to lower hemodynamic effect caused by superficial blood circulation providing a more dominant effect of brain hemodynamics at 5 cm. This could address the possible temporal effect of the extracerebral tissues on the timing characteristics of brain hemodynamics. However, more statistical analysis is needed to be conducted.

The primary application of this study may be the simplification of fNIRS hardware and software, since short-distance detectors require additional hardware solely for correcting superficial (skin) effects.

Another possible application could be in tomographic systems, Diffuse Optical Tomography (DOT) where multiple long separations combined with shorts could improve depth localization. As mentioned before, at longer separations (e.g., 4–5 cm), a larger fraction of detected photons has interacted with cortical tissue, and the relative contribution of scalp hemodynamic decreases. Even though the total signal is weaker, the brain-to-scalp sensitivity ratio improves, which can be valuable in DOT analyses.

The future plan for this study includes recruiting more participants with a wider range of ages and genders to investigate the consistency of the observed phenomena. Moreover, possible simulation studies will be considered if they could contribute to a better understanding of the problem.

Acknowledgments. The study was financed by BF PHOTON-WEAR (3285/31/2023).

Disclosure of Interests. he authors declare that they have no known competing financial interests or personal relationships that could have appeared to influence the work reported in this paper.

References

1. Korhonen, V.O., et al.: Light propagation in NIR spectroscopy of the human brain. IEEE J. Selected Top. Quantum Electron. **20**, 289–298 (2013)
2. Photon migration in the presence of a single defect: a perturbation analysis (2025). https://opg.optica.org/ao/viewmedia.cfm?uri=ao-34-19-3826. Accessed 3 Dec
3. Zahida, G., Lin, S., Toronov, V., Guerouah, Z., Lin, S., Toronov, V.: Measurement of adult human brain responses to breath-holding by multi-distance hyperspectral near-infrared spectroscopy. Appl. Sciences **12** (2021).https://doi.org/10.3390/app12010371
4. Re, R., et al.: Reliable fast (20 Hz) acquisition rate by a TD fNIRS device: brain resting-state oscillation studies. Sensors (Basel, Switz.) **23**, 196 (2022). https://doi.org/10.3390/s23010196
5. SM322 datasheet,ElFys SM322 photodetector datasheet (2026). https://cdn.prod.websitefiles.com/655b41cb143610f766b510cb/65cb4a1826b0d2220a1cb2d2_sm322-datasheet.pdf

6. Si PIN photodiode S5971/S5972/S5973 series (2026). https://www.hamamatsu.com/content/dam/hamamatsu-photonics/sites/documents/99_SALES_LIBRARY/ssd/s5971_etc_kpin1025e.pdf. Accessed 3 Feb
7. Technical note for Si photodiodes by HAMAMATSU. https://www.hamamatsu.com/content/dam/hamamatsu-photonics/sites/documents/99_SALES_LIBRARY/ssd/si_pd_kspd9001e.pdf

Continuous Measurement of Cardiovascular Markers Using SCG During Cycle Ergometer Test

Aleksandra Zienkiewicz[1(✉)], Mikko Tulppo[2], Rasmus Valtonen[2], and Teemu Myllylä[1,3]

[1] Optoelectronics and Measurement Techniques Research Unit, University of Oulu, Oulu, Finland
aleksandra.zienkiewicz@oulu.fi

[2] Research Unit of Biomedicine and Internal Medicine, University of Oulu, Oulu, Finland

[3] Research Unit of Medical Imaging, Physics and Technology, University of Oulu, Oulu, Finland

Abstract. Seismocardiography (SCG) provides a noninvasive measure of cardiac mechanical activity using chest-mounted inertial sensors. While SCG has shown promise under resting and moderate activity conditions, its behavior during high-intensity exercise, particularly near volitional exhaustion, remains insufficiently characterized. This study investigated the feasibility and behavior of SCG during an incremental cycle ergometer test to voluntary exhaustion using an SCG-only measurement approach, with emphasis on heart rate tracking and waveform morphology. Six adult participants performed an incremental workload cycling protocol to voluntary exhaustion. SCG signals were continuously acquired using a sternal accelerometer throughout rest and exercise. SCG-derived HR closely followed the expected response throughout the exercise protocol, including near-exhaustive conditions, indicating preserved cardiac mechanical periodicity despite increasing motion and respiratory influence. Peak-to-peak SCG amplitude exhibited systematic changes with increasing workload. These findings demonstrate that SCG remains analyzable during maximal incremental cycling using a standalone sensor and that morphology-based features capture meaningful exercise-induced changes. The results support further investigation of SCG waveform analysis for cardiomechanical monitoring during high-intensity exercise and motivate future work exploring advanced physiological metrics using minimal sensor configurations.

Keywords: exercise · signal morphology · seismocardiography

1 Introduction

Incremental exercise testing to voluntary exhaustion, most commonly performed using a cycle ergometer, is frequently used in exercise physiology and cardiopulmonary assessment. It provides a controlled environment that taxes body systems simultaneously, with

M. Säreströniemi et al. (Eds.): NCDHWS 2026, CCIS 3010, pp. 212–224, 2026.
https://doi.org/10.1007/978-3-032-28819-6_14

heart rate (HR), stroke volume, cardiac output, and ventilatory responses all changing with increasing workload, as the cardiovascular system must adapt to meet heightened metabolic demand [1]. Such modification enables quantification of functional capacity, endurance, and health status [1–3]. However, many conventional measurements used in exercise testing—such as cuff-based blood pressure (BP) readings—offer limited insight into the cardiac processes due to their intermittent nature. Wearable, unobtrusive technologies capable of capturing bio-signals continuously and noninvasively during exercise are therefore in demand.

Seismocardiography (SCG) is rarely considered for the purpose, despite its use in the passive measurements. SCG is an emerging non-invasive technology that measures cardiac activity from heart-induced vibrations at the chest wall, using an accelerometer [4–6]. Multiple studies have linked the SCG signal to cardiac function [7], artery disease [8], cardiorespiratory fitness [9–11], and blood pressure [12–14]. SCG has been used both individually and in combination with other biosignals, such as ECG and PPG. However, due to the complex nature of SCG signals, and their high susceptibility to motion artifacts and confounding effects from respiration and posture changes, the application in dynamic exercise seems to be limited. Motion-induced signal distortion and respiratory influence on chest wall movement can both alter SCG morphology and complicate interpretation under high-intensity conditions. Nevertheless, recent investigations have shown that interpretable SCG signals can be acquired during physical activity with appropriate sensor placement and processing pipelines, highlighting the potential for SCG to capture meaningful mechanical data even in the presence of motion [8, 15].

Among dynamic exercise modalities, cycle ergometry presents unique advantages for SCG recording. Unlike treadmill protocols, cycling constrains the body in a seated position and reduces large-amplitude upper-body motion, which can help mitigate motion artifact in accelerometer-based measurements while still producing a high cardiovascular load [1]. This makes incremental cycling an appealing platform for studying SCG under gradually increasing physiological stress, including near exhaustion. Advances in sensor technology, signal processing, and machine learning have made it feasible to collect and analyze SCG signals with improved signal-to-noise ratios and to begin relating them to functional cardiovascular parameters.

Much of the existing SCG literature has focused on resting measurements or submaximal activity, and in some cases used SCG in conjunction with auxiliary signals or models to estimate parameters such as peak oxygen uptake (VO_2max) or cardiorespiratory fitness [9, 10]. These studies provide evidence that SCG morphology and derived features correlate with functional cardiovascular measures. However, there remains limited investigation of continuous SCG morphology and feature evolution during the full intensity spectrum of an incremental exercise test performed to exhaustion. In particular, systematic analysis of how SCG waveform shape and repeatable morphological features behave from rest through maximal exercise—in the absence of other biosignals (e.g., ECG or PPG)—is currently sparse.

The present study therefore investigates SCG changes during an incremental cycle ergometer test performed to voluntary exhaustion, using a chest-mounted accelerometer to continuously acquire SCG signals without reliance on auxiliary sensors. The analysis focuses on SCG waveform morphology and how key signal features evolve as exercise intensity increases. By examining SCG signal shape across a gradient of workloads, this work aims to determine whether SCG provides reliable and meaningful cardiomechanical information under high-intensity conditions.

2 Materials and Methods

2.1 Subjects

Data were collected from six (4 female, 2 male) volunteers, recruited from the University of Oulu and consisted of students and exchange students. Participants were recruited by introducing the research during lectures. Exclusion criteria included having a condition that prevents from performing hard/exhaustive physical activities and cognitive/sensory difficulties or insufficient command of the language that, in the opinion of the recruiting professional, made it difficult to understand the questions raised in the surveys, scales or instruments used in the study. Basic information such as height, weight, and current health status was collected with a questionnaire. Before the exercise test, body composition was assessed using a bioelectrical impedance analyzer (InBody 720, Biospace Co., Ltd., South Korea). Participants then rested in a seated position in a quiet environment, after which resting BP was measured three times at two-minute intervals using an automated sphygmomanometer (Schiller BP-200 Plus, Schiller AG, Switzerland). The mean of the three measurements was recorded. Subject characteristics are shown in the Table 1.

Table 1. Subject (n = 6) characteristics and baseline physiological levels. SBP: systolic blood pressure, DBP: diastolic blood pressure, HR: heart rate. Data are shown as mean (SD).

Characteristic	Value	Physiological marker	Baseline value
Age	24.67 (5.72)	SBP (mmHg)	134 (124–141)
Sex	4F, 2M	DBP (mmHg)	80 (78–84)
Height	168.17 (9.37)	HR (bpm)	93 (84–97)
Weight	62.28 (7.22)		
Fat (%)	25.76 (5.95)		
Muscle (%)	27.30 (3.73)		

2.2 Measurement Procedure

SCG signals were collected using the chest-worn accelerometer connected to the wearable monitoring device developed in the University of Oulu [16–19]. The test was performed on a cycle ergometer using an incremental protocol until voluntary exhaustion. The test began with a 5-min warm-up at 0 W, followed by an initial workload of 50 W. Thereafter, workload was increased every 3 min by 25 W in men and 20 W in women. Participants maintained a constant pedaling cadence throughout the test, which was terminated at subjective exhaustion.

At the end of each workload stage, BP was measured using an automated sphygmomanometer (Schiller BP-200 Plus, Schiller AG, Switzerland), capillary blood samples were obtained from the fingertip for lactate analysis using a portable analyzer (Lactate Scout+, SensLab GmbH, Germany), and perceived exertion was assessed using the Borg Rating of Perceived Exertion scale (6–20).

After completion of the incremental phase, participants performed a 5-min active recovery at 50 W, after which blood pressure was measured. All lactate measurements were performed by the same investigator supervising the exercise protocol.

One of the subjects underwent an additional measurement using a standard three-lead ECG, which was utilized for HR comparison. ECG signals collected from the other subjects were not usable due to electrode failure.

2.3 Signal Processing

Signal analysis was performed using MATLAB (Mathworks 2023b). SCG signals were sampled with 250 Hz rate and filtered with a Butterworth bandpass filters of 3rd order, cutoff frequencies of 10 and 35 Hz, as suggested in [12] and sensor-specific recommendations reported in [20], which align with the frequency range of the systolic SCG components along the dorsoventral axis [21–23]. This bandwidth selection effectively suppresses low-frequency baseline drift related to respiration as well as high-frequency noise and artifacts associated with valve-closure acoustics, while maintaining the essential morphological characteristics of the SCG waveform. SCG peaks detected in intervals deviating by 300 ms from a local moving average (window 29 samples) were removed to obtain a consistent sequence of physiological beats. ECG signal was sampled with 250 Hz. After pre-processing with a 0.8 Hz high-pass Butterworth filter (order = 5), the R-peak detection in the ECG signal was conducted using the Pan–Tompkins algorithm.

2.4 Performance Steps

To be able to compare data across participants, five characteristic physiological states were defined and the corresponding data at those points were extracted from the dataset, as suggested in [24].

- PRE: value at rest before the cycling.
- WARM UP: value during initial 5 min warm-up with 0 W workload. The last completed BP measurement with the corresponding HR and lactate were used.
- THR: values at 4.0 mmol/L as an indication of lactate threshold. The first completed BP measurement with the corresponding HR and watt values after passing thresholdof 4.0 mmol/L was extracted.
- MAX: values when exhaustion was reported, maximum HR stage.
- POST: values measured after test, during 5 min active recovery cycling with 50 W workload.

Performance steps and example of corresponding HR are visualised in Fig. 1.

2.5 Statistical Analysis

To assess differences between performance stages (Warm-up, Threshold, Max, and Post), linear mixed-effects models were used, with stage included as a fixed effect and subject as a random intercept to account for repeated measurements within individuals and to accommodate missing values across stages. Omnibus effects of stage were evaluated using F-tests derived from fixed-effect contrasts of the mixed-effects models. When a significant main effect of stage was detected, pairwise comparisons between stages were performed using model-based contrasts with Bonferroni correction for multiple comparisons. Results are reported as $F(\mathrm{df}_1, \mathrm{df}_2)$ test statistics with corresponding p-values. Descriptive statistics are presented as mean ± standard deviation (SD), and statistical significance was defined as $p < 0.05$.

3 Results

3.1 Physiological Profiles

All participants completed the incremental exercise protocol to individual exhaustion. Following a standardized warm-up at 0 W, the initial workload was set to 50 W and subsequently increased in fixed increments until termination of the test. The mean number of exercise stages performed at non-zero workload was 5.6 (1.6). Visualisation of the protocol stages is shown on Fig. 1.

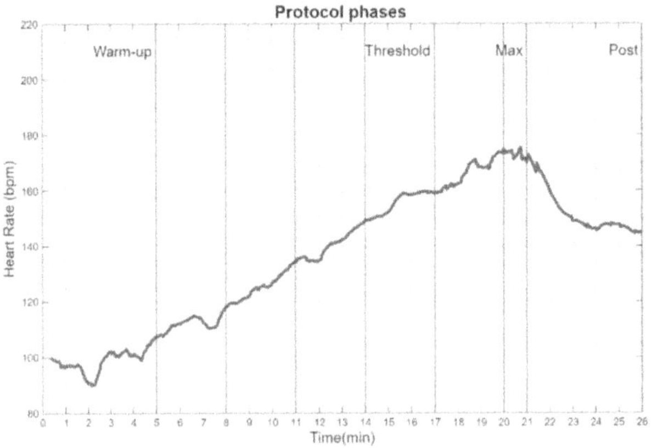

Fig. 1. Protocol phases. Red lines indicate the change of the workload.

Stage-specific physiological responses are summarized in Table 2, with corresponding plots shown on Fig. 2.

Table 2. Median (interquartile range) values of workload and physiological variables across exercise stages.

Protocol stage	SBP (mmHg)	DBP (mmHg)	Lactate	HR (bpm)
Pre	134 (124–141)	80 (78–84)	-	93 (84–97)
Warm-up	147 (139–149)	81 (74–83)	1.9 (1.7–2.1)	113 (103–128)
Threshold	161 (152–171)	85 (79–97)	4.7 (3.6–5.7)	175 (157–178)
Max	171 (150–176)	87 (70–96)	10.7 (8.7–11)	186 (173–200)
Post	146 (130–149)	79 (73–83)	1.7 (1.7–4.3)	141 (137–144)

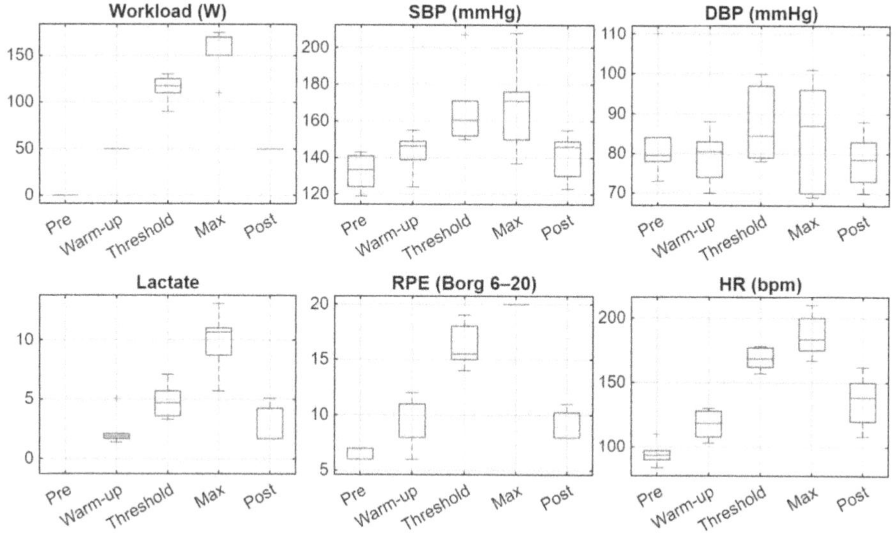

Fig. 2. Boxplots of workload and physiological responses across exercise stages, showing median and interquartile range for each variable.

3.2 Single-Subject SCG Signal Characteristics

Calculating the average shape of the heartbeat response indicated its high dependence on the protocol stage (see Fig. 3).

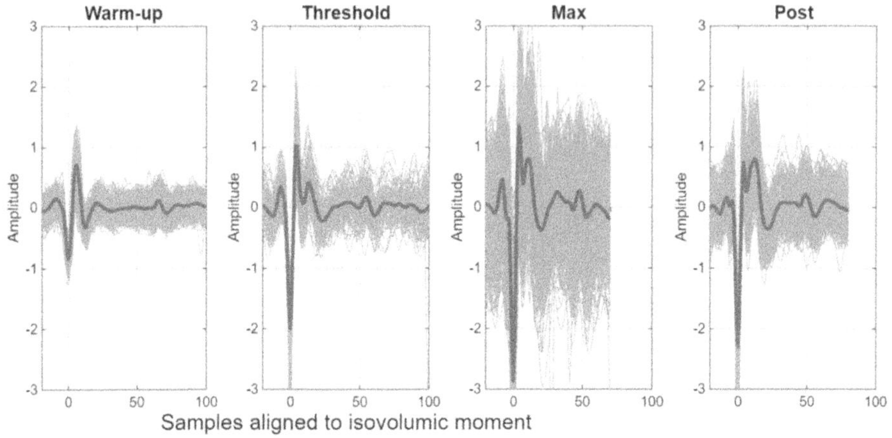

Fig. 3. Average SCG peak shape in different protocol stages. Peaks were aligned to the isovolumic moment (minimal point). Presented are results for Subject 1. Red line indicates average.

When analyzing power spectral density (PSD) of raw SCG in the same subject (see Fig. 4), exercise induces a broadband increase in raw-signal spectral power from warm-up to maximal workload, while preserving the overall spectral structure; post-exercise power remains elevated, indicating incomplete physiological recovery.

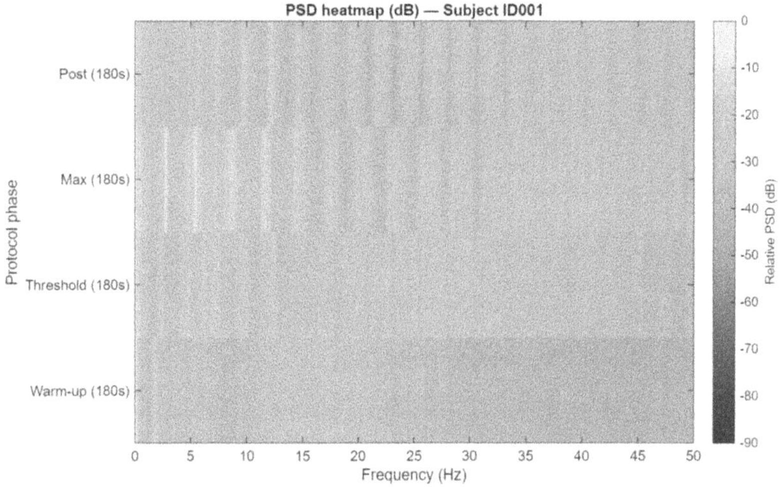

Fig. 4. PSD heatmap of raw SCG signal in different protocol stages.). Presented are results for Subject 1

For Subject 1, SCG derived HR was tested against reference ECG-based HR using correlation and Bland–Altman analysis (see plots in Fig. 5), showing an excellent agreement between values (SCG HR = 0.999 × ECG HR + 0.189, r2 = 0.9982). Bland–Altman analysis demonstrated a small increase in dispersion at higher heart rates, suggesting minor proportional differences between SCG- and ECG-derived estimates. Nevertheless, limits of agreement stayed between −2.5 to + 2.5 bpm across 3120 paired samples, which indicated overall high beat-to-beat consistency between modalities. After confirming that SCG-derived HR accuracy was satisfactory, all subsequent analyses were performed solely based on SCG measurements.

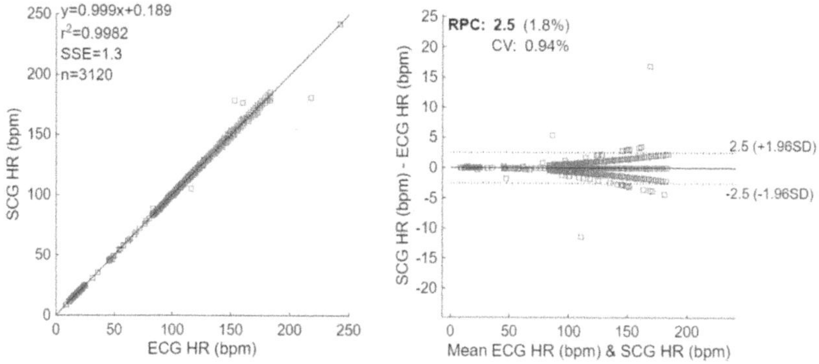

Fig. 5. The regression and Bland–Altman plots for Subject 1. r2: Pearson's r-value squared, SSE: sum of squared error, n: number of data points used, 'RPC(%): reproducibility coefficient and % of mean values, CV: coefficient of variation (SD of mean values in %).

3.3 Exercise Stage Effects on SCG Amplitude and HR

HR and peak-to-peak SCG amplitude were quantified for all subjects. These measures were subjected to signal-specific quality control and temporal normalization prior to stage-wise analysis across the exercise protocol (Fig. 6). Corresponding numerical values are shown in Table 3.

Table 3. Stage-wise summary statistics of systolic timing indices and heart rate. Values are reported as mean (SD) of subject-level means.

Protocol stage	Peak-to-peak (a.u.)	HR (bpm)
Warm-up	56.3 (48.5)	100.0 (13.4)
Threshold	145.2 (75.6)	147.6 (7.0)
Max	182.1 (100.2)	176.7 (20.2)
Post	158.2 (77.6)	168.1 (19.3)

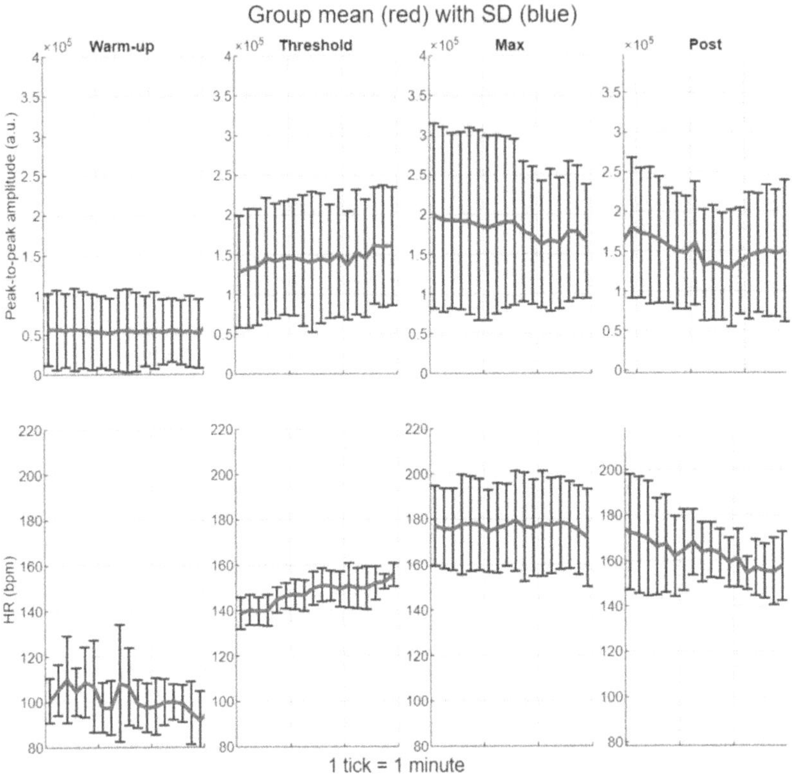

Fig. 6. Stage-aligned group-average time courses of systolic timing indices and HR during the incremental exercise protocol. Mean ± SD traces are shown across five protocol stages.

Exercise stage had a significant effect on both peak-to-peak amplitude and HR, as assessed using linear mixed-effects models with stage as a fixed effect and subject as a random intercept (Peak-to-peak amplitude: $F(3, 19) = 16.11$, $p < 0.001$; HR: $F(3, 19) = 39.10$, $p < 0.001$), see Fig. 7.

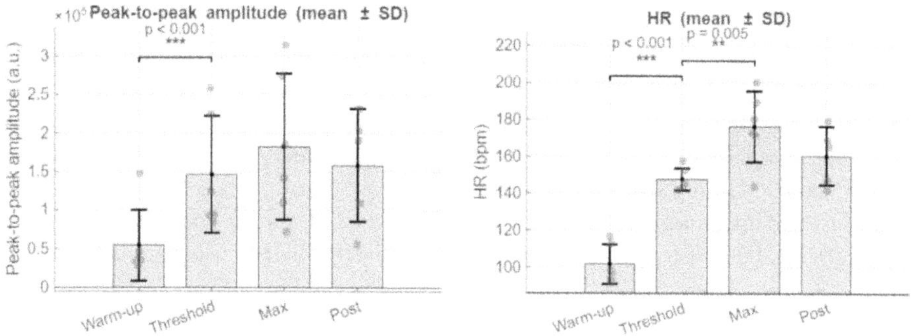

Fig. 7. Stage-wise changes in peak-to-peak amplitude and heart rate (HR) across the exercise protocol. Bars represent group means and error bars indicate standard deviations (mean ± SD), with individual subject values shown as gray dots.

4 Discussion

This study examined SCG-only response during an incremental cycle ergometer test to voluntary exhaustion. The results demonstrate that SCG signals remain analyzable across increasing exercise intensity, supporting the feasibility of capturing cardiomechanical information during high-intensity cycling without auxiliary biosignals.

SCG-derived HR closely followed the expected HR response throughout the protocol, including near exhaustion (see Figs. 2 and 6). When compared to ECG-derived HR, the differences were increasing with HR, but still within the − 2.5 to +2.5 bpm limits of agreement (Fig. 5). This indicates that the dominant periodic structure of the SCG signal is preserved despite increasing motion, respiratory influence, and signal non-stationarity. In addition, peak-to-peak SCG amplitude exhibited systematic changes with increasing workload (Fig. 6), which might suggest that SCG waveform morphology reflects underlying cardiomechanical adaptation to rising cardiovascular demand. This finding supports the growing emphasis in recent literature on morphology-based SCG features [11, 12, 25].

Changes in SCG waveform shape are likely influenced not only by cardiac mechanics but also by respiration. The progressive increase in breathing frequency and depth during the ramp test alters intrathoracic pressure and chest wall motion, contributing to amplitude modulation and morphological variability (Fig. 4). The increasing spectral overlap between respiratory and cardiac components near exhaustion further complicates interpretation and underscores respiration as a key factor shaping SCG signals during high-intensity exercise. An important implication of the observed morphology changes is the potential relevance of SCG for BP–related investigations. While BP was not estimated in this study, utilizing the sensitivity of SCG waveform characteristics, without additional ECG or PPG sensors, would be particularly attractive for wearable and exercise-based monitoring, though this remains a topic for future targeted studies.

Several limitations should be considered. The sampling frequency was insufficient to support reliable extraction of fine intra-beat timing features, constraining the analysis to morphology-based descriptors. Additionally, the relatively small sample size limits generalizability and precludes detailed assessment of inter-individual variability. Finally, the absence of reference measurements restricts physiological interpretation of specific waveform changes, though this design choice was consistent with the goal of evaluating SCG as a standalone modality.

In summary, this work demonstrates that SCG can not only track HR but also exhibit systematic morphology changes during an incremental cycle ergometer test to exhaustion using an SCG-only setup. The findings support morphology-based SCG analysis as a practical and informative approach under high-intensity exercise conditions and motivate future studies exploring advanced cardiocirculatory metrics using minimal sensor configurations.

Acknowledgments. The authors want to thank Mr. Jari Paunonen and Mr. Eerik Jaakola for the data collection. This work was supported by 6GBRIDGE - Next generation healthcare and wearable diagnostics utilizing 6 G project (11,146/31/2022).

Disclosure of Interests. The authors have no competing interests to declare that are relevant to the content of this article.

References

1. Glaab, T., Taube, C.: Practical guide to cardiopulmonary exercise testing in adults. Respir. Res. **23**, 9 (2022). https://doi.org/10.1186/S12931-021-01895-6/TABLES/2
2. Puttini, F., Pezzuto, B., Vignati, C.: Cardiopulmonary exercise testing in the prognostic assessment of heart failure: from a standardized approach to tailored therapeutic strategies. Medicina (Lithuania) **61** (2025).https://doi.org/10.3390/medicina61101770
3. MF, P., U, C., PG, A., et al.: Statement on cardiopulmonary exercise testing in chronic heart failure due to left ventricular dysfunction: recommendations for performance and interpretation. Part I: definition of cardiopulmonary exercise testing parameters for appropriate use in chronic heart failure. Eur. J. Cardiovasc. Prev. Rehabil. **13**, 150–164 (2006). https://doi.org/10.1097/01.HJR.0000209812.05573.04
4. Balali, P., Rabineau, J., Hossein, A., et al.: Investigating cardiorespiratory interaction using ballistocardiography and seismocardiography—a narrative review. Sensors **22**, 9565 (2022)
5. Rai, D., Thakkar, H.K., Rajput, S.S., et al.: A comprehensive review on seismocardiogram: current advancements on acquisition, annotation, and applications. Mathematics **9**, 2243 (2021)
6. Taebi, A., Solar, B.E., Bomar, A.J., et al.: Recent Advances in Seismocardiography. Vibration **2**, 64–86 (2019).https://doi.org/10.3390/vibration2010005
7. Ganti, V.G., Gazi, A.H., An, S., et al.: Wearable seismocardiography-based assessment of stroke volume in congenital heart disease. J. Am. Heart Assoc. **11**, e026067 (2022). https://doi.org/10.1161/JAHA.122.026067
8. Dehkordi, P., Bauer, E.P., Tavakolian, K., et al.: Identifying patients with coronary artery disease using rest and exercise seismocardiography. Front. Physiol. **10**, 472815 (2019). https://doi.org/10.3389/FPHYS.2019.01211/BIBTEX
9. Hansen, M.T., Rømer, T., Højgaard, A., et al.: Validity and reliability of seismocardiography for the estimation of cardiorespiratory fitness. Cardiovasc Digit Health J **4**, 155–163 (2023)
10. Schulenburg, R., Schmidt, S.E., Schröder, J., et al.: Evaluating seismocardiography as a non-exercise method for estimating maximal oxygen uptake. Healthcare **12**, 2162 (2024). https://doi.org/10.3390/HEALTHCARE12212162

11. Sorensen, K., Poulsen, M.K., Karbing, D.S., et al.: A clinical method for estimation of VO 2max using seismocardiography. Int. J. Sports Med. **41**, 661–668 (2020). https://doi.org/10.1055/A-1144-3369/ID/R7933-0016/BIB
12. Zienkiewicz, A., Korhonen, V., Kiviniemi, V., Myllylä, T.: Continuous estimation of blood pressure by utilizing seismocardiogram signal features in relation to electrocardiogram. Biosensors (Basel) **14**, 621 (2024)
13. Zienkiewicz, A., Favre, M., Ferdinando, H., et al.: Blood pressure wave propagation—a multisensor setup for cerebral autoregulation studies. Physiol. Meas. **42**, 115007 (2021)
14. Myllylä, T., Zacharias, N., Korhonen, V., et al.: Multimodal brain imaging with magnetoencephalography: a method for measuring blood pressure and cardiorespiratory oscillations. Sci. Rep. **7**, 172 (2017)
15. Dhar, R., Darwish, S.E., Darwish, S.A., et al.: Effect of respiration and exercise on seismocardiographic signals. Comput. Biol. Med. **185** (2025).https://doi.org/10.1016/J.COMPBIOMED.2024.109600
16. Ilvesmäki, M., Moradi, S., Paunonen, J., et al.: Spectral entropy of cerebral fluids during human sleep measured by wearable fNIRS device **12841**, 23–27 (2024). https://doi.org/10.1117/12.3005675
17. Ferdinando, H., Moradi, S., Korhonen, V., et al.: Altered cerebrovascular-CSF coupling in Alzheimer's Disease measured by functional near-infrared spectroscopy. Sci. Rep. **13**(1), 22364 (2023). https://doi.org/10.1038/s41598-023-48965-x
18. Myllylä, T., Korhonen, V.: Functional near-infrared spectroscopy in cancer diagnostics. Multimodal Opt. Diagn. Cancer 195–207 (2020).https://doi.org/10.1007/978-3-030-44594-2_5
19. Mannini, F.: Glymphometer device validation through EEG and fNIRS signals acquisition and processing for functional brain analysis (2023)
20. Myllylä, T.S., Elseoud, A.A., Sorvoja, H.S.S., et al.: Fibre optic sensor for non-invasive monitoring of blood pressure during MRI scanning. J. Biophotonics **4**, 98–107 (2011)
21. Romano, C., Schena, E., Formica, D., Massaroni, C.: Comparison between chest-worn accelerometer and gyroscope performance for heart rate and respiratory rate monitoring. Biosensors (Basel) **12**, 834 (2022)
22. Shafiq, G., Tatinati, S., Veluvolu, K.C.: Automatic annotation of peaks in seismocardiogram for systolic time intervals. In: 2016 38th Annual International Conference of the IEEE Engineering in Medicine and Biology Society (EMBC), pp 2672–2675 (2016)
23. Sieciński, S., Kostka, P.S., Tkacz, E.J.: Heart rate variability analysis on electrocardiograms, seismocardiograms and gyrocardiograms on healthy volunteers. Sensors **20**, 4522 (2020)
24. Heimark, S., Eitzen, I., Vianello, I., et al.: Blood pressure response and pulse arrival time during exercise testing in well-trained individuals. Front. Physiol. **13** (2022).https://doi.org/10.3389/fphys.2022.863855
25. Chen, C.-H., Lin, W.-Y., Lee, M.-Y.: Computer-aided detection of fiducial points in seismocardiography through dynamic time warping. Biosens. (Basel) **12**, 374 (2022)

Lightweight, Explainable, and Efficiency-Aware Deep Learning for Early Sepsis Prediction from Structured Electronic Health Record Time-Series

Attaphongse Taparugssanagorn[1(✉)], Mariella Säreströniemi[2,3], Matti Hämäläinen[3], and Jari Iinatti[3]

[1] Asian Institute of Technology, Pathumthani 12120, Thailand
attaphongset@ait.asia
[2] Health Science and Technology, Faculty of Medicine and InfoTech Oulu, Oulu 90014, Finland
mariella.sarestoniemi@oulu.fi
[3] Centre for Wireless Communications, University of Oulu, Oulu 90014, Finland
{matti.hamalainen,jari.iinatti}@oulu.fi
https://ait.ac.th/, https://www.oulu.fi/

Abstract. Early detection of sepsis in Intensive Care Units (ICUs) is critical, as delayed intervention significantly increases mortality risk. This study investigates early sepsis prediction using multivariate physiological time-series data from the PhysioNet 2019 dataset, comprising 40 structured Electronic Health Record (EHR) variables recorded hourly. We evaluate lightweight deep learning models, including 1D-CNN, GRU, TCN, and a lightweight CNN–ViT hybrid, under a unified protocol targeting prediction up to 6 h before sepsis onset. This prediction horizon follows the PhysioNet 2019 benchmark and represents a clinically meaningful early-warning window that balances actionable intervention time with sufficient predictive signal. The results show that effective temporal modeling is key for early detection. The TCN achieves the most favorable balance between predictive performance and efficiency, with the highest recall (0.778), tied highest F1-score (0.495), highest AUPRC (0.50), and highest AUC (0.907 ± 0.010). It also records the lowest inference latency (0.62 s total over the test set under a CPU-only setting), supporting real-time applicability. In contrast, CNN–ViT achieves competitive performance (AUC 0.906 ± 0.011) but incurs substantially higher computational cost (44.34 s). Explainability using SHAP highlights clinically plausible indicators, including blood pressure, heart rate, oxygen saturation, and lactate. Overall, lightweight temporal models offer a practical and clinically meaningful solution for early sepsis prediction under real-time constraints.

M. Säreströniemi et al. (Eds.): NCDHWS 2026, CCIS 3010, pp. 225–244, 2026.
https://doi.org/10.1007/978-3-032-28819-6_15

Keywords: Early sepsis prediction · Explainable AI · Lightweight deep learning · Clinical time-series · Temporal modeling

1 Introduction

Sepsis remains a leading cause of critical illness and mortality in Intensive Care Units (ICUs), with outcomes strongly dependent on timely recognition and intervention. Once the inflammatory response becomes dysregulated, patient deterioration can occur rapidly, leaving a narrow window for effective treatment. In ICU settings, even highly accurate predictive models have limited clinical value if alerts are not generated within clinically actionable time windows. Recent surveys, including the work by Islam et al. (2023), highlight the increasing adoption of Machine Learning (ML) and Deep Learning (DL) techniques to improve early sepsis detection using Electronic Health Records (EHRs) [1].

In this study, the term EHR refers to structured clinical time-series data derived from ICU settings, comprising both hourly recorded ICU physiological variables (e.g., heart rate, oxygen saturation) and intermittently recorded laboratory measurements. While traditional EHR systems are not strictly real-time, modern ICU environments integrate monitoring systems that generate high-frequency physiological data streams alongside clinical records.

Traditional clinical assessment tools, such as the Sequential Organ Failure Assessment (SOFA) score and the Systemic Inflammatory Response Syndrome (SIRS) criteria, remain widely used in ICU practice but suffer from inherent limitations. These rule-based systems rely on intermittently sampled measurements and predefined thresholds, making them insensitive to subtle or evolving physiological changes. Their static nature limits adaptability to individual patient trajectories, often resulting in delayed alerts or excessive false positives, particularly in complex or atypical cases.

Prior studies have shown that fine-grained temporal patterns in vital signs, such as blood pressure and heart rate variability, contain predictive information that precedes overt clinical deterioration [2]. However, exploiting such dynamics requires continuous monitoring and computational models capable of learning from multivariate time-series data. This need has motivated the use of advanced DL architectures, including Long Short-Term Memory (LSTM) networks, Gated Recurrent Units (GRU), and Transformer-based models, which have demonstrated improved performance over traditional approaches [3–5].

Despite these advances, most existing DL-based sepsis prediction systems are designed primarily to maximize predictive accuracy, with limited consideration of computational efficiency or deployment constraints. Many state-of-the-art models rely on deep recurrent stacks or full self-attention mechanisms, resulting in high parameter counts, increased inference latency, and substantial memory and power requirements. Such characteristics may limit their ability to generate predictions within clinically actionable time windows, particularly in resource-constrained ICU or edge-based environments.

Early sepsis detection requires models to process continuously updated patient data and deliver predictions within minutes to hours before clinical onset, enabling timely intervention. In modern ICUs, predictive models are increasingly expected to operate continuously, close to the data source, and under strict timing constraints. In this work, we adopt a 6-hour prediction horizon, consistent with the PhysioNet 2019 benchmark, as it represents a clinically actionable early-warning window that balances sufficient lead time for intervention with the availability of reliable predictive signals in structured ICU time-series data. This shift toward edge and near-edge intelligence further necessitates lightweight architectures that can deliver timely predictions without dependence on centralized high-performance computing resources. Consequently, model efficiency becomes an important design objective alongside predictive performance.

In parallel, the growing emphasis on eXplainable Artificial Intelligence (XAI) has addressed another key barrier to clinical adoption. Methods such as SHapley Additive exPlanations (SHAP) provide patient-specific insights into feature relevance and temporal importance, supporting clinical interpretability and trust. However, explainability techniques are rarely integrated into efficiency-aware architectures, leaving a gap between transparent modeling and deployable system design.

Motivated by these challenges, this work focuses on lightweight deep learning architectures for early sepsis prediction from structured EHR time-series data. By explicitly modeling structured ICU time-series that combine continuously monitored vital signs and clinical measurements, the proposed framework balances predictive performance, computational efficiency, and interpretability, targeting practical deployment in ICU and edge-based clinical monitoring environments.

1.1 Related Works and Research Gap

Machine learning and deep learning methods have been widely explored for early sepsis detection in ICU settings. Early studies demonstrated that models trained on structured electronic health record time-series variables can outperform traditional rule-based clinical scores such as SOFA and SIRS in early sepsis identification [4]. These works established the feasibility of data-driven sepsis prediction using routinely collected ICU measurements, including vital signs and laboratory values.

Subsequent research introduced more complex temporal modeling techniques, including recurrent neural networks, attention-based models, and transformer architectures, to capture long-range dependencies in patient trajectories [5,6]. While these approaches often report improved predictive performance, they typically rely on computationally intensive architectures with large parameter counts and high inference latency, limiting their suitability for real-time or bedside deployment in resource-constrained clinical environments.

Parallel research directions have investigated multimodal integration, incorporating unstructured clinical notes or high-resolution physiological waveforms such as electrocardiograms and arterial blood pressure signals [2,3]. Although these modalities can provide complementary clinical information, their practical adoption is hindered by challenges related to data availability, synchronization, noise sensitivity, and substantially increased computational and storage requirements. As a result, many multimodal and waveform-based systems remain confined to retrospective analyses or offline settings and are difficult to deploy in operational ICU workflows.

Another persistent challenge concerns model interpretability. While explainability techniques such as SHAP and attention visualization have been increasingly adopted, they are often applied post hoc or qualitatively, without explicit integration into lightweight temporal architectures or clear linkage to patient-specific time-series dynamics. This limits their clinical utility, particularly in time-critical decision support scenarios.

Taken together, existing literature reveals a clear research gap: the lack of efficiency-aware deep learning frameworks that achieve competitive early sepsis prediction performance using only structured EHR time-series data, while maintaining low computational complexity, fast inference, and clinically meaningful interpretability. Addressing this gap is essential for enabling practical, real-time deployment of sepsis prediction models in ICU environments. Recent surveys have also highlighted that many deep learning approaches for EHR analysis prioritize predictive performance over computational efficiency, limiting real-time clinical adoption [7].

1.2 Our Contributions

This work addresses the gap between predictive performance and practical deployability in deep learning approaches for early sepsis prediction from structured clinical time-series data. While prior studies often emphasize predictive accuracy using complex architectures, they frequently overlook computational efficiency, inference latency, and interpretability, which are critical for time-sensitive ICU decision support. The main contributions of this study are summarized as follows.

First, we propose an efficiency-aware evaluation framework for early sepsis prediction using structured EHR time-series data. The framework is designed to balance predictive performance with computational efficiency, enabling timely predictions within clinically relevant intervention windows under CPU-based deployment conditions.

Second, we conduct a systematic comparison of lightweight architectures, including one-dimensional Convolutional Neural Networks (1D-CNN), Gated Recurrent Units (GRU), and Temporal Convolutional Networks (TCN). These models are evaluated under a unified experimental setup to ensure fair comparison and to assess their suitability for low-latency clinical deployment.

Third, we introduce a lightweight CNN–Vision Transformer (CNN–ViT) architecture tailored for structured time-series data. By combining convolutional temporal feature extraction with shallow self-attention, the model captures both local and global temporal dependencies, albeit at a higher computational cost compared to purely convolutional or recurrent models.

Fourth, beyond predictive accuracy, we evaluate model efficiency using inference latency under a consistent CPU-based evaluation protocol, enabling transparent analysis of performance–efficiency trade-offs in real-time ICU monitoring scenarios.

Finally, we incorporate model interpretability using SHapley Additive exPlanations (SHAP), providing clinically plausible temporal feature attributions that enhance transparency and support clinical trust.

Overall, this work demonstrates that lightweight temporal models can achieve competitive predictive performance while satisfying practical efficiency and deployment constraints in ICU environments.

2 Dataset and Preprocessing

2.1 Dataset Description

This study employs the Prediction of Sepsis dataset from the PhysioNet/Computing in Cardiology Challenge 2019, distributed via Kaggle [8]. The dataset is derived from real Intensive Care Unit (ICU) admissions and provides hourly structured Electronic Health Record (EHR) data for sepsis prediction up to six hours before clinical diagnosis. It includes 40 physiological and laboratory variables, such as heart rate, blood pressure, respiratory rate, oxygen saturation, white blood cell count, lactate, creatinine, and demographic information including age and gender. All patient records are organized into temporally aligned files, where each row corresponds to one hour of observations, enabling direct construction of multivariate time-series samples for supervised learning.

Vital signs and laboratory measurements are recorded at hourly intervals, reflecting aggregated clinical observations rather than continuous waveform signals. This combination captures both rapid physiological fluctuations and slower metabolic trends relevant to early sepsis progression. The dataset provides structured and consistently formatted clinical time-series, making it suitable for benchmarking machine learning and deep learning models for early sepsis prediction. In this study, we focus on lightweight deep learning architectures to evaluate the trade-off between predictive performance and computational efficiency. The dataset contains only structured EHR variables (no raw waveform data), and is therefore treated as a single multivariate time-series modality.

Each patient record consists of hourly measurements with missing values, reflecting real-world clinical documentation practices.

2.2 Data Preprocessing and Feature Extraction

All structured variables undergo standardized preprocessing prior to model training. Missing values in the hourly time-series are handled using forward filling for physiological measurements and median imputation for laboratory variables, ensuring temporal continuity while avoiding unrealistic signal artifacts. All numerical features are normalized to zero mean and unit variance using statistics computed from the training set only, and then applied to validation and test sets.

To prevent data leakage, patient-level separation is strictly enforced before any preprocessing or window generation. The data set is first divided into training, validation, and test sets based on unique patient identifiers. Sliding windows are then constructed independently within each subset.

To construct uniform learning samples, patient records are segmented into fixed-length hourly time windows with 50% overlap. This windowing strategy balances temporal resolution with computational efficiency and increases the number of training samples while preserving temporal structure. Sequences shorter than the required window length are zero-padded, while longer records are truncated, resulting in consistent input dimensions across all models.

No handcrafted spectral features or frequency-domain transformations are applied. Instead, raw normalized time-series are directly provided to the learning models, allowing convolutional and attention-based layers to automatically learn relevant temporal patterns. This design choice aligns with the lightweight modeling objective, avoiding costly preprocessing steps such as short-time Fourier transforms, wavelet decompositions, or feature selection pipelines.

Local temporal dynamics, such as abrupt changes in vital signs or gradual laboratory trends, are captured implicitly by one-dimensional convolutional layers in CNN-based and hybrid architectures, while longer temporal dependencies are modeled using recurrent units, temporal convolutions, or lightweight self-attention mechanisms.

Given the inherent class imbalance between sepsis and non-sepsis cases, class-weighted loss functions are applied during training to improve sensitivity to minority cases.

Through minimal yet robust preprocessing and end-to-end learning from structured time-series data, this pipeline supports efficient training, low inference latency, and fair evaluation of lightweight deep learning architectures for early sepsis prediction.

3 Proposed Lightweight Hybrid Framework

3.1 Overview of the Framework

The proposed framework targets early sepsis prediction using structured multivariate time-series data collected from intensive care unit electronic health records. The objective is to design an efficiency-aware deep learning system that captures both short-term physiological variations and long-range temporal dependencies while maintaining low computational complexity.

In this context, real-time refers to generating predictions within seconds, which is negligible compared to the hourly update frequency of ICU data and enables timely clinical decision support. This notion of real-time performance is related to inference latency and system efficiency, rather than the prediction horizon.

Formally, the prediction task is defined as

$$y = f_{\theta}(X), \tag{1}$$

where $X \in \mathbb{R}^{T \times F}$ denotes a fixed-length sequence of F structured clinical variables observed over T hourly time steps, and $y \in \{0, 1\}$ represents the binary sepsis label. The prediction target is defined at a 6-hour horizon prior to sepsis onset, consistent with the PhysioNet 2019 benchmark. This horizon specifies how far in advance sepsis is predicted and reflects a clinically meaningful early-warning window, independent of the real-time inference requirement.

This study focuses on structured EHR time-series data to ensure reproducibility, computational efficiency, and compatibility with routinely collected ICU data. The framework is modular and supports multiple lightweight architectures under a unified preprocessing and evaluation protocol, enabling systematic comparison of efficiency–accuracy trade-offs.

3.2 Deep Learning Architectures

Convolutional Feature Extraction. One-dimensional convolutional layers serve as the primary feature extractors across all CNN-based and hybrid models. Given an input sequence $x = \{x_t\}_{t=1}^{T}$, a convolutional operation is defined as

$$h_t = \sigma\left(\sum_{i=0}^{k-1} w_i \, x_{t+i} + b\right), \tag{2}$$

where k is the kernel size and $\sigma(\cdot)$ denotes a nonlinear activation. This operation captures local temporal patterns such as abrupt changes in vital signs or short-term laboratory fluctuations that often precede sepsis onset.

Recurrent and Temporal Convolutional Modeling. To model longer-term physiological trends, recurrent and temporal convolutional architectures are evaluated. Gated Recurrent Units (GRU) are employed as a lightweight alternative to LSTMs, offering reduced parameter count while retaining the ability to model sequential dependencies:

$$h_t = \mathrm{GRU}(h_{t-1}, x_t). \tag{3}$$

Temporal Convolutional Networks (TCN) extend standard CNNs using dilated causal convolutions,

$$h_t = \sigma\left(\sum_{i=0}^{k-1} w_i \, x_{t-d\cdot i}\right), \tag{4}$$

where d is the dilation factor. This design enables exponentially expanding receptive fields without recurrent computation, making TCNs well-suited for efficient modeling of long ICU time-series.

Attention-Based Architectures. Transformer-based models are evaluated to capture global temporal dependencies. Given query, key, and value matrices $\mathbf{Q}$, $\mathbf{K}$, and $\mathbf{V}$, self-attention is computed as

$$\mathrm{Attention}(\mathbf{Q}, \mathbf{K}, \mathbf{V}) = \mathrm{softmax}\left(\frac{\mathbf{Q}\mathbf{K}^\top}{\sqrt{d_k}}\right)\mathbf{V}. \tag{5}$$

To reduce the computational overhead of standard Transformers, the proposed CNN–Vision Transformer (CNN–ViT) applies self-attention to temporally compressed convolutional feature tokens rather than raw time steps. Specifically, CNN-extracted embeddings are grouped into non-overlapping temporal patches and projected into token representations,

$$\mathbf{z}_0 = [\mathbf{x}_p^1\mathbf{E};\, \mathbf{x}_p^2\mathbf{E};\, \ldots;\, \mathbf{x}_p^N\mathbf{E}] + \mathbf{E}_{\text{pos}}, \tag{6}$$

where $\mathbf{E}$ is a linear projection matrix and $\mathbf{E}_{\text{pos}}$ denotes the positional encoding matrix. A classification token aggregates global contextual information for final prediction.

Hybrid Architectures. Hybrid architectures combine complementary modeling mechanisms to balance predictive expressiveness and computational efficiency. In this study, we focus on lightweight hybrid designs operating on structured EHR time-series data without incorporating additional modalities such as high-resolution waveforms or clinical text.

In the CNN–ViT model, convolutional features are first compressed into compact temporal representations and then transformed into token embeddings for lightweight self-attention. This enables global temporal dependency modeling while maintaining controlled computational cost, making it suitable for near real-time ICU decision support.

In the CNN–GRU architecture, convolutional embeddings serve as inputs to the recurrent layer,

$$\mathbf{h}_t = \text{GRU}(\mathbf{H}_t^{\text{CNN}}, \mathbf{h}_{t-1}), \tag{7}$$

allowing efficient modeling of sequential dependencies with reduced parameter complexity compared to deeper recurrent architectures.

Unlike full Transformer models applied directly to raw sequences, these hybrid designs reduce sequence length prior to attention, significantly lowering computational overhead while preserving clinically relevant temporal structure.

Overall, the architectural design reflects the multi-scale nature of sepsis progression: short-term deviations are captured by convolutions, medium-term trends by recurrent or dilated temporal modeling, and long-range interactions by attention-based aggregation.

3.3 Explainable AI Integration

Model interpretability is incorporated using SHapley Additive exPlanations (SHAP), a post hoc feature attribution method that quantifies the contribution of each input variable to the model prediction. For a prediction $y = f_\theta(X)$, SHAP decomposes the output as

$$f_\theta(X) = \phi_0 + \sum_{i=1}^{M} \phi_i, \tag{8}$$

where ϕ_i represents the marginal contribution of feature i relative to a baseline expectation. In this study, SHAP is applied to structured EHR time-series inputs, enabling feature-level interpretation across physiological variables and time steps.

For the CNN–ViT model, SHAP values are computed with respect to the final prediction output, allowing attribution of both temporal segments and clinical variables without requiring additional alignment heuristics. This design supports consistent comparison of feature importance across different model architectures.

Analysis of SHAP attributions indicates that key clinical variables, including heart rate, mean arterial pressure (MAP), respiratory rate, oxygen saturation, lactate levels, and white blood cell (WBC) count, consistently contribute to early sepsis predictions. These variables align with established clinical indicators of infection and organ dysfunction, reinforcing the clinical plausibility of the learned representations.

While attention mechanisms in Transformer-based models can highlight influential temporal regions, they are not treated as standalone explanations. Instead, SHAP serves as the primary interpretability tool, providing theoretically grounded and model-agnostic explanations.

Overall, the integration of SHAP enables identification of clinically relevant temporal patterns and supports transparent, interpretable, and deployment-oriented decision-making in ICU environments.

3.4 Efficiency Evaluation Setup

Inference latency is measured on a CPU-only environment using TensorFlow/Keras, without GPU acceleration. For each model, the total inference time is recorded over the entire test set and subsequently normalized to obtain the average per-sample latency.

All evaluations are conducted using a batch-processing approach (batch size determined automatically by the framework), reflecting practical deployment conditions where multiple patient samples may be processed efficiently in parallel.

To ensure fair comparison, all models are implemented within the same software framework and evaluated under identical hardware and runtime conditions. Therefore, observed differences in inference time primarily reflect architectural efficiency rather than implementation bias.

3.5 Evaluation Metrics

Early sepsis prediction is a highly imbalanced classification task, requiring evaluation metrics that reflect clinical priorities rather than overall class frequency. Accuracy alone is therefore insufficient, as it is dominated by the majority non-sepsis class and can obscure clinically critical failure modes [9].

Precision and recall provide complementary perspectives: precision reflects the reliability of sepsis alerts and is important for reducing alarm fatigue, while recall measures the ability to identify true sepsis cases, directly aligning with the goal of minimizing missed detections [10]. The F1-score balances these objectives and serves as a stable summary metric under class imbalance [11].

To provide a threshold-independent assessment, the Area Under the Receiver Operating Characteristic Curve (AUC) is also reported. In addition, given the class imbalance, the Area Under the Precision–Recall Curve (AUPRC) is considered to better reflect performance on the minority (sepsis) class. Where applicable, performance metrics are reported with 95% confidence intervals to assess statistical robustness and support reliable comparison between models.

In addition to predictive performance, inference latency is evaluated as a key deployment constraint. In the PhysioNet 2019 setting, predictions are generated at hourly intervals, but must be computed within clinically actionable time windows (e.g., seconds to minutes) to support timely intervention. In ICU practice, even highly accurate models have limited value if predictions cannot be delivered within such operational constraints [12].

To assess generalization, models are evaluated on a held-out test set with patient-level separation, ensuring that data from the same patient does not appear in both training and testing sets. A leave-one-unit-out cross-unit validation protocol is further employed to capture distribution shifts across ICU units, including differences in patient populations, measurement frequency, and clinical practices.

Confusion matrices are used to provide detailed insight into class-specific performance. In addition, low-dimensional visualization via Principal Component Analysis (PCA) highlights substantial overlap between early sepsis and non-sepsis trajectories, illustrating the intrinsic difficulty of the task and explaining residual classification ambiguity even for advanced models [12,13].

3.6 Baseline and Comparative Models

The comparative evaluation includes both single-mechanism and hybrid architectures to provide a balanced assessment of predictive performance and computational efficiency for structured EHR time-series data. The selected models reflect commonly used approaches in the literature while remaining compatible with deployment-oriented constraints.

Baseline models include 1D-CNN, GRU, and TCN, each capturing different temporal characteristics of ICU data. CNN-based models efficiently detect localized physiological variations but lack explicit mechanisms for long-range dependency modeling. Recurrent architectures such as GRU capture temporal evolution but may introduce higher computational cost and sequential processing constraints. TCNs extend temporal coverage through dilated convolutions, enabling efficient modeling of longer temporal contexts while maintaining parallel computation.

Hybrid architectures, including CNN–GRU and CNN–ViT, are introduced to combine local feature extraction with longer-range temporal modeling. The CNN–ViT model applies lightweight self-attention to temporally compressed convolutional representations, enabling global dependency modeling with reduced computational overhead compared to standard Transformer architectures.

Experimental results indicate that models capturing longer temporal dependencies, particularly TCN and CNN–ViT, achieve strong recall and AUC performance, highlighting the importance of extended temporal context in early sepsis detection. Among the evaluated models, TCN achieves the best overall balance between predictive performance (AUC = 0.907, recall = 0.778) and inference latency (0.62 s), while CNN–ViT provides competitive AUC (0.906) at higher computational cost.

These results demonstrate that performance gains are not solely dependent on architectural complexity, but on the ability to efficiently model temporal dependencies under practical constraints. Persistent overlap between sepsis and non-sepsis trajectories further indicates that classification performance is limited not only by model capacity but also by intrinsic physiological ambiguity in early-stage sepsis.

All models are evaluated under a consistent experimental setup. Inference latency is measured per sample under the same hardware and software configuration (specified in Section X), ensuring fair comparison of computational efficiency. Given that predictions are generated at hourly intervals, inference times on the order of seconds are considered compatible with clinically actionable decision support in ICU settings.

Table 1. Predictive performance, AUPRC, and inference latency of evaluated models (mean ± 95% CI). Accuracy is reported for completeness but interpreted cautiously due to class imbalance.

Model	Acc	Prec	Recall	F1-score	AUC	AUPRC	Time (s)
1D-CNN	0.927	0.386	0.694	0.495 ± 0.024	0.901 ± 0.012	0.42	23.57
GRU	0.931	0.334	0.744	0.467 ± 0.021	0.903 ± 0.011	0.45	1.66
TCN	**0.936**	0.361	**0.778**	**0.495** ± 0.020	**0.907** ± 0.010	**0.50**	**0.62**
CNN–ViT	0.932	0.362	0.725	0.483 ± 0.022	0.906 ± 0.011	0.47	44.34

Notes: Precision, recall, and F1-score reflect class imbalance effects. AUPRC provides a more informative measure for minority-class (sepsis) detection, where baseline performance is close to the positive class prevalence. TCN achieves the best balance between sensitivity, discrimination, and computational efficiency. CNN–ViT achieves competitive AUC and AUPRC but incurs substantially higher inference latency.

4 Results

4.1 Baseline and Comparative Models

Table 1 summarizes the predictive performance and inference latency of all evaluated models. Although accuracy is reported for completeness, it is interpreted cautiously due to the strong class imbalance, where non-sepsis samples dominate. Consequently, recall, precision, F1-score, AUC, and AUPRC provide more clinically meaningful indicators of early sepsis detection performance.

Across all models, high accuracy values (above 0.92) primarily reflect correct classification of the majority class. More informative distinctions emerge when considering recall and precision. In particular, recall highlights the ability to detect true sepsis cases, while precision reflects the reliability of alerts and the potential to mitigate alarm fatigue. The F1-score provides a balanced summary of these competing objectives.

Among all architectures, the Temporal Convolutional Network (TCN) achieves the best overall balance between predictive performance and computational efficiency. TCN attains the highest recall (0.778), highest AUPRC (0.50), and top AUC (0.907), while achieving a tied-best F1-score (0.495). These results indicate strong discrimination of the minority (sepsis) class. In addition, TCN exhibits the lowest inference latency (0.62 s per sample), making it well suited for ICU deployment where predictions are generated at hourly intervals but must be computed within clinically actionable time windows (e.g., seconds to minutes).

The GRU model achieves competitive recall (0.744) and moderate AUPRC performance (0.45), but incurs higher inference latency due to sequential processing. The 1D-CNN model achieves comparable F1-score (0.495) and reasonable AUPRC (0.42), but shows substantially higher inference time in our implementation. This discrepancy likely reflects differences in model configuration, sequence length, and execution environment, underscoring the importance of reporting implementation details for fair efficiency comparisons.

The CNN–ViT hybrid model achieves competitive predictive performance (AUC = 0.906, F1-score = 0.483) and strong AUPRC (0.47), demonstrating its ability to capture global temporal dependencies. However, its substantially higher inference latency (44.34 s per sample) limits its suitability for time-constrained deployment. Instead, CNN–ViT is better interpreted as a high-capacity reference model that supports interpretability through attention mechanisms.

Across all models, AUPRC values (0.42–0.50) are substantially higher than the baseline prevalence of sepsis, confirming effective discrimination of the minority class despite severe imbalance. Nevertheless, recall remains consistently lower than accuracy, highlighting the inherent difficulty of early sepsis detection due to overlapping physiological patterns and class imbalance.

Performance metrics are reported with 95% confidence intervals (see Table 1) to quantify statistical variability and support reliable comparison between models. Results are obtained using a held-out test set with patient-level separation, ensuring no overlap of patient records between training and testing data. Additional leave-one-unit-out validation confirms that performance trends remain consistent under distribution shifts across ICU units.

The confusion matrix of the best-performing model (Fig. 1) provides detailed insight into class-specific performance. The model correctly identifies the majority of non-sepsis and sepsis cases; however, both false positives and false negatives

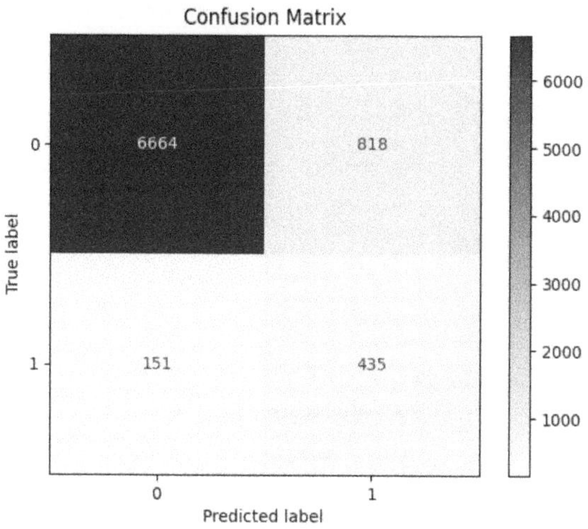

Fig. 1. Confusion matrix of the best-performing model (TCN) on the held-out test set. The model achieves high sensitivity, but false negatives remain, reflecting the intrinsic difficulty of early sepsis detection under class imbalance and overlapping physiological patterns.

remain. In particular, false negatives indicate that a subset of early sepsis cases exhibits physiological patterns similar to non-sepsis trajectories, making them difficult to distinguish.

These observations are consistent with the overall performance trends, where achieving high sensitivity remains challenging due to class imbalance and overlapping physiological signals. Confusion matrices for other models show similar patterns and are omitted for brevity.

Furthermore, the PCA visualization (Fig. 2) illustrates the distribution of learned feature representations. Although partial class separation is achieved, a substantial overlap persists near the decision boundary, highlighting the intrinsic difficulty of early sepsis detection and explaining residual classification ambiguity even for advanced architectures.

Overall, these results demonstrate that (i) accuracy alone is insufficient for evaluating early sepsis prediction, (ii) sensitivity-oriented metrics such as recall and AUPRC are critical for clinical relevance, and (iii) efficient temporal modeling, as achieved by TCN, enables a favorable balance between predictive performance and deployment feasibility.

4.2 Interpretability Analysis

Explainable AI (XAI) techniques are incorporated to enhance model transparency and support clinical trust in sepsis prediction. While the TCN achieves the best overall predictive performance in terms of accuracy, recall, F1-score, and AUC (Table 1), interpretability analysis is conducted on the CNN–ViT model.

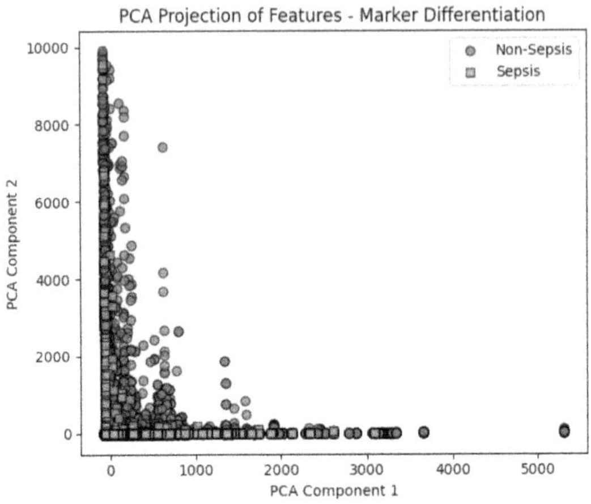

Fig. 2. PCA projection of learned representations from the CNN–ViT model onto the first two principal components. While partial separation between sepsis and non-sepsis samples is observed, substantial overlap remains, indicating limited separability and explaining residual classification errors.

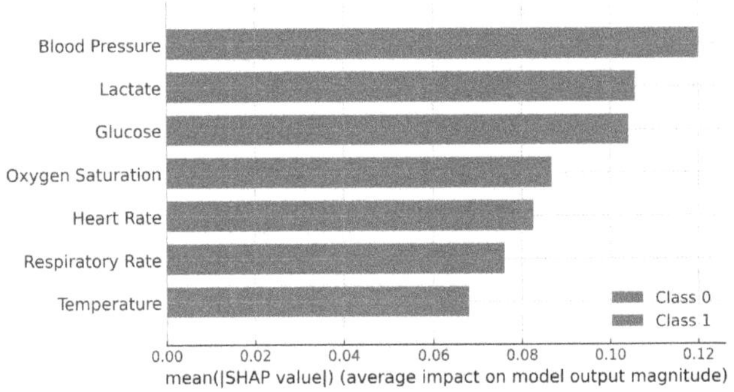

Fig. 3. SHAP summary plot for the CNN–ViT model illustrating global feature importance. Vital signs dominate the predictive contribution.

Although TCNs are effective at capturing long-range temporal dependencies through dilated convolutions, their hierarchical convolutional structure makes fine-grained, global feature attribution less straightforward. In contrast, the CNN–ViT architecture operates on explicit tokenized representations with self-attention mechanisms, which are inherently well suited for post-hoc attribution methods such as SHapley Additive exPlanations (SHAP).

Therefore, SHAP is applied to the CNN–ViT model to analyze the relative contribution of clinical features across temporal tokens, providing intuitive and clinically interpretable insights into model decision-making. This approach reflects a practical trade-off between predictive optimality and interpretability, emphasizing transparency and explanatory clarity without undermining the comparative performance analysis of the TCN.

Figure 3 presents the SHAP summary plot for CNN–ViT, highlighting the most influential clinical features contributing to sepsis prediction. Key vital signs and laboratory variables, including blood pressure, lactate, glucose, oxygen saturation, and heart rate, consistently emerge as dominant predictors. Feature values are color-coded to indicate magnitude, enabling interpretation of both importance and directional effects. Deviations from normal physiological ranges, whether elevated or suppressed, are strongly associated with increased sepsis risk, aligning well with established clinical knowledge.

To assess robustness, SHAP analyses are conducted across multiple stratified folds and leave-one-unit-out validation settings. Feature importance rankings remain stable across ICU units, indicating that learned representations are not artifacts of specific data splits. Temporal SHAP trajectories further reveal that feature contributions intensify in the hours preceding sepsis onset, supporting the role of deep temporal models as early-warning systems rather than retrospective classifiers.

While CNN–ViT does not achieve the highest predictive performance and exhibits higher inference latency, its interpretability offers valuable clinical insight into feature relevance and temporal dynamics. These findings complement the strong empirical performance and deployment efficiency of TCN, which is identified as the most suitable model for real-time clinical implementation in this study.

Table 2. Ablation study results for CNN–ViT. Performance differences are reported relative to the full model evaluated under the same test protocol as Table 1.

Ablation Scenario	F1-score	Δ F1
Full CNN–ViT	0.483	–
Without structured EHR features	0.460	−0.023
Without temporal sequences	0.455	−0.028
Without CNN backbone	0.467	−0.016
Without Transformer blocks	0.468	−0.015

4.3 Ablation Studies

Ablation experiments are conducted to analyze the contribution of individual components within the CNN–ViT architecture (Table 2). Although TCN achieves the best overall predictive performance and efficiency, this analysis focuses on understanding the internal behavior of the hybrid CNN–ViT model.

All ablated variants are evaluated under an identical experimental protocol and patient-level test set to ensure fair comparison. The full CNN–ViT configuration serves as the reference model. The F1-score is used as the primary evaluation metric due to class imbalance in early sepsis prediction.

Performance differences are defined as:

$$\Delta F1\text{-}score = F1_{\text{ablated}} - F1_{\text{full}}. \tag{9}$$

As shown in Table 2, removing temporal sequences leads to the largest performance degradation, highlighting the importance of longitudinal modeling. Removing structured EHR features also reduces performance, confirming their complementary role.

Further ablations indicate that both convolutional layers and Transformer blocks contribute meaningfully to performance. The CNN backbone captures local temporal patterns, while the Transformer component models long-range dependencies. Their combination enables effective hybrid representation learning.

Overall, the results show that CNN–ViT benefits from the synergy between convolutional feature extraction, attention-based global modeling, and structured EHR integration, even though it is not the most efficient or best-performing model in the overall comparison.

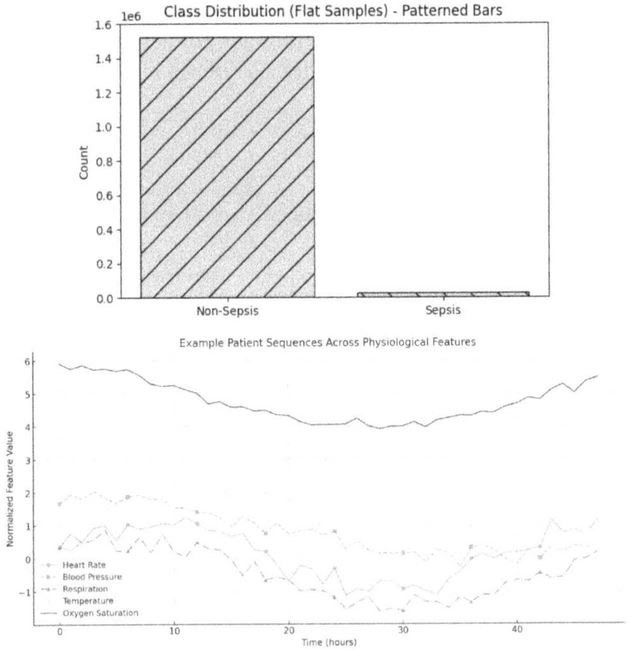

Fig. 4. Class distribution of sepsis versus non-sepsis patients (top), highlighting severe class imbalance, and example normalized physiological time-series from a representative patient (bottom), illustrating intra-patient temporal variability and inter-patient heterogeneity across vital signs.

4.4 Discussion: Data Characteristics and Learned Representations

Figure 4 highlights two key challenges in early sepsis prediction. First, the dataset exhibits strong class imbalance, where non-sepsis cases dominate the population. This imbalance limits the interpretability of accuracy and motivates the use of recall-, F1-, and AUPRC-based evaluation metrics.

Second, the example patient trajectories illustrate substantial intra-patient variability and inter-patient heterogeneity across physiological signals. Early sepsis progression is therefore not characterized by abrupt changes, but rather by subtle and time-varying deviations in multiple vital signs. This property makes the prediction task inherently challenging, particularly under the 6-hour prediction horizon considered in this study, where early physiological indicators may be weak and partially overlapping with non-sepsis patterns. This reinforces the need for models capable of capturing long-range temporal dependencies.

To better understand the structure of the learned feature space, we refer to the latent representation analysis of the CNN–ViT model presented in Fig. 2. The projected embeddings indicate improved separation between sepsis and non-sepsis cases compared to raw input space, suggesting that the model learns higher-level temporal and cross-variable interactions. However, a non-negligible overlap remains near the decision boundary, reflecting clinically ambiguous early-stage cases and partially explaining the saturation in predictive performance across models.

Although the CNN–ViT model is not the best-performing architecture in terms of efficiency or overall predictive performance, it provides a useful intermediate representation for analysis. Its hybrid design enables structured feature learning that supports both performance evaluation and interpretability analysis. In this work, it is therefore used primarily as an analytical reference model to complement the stronger deployment-oriented performance of the TCN.

5 Conclusion and Future Work

This study presented a lightweight and efficiency-aware deep learning framework for early sepsis prediction using structured Electronic Health Record (EHR) time-series data. The primary objective is to model clinically meaningful temporal dynamics under severe class imbalance while maintaining computational efficiency suitable for time-sensitive ICU environments. The prediction task is defined at a 6-h horizon prior to sepsis onset, reflecting a clinically actionable early-warning window consistent with the PhysioNet 2019 benchmark.

Across all evaluated methods, results consistently demonstrate that modeling temporal dependencies is critical for early sepsis detection. Architectures capable of capturing longer-range temporal structure outperform those relying solely on local feature extraction or short-term temporal modeling. This confirms that early sepsis progression is better characterized by gradual physiological deterioration rather than abrupt changes, particularly when predictions are required several hours before clinical onset.

Among all compared models, the Temporal Convolutional Network (TCN) demonstrates the most favorable trade-off between predictive performance and computational efficiency. It achieves the highest recall, F1-score (tied), AUC, and AUPRC, indicating strong and consistent discrimination of the minority (sepsis) class. Notably, TCN also records the lowest inference latency under a CPU-based evaluation setting, highlighting its efficiency even without hardware acceleration. This combination of high sensitivity and low computational overhead makes TCN particularly well suited for real-time clinical decision support in intensive care environments, where timely and reliable predictions are critical.

In contrast, hybrid architectures such as CNN–ViT provide complementary insights into representation learning. While not the best-performing model in terms of efficiency or deployment suitability, CNN–ViT captures structured temporal dependencies through the combination of convolutional feature extraction and attention-based modeling. Its learned representations demonstrate improved separability compared to raw input space, making it valuable for interpretability and ablation analysis rather than primary deployment.

Interpretability analysis using SHAP further confirms that model predictions are strongly influenced by clinically established biomarkers, including heart rate, blood pressure, oxygen saturation, and lactate levels. These findings align with known physiological indicators of sepsis and support the clinical validity of the learned models. In addition, ablation studies demonstrate that removing either structured EHR features or waveform signals consistently degrades performance, confirming the importance of temporal and multivariate information.

Several limitations should be acknowledged. First, the retrospective nature of the dataset may limit external generalizability across institutions and ICU protocols. Second, despite strong overall discriminative performance, precision remains constrained by class imbalance, which is a known challenge in early sepsis prediction. Third, while the proposed TCN model is computationally efficient, deployment in real ICU systems still requires careful validation under real hardware and streaming constraints. In addition, the fixed 6-hour prediction horizon may not capture all clinically relevant scenarios, and evaluating multiple prediction horizons remains an important direction for future work.

Future work will focus on improving robustness and clinical applicability. This includes exploring more efficient multimodal fusion strategies, such as lightweight cross-modal attention and hierarchical temporal modeling. Additional data modalities, including laboratory trajectories, medication records, and clinical notes, may further enhance predictive performance. Moreover, uncertainty-aware and calibration-aware modeling techniques will be investigated to improve reliability in high-stakes clinical environments.

In summary, this work demonstrates that lightweight temporal modeling using TCN provides an effective and clinically meaningful solution for early sepsis prediction, achieving a strong balance between predictive accuracy, interpretability, and computational efficiency.

Acknowledgments. This work was partly supported by 6G Flagship (Grant Number 369116) funded by the Research Council of Finland.

References

1. Islam, K.R., et al.: Machine learning-based early prediction of sepsis using electronic health records: a systematic review. J. Clin. Med. **12**(17), pp. 1–29 (2023). https://doi.org/10.3390/jcm12175658
2. Shashikumar, S.P., et al.: Early sepsis detection in critical care patients using multiscale blood pressure and heart rate dynamics. J. Electrocardiol. **50**(6), 739–743 (2017). https://doi.org/10.1016/j.jelectrocard.2017.08.013
3. Yang, Z., Cui, X., Song, Z.: Predicting sepsis onset in ICU using machine learning models: a systematic review and meta-analysis. BMC Infect. Dis. **23**(1), 1–21 (2023). https://doi.org/10.1186/s12879-023-08614-0
4. Desautels, T., et al.: Prediction of sepsis in the intensive care unit with minimal electronic health record data: a machine learning approach. JMIR Med. Inform. **4**(3), e28 (2016). https://doi.org/10.2196/medinform.5909
5. Diwan, S., Gandhi, V., Baidya Kayal, E., Khanna, P., Mehndiratta, A.: Explainable machine learning models for mortality prediction in patients with sepsis in tertiary care hospital ICU in low- to middle-income countries. Intensive Care Med. Exp. **13**(1), 1–13 (2025). https://doi.org/10.1186/s40635-025-00765-5
6. Vagliano, I., et al.: Prognostic models of in-hospital mortality of intensive care patients using neural representation of unstructured text: a systematic review and critical appraisal. J. Biomed. Inform. **146**, 1–11, 104504 (2023). https://doi.org/10.1016/j.jbi.2023.104504
7. Shickel, B., Tighe, P.J., Bihorac, A., Rashidi, P.: Deep EHR: a survey of recent advances in deep learning techniques for electronic health record analysis. IEEE J. Biomed. Health Inform. **22**(5), 1589–1604 (2018). https://doi.org/10.1109/JBHI.2017.2767063
8. Reyna, M.A., et al.: Early prediction of sepsis from clinical data: the PhysioNet/computing in cardiology challenge 2019. Crit. Care Med. **48**(2), 210–217 (2020). https://doi.org/10.1097/CCM.0000000000004145
9. Rainio, O., Teuho, J., Klén, R.: Evaluation metrics and statistical tests for machine learning. Sci. Rep. **14**, 6086 (2024). https://doi.org/10.1038/s41598-024-56706-x
10. Sokolova, M., Lapalme, G.: A systematic analysis of performance measures for classification tasks. Inf. Process. Manage. **45**(4), 427–437 (2009). https://doi.org/10.1016/j.ipm.2009.03.002
11. Christen, P., Hand, D.J., Kirielle, N.: A review of the F-measure: its history, properties, criticism, and alternatives. ACM Comput. Surv. **56**(3), 1–24 (2023). https://doi.org/10.1145/3606367. Article 73
12. Muşat, F., et al.: Machine learning models in sepsis outcome prediction for ICU patients: integrating routine laboratory tests—a systematic review. Biomedicines **12**(12), 2892 (2024). https://doi.org/10.3390/biomedicines12122892
13. Rao, R.S., Dewangan, S., Mishra, A., Gupta, M.: A study of dealing class imbalance problem with machine learning methods for code smell severity detection using PCA-based feature selection technique. Sci. Rep. **13**, 16245 (2023). https://doi.org/10.1038/s41598-023-43380-8

Attitudes Towards Workplace Data Collection Among Factory Workers: Results from a Finnish Survey

Milla Immonen[1,2], Satu-Marja Mäkelä[2], Eija Kaasinen[2], Elina Annanperä[3], Anna Rohunen[3], Kari Hiekkanen[4], Anu-Hanna Anttila[5], and Pekka Siirtola[3](✉)

[1] Lapland University of Applied Sciences, Jokiväylä 11 C, 96300 Rovaniemi, Finland
milla.immonen@lapinamk.fi
[2] VTT Technical Research Centre of Finland, Kaitoväylä 1, P.O. Box 1100, 90571 Oulu, Finland
{milla.immonen,satu-marja.makela,eija.kaasinen}@vtt.fi
[3] University of Oulu, P.O. Box 8000, 90014 Oulu, Finland
{elina.annanpera,anna.rohunen,pekka.siirtola}@oulu.fi
[4] Haaga Helia University of Applied Sciences, Ratapihantie 13, 00520 Helsinki, Finland
kari.hiekkanen@haaga-helia.fi
[5] Finnish Industrial Union, Hakaniemenranta 1A, P.O. Box 107, 00531 Helsinki, Finland
anu-hanna.anttila@teollisuusliitto.fi

Abstract. This study examines the attitudes of factory workers' towards the collection and use of data on the factory floor to support worker well-being. The study is based on a survey of 385 members of The Finnish Industrial Union who work as shop stewards or labor protection representatives. The survey was adapted from earlier study conducted for construction site workers [20]. Developing data-intensive solutions to improve work conditions, such as well-being and safety, requires increasing amounts of data collected from workers. The results of the study show that, in general, workers have positive attitudes towards collecting data on the factory floor. Workers are interested in their personal well-being and would like to obtain information about their physical strain, ergonomics, and emotional stress. However, respondents had concerns about unauthorized access to the data or the use of the information against them by the employer or colleagues. No statistically significant correlation was found between attitudes and work experience in years. The study suggests that involving workers in the decision-making process regarding data use is essential to increase acceptance. The study concludes that the introduction of new data-based technologies in factories requires open communication with workers, including clear explanations of the purposes of data collection and how the data will be used.

Keywords: Factory work · well-being · data collection · factory floor · data-based technologies · acceptance

Eija Kaasinen—Retired.

M. Särestöniemi et al. (Eds.): NCDHWS 2026, CCIS 3010, pp. 245–262, 2026.
https://doi.org/10.1007/978-3-032-28819-6_16

1 Introduction

Industry 4.0 transformation is expected to qualitatively enrich factory work by providing a more interesting working environment, greater autonomy, and increased opportunities for self-development [1]. Smart factories aim to adapt to workers with different skills, capabilities, and preferences [2]. Industry 5.0 complements the techno-economic vision of the Industry 4.0 paradigm by emphasizing the societal role of industry. It calls for human-centric solutions that adapt production processes to the needs of the worker, compensating for physical and cognitive capacity throughout the entire work career [3]. As IoT and current AI trends converge, IoT data is now more important than ever, with the rising utilisation of AI solutions. AI transforms sensor data from connected devices into autonomous real-time decisions in real - time that make systems more efficient, predictive, and personalized, thereby optimizing operations, maintenance, and productivity.

To adapt smart factories and work tasks to the needs of individual workers, relevant and up-to-date information is required from each worker. This creates a growing need to monitor, collect, and analyze worker-related data. The concept of a human digital twin has been introduced to collect and represent worker data for various purposes. Digital twin systems incorporating human elements have been used, for example, to ensure safe human movement around robots [4], to enhance operator safety in process plants [5], and to coordinate robot assembly tasks alongside humans [6]. Contemporary worker model concepts target an increasingly broad set of personal information and capabilities, such as workload and task history data, which are collected to determine factors like worker fatigue [7–9] or mental workload [10].

Beyond personal information and capabilities, worker data have also been used to capture implicit knowledge related to task execution. Examples include linking virtual tasks to their physical counterparts through motion capture [11], the use of interactive tool digital twins [12], and human digital twins that negotiate with workstation digital twins to determine whether the requirements of the worker and the workstation are aligned [13]. These solutions have the potential to enhance worker comfort and productivity and to provide digital training opportunities for novice workers. Consequently, modeling human well-being, including ergonomic aspects, must be taken into account in the future development of workforce planning systems [14].

Early research on human digital twins was based on the idea that employee properties need to be constructed using profiles, preferences, or recorded behavioral patterns creating a digital model of human attributes, i.e., a digital representation of the individual person [14–17]. Since then, research has moved towards the use of data from company databases, related to the manufacturing process, and the monitoring of workers' activities, movements, and physiological phenomena using wearables and environmental sensors to obtain feedback and characterize both workers and tasks of work [18,19].

Despite the potential benefits [2,20], measuring workers and maintaining worker digital twins remain highly sensitive issues due to multiple ethical concerns. If self-tracking at work is proposed by an employer, it may become a form of pushed self-tracking, which can be difficult to refuse and may involve risks of exclusion or stigmatization when opting out [21,22]. Although workers should be given the opportunity to define what information is collected from them, an excessive number of choices may increase stress and complicate the adoption of new technologies [23]. Solutions that monitor workers' well-being and/or work performance should therefore be voluntary [23,24]. Particular attention should be paid to providing positive and encouraging feedback [25]. Data protection and ethical challenges must be addressed at both societal and workplace levels in order to establish ethically sound conditions for data use [24]. For instance, [20] indicates that construction site workers are willing to use wearables and hold positive attitudes toward sharing data to improve occupational safety.

Artificial intelligence (AI)-based solutions provide new opportunities to analyze worker digital twin data and factory process data to gain insights related to well-being, occupational safety, and production efficiency. Recent work has also explored AI-driven human digital twins that integrate heterogeneous data streams and support higher-level interpretation and interaction, for example through large language modelâĂŞbased digital twin architectures [26]. However, the adoption of such technologies also raises concerns among workers. Del Giudice et al. examined employees' acceptance of AI in organizations [27] and found that acceptance is closely linked to general attitudes toward technology, which are influenced by personal traits such as rational, emotional, and cognitive dimensions. Furthermore, an organizational culture that supports technological adoption and automation can reduce employee concerns and improve acceptance through re-skilling and up-skilling of competencies and knowledge. Similar findings were reported by Rueckert et al., who studied the acceptance of AI in production environments [28]. They emphasized the importance of up-skilling and knowledge sharing and noted that employee involvement from the early stages of technology adoption, consideration of individual needs, and transparent communication about opportunities and risks are essential for maximizing acceptance. Several studies also suggest that when the purpose of data collection is clearly defined, properly explained, and perceived as meaningful–particularly in relation to safety—employees are more willing to participate in data collection and share their data [29,30].

Despite the growing body of research on worker digital twins, IoT-based monitoring, and AI adoption in industrial environments, there is still limited empirical evidence on how factory-floor employees perceive the collection and use of worker-related data.

This article focuses on examining factory workers' attitudes and acceptance toward data-intensive solutions, including the collection of IoT- and well-being-related data on the factory floor and their use for enhancing work organization, ergonomics, occupational safety, and well-being. Shop stewards and labor protection representatives responded to the survey from their professional roles, which provide a broader and more general perspective than that of individual workers. In addition, this study aims to identify factors that promote the adoption of data-based technologies. The findings contribute to the design and implementation of data-driven services for factory environments. One example of such services is the AI Foreman concept, which was studied in parallel with this digital survey. The AI Foreman is an automated assistant for production planning and scheduling in factory environments, utilizing workers' personal data such as competencies, personal preferences, and health and well-being status [37]. Additionally, data-based solutions can be developed to support factory workers' well-being, for example by managing workload or improving work ergonomics.

2 Material and Methods

An anonymous digital survey was conducted in June 2020 in Finland and the invitation with a link to the digital survey was sent via e-mail to shop stewards and labor protection representatives of The Finnish Industrial Union. The number of recipients on the mailing list was 2022. The recipients were reminded once to complete the survey. Participation was voluntary.

The survey included multiple choice questions as well as open text field questions. To ensure respondent anonymity, the survey did not include any personal or identifiable questions. For this reason, variables such as educational or social status were intentionally excluded from the questionnaire.

The research group designed the digital survey to focus on wearables and the utilization of personal data in industrial work. The survey had a partially similar structure to earlier survey for construction site workers [20], but was adapted to support needs of this study. In addition, the survey items were designed to align with data intensive use cases relevant to the AI Foreman concept and were informed by privacy calculus thinking, in which individuals weigh potential benefits against perceived risks when considering the disclosure of personal data [31]. In this study, potential benefits included improvements in occupational safety, ergonomics, and work conditions, while risk related items captured privacy concerns as well as possible disruptions to work tasks caused by data collection.

The survey covered questions related to attitudes and acceptance toward data-intensive new solutions and collecting IoT and well-being data on the factory floor and their utilization to improve the work circulation, ergonomics, work safety and well-being. The survey was carried out in Finland, where the official and most used languages are Finnish and Swedish. The original survey was written in Finnish and was translated by a professional translator into Swedish. The respondents were allowed to choose the language they prefer. The recipients of the survey e-mail were informed in the cover letter, that the aim of the survey is to obtain information about workers' perspectives in utilizing data collected with smart devices and sensors in the factory floor. The survey included questions related to background of the respondents (items 1–4), work characteristics (items 5–7), experiences of data-collection devices (items 8–10), interest in utilizing information collected by different devices (item 11) and willingness to share data to employer, third party (such as occupational healthcare) or automatic work planning (item 12–14), wishes for receiving information about work and well-being during the workday (items 15–16) and worries of misuse of information (item 17). The survey items are described in more detail in Appendix Table 3.

The survey included several types of response options depending on the nature of each item. In most Likert-type statements, a neutral midpoint option (e.g., 'no significance for me' or 'neither agree nor disagree') was placed at the center of the response scale (items 6, 11a-d, 12, 12a-d). In addition, some items included the option 'I don't know', which was intentionally positioned outside the main response scale to distinguish uncertainty from neutrality (items 12, 12a-d, 13, 14, 15, 15a-b, 17, 17a-d). Items 12 and 12aâĂŞd included both a neutral option and an 'I don't know' option to ensure that the neutral choice reflected an actual midpoint in the respondent's attitude, while uncertainty or lack of knowledge could be expressed separately. For the statistical analyses, neutral midpoint responses were treated as valid scale values, whereas 'I don't know' responses were excluded from analyses in cases where they could not be interpreted as a meaningful position on the underlying attitude dimension.

The analysis of both the quantitative and qualitative questions was performed with quantitative analytics methods. SPSS was used for statistical analysis. The analysis methods included descriptive statistical analysis and calculating mean, standard deviation, and median of responses in the survey. For those questions that the "I don't know" -option cannot be interpreted as a neutral response, the statistical analyses were performed by excluding responses with that selection. The correlation between work experience in years and attitude was studied using Spearman correlation analysis. The responses to the open ended questions were analyzed by quantifying their content. Two researchers independently categorized all open ended responses based on their thematic content, assigning each response up to two categories, a primary and a secondary theme. The researchers then compared and harmonized their categorizations, which showed a high degree of agreement. Finally, the number of responses within each category was summed.

3 Results

Altogether 358 shop stewards and labor protection representatives of The Finnish Industrial Union (response rate 19%) answered the survey. The response rate was (19%), which is considered good for this type of digital survey. The characteristics of the respondents are shown in Table 1, the items are described in more detail in Appendix Table 3. Large majority of the participants responded as being employed (98.3%) and three thirds of the respondents (77.1%) worked in regular day shift when answering the survey. Industrial fields of manufacture of fabricated metal products and manufacturing of machinery and equipment were well presented among the respondents and most of the respondents had worked over 10 years. Because all invited participants were members of the same industrial union and worked in comparable occupational roles, it is likely that the non-respondents shared broadly similar demographic and work-related characteristics with the respondents. However, as no direct data are available for the non-respondents, potential differences cannot be fully ruled out.

Altogether 21 respondents wrote additional details to the open field question about the questions related to employment status, work circumstances, and workload. Seven respondents wrote that competence development or having an education or training is not possible or prohibited at their workplaces. One respondent commented that competence development is allowed in their workplace. Five comments dealt with the lack of work circulation, but one respondent mentioned that there is a successful work circulation in their workplace. Two comments were about hurry at work, one about poor leadership and one about poor communication. Two respondents wanted to explain that their comments are from the perspective of their roles as shop stewards and labor protection representatives and one explained that they had responded from the perspective of a worker, even though they are a shop steward. Three respondents gave more specific information about workload from their personal perspective.

Technology Use and Data Sharing
Nearly half of the respondents currently use technologies for measuring their well-being. Activity wristband, smart ring, smart phone, or heart rate sensor was used for measuring movement or physical functions by 48.9% and for measuring sleep by 22.9% of the respondents, items 8a -8b. Altogether 47.5% responded that they had used an activity wristband, a smart ring, a smart phone, or a heart rate sensor during the workdays for measuring movement or physical functions, item 9. More than half of the respondents thought that the information gathered by activity wristband, smart ring, smart phone, or heart rate sensor is reliable, item 10; fully reliable (1.7%) or somewhat reliable (54.2%). Neutral attitude was responded by 17.9% participants (not reliable and not unreliable). Of the participants, 5.9% thought that the information gathered with the technologies is rather unreliable and 0.3% fully unreliable. Fifth of the participants (20.1%) responded that they don't know or that they don't have experience of the reliability aspect. Interest in utilizing information collected from the work environment during the working day was positive towards wearables, environmental and movement sensors, but negative towards cameras, see Fig. 1 for more details.

Majority of the respondents agreed or somewhat agreed to giving access to data to the employer to be able to improve occupational safety, identify individual health risks, diversify workload, and plan work tasks, more details are shown in Fig. 2. However, more than half of the respondents expressed their concern that their employer or coworkers might use the collected information against them, that the employer might learn private or sensitive information about the employees, or that someone might gain an unauthorized access to data. Majority of the respondents were not worried about data collection disturbing their work, see Fig. 3.

Giving access to data for a third party, such as occupational health care, who would not pass the information further to the employer, would be acceptable to

Table 1. Employment status, work circumstances and workload, items 1–7

Characteristic	Category	Amount	Percentage
Employment	Employed	352	98.3%
	Laid off	5	1.4%
	Unemployed	1	0.3%
Work shifts	Regular day work	276	77.1%
	Two shifts	64	17.9%
	Three shifts	18	5.0%
	Regular evening work	0	0.0%
	Regular night work	0	0.0%
	Regular weekend work	0	0.0%
Field of industry	Manufacturing of fabricated metal products	140	39.1%
	Manufacturing of machinery and equipment	74	20.7%
	Electrical and electronics industry	41	11.5%
	Service and maintenance	31	8.7%
	Metal processing	15	4.2%
	Manufacture of transport equipment	12	3.4%
	Foundry industry	8	2.2%
	Sheet metal and industrial insulation	6	1.7%
	Mining industry	2	0.6%
	Other	29	8.1%
Experience in the current field	0–4 years	9	2.5%
	5–9 years	25	7.0%
	10–19 years	127	35.5%
	20–29 years	125	34.9%
	Over 30 years	72	20.1%
Factors affecting workload	Physical	276	77.1%
	Safety	145	40.5%
	Work-related	215	60.1%
	Interaction	182	50.8%
	Worktime	72	20.1%
Able to develop own skills at work	Fully disagree	16	4.5%
	Somewhat disagree	87	24.3%
	Neither agree nor disagree	56	15.6%
	Somewhat agree	168	46.9%
	Fully agree	31	8.7%
Appropriate task rotation	Fully disagree	15	4.2%
	Somewhat disagree	69	19.3%
	Neither agree nor disagree	48	13.4%
	Somewhat agree	174	48.6%
	Fully agree	52	14.5%

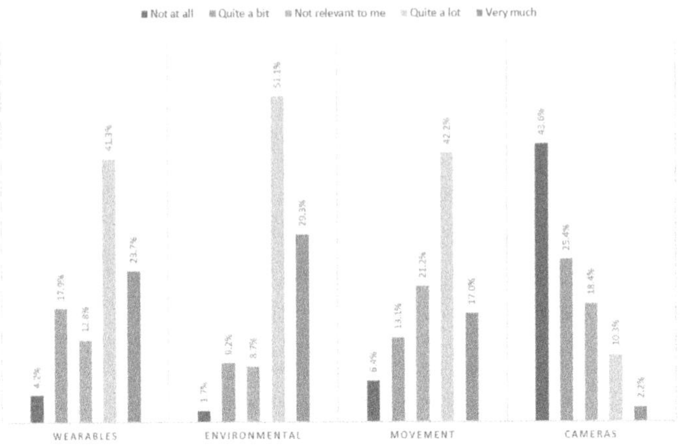

Fig. 1. Interest in utilizing information collected by different device, items 11a–d.

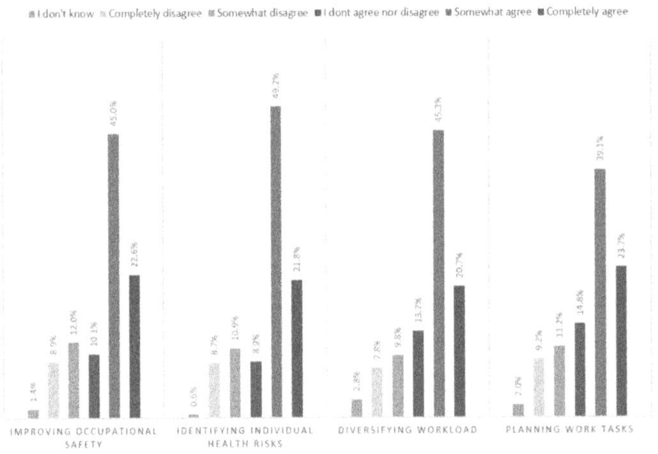

Fig. 2. Willingness to share data to employer, third body or automatic work planning, items 12a–d.

68.4% of the respondents, would not be acceptable to 14.0%, and 17.6% were not able to tell their opinion to the question, item 13. In addition, more than half of the respondents (57%) would allow access to data for enabling automatic work planning, if it would enhance work-related matters (hurry, goals, amount of work), 60.6% if it would enhance interaction and 57.8% if it would enhance work time planning. Respectively, about fifth of the respondents would not allow using the data for these purposes and about fifth answered "I don't know", see Fig. 4.

Most respondents answered that seeing measured information of themselves during the workday somewhat interest them (59%) and interest a lot (22.9%). If the measured information would be combined with measured information from

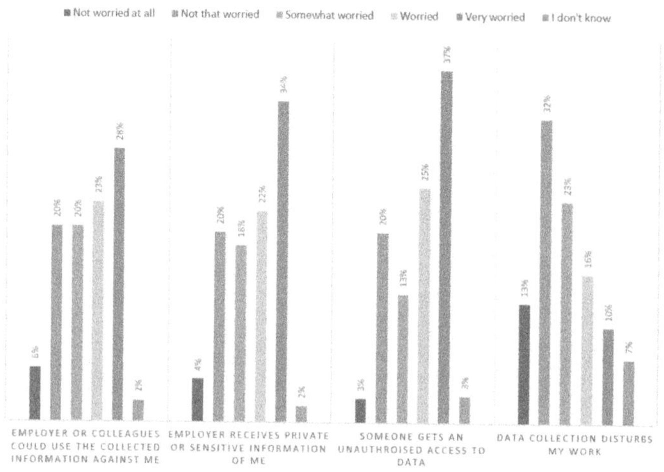

Fig. 3. Worries of misuse of information from physical functions, item 17a–d.

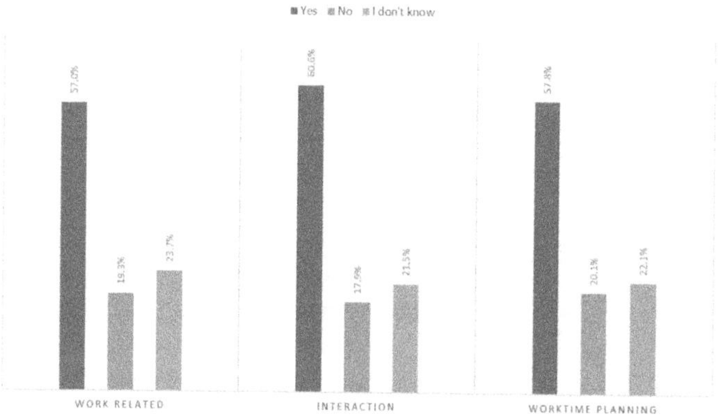

Fig. 4. Willingness to share collected data for automatic work planning, item 14.

free time the respondents' answered somewhat interest them (54%) and interest a lot (26.5%), see Fig. 5. Figure 6 shows respondents' selections to question "What kind of information would you like to see during the workday?". Most of the respondents would like to be informed about unergonomic working postures and physical strain, as well as emotional stress.

Spearman correlation analysis didn't show statistically significant correlation ($p<.005$) between work experience and attitudes of interest using technology during the day, giving access to data to employer or worries against utilizing data collected from physical functions during the workday, the results are shown in Table 2.

Altogether, 33 respondents wrote a comment to the open field at the end of the survey. Over one third of the comments (12) included concerns of misuse

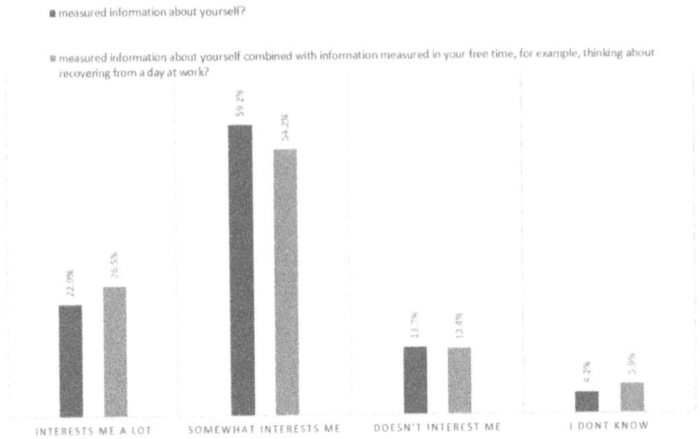

Fig. 5. Interested of seeing measured information during the workday and combined with measured information from free time, items 15a–b.

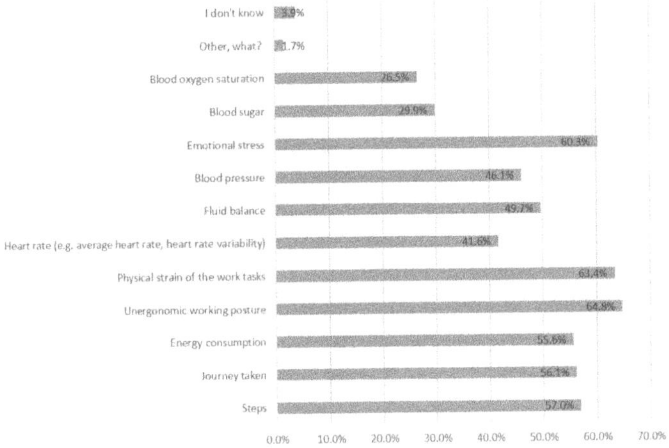

Fig. 6. Interest to see specific information related to well-being during the work shift, item 16.

data collected at workplace, and nearly as many (9) about privacy concerns. Three of the comments mentioned that the data should be only accessible by occupational health or other similar third party. Furthermore, three comments mentioned that the workers should be able to define, who can access their data. Two comments referred to Orwell's 1984. Additionally, there were six participants who were willing to prohibit using sensors or cameras for measuring workers. Five participants wanted to clarify the workload or working circumstances at their workplaces. Four comments included experiences from previous measurements at work and one comment gave feedback about the survey and hoped that this survey helps enhancing the work circumstances.

Table 2. Relationships between work experience and attitudes towards technology use and data sharing

Item	fN	Correlation coefficient	Significance
Correlation between work experience and interest in using technologies during the workday			
Wearables	312	−0.124	0.019
Environmental sensors	327	−0.132	0.017
Movement sensors	282	−0.072	0.225
Cameras	292	−0.045	0.449
Correlation between work experience and giving access to data to the employer			
Safety	353	−0.020	0.709
Personal health risks	356	0.020	0.707
Adjusting workload	348	0.013	0.811
Work planning	351	−0.008	0.881
Correlation between work experience and worries about utilizing data collected from physical functions during the workday			
Employer using information against me	350	0.035	0.512
Employer could obtain private or sensitive information	352	0.006	0.908
Unauthorized access to my data	348	−0.040	0.461
Data collection disturbs my work	334	−0.051	0.353

4 Discussion and Conclusion

This study provides a novel contribution by offering a systematic examination of factory-floor data practices from the viewpoint of shop stewards and labor protection representatives. This perspective has been largely overlooked in prior research, which has predominantly focused on individual employees or technical implementations of data-intensive solutions. By capturing the attitudes of worker representatives, who formally negotiate and oversee data related practices in industrial environments, the study extends current knowledge on the organizational, ethical, and social conditions that shape the acceptance of worker related data collection.

The study examined the attitudes of shop stewards and labor protection representatives of the Finnish Industrial Union toward collecting data on the factory floor and utilizing such data to improve work-related well-being. In summary, the survey revealed four main findings. First, shop stewards and labor protection representatives generally expressed positive attitudes toward factory-floor data collection, with the notable exception of camera-based monitoring. Second, acceptance of data use increased when the purpose was clearly connected to well-being, safety, or health-related improvements, and was lower when the data were associated with performance monitoring or work organization. Third, respondents emphasized concerns related to privacy, unauthorized access, and potential misuse, while also highlighting the importance of transparency and clear communication. Fourth, interest in using technology and willingness to share data were not associated with years of work experience, indicating that attitudes were relatively consistent across experience levels.

These findings indicate that union representatives generally hold favorable attitudes toward worker-related data collection, except in the case of camera-based monitoring. Nearly half of the respondents were already using personal devices to track their own well-being, and more than half viewed the information from wearable devices as reliable—although a substantial minority selected the neutral option, suggesting uncertainty about the accuracy of such data. When asked to consider a hypothetical scenario in which collected worker data would be used to enhance occupational safety, identify individual health risks, or improve working conditions, most respondents were willing to grant employers access to the data. At the same time, they expressed strong concerns about unauthorized access and the potential misuse of information by employers or colleagues, as reflected also in the open-ended responses. Acceptance was higher for data access by third parties, such as occupational healthcare services, and for automatic work-planning systems, although the relatively high number of "I don't know" responses suggests that these roles may be difficult to conceptualize or require further clarification.

Overall, the results indicate that workers are interested in receiving feedback on their well-being, including information on physical strain, ergonomics, and emotional stress. Importantly, work experience did not appear to influence attitudes toward technology use or data sharing. Privacy concerns, however, were prevalent across respondents and were reinforced by themes emerging from the open-ended responses.

Privacy concerns were prevalent among respondents, and these were confirmed by the open-ended responses. Similar privacy-related concerns regarding worker monitoring have been identified in previous studies [20,32]. Transparency and trust in data collection systems are key approaches for addressing these concerns. Individuals contributing to the data should have access to aggregated views of their data and clear information about how it is used. In addition, user interfaces should be designed to support trust by being intuitive and by clearly explaining how data are interpreted and applied [33,34].

Jacobs et al. examined the acceptance of wearable use cases in the workplace and found that use cases focusing on safety, with data collection limited strictly to work-related contexts, achieved the highest acceptance. In contrast, tracking information during and outside of work to improve productivity received the lowest acceptance [29], which aligns with the findings of this study. Tailoring AI-based systems to the anticipated user group is also important for achieving higher acceptance [35]. Furthermore, le Feber et al. emphasized that all individuals affected by workplace sensors or data collection should be involved in decision-making processes [30].

The findings of this study are also consistent with earlier research on Finnish construction site workers [20]. Interest in using technology during the workday was generally high, except for camera-based technologies. Similarly, acceptance of data sharing was higher when the purpose was related to well-being or occupational safety than when it involved work organization. Measurements related to work performance may be associated with productivity, efficiency, and monitoring of performance, which are particularly sensitive topics for workers. Therefore, communication between employers and employees should be open and transparent regarding work-related measurements and the development of new applications to avoid misunderstandings and unnecessary barriers.

Data-intensive solutions are rapidly evolving into AI-enabled applications. In industrial environments, the effectiveness of AI relies on both the availability and quality of shared data. Developing next-generation solutions, such as those aimed at enhancing well-being and safety, requires the aggregation of data collected from workers. This approach aligns with the human-centric ideals of Industry 5.0 and necessitates the collection and sharing of measured worker data.

Employees' acceptance of data sharing, AI and related techonologies depends largely on their individual attitudes toward technology, which are influenced by personal traits such as rational, emotional, and cognitive dimensions [27]. Braganza et al. conducted a survey in West London, UK, and found that AI adoption weakens the positive relationship between psychological contracts and job engagement, while having no significant impact on employees' trust in their employer [36]. Rueckert et al. highlighted the importance of informing employees about the opportunities and risks associated with AI and involving them from the early stages of introducing disruptive technologies [28]. They also emphasized the need to involve all organizational levels in AI development at an early stage [28].

AI-based systems for worker management, such as the aforementioned AI Foreman [37], may incorporate gamified features, including rewards, to improve productivity and employee satisfaction. Such systems can also support decision-making, people analytics, and occupational health and safety. However, the use of AI in worker management may also lead to risks such as dehumanization, nudging practices, and the datafication of the workplace, potentially limiting workers' autonomy, privacy, and creativity [38]. It has also been suggested that AI may lead to "gigification", whereby remaining jobs in supply chains acquire characteristics of gig work [39]. As AI-driven decision-making systems become increasingly common, it is essential that data representing factory workers are presented in diverse and balanced ways. At the same time, the use of worker-generated data must always be designed in an ethical and unbiased manner, with the goal of improving working conditions rather than contributing to dehumanization.

This AI-based application design can be guided by addressing ethical questions, assessing the ethical impacts of information technology [22,40], identifying and responding to the values of target users [41], or adhering to established ethical guidelines and principles [42,43]. An ethics-by-design approach ensures that ethical issues are identified early in the development process and that the focus remains on creating ethically sound solutions from the outset, rather than addressing problems retrospectively [43].

Introducing new technologies in factory environments requires open communication with workers, including clear explanations of the purposes of data collection, how the data are used, by whom, and what benefits may be achieved. Workers' rights to participate in decisions regarding data use must be respected, and data collection should not distract workers or disrupt workflows. At the same time, the appropriate use of data can offer significant benefits to workers, including improvements in overall well-being and well-being at work.

This study has several limitations. The digital survey was distributed to shop stewards and labor protection representatives of the Finnish Industrial Union, whose perspectives may differ from those of individual factory workers, and who may also view workplace data practices more critically due to their participation in workplace disputes and personnel issues. In addition, individuals in these roles are typically more aware of regulations and ethical considerations related to workers' rights. Information on the educational or social background of the respondents was not collected to maintain anonymity, and therefore potential biases arising from such differences could not be assessed. Finland is considered a high-trust society, where citizens generally trust the parliamentary and legal system [44], and where the role of worker unions has historically been strong in traditional industries. The study was conducted during the COVID-19 pandemic; although infection rates in Finland were relatively low at the time, the pandemic may nevertheless have influenced industrial employment and lay-offs.

Finally, it should be noted that workers' attitudes toward data collection are not the sole consideration, as such practices are also regulated by law. In the context of this study, relevant regulations include the EU General Data Protection Regulation (GDPR), national data protection legislation, and the Finnish Act on the Protection of Privacy in Working Life. While the GDPR establishes important safeguards for the protection of personal data and employees' rights, it does not automatically generate trust. Regulatory frameworks are necessary to protect employees in their subordinate position relative to employers and to minimize the risk of data misuse. Therefore, before applying the findings of this study in practice, the challenges associated with legislative requirements must also be carefully considered.

Our findings also connect directly to the requirements of the GDPR and the Finnish Act on the Protection of Privacy in Working Life. Respondents' concerns about unauthorized access, misuse of data, and unclear purposes for data processing mirror core GDPR principles, including purpose limitation, data minimization, and security of processing. The emphasis placed by respondents on transparency, meaningful explanations, and control over one's own data aligns with GDPR obligations for informed consent, the right to access personal data, and the requirement for clear communication about processing activities. Moreover, the stronger acceptance of data use by third parties such as occupational healthcare services is consistent with the legal requirement that processing must be justified by a legitimate purpose and, in workplace contexts, typically tied to safety or health rather than performance monitoring. These parallels suggest that the attitudes expressed by worker representatives are not only ethical or practical concerns but also reflect legally grounded expectations that employers must address when designing data-intensive solutions.

Acknowledgement. This work was supported by the Business Finland, the national Finnish funding agency.

A Appendix

Table 3. Survey concepts, items, and response options

Concept measured	Item	Concept	Response options
Background information (Items 1–7)	1	Which field do you work in?	Service and maintenance; mining industry; machinery and equipment manufacture; vehicle manufacture; metal processing; manufacture of fabricated metal products; sheet metal and industrial insulation; electrical and electronics industry; foundry industry; other (specify)
	2	Are you currently employed, laid off from employment, or unemployed?	Employed; laid off from employment; unemployed
	3	What kind of working time do you have?	Two-shift; three-shift; regular daytime work; regular evening work; regular night work; regular weekend work
	4	How long is your work experience in the field?	0–4 years; 5–9 years; 10–19 years; 20–29 years; 30 years or more
	5	Which factors cause workload in your work? (Multiple choice)	Physical factors; safety-related factors; work-related factors; interaction-related factors; work time-related factors
	6	I get to develop my skills at work and my job responsibilities vary at a suitable level	Strongly disagree; somewhat disagree; neither agree nor disagree; somewhat agree; strongly agree
Optional comment	7	Optional comments on the above questions	Open field
Experiences of data-collection devices (Items 8–10)	8a	Use of devices to track physical activity	Yes / No
	8b	Use of devices to monitor sleep	Yes / No
	9	Use of devices during the workday	Yes / No
	10	Perceived reliability of device-generated information	Likert scale
Interest in utilizing collected information (Item 11)	11a	Interest in using wearable devices to track physical activity	Very much; quite a lot; not relevant; quite a little; not at all
	11b	Interest in using environmental sensor data at work	Same as above
	11c	Interest in using motion sensor data at work	Same as above
	11d	Interest in using camera-based data at work	Same as above
Willingness to share data (Items 12–14)	12	Willingness to allow employer to use collected data	Fully agree; somewhat agree; neither agree nor disagree; somewhat disagree; fully disagree; I don't know
	12a	Data use for improving safety	Same as above
	12b	Data use for identifying personal health risks and well-being	Same as above
	12c	Data use for balancing workload	Same as above
	12d	Data use for planning work tasks	Same as above
	13	Willingness to share data with a third party (non-identifiable)	Yes; No; I don't know
	14	Willingness to share data for automatic work planning	Yes; No; I don't know
Wishes for receiving information (Items 15–16)	15	Interest in receiving information during the workday	Interests me a lot; somewhat interests me; does not interest me; I don't know
	15a	Interest in receiving measured personal data	Same as above
	15b	Interest in receiving combined workday and free-time data	Same as above
	16	Types of information of interest during the workday	Multiple selection
Worries about misuse of information (Item 17)	17	Concerns related to measuring physical functions at work	Not worried at all; not worried; somewhat worried; worried; extremely worried; I don't know
	17a	Data used against me	Same as above
	17b	Employer accessing private information	Same as above
	17c	Unauthorized access to data	Same as above
	17d	Data collection disturbing work	Same as above

References

1. Gorecky, D., Schmitt, M., Loskyll, M., Zühlke, D.: Human-machine-interaction in the industry 4.0 era. In: Proceedings of 12th IEEE International Conference Industrial Informatics (INDIN), pp. 289–294 (2014). https://doi.org/10.1109/INDIN.2014.6945523
2. Kaasinen, E., et al.: Empowering and engaging industrial workers with Operator 4.0 solutions. Comput. Ind. Eng. **139**, 105678 (2020). https://doi.org/10.1016/j.cie.2019.01.052
3. Breque, M., De Nul, L., Petridis, A.: Industry 5.0 – Towards a sustainable, human-centric and resilient European industry (2021). https://research-and-innovation.ec.europa.eu/, Accessed 7 June 2023
4. Dröder, K., Bobka, P., Germann, T., Gabriel, F., Dietrich, F.: A machine learning-enhanced digital twin approach for human-robot-collaboration. Procedia CIRP **76**, 187–192 (2018). https://doi.org/10.1016/J.PROCIR.2018.02.010
5. Bevilacqua, Met al.: Digital twin reference model development to prevent operators' risk in process plants. Sustainability **12**, 1088 (2020). https://doi.org/10.3390/SU12031088
6. Bilberg, A., Malik, A.A.: Digital twin driven human–robot collaborative assembly. CIRP Ann. **68**, 499–502 (2019). https://doi.org/10.1016/J.CIRP.2019.04.011
7. Vernim, S., Walzel, H., Knoll, A., Reinhart, G.: Towards capability-based worker modelling in a smart factory. IEEE Int. Conf. Ind. Eng. Eng. Manag. 1576–1580 (2018). https://doi.org/10.1109/IEEM.2017.8290158
8. Peruzzini, M., Grandi, F., Pellicciari, M.: Exploring the potential of Operator 4.0 interface and monitoring. Comput. Ind. Eng. **139**, 105600 (2020). https://doi.org/10.1016/J.CIE.2018.12.047
9. Ruppert, T., Jaskó, S., Holczinger, T., Abonyi, J.: Enabling technologies for operator 4.0: a survey. Appl. Sci. **8**, 1650 (2018). https://doi.org/10.3390/app8091650
10. Mach, S., Storozynski, P., Halama, J., Krems, J.F.: Assessing mental workload with wearable devices. Appl. Ergon. **105**, 103855 (2022). https://doi.org/10.1016/j.apergo.2022.103855
11. Nikolakis, N., Alexopoulos, K., Xanthakis, E., Chryssolouris, G.: The digital twin implementation for linking virtual and physical human-based production tasks. Int. J. Comput. Integr. Manuf. **32**, 1–12 (2018). https://doi.org/10.1080/0951192X.2018.1529430
12. Wang, Q., Jiao, W., Wang, P., Zhang, Y.: Digital twin for human-robot interactive welding and welder behavior analysis. IEEE/CAA J. Autom. Sin. **8**, 334–343 (2021). https://doi.org/10.1109/JAS.2020.1003518
13. Graessler, I., Poehler, A.: Integration of a digital twin as human representation in scheduling in CPS. IEEE Int. Conf. Ind. Eng. Eng. Manag. 289–293 (2018). https://doi.org/10.1109/IEEM.2017.8289898
14. Othman, M., Bhuiyan, N., Gouw, G.J.: Integrating workers' differences into workforce planning. Comput. Ind. Eng. **63**, 1096–1106 (2012). https://doi.org/10.1016/j.cie.2012.06.015
15. Graessler, I., Poehler, A.: Intelligent control of an assembly station via a worker digital twin. Procedia Manuf. **24**, 185–189 (2018). https://doi.org/10.1016/J.PROMFG.2018.06.041
16. Mawanda, H.J.: Beyond Technology. ProQuest LLC (2012)
17. Pearce, M., Mutlu, B., Shah, J., Radwin, R.: Optimizing makespan and ergonomics in collaborative robotics. IEEE Trans. Autom. Sci. Eng. **15**, 1772–1784 (2018). https://doi.org/10.1109/TASE.2018.2789820

18. Uhlemann, T.H.J., Lehmann, C., Steinhilper, R.: The digital twin. Procedia CIRP **60**, 335–340 (2017). https://doi.org/10.1016/j.procir.2016.11.152
19. Yang, Z., Zhang, P., Chen, L.: RFID-enabled indoor positioning for MES. Neurocomputing **174**, 121–133 (2016). https://doi.org/10.1016/j.neucom.2015.05.120
20. Häikiö, J., Kallio, J., Mäkelä, S.-M., Keränen, J.: IoT-based safety monitoring. Int. J. Occup. Environ. Saf. **4**, 1–14 (2020). https://doi.org/10.24840/2184-0954_004.001_0001
21. Lupton, D.: The diverse domains of quantified selves. Econ. Soc. **45**, 101–122 (2016). https://doi.org/10.1080/03085147.2016.1143726
22. Moore, P., Piwek, L.: Regulating wellbeing in the quantified workplace. Empl. Relations **39**, 308–316 (2017). https://doi.org/10.1108/ER-06-2016-0126
23. Heikkilä, P., Schmalfuß, F., Honka, A., Kaasinen, E., Mach, S., Väänänen, K.: Quantified Factory Worker. In: ACM International Conference on Proceedings of Ser., pp. 202–211 (2018). https://doi.org/10.1145/3275116.3275119
24. ACE-Factories White Paper: Human Centered Factories (2019). https://drive.google.com/, Accessed 4 May 2020
25. Kaasinen, E., Anttila, A.-H., Heikkilä, P.: New Industrial Work. Human-Technol. Interact. 271–301 (2023). https://doi.org/10.1007/978-3-030-99235-4_11
26. Sprint, G., Schmitter-Edgecombe, M., Cook, D.: Building a human digital twin (HDTwin) using large language models for cognitive diagnosis: algorithm development and validation. JMIR Form. Res. **8**, e63866 (2024). https://doi.org/10.2196/63866
27. Del Giudice, M., Scuotto, V., Orlando, B., Mustilli, M.: Human-centered acceptance of AI. Hum. Resour. Manag. Rev. (2021). https://doi.org/10.1016/J.HRMR.2021.100856
28. Rueckert, P., Papenberg, B., Sievers, T.S., Tracht, K.: On-Site Learning Factories for AI Adoption. SSRN (2021). https://doi.org/10.2139/SSRN.3864445
29. Jacobs, J.V., Hettinger, L.J., Huang, Y.H., et al.: Employee acceptance of wearables. Appl. Ergon. **78**, 148–156 (2019). https://doi.org/10.1016/J.APERGO.2019.03.003
30. Le Feber, M., Jadoenathmisier, T., Goede, H., Kuijpers, E., Pronk, A.: Ethics and privacy before workplace sensors. Ann. Work Expo. Heal. **65**, 3–10 (2021). https://doi.org/10.1093/ANNWEH/WXAA093
31. Laufer, R.S., Wolfe, M.: Privacy as a concept and a social issue: A multidimensional developmental theory. J. Soc. Issues **33**(3), 22–42 (1977)
32. Pütz, S., Rick, V., Mertens, A., Nitsch, V.: IoT monitoring of mental workload. Appl. Ergon. **102**, 103739 (2022). https://doi.org/10.1016/J.APERGO.2022.103739
33. Vilaza, G.N., Bardram, J.E.: Sharing access to behavioral and health data. PervasiveHealth 346–350 (2019). https://doi.org/10.1145/3329189.3329229
34. Choe, E.K., Lee, N.B., Lee, B., Pratt, W., Kientz, J.A.: Quantified-selfers' practices. In: CHI Proc., pp. 1143–1152 (2014). https://doi.org/10.1145/2556288.2557372
35. Hosselet, P.F.: The acceptance of AI-enabled DSS (2018)
36. Braganza, A., Chen, W., Canhoto, A., Sap, S.: AI adoption and psychological contracts. J. Bus. Res. **131**, 485–494 (2021). https://doi.org/10.1016/J.JBUSRES.2020.08.018
37. Bomström, H., Annanperä, E., Kelanti, M., et al.: Digital Twins about Humans. J. Comput. Inf. Sci. Eng. **22** (2022). https://doi.org/10.1115/1.4054270/1140039
38. van den Broek, E.L.: Monitoring technology for well-being. EU-OSHA (2017)

39. Braganza, A., Chen, W., Canhoto, A., Sap, S.: Gigification & AI. Prod. Plan. Control (2021). https://doi.org/10.1080/09537287.2021.1882692
40. Wright, D.: Ethical impact assessment of IT. Ethics Inf. Technol. **13**, 199–226 (2011). https://doi.org/10.1007/s10676-010-9242-6
41. Friedman, B., Kahn, P.H., Borning, A., Huldtgren, A.: Value Sensitive Design. In: Springer, Dordrecht, pp. 55–95 (2013). https://doi.org/10.1007/978-94-007-7844-3_4
42. European Commission: Ethics Guidelines for Trustworthy AI (2019). https://ec.europa.eu/, Accessed 4 May 2020
43. Kosta, E., Pitkänen, O., Niemelä, M., Kaasinen, E.: Ethical challenges in ambient intelligence for health care. Sci. Eng. Ethics **16**, 303–323 (2010). https://doi.org/10.1007/s11948-009-9150-5
44. Bäck, M., Karv, T., Kestilä-Kekkonen, E.: Finland: a country of high political trust and weak political self-efficacy. In: Political Behaviour in Contemporary Finland: Studies of Voting and Campaigning in a Candidate-Oriented Political System, Vol. 1, pp. 30–42 (2024). https://doi.org/10.4324/9781003452287-4

Robust Running Cadence Estimation Using Multi-axis IMU in Different Body Locations

Nastaran Taefi Aghdam[1(✉)], Kai Noponen[1], Timo Hyart[1], Ahmed Shaheen[1], Rasmus Valtonen[2], Mikko Tulppo[2], and Tapio Seppänen[1]

[1] Center for Machine Vision and Signal Analysis (CMVS), Faculty of Information Technology and Electrical Engineering, University of Oulu, Oulu, Finland
Nastaran.TaefiAghdam@oulu.fi

[2] Research Unit of Biomedicine and Internal Medicine, Faculty of Medicine, University of Oulu, Oulu, Finland

Abstract. Accurate running cadence rate estimation offers great value for performance assessment, gait analysis, and injury prevention. While this can be done using wearable inertial sensors, challenges such as motion artifacts, sensor orientation, placement and harmonics ambiguity in periodic motion signals make robust cadence detection challenging. To overcome these challenges, a method is proposed to use frequency domain analysis along with dynamic programming (DP) to estimate cadence from multi-axis Inertial Measurement Units (IMU) data. The proposed method uses scoring of the detected spectral peaks across accelerometers and gyroscope channels to distinguish different harmonics which appear on the running frequency band-limited spectrum. Then by tracking only fundamental harmonics and preventing switching between different harmonics, the cadence trajectory will be estimated accurately. The estimated cadence values are compared to a reference signal collected from shoe mounted sensors. The method is tested in multiple locations of sensor placement over the body and demonstrates a robust performance with a low mean absolute error of 0.31 ± 0.08 steps per minute across all locations. The proposed method is suitable for real-time applications, offering a practical solution for wearable gait monitoring.

Keywords: Cadence · Step Rate · Motion sensors · Running Gait Analysis

1 Introduction

Cadence, defined as the number of steps per minute (spm), is a key parameter in gait analysis and useful for performance monitoring, rehabilitation, and injury prevention during running. In wearable systems, cadence estimation can be performed using accelerometers or Inertial Measurement Units (IMUs) that record linear acceleration and angular velocity along three orthogonal axes. These sensors capture periodic patterns associated with limb movements during walking or running [1]. IMU-based manners have enabled cadence estimation outside laboratory settings in a compact and cost-effective manner and are increasingly in demand for continuous monitoring in sports, health tracking, and mobile clinical assessments [2, 3].

M. Särestöniemi et al. (Eds.): NCDHWS 2026, CCIS 3010, pp. 263–279, 2026.
https://doi.org/10.1007/978-3-032-28819-6_17

In this study, cadence refers to the total step rate during running. Stride frequency refers to the frequency of complete gait cycles of a single leg, where one stride consists of two steps. Accordingly, cadence is equal to twice the stride frequency. Cadence can be detected using time-domain techniques such as peak detection or zero-crossing of periodic acceleration signals. These are computationally efficient and suitable for embedded systems, yet can be sensitive to motion artifacts, changes in sensor orientation or user variabilities [6]. To address these limitations, frequency-domain methods have been introduced. These methods identify the dominant periodicity of gait by locating spectral peaks in the Fourier-transformed IMU signal [4]. By applying the Fast Fourier Transform (FFT) to segments of accelerometer or gyroscope data, the dominant frequency component corresponding to step cycles can be identified. This approach is relatively robust to noise and is commonly used for both torso-mounted and foot-mounted sensors. Filtering the signal within a cadence-relevant band (typically 1–4 Hz) is crucial to isolate step-related motion from background noise [5]. However, harmonic dominance can cause confusion between stride and step frequencies [6]. An alternative approach involves identifying periodic peaks in the acceleration signal along the vertical or anterior-posterior axis, depending on the sensor location. Peak detection methods are computationally efficient and can work well in smooth motion scenarios but are more sensitive to noise and variable stride lengths [7]. Both time domain and spectral approaches show comparable results with their own limitations. A hybrid approach can complement each other's shortcomings [8, 9].

Cross correlation has been utilized to detect the best combination of IMU axis to detect the cadence rate. Combining multiple inertial channels (e.g., vertical, lateral, and sagittal axes of acceleration and rotation) and aggregating spectral peak estimates across axes helps improve the robustness to orientation and accuracy of cadence estimation [10–13].

Adaptive frequency oscillators have been proposed to dynamically track cadence by synchronizing with the rhythmic gait signal [14, 15]. These methods adapt to tempo changes and are resilient to noise but require careful parameter tuning and could be computationally intensive. LSTM is also utilized in different approaches, for example a deep LSTM-based step-counting algorithm which uses an IMU embedded in a running shoe's sole and an attention-based LSTM approach framing step counting as a sequence-to-one regression which predicts total steps from an entire accelerometer time-series [16, 17]. In addition, supervised machine learning with traditional models and deep learning networks have been applied on IMU-derived features for gait recognition [18]. While it is accurate under controlled conditions, such models typically demand extensive labeled training data.

On the other hand, the accuracy of cadence estimation depends on sensor placement [6]. Sensor placement varies based on the focusing area, for instance sensors mounted on the lower limbs are preferred to study the leg movements [19]. The sensor placement and orientation have been studied, investigating gait analysis algorithms via different locations including wrist, pelvis, foot, head, thigh, shank, etc. [20–23].

However, based on the studies, while sensor placement is important, the best performing location can be different based on the algorithm. For instance, in one study ankle-mounted sensors provided better performance than those mounted on the wrist

[24], while arm mounted sensor outperforms ankle mounted sensor [23], or foot-mounted sensors yield more precise step timing in different studies [25].

Despite these advancements, accurately estimating cadence under variable conditions—such as changing speeds, surface irregularities, and diverse sensor placements (e.g., foot, waist, chest, or smartphone pocket)—remains an open problem. Although the current algorithms generally perform well, a major challenge arises from harmonic dominance, where the second or third harmonic overtakes the true fundamental [6]. Notably, the tendency to switch between harmonics can produce physiologically implausible or temporally inconsistent cadence profiles. Hybrid methods that combine spectral analysis with temporal modeling have also gained attention. Dynamic programming (DP), commonly used in speech and music signal processing, has been adapted to track spectral peaks over time while enforcing temporal continuity [26]. For instance, Viterbi Algorithm is used to find the most likely sequence of hidden states in a Hidden Markov Model (HMM), based on observed data. It solves a global optimization problem using local (recursive) decisions and backtracking. This strategy helps resolve ambiguous peaks caused by noise or harmonic confusion, offering a principled way to impose trajectory smoothness and physiological plausibility [27, 28].

In this work, we present a robust frequency-domain cadence estimation method using a DP framework that explicitly tracks the fundamental harmonic. By aggregating spectral evidence across IMU axes and imposing temporal smoothness constraints, the proposed method avoids harmonic switching and generates stable cadence trajectories suitable for real-time deployment.

Moreover, while most studies focus on a deeper understanding of gait events and gait analysis, this study focuses on cadence rate detection and proposes a method to estimate cadence rate which can be used for multiple locations without sensitivity to the orientation of sensors.

In conclusion, although multiple strategies exist for cadence estimation from wearable IMUs, each exhibits trade-offs between accuracy, robustness, and real-time feasibility. Our proposed method enhances frequency-based cadence tracking by combining harmonic evidence scoring with DP-based trajectory optimization, ensuring stable and accurate estimation across various sensor placements and running conditions.

2 Materials and Methods

2.1 Data Acquisition and Preprocessing

This study utilized a dataset collected from subjects running on a treadmill at different speeds. The data set was collected in the exercise physiology research laboratory of the Research Unit of Biomedicine and Internal Medicine, Faculty of Medicine, University of Oulu, Finland. Ethical statement was acquired from The Regional Medical Research Ethics Committee of the Wellbeing Services County of North Ostrobothnia.

The measurements were conducted over two separate days: 22 subjects participated (11 males, 11 females; age: 25.2 ± 6.0 years; height: 173.5 ± 10.4 cm; weight: 69.5 ± 11.9 kg) on Day 1, and 20 of them returned for Day 2. On the first day of measurement, subjects went through a maximal exercise test where each subject ran up to the fastest speed they can, ranging from 7 to 18 km/h. However, the maximum speed is different for each participant based on their ability. Participants run at each speed for 3 min by a progressive increase in speed by 1 km/h, with 20-s rest-intervals between each stage, however the rest intervals have been excluded from the data in analysis. And during the second day, they ran at predefined running speeds corresponding to 60%, 80%, 100%, and 120% of their ventilatory threshold [29], for 5 min at each speed.

Data was acquired using a wearable inertial measurement unit (Verity Sense, Polar Electro Ltd). The device had custom firmware to allow higher sampling rates. The IMU unit comprises a tri-axial accelerometer, gyroscope and magnetometer, providing six channels of motion data (X, Y, Z axes for acceleration, angular velocity and magnetic field strength). The device was worn on multiple locations including chest, pelvic, upper and lower arms, thighs and shanks and feet, and signals were resampled at 32 Hz. To prepare the data for frequency-domain analysis, each signal was segmented into 8-s overlapping windows with 6-s overlapping. We choose an 8-s window length, which provides sufficient duration to resolve low-frequency stride patterns while still responding to changes in cadence. Consecutive windows overlap substantially to ensure frequent updates and smooth tracking over time.

2.2 Cadence Detection and Harmonic Support Score Algorithm

Within each 8-s window of data, all six signal channels are passed through a zero-phase 3rd-order Butterworth bandpass filter with cutoff frequencies between 1.5 and 4 Hz to isolate cadence rate limit for running and suppress high and low-frequency noise. The lower cutoff reduces lower movements or sensor drift frequencies, and the upper cutoff reduces high-frequency noise and other motions not related to cadence. The filtered data are then zero-padded to 4096 samples per window and transformed via FFT. The zero-padding increases the frequency resolution of the subsequent spectral analysis without adding new information, allowing for more precise locating of peak frequencies. It results in spectrum interpolation with finer grid and allows to use the discretized spectrum to locate the peak frequency of an isolated spectral peak more accurately [30]. Finally, only the magnitude of the positive frequency spectrum is retained and converted from Hz to steps per minute (spm).

The magnitude spectra from all six channels are normalized using L2 normalization. For each time window k, the magnitude spectrum for each channel c is calculated (Eq. (1)) and normalized (Eq. (2))

$$S_c^{(k)}(f) = \mid \mathrm{FFT}(x_c^{(k)}(t)) \mid \tag{1}$$

$$\hat{S}_c^{(k)}(f) = \frac{S_c^{(k)}(f)}{\|S_c^{(k)}\|_2 + \varepsilon} \tag{2}$$

where $x_c^{(k)}(t)$ is time-domain signal from the c-th IMU channel in k-th time window, $S_c^{(k)}(f)$ is the magnitude spectrum at frequency f, $\|S_c^{(k)}\|_2$ is the L2 norm of the magnitude spectrum, ε is a small positive constant to prevent division by zero and $\hat{S}_c^{(k)}(f)$ is the normalized magnitude spectrum.

To combine information from the accelerometer and gyroscope axes, one composite spectrum is produced as the sum of normalized magnitude spectra of all channels, shown inequation (3) where $S^{(k)}_{\text{composite}}(f)$ is the composite spectrum. The result is a single aggregated spectrum representing the overall periodic motion content at each frequency within the window. Peaks that consistently appear across multiple axes will reinforce each other, while random noise or axis-specific artifacts tend to average out.

$$S^{(k)}_{\text{composite}}(f) = \sum_{c=1}^{C} \hat{S}_c^{(k)}(f) \tag{3}$$

The composite spectral curve typically shows a dominant peak around the runner's step frequency or stride frequency, along with potential harmonic peaks. As shown in Fig. 1 each IMU channel exhibits a prominent peak corresponding either to the cadence or one of its harmonics. Considering the possibility of changing the sensor orientation, this approach will make the algorithm robust against changes in orientation.

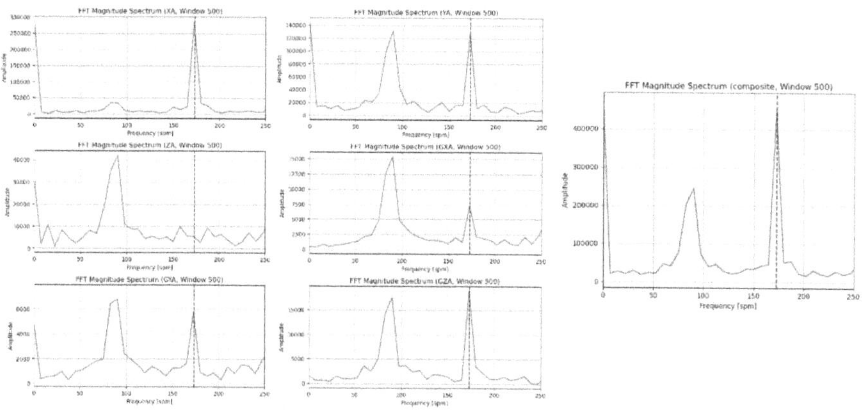

(a) 3 axes acceleration – XA, YA, ZA- and 3 axes angular velocity -GXA, GYA, GZA- power spectrum of an 8s Window.

(b) composite power spectrum of an 8s Window.

Fig. 1. An example of different axes of acceleration and angular velocity power spectrum (A) and the composite power spectra (B) (True cadence rate is shown by vertical red dotted line).

Next, peak detection and harmonic candidate identification are performed on the composite power spectrum. In this step, peaks are defined as local maxima by setting a minimum peak distance threshold (2 frequency bins) and limiting the number of peaks (6 peaks) to focus on relevant candidates and keep computation efficient. Each detected peak has a frequency value f (in Hz) corresponding to a hypothesized oscillatory component in the motion. Due to the dynamics of running, these peaks often include the fundamental stride frequency, which is defined as one-leg step frequency, and its harmonics. For example, if the runner's one-leg stride frequency is s, the IMU signals often contain a strong component at the cadence frequency 2 × s. Because each foot impact creates motion at twice the stride rate. And sometimes a component at 3 × s, a third harmonic, possibly from higher-frequency body oscillations or impact transients.

For each found spectral peak frequency (f_{peak}), the algorithm generates candidates for fundamental frequency as s_0 by assuming that f_{peak} could be the 1st, 2nd, or 3rd harmonic of the underlying stride rate (see Eq. (4)):

$$s_0 = \frac{f_{peak}}{m}, m \in \{1,2,3\} \tag{4}$$

If the peak is considered the first harmonic (fundamental), then a candidate fundamental frequency is $s_0 = f_{peak}$, If the peak is assumed to be the second harmonic, then the underlying fundamental stride frequency would be $s_0 = \frac{f_{peak}}{2}$. And similarly, if the peak is assumed to be the third harmonic, the candidate fundamental would be $s_0 = \frac{f_{peak}}{3}$. Then, all such candidates will be considered if they satisfy a simple rule that after dividing, s_0 should still lie within the running frequency band; if it falls outside, that candidate will be discarded.

This way, even if the most prominent peak in the spectrum is the runner's step rate/cadence (which is 2 × stride), the correct stride frequency as a candidate will be considered as half of that peak's frequency. Similarly, if a third-harmonic overtone appears strongly, one-third of that frequency will be considered as a possible fundamental.

Then a harmonic support score for each candidate fundamental frequency (s) is defined that reflects how well the spectrum supports s being the true stride frequency. The score is based on the presence and strength of harmonically related peaks in the composite spectrum. The candidate's score is calculated as a weighted sum of these harmonic magnitudes as shown in the Eq. (5).

$$\text{score}(s_0) = w_1 \cdot S_{\text{pool}}(s_0) + w_2 \cdot S_{\text{pool}}(2s_0) + w_3 \cdot S_{\text{pool}}(3s_0) \tag{5}$$

With $w_1 = 1.0, w_2 = 0.8$, and $w_3 = 0.35$ which are empirical weights. After exhaustive experimentation, these values were tuned based on expected relative strengths of fundamental frequency and its harmonics to achieve best results. We retain top candidates per window, based on these scores. Here the fundamental frequency is weighted more heavily than higher harmonics, since a true fundamental should ideally have a clear peak at its own frequency. This approach is robust as it gives a high score if all harmonics are consistently present, but even if one or two are weaker, a strong fundamental and second harmonic can still yield a good score for the candidate.

After this step, the window's data is reduced to a set of candidate stride frequencies each with an associated harmonic support score. Candidates too close in frequency are pruned by keeping only the highest-scoring entry. If no peaks are found in the spectrum, fallback candidates are generated by exhaustive scanning within the running frequency range using the same scoring method.

2.3 Cadence Tracking via Dynamic Programming

To produce a smooth, robust estimate of cadence over time, the algorithm tracks the fundamental frequency across consecutive windows using a dynamic programming (DP) approach inspired by the Viterbi algorithm application in ECG analysis [31]. Each window provides a set of candidate stride frequencies with their scores, which reflect how well that frequency fits the current data. However, simply choosing the top candidate in each window independently can result in sudden jumps if a wrong peak temporarily looks stronger. Instead, the sequence of windows is considered as a time series to find the best continuous frequency trajectory through them, balancing the per-window spectral evidence with temporal consistency constraints.

The state space is defined by considering each candidate for a fundamental frequency, $s_i^{(k)}$, at time window k as a possible state. Then the harmonic support score is considered as the observation score for that state, higher score means that frequency is strongly supported by the spectrum in that window.

A transition cost is also defined as penalizing sudden changes in the frequency from one window to the next. Between window k and *k-1*, if we have a candidate frequency $s_i^{(k)}$ in window k and $s_j^{(k1)}$ in window *k-1*, the transition cost is considered as a coefficient (λ) of the absolute difference $s_i^{(k)} - s_j^{(k1)}$. The constant λ is tuned so that large changes in cadence in a short time are considered unlikely. In practice, because runners cannot change stride frequency instantaneously by large amounts, this transition penalty guides the algorithm to favor gradual changes consistent with real motion, in fact stride frequency might change only a few percent per second at most, unless the runner abruptly starts or stops.

Let $J_k(i)$ be the best cumulative score ending at the i-th candidate in window k, to track the optimal sequence of stride frequency (half-cadence) values $s_0^{(k)}$ across windows $k = 1,2,\ldots,N$. The recurrence is calculated as shown in Eq. (6).

$$J_k(i) = \max_j \left[J_{k-1}(j) - \lambda \cdot |\mathrm{s}_\mathrm{i}^{(\mathrm{k})} - \mathrm{s}_\mathrm{j}^{(\mathrm{k1})}| \right] + score_i^{(k)} \quad (6)$$

where $s_i^{(k)}$ is the i-th candidate half-cadence in window k, and λ is a jump penalty (chosen as 0.12 by experiment), discouraging abrupt cadence changes. Then, the optimal sequence path is obtained via forward pass, and backtracking yields the sequence of half-cadence estimates as $\hat{s}_0^{(1)}, \hat{s}_0^{(2)}, \ldots, \hat{s}_0^{(N)}$. This non-switching approach ensures that only one harmonic track is followed, avoiding transient jumps between the fundamental, second, and third harmonics. The final cadence estimate (both legs) is computed as shown in Eq. (7).

$$Cadence^{(k)} = 2 \cdot \hat{s}_0^{(k)} \quad (7)$$

Additionally, third harmonic estimate $3 \cdot \hat{s}_0^{(k)}$ and harmonic sources are extracted for analysis and visualization. Figure 2 demonstrates a sample of defined scores on the detected candidates, and how the path follows the higher scores consistently. The bigger circle means higher score.

For evaluation, the estimated cadence is compared against the reference obtained from shoe mounted sensor $c_{\mathrm{ref}}^{(k)}$. MAE is calculated between the estimated and reference cadence trajectories as shown in Eq. (8).

$$\mathrm{MAE} = \frac{1}{N} \sum_{k=1}^{N} |\ \mathrm{Cadence}^{(k)} - c_{\mathrm{ref}}^{(k)}\ | \quad (8)$$

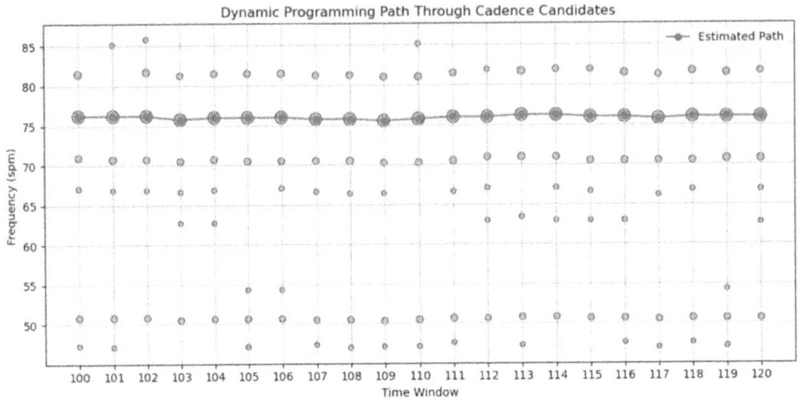

Fig. 2. Detected fundamental frequency candidates (gray circles) across time windows from the wrist sensor. The circle size reflects the candidate's spectral score, with larger circles indicating stronger evidence. The red path highlights the optimal cadence trajectory estimated via dynamic programming. Frequency is shown in steps per minute (spm).

Overall, this approach provides a robust estimation of running cadence by combining multi-axis inertial data, frequency-domain analysis, harmonic peak identification, and dynamic programming-based temporal smoothing. It effectively distinguishes the true fundamental stride rate from its harmonics and noise, yielding an accurate, smooth cadence tracking suitable for real-time feedback in running applications. This method is modular and applicable across various sensor placements.

After a careful analysis of the spectrogram structures and the biomechanics of running, the proposed method is identified as the best-performing approach in this study. The algorithm is implemented in Python using NumPy and SciPy for signal processing. Processing is vectorized for efficiency and can be executed in real-time, with a processing time of 0.513 s for a segment containing 100 windows (each 8 s long). All hyperparameters including window length, FFT size, frequency bounds, harmonic weights, peak detection thresholds, and DP penalties were empirically tuned on first day of measurement. The hyperparameter selection was guided by prior knowledge of running cadence physiology together with empirical evaluation of spectral separability and temporal tracking stability. Specifically, the frequency bounds were chosen to cover the physiologically plausible cadence range during running, considering the used data variability and running frequency limits mentioned on other studies, a relatively wide range is defined to make sure the running cadence is preserved [32][33]. The window length and FFT size were selected to balance frequency resolution against temporal responsiveness. Harmonic weights and dynamic programming (DP) transition penalties were adjusted to promote stable tracking of the fundamental cadence frequency while reducing harmonic switching. No subject-specific tuning was performed. Once determined, all parameters were fixed and applied unchanged to the independent validation data from the second measurement day. (See Sect. 2.1. Data Acquisition and Preprocessing).

3 Results

The proposed cadence rate estimation pipeline is evaluated against reference, computed and manually validated using the foot mounted IMU sensor. The primary metric, used for evaluation is MAE between the estimated and reference cadence trajectories.

The results in Table 1 presents the MAE of estimated cadence rate, averaged over subjects, in different sensor placements over body, number of samples refers to number of participants with available data at each location. It shows high temporal alignment between the estimated cadence and ground truth, with average MAE of 0.31 ± 0.08 spm across all locations. The dynamic programming tracker maintained smooth cadence rate transitions and successfully rejected spectral distractions caused by stronger second or third harmonics. The number of samples at each location is different due to occasional failures, where data is not available due to technical problems during measurement. However, assuming a comparable number of subjects across all locations, among the evaluated sensor placements, the pelvis and left arm exhibited the lowest average MAE (0.28 spm), while the right wrist showed the highest variability (MAE = 0.33 ± 0.13 spm). Time–frequency visualizations of the FFT spectrum confirmed that the estimated cadence curve followed the true fundamental across windows. To take a closer look at the effect of sensor placement, the algorithm is also evaluated across 5 grouped anatomical regions, including torso (chest and pelvis), wrist, arm, thigh and shank without separating left and right limbs. Table 2 summarizes the results for each group which approve the torso area as the best performing with the lowest average MAE (0.29 spm) and variability (±0.07).

Table 1. Cadence Estimation Mean Absolute Error at Different Sensor Placements

Location	Average MAE ± SD (spm)	Number of Samples
Chest	0.30 ± 0.09	18
Pelvis	0.28 ± 0.04	9
Right Wrist	0.34 ± 0.13	6
Left Wrist	0.33 ± 0.09	16
Right Arm	0.31 ± 0.09	16
Left Arm	0.28 ± 0.03	6
Right Thigh	0.33 ± 0.11	10
Left Thigh	0.30 ± 0.06	15
Left Shank	0.32 ± 0.08	18

Table 2. Cadence Rate Estimation Mean Absolute Error at Grouped Regions.

Location	Average MAE ± SD (spm)	Number of Samples
Torso	0.29 ± 0.07	27
Wrist	0.33 ± 0.10	22
Arm	0.31 ± 0.08	22
Thigh	0.31 ± 0.08	25
Shank	0.32 ± 0.08	18

Figure 3, Fig. 4 and Fig. 5 demonstrate some examples of estimated cadence rate in comparison with true cadence over different speeds and sensor locations over body. These figures indicate stable MAE across treadmill speeds, suggesting consistent estimation of performance under varying running intensities.

Moreover, Fig. 6 is provided to visualize the performance in overcoming the harmonics. It presents a time–frequency visualization of the composite spectrum, constructed by summing normalized magnitude spectra across all six IMU axes. This representation highlights dominant frequency components over time. The cadence tracking algorithm robustly follows the true cadence (black stars), accurately identifying the fundamental stride frequency (blue dashed) and rejecting confounding peaks from second and third harmonics. The final estimated cadence (red dashed) consistently aligns with the ground truth across varying running speeds, demonstrating the stability of the approach.

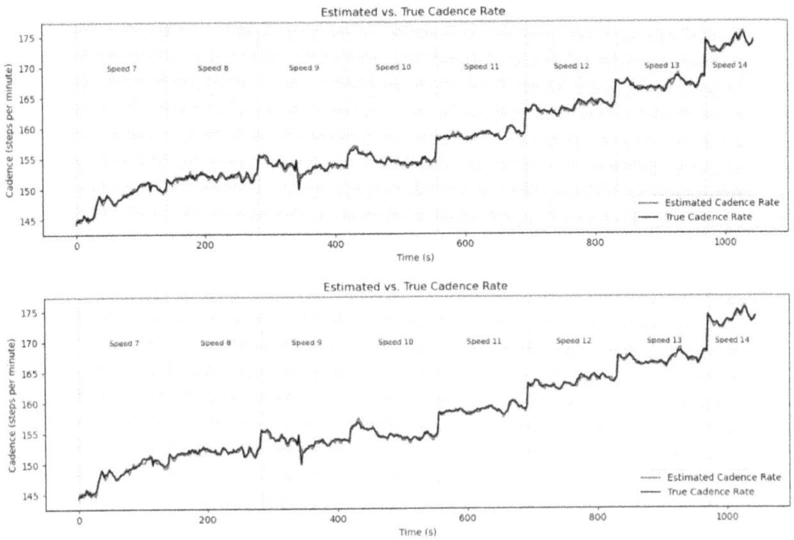

(a)

(b)

Fig. 3. Comparison of Estimated Cadence VS True Cadence across Running Speeds (in km/h), marked on plot. Results shown for Wrist (a) and Chest (b) sensor placements for Subject 1.

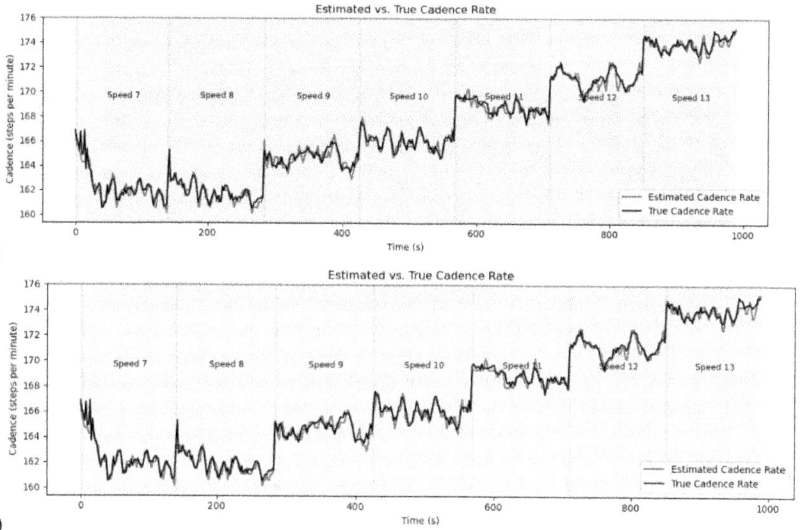

(a)

(b)

Fig. 4. Comparison of Estimated Cadence VS True Cadence across Running Speeds (in km/h), marked on plot. Results shown for Arm (a) and Thigh (b) sensor placements for Subject 2.

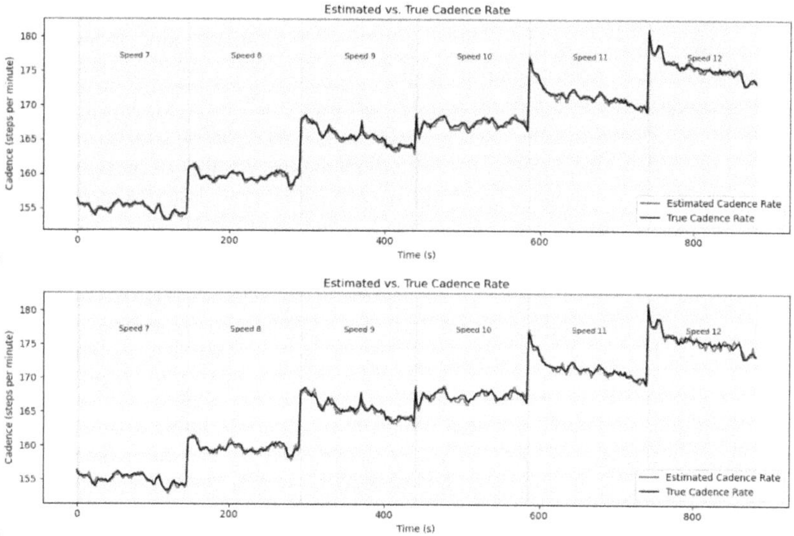

(a)

(b)

Fig. 5. Comparison of Estimated Cadence VS True Cadence across Running Speeds (in km/h), marked on plot. Results shown for Pelvis (a) and Shank (b) sensor placements for Subject 3.

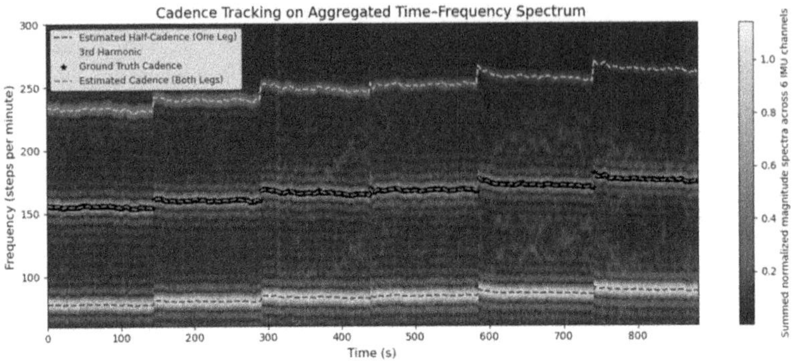

Fig. 6. Time-frequency spectrogram of the composite signal, showing the estimated cadence and its harmonics vs. true cadence.

4 Discussion

This study introduces a robust cadence estimation method that avoids common challenges such as harmonic confusion and temporal missing the true cadence rate. By focusing the DP search on the fundamental harmonic and incorporating multi-channel spectral information, the method generates physiologically plausible cadence trajectories. The algorithm is evaluated on different body locations and results indicate that cadence estimation performance varied slightly across sensor placements. The pelvis (0.28 ± 0.04 spm, n = 9) and left arm (0.28 ± 0.03 spm, n = 6) achieved the lowest mean errors, while the chest (0.30 ± 0.09 spm, n = 18) and left thigh (0.30 ± 0.06 spm, n = 15) also demonstrated strong performance with larger sample size. It is worth noting that the number of samples between placements (number of participants per sensor location) varied due to occasional sensor failures, which should be considered when comparing locations with limited data. Thus, when considering only sensor locations with sufficient data ($\geq$ 15 samples), the cadence estimation algorithm maintained consistent and low error rates across all sensor locations. The average MAE ranges from 0.30 to 0.34 spm with standard deviation below 0.13 spm. This narrow error indicates that the proposed method performance is reliable and consistent across the commonly used sensor placements. Although some locations such as left wrist and left shank with 16 and 18 samples had slightly higher MAE and variability, they remained comparable suggesting the method is robust even under more dynamic limb movements.

Evaluation of the grouped locations demonstrates that the torso region yielded the lowest average MAE at 0.29 spm, followed closely by the arm and thigh groups (both 0.31 spm), and the shank (0.32 spm). The wrist showed the highest error at 0.33 spm with greater variability (SD = 0.10), which may reflect increased motion variability during running. Overall, the results indicate that the proposed algorithm maintains consistent performance across different body segments, with minimal degradation at more dynamic placements. Considering all limitations, the method consistently achieved cadence errors below 0.5 spm across all locations, demonstrating strong robustness and adaptability to various sensor configurations.

Moreover, the cadence estimation algorithm demonstrates consistent performance across varying treadmill running speeds as shown in Fig. 3-Fig. 5, maintaining low and stable error rates with no substantial degradation during speed transitions. This robustness under dynamic conditions suggests strong generalizability across a wide range of running intensities, making it suitable for real-world applications where pace fluctuates.

Compared to traditional time-domain peak detectors and learning-based classifiers, the proposed method is interpretable, generalizable, and computationally efficient. It can be deployed on mobile hardware for real-time running feedback without requiring individual-specific training data. Wu et al. (2025) Proposed "VibRun," a deep-learning Transformer approach using a treadmill-mounted IMU (vibration sensor) to estimate running cadence (plus other gait metrics). Tested with 17 runners at varied treadmill speeds (3–6 mph). Produced cadence within 1.7 spm ($\approx$2.4%) of ground-truth, on average, across 83% of instances with zero error, demonstrating high accuracy and robustness [34]. Nie et al. (2024) developed an acoustic sensing system which achieved 3.74 spm for cadence estimation. They also reported Apple Watch MAE of about 10.69 spm, and foot-mounted sensors like RunScribe around 1.54 spm [35]. Ducharme et al. (2021) developed a "transparent" step detection algorithm using calibrated optimal acceleration peak thresholds for waist vs. wrist accelerometers (0.027 g and 0.036 g on vector-magnitude signals), it was validated on 75 adults performing everyday activities and treadmill walking/running from 0.22 to 2.2 m/s (~0.8–7.9 km/h). The tuned thresholds yielded RSME on waist around 2.3 steps/min and on wrist around 6.5 steps/min [36]. Khan & Abedi (2022) Proposed an attention-based LSTM approach framing step counting as a sequence-to-one regression which predicts total steps from an entire accelerometer time-series. Unlike typical step-by-step detectors, it doesn't require labeling each step or setting sliding windows. Evaluated on 3 public datasets with walking and running data, the model automatically learned step patterns and achieved MAE of 1.25 spm for their proposed attention based LSTM and 2.51 spm for only LSTM [17]. These studies are summarized in Table 3. While most methods result in comparable errors, they have some limitations including requiring specific sensor location and computational cost. Moreover, none of these methods address the harmonics challenge directly.

The main limitation of the current work lies in its validation scope, which was confined to treadmill running under controlled speed and consistent terrain. While effective under controlled running conditions, further validation is required across a broader range of running speeds and terrains. To extend the solution into more dynamic and real-world conditions, the future work may tune the hyperparameters or investigate generalization across activities by incorporating the automatic activity detection and threshold setting. Moreover, stride length and gait phase detection modules can be analyzed by further computations relying on the accurate and robust baseline for detection step rates therefore the step phases.

Table 3. Summary of Cadence Estimation Methods for Running Activities

Reference	Sensor location	Method	Activity	Results (MAE)1
Nie et al. (2024) [35]	Wrist	Apple Watch	Running	10.69 spm
Nie et al. (2024) [35]	foot-mounted on both shoes	RunScribe	Running	~ 1.54 spm
Nie et al. (2024) [35]	On the treadmill	acoustic sensing system	Running	3.74 spm
Wu et al. (2025) [34]	treadmill-mounted IMU	deep-learning Transformer	Running	1.7 spm
Ducharme et al. (2021) [36]	waist and wrist	acceleration peak threshold	Everyday activities/ Treadmill walking/Running	~ 4.4 spm (RSME)1
Khan & Abedi (2022) [17]	multiple placements	LSTM	Walking/ Running	2.51 spm
Khan & Abedi (2022) [17]	multiple placements	attention-based LSTM	Walking/ Running	1.25 spm
Proposed method	**Multiple locations**	**DP tracker**	**Running**	**0.31 ± 0.08 spm**

[1] Mean Absolute error is reported to compare results, however, for one study the reported metric was different, mentioned in table

5 Conclusion

This study presents a robust and interpretable dynamic programming (DP)–based cadence estimation framework leveraging time–frequency analysis to track the true fundamental step frequency while suppressing harmonic artifacts. By avoiding switching between harmonics and smoothing temporal variations, the method delivers accurate cadence estimates suitable for real-time feedback and long-term gait monitoring. Evaluated across multiple sensor locations during controlled running conditions, the method achieved a low mean absolute error of 0.31 ± 0.08 spm, outperforming or matching the accuracy of many recent methods, including deep learning and spectral approaches. Sensor location analysis further confirmed that the proposed method performs reliably across multiple placements, with optimal accuracy at pelvis, chest, and left arm, yet still maintaining acceptable error margins at more variable locations like the wrist and thighs. The performance is also monitored, which indicates the consistent performance of the proposed method over different running speeds from 7 to 18 km/h. This flexibility supports the practical deployment of the algorithm across different wearable configurations, without requiring strict sensor placement.

Compared to state-of-the-art techniques—such as attention-based LSTMs, Transformer-based models like VibRun, and dual-threshold rule-based methods—the proposed algorithm offers a unique advantage by directly addressing harmonic confusion, a common yet under-explored challenge in cadence estimation. Its computational efficiency and generalizability make it well-suited for real-time deployment on mobile hardware, without requiring user-specific calibration or large training datasets.

Future work should expand to varying terrains, inclines, and outdoor running, and integrate automatic activity segmentation and gait phase detection. The presented framework provides a strong foundation for these extensions, anchored by reliable cadence tracking across body locations.

Acknowledgments. This study was funded by Business Finland project BIOFUSION (grant number 5311/31/2022).

Disclosure of Interests. he authors have no competing interests to declare that are relevant to the content of this article.

References

1. Lin, S., et al.: A review of gait analysis using gyroscopes and inertial measurement units. Sensors **25**(11), 3481 (2025). https://doi.org/10.3390/s25113481
2. Aminian, K., Najafi, B.: Capturing human motion using body-fixed sensors: outdoor measurement and clinical applications. Computer Animation and Virtual Worlds (2004)
3. Kobsar, D., Charlton, J.M., Tse, C., et al.: Validity and reliability of wearable inertial sensors in healthy adult walking: a systematic review and meta-analysis. J. NeuroEng. Rehabil. **17**, 62 (2020). https://doi.org/10.1186/s12984-020-00685-3
4. Salarian, P., et al.: Gait assessment in Parkinson's disease using a wearable system. IEEE Trans. Biomed. Eng. **51**(8) (2004)
5. Mannini, A., Sabatini, A.M.: Machine learning methods for classifying human physical activity from on-body accelerometers. Sensors (Basel) **10**(2), 1154–1175 (2010). https://doi.org/10.3390/s100201154. Epub 2010 Feb 1. PMID: 22205862; PMCID: PMC3244008
6. Karuei, I., Schneider, O.S., Stern, B., Chuang, M., MacLean, K.E.: RRACE: Robust realtime algorithm for cadence estimation. Pervasive Mob. Comput. **13**, 52–66 (2014). https://doi.org/10.1016/j.pmcj.2013.09.006. ISSN 1574–1192
7. Trojaniello, D., et al.: Estimation of step-by-step spatio-temporal parameters of normal and impaired gait using shank-mounted magneto-inertial sensors: application to elderly, hemiparetic, parkinsonian and choreic gait. J. Neuroeng. Rehabil. **11**(11), 152 (2014). https://doi.org/10.1186/1743-0003-11-152
8. Tarashansky, A., Vathsangam, H., Sukhatme, G.S.: A study of position independent algorithms for phone-based gait frequency detection. In: 2014 36th Annual International Conference of the IEEE Engineering in Medicine and Biology Society, pp. 5984–5987. Chicago, IL, USA, (2014). https://doi.org/10.1109/EMBC.2014.6944992
9. Brajdic, A., Harle, R.: Walk detection and step counting on unconstrained smartphones. In: Proceedings of the 2013 ACM international joint conference on Pervasive and ubiquitous computing (UbiComp '13). Association for Computing Machinery, pp. 225–234. New York, NY, USA (2013). https://doi.org/10.1145/2493432.2493449
10. van Oeveren, B.T., de Ruiter, C.J., Beek, P.J., Rispens, S.M., van Dieën, J.H.: An adaptive, realtime cadence algorithm for unconstrained sensor placement. Med. Eng. Phys. **52**, 49–58 (2018). https://doi.org/10.1016/j.medengphy.2017.12.007

11. McCamley, J., Donati, M., Grimpampi, E., Mazzà, C.: An enhanced estimate of initial contact and final contact instants of time using lower trunk inertial sensor data. Gait Posture **36**(2), 316–318 (2012). https://doi.org/10.1016/j.gaitpost.2012.02.019. Epub 2012 Mar 31 PMID: 22465705
12. Femiano, R., Werner, C., Wilhelm, M., Eser, P.: Validation of open-source step-counting algorithms for wrist-worn tri-axial accelerometers in cardiovascular patients, Gait & Posture, Vol. 92, Pp. 206–211 (2022). https://doi.org/10.1016/j.gaitpost.2021.11.035 ISSN 0966–6362
13. Hannink, J., Kautz, T., Pasluosta, C.F., Gaßmann, K.-G., Klucken, J., Eskofier, B.M.: Sensor-based gait parameter extraction with deep convolutional neural networks. IEEE J. Biomed. Health Inform. **21**(1), 85–93 (2017). https://doi.org/10.1109/JBHI.2016.2636456
14. Seo, K., Hyung, S., Choi, B.K., Lee, Y., Shim, Y.: A new adaptive frequency oscillator for gait assistance. In: 2015 IEEE International Conference on Robotics and Automation (ICRA), pp. 5565–5571. Seattle, WA, USA (2015). https://doi.org/10.1109/ICRA.2015.7139977
15. Tomc, M., Matjačić, Z.: Real-time gait event detection with adaptive frequency oscillators from a single head-mounted IMU. Sensors (Basel). **23**(12), 5500 (2023). https://doi.org/10.3390/s23125500
16. Lucot, Q., Beurienne, E., Behr, M.: Multi-activity step counting algorithm using deep learning foot flat detection with an IMU inside the sole of a shoe. Sens. (Basel). **24**(21), 6927 (2024). https://doi.org/10.3390/s24216927
17. Shehroz, K., Ali, A.: Step Counting with Attention-based LSTM (2022). https://doi.org/10.48550/arXiv.2211.13114
18. Alharthi, A.S., Yunas, S.U., Ozanyan, K.B.: Deep learning for monitoring of human gait: a review. IEEE Sens. J. **19**(21), 9575–9591 (2019). https://doi.org/10.1109/JSEN.2019.2928777
19. Godfrey, A., Conway, R., Meagher, D., OLaighin, G.: Direct measurement of human movement by accelerometry. Med Eng Phys. **30**(10), 1364–1386 (2008). https://doi.org/10.1016/j.medengphy.2008.09.005. Epub 2008 Nov 8. PMID: 18996729
20. Kim, Y.K., et al.: Leveraging deep learning and wearables for automatically identifying gait event: effects of age and location of sensors on the assessment of gait events. IEEE Sens. J. **25**, 792–802 (2025)
21. Anaya-Campos, L.E., Sanchez-Fernandez, L.P., Quinones-Uriostegui, I.: Motion smoothness analysis of the gait cycle, segmented by stride and associated with the inertial sensors' locations. Sensors **25**, 368 (2025)
22. Vittoria Guerra, B.M., Sozzi, S., Pizzocaro, S., De Nunzio, A.M., Schmid, M.: AI processing of wearable IMU data for exoskeleton gait analysis. In: Proceedings of the 2024 IEEE 8th Forum on Research and Technologies for Society and Industry Innovation (RTSI), pp. 380–384. Milan, Italy (2024)
23. Isaia1, C., Michaelides, M.P: Step counting by optimum fusion of IMU sensor measurements. In: IPIN-WCAL 2025: Workshop for Computing & Advanced Localization at the Fifteenth International Conference on Indoor Positioning and Indoor Navigation, September 15–18, 2025, Tampere, Finland (2025)
24. Rhudy, M.B., Mahoney, J.M.: A comprehensive comparison of simple step counting techniques using wrist- and ankle-mounted accelerometer and gyroscope signals. J. Med. Eng. Technol. **42**(3), 236–243 (2018). https://doi.org/10.1080/03091902.2018.1470692
25. Meingast, T., Carrier, B., Melvin, A., Kozloff, K.M., DeJong Lempke, A.F., Lepley, A.S.: Limited interchangeability of smartwatches and lace-mounted IMUs for running gait analysis. Sensors **25**(17), 5553 (2025). https://doi.org/10.3390/s25175553
26. de Cheveigné, A., Kawahara, H.: YIN, a fundamental frequency estimator for speech and music, J. Acoust. Soc. Am. **111**(4) (2002)
27. Viterbi, A. J.: Viterbi algorithm. Scholarpedia **4**(1), 6246 (2009)

28. Holkeri A, et al.:. Experiences in digitizing and digitally measuring a paper-based ECG archive. J Electrocardiol. **51**(1):74–81 (2018). https://doi.org/10.1016/j.jelectrocard.2017.09.007. Epub 2017 Sep 27. PMID: 29031413
29. Contreras-Briceño, F., Cancino, J., Espinosa-Ramírez, M. et al.: Estimation of ventilatory thresholds during exercise using respiratory wearable sensors. npj Digit. Med. **7**, 198 (2024). https://doi.org/10.1038/s41746-024-01191-9
30. Lindsten, F.: A remark on zero-padding for increased frequency resolution (2010). Sitio web: http://goo.gl/uBMFTw
31. Noponen, K.: Viterbi algorithm application in ECG analysis (personal communication)
32. Figueiredo, I., Reis, E., Silva, M., Sousa, J.E.: The influence of running cadence on biomechanics and injury prevention: a systematic review. Cureus **17**(8), e90322 (2025). https://doi.org/10.7759/cureus.90322. PMID: 40964543; PMCID: PMC12440572
33. Vincent, H.K., et al.: Cadence impact on cardiopulmonary, metabolic and biomechanical loading during downhill running. Gait Posture **71**, 186–191 (2019). https://doi.org/10.1016/j.gaitpost.2019.04.022. Epub 2019 May 2 PMID: 31075662
34. Wu, T., et al.: VibRun: Real-time Unobtrusive Gait Analysis for Treadmill Running via Footstep Vibrations. In: Proceeedings ACM Interact. Mob. Wearable Ubiquitous Technology, Vol. 9, no. 3, 141 (September 2025), p. 25 (2025). https://doi.org/10.1145/3749539
35. Nie, J., Fan, Y., Xuan, Z., Preindl, M., Jiang, X.: Real-time non-contact estimation of running metrics on treadmills using smartphones. In: Proceedings of the 30th Annual International Conference on Mobile Computing and Networking (ACM MobiCom '24). Association for Computing Machinery, pp. 1644–1646. New York, NY, USA (2024). https://doi.org/10.1145/3636534.3697446
36. Ducharme, S.W., et al.: A transparent method for step detection using an acceleration threshold. J Meas Phys Behav. **4**(4), 311–320 (2021). https://doi.org/10.1123/jmpb.2021-0011. Epub 2021 Oct 25. PMID: 36274923; PMCID: PMC9586317

Multimodal Driver State Monitoring in a Simulated Environment: A Health-Oriented, Human-in-the-Loop Evaluation

Prabhash Rathnayake(✉), Sameera Gamage, Akke-Pekka Törmänen, and Ella Peltonen

University of Oulu, Oulu, Finland

Abstract. Continuous monitoring of human cognitive and physiological state is a key challenge in digital health, particularly in safety-critical environments such as driving. This paper presents a multimodal driver-state monitoring framework integrating electroencephalography (EEG), wearable physiological sensing, and posture-based vision analysis. The proposed system enables synchronised, window-based analysis of cognitive workload and fatigue-related indicators across varying driving scenarios. We report preliminary results from a simulator-based pilot study, showing that the sensing modalities capture complementary aspects of driver state: EEG is sensitive to rapid cognitive changes, wearables reflect slower physiological trends related to fatigue and stress, and posture features capture behavioural adaptation. The study demonstrates the feasibility of multimodal integration while highlighting practical challenges, including sensor intrusiveness, movement-related noise, and inter-individual variability. Rather than proposing deployable algorithms, this work provides methodological insights to inform future real-vehicle implementations and illustrates how human-state awareness can be integrated into software-defined vehicle architectures to support health-aware, human-in-the-loop adaptation in future intelligent vehicles.

Keywords: Multimodal sensing · Driver monitoring · Digital health · Software-defined vehicles

1 Introduction

Digital health systems are increasingly focusing on continuous monitoring of people's cognitive, physical, and behavioural states. This proactive approach supports prevention, enables early interventions, and facilitates adaptive decision-making in everyday situations. In driving, fatigue, drowsiness, and mental workload pose safety risks and indicate cognitive strain and long-term well-being. In parallel, modern vehicles are evolving from hardware-centric machines into software-defined platforms capable of over-the-air updates, adaptive algorithms, and real-time diagnostics [8]. While this transformation enables continuous improvement in vehicle functionality, significantly less emphasis has been placed

M. Säreståniemi et al. (Eds.): NCDHWS 2026, CCIS 3010, pp. 280–296, 2026.
https://doi.org/10.1007/978-3-032-28819-6_18

on integrating the human driver as an active component within software-defined vehicle (SDV) architectures. In most of the monitoring systems, driver state remains largely external to vehicle decision-making and control logic [13].

Conversely, road traffic accidents persist as a major global safety challenge. According to the World Health Organisation, approximately 1.19 million people die each year due to road traffic injuries worldwide [18]. Among the contributing human factors, driver fatigue, mental load and drowsiness are widely recognised causes of degraded driving performance, leading to reduced vigilance, delayed reaction times, and impaired decision-making [14,15].

These risks also exist in automated driving situations, where drivers may remain disengaged for extended periods yet are still expected to resume control when required. Studies have highlighted driver drowsiness as a critical factor affecting takeover performance in automated driving. This emphasises the need for more comprehensive physiological and behavioural measurements to understand the underlying mechanisms during control transitions [12]. Together, these findings indicate that safe human-automation interaction depends not only on system capabilities but also on the driver's cognitive, physiological, and behavioural state during critical moments.

To address these challenges, we propose Human-in-the-Loop Automotive Sensing (HiLAS). This multimodal framework estimates driver attention, workload, and fatigue by integrating EEG, wearable physiological sensors, and vision-based posture analysis. Each modality contributes complementary information. HiLAS is designed within the context of SDV, where human-state estimates can be fed into the vehicle software layer for adaptive warnings, improved human-machine interface (HMI) behaviour, and safer navigation assistance. Through a simulator-based pilot study, this research evaluates the feasibility of multimodal human-state sensing and offers methodological insights into system integration, data fusion, and the practical challenges of applying these approaches to future in-vehicle systems. We address the following research questions:

RQ1: How can multimodal sensing be utilised to evaluate cognitive workload, engagement levels, and fatigue-related states during driving?
RQ2: What complementary insights do EEG, wearable sensing, and posture tracking offer, and what challenges might hinder their effective application in automotive settings?

1.1 Mental Workload, Fatigue, and Drowsiness

Driver state is commonly described using three related but distinct concepts: mental workload, fatigue, and drowsiness. Mental workload refers to the immediate cognitive demand placed on the driver by the driving task and the surrounding environment. It changes rapidly with traffic density, intersections, or secondary tasks, and mainly reflects short-term demands on attention and decision-making [9]. Fatigue is a slower, cumulative state that develops over time on task. It is associated with reduced alertness, slower reaction times, and physiological changes related to prolonged effort [6]. Drowsiness represents a more severe fatigue-related condition, closer to falling asleep, and is typically characterised by reduced vigilance, prolonged eye closure, and degraded vehicle control [16]. While driving, these states can occur simultaneously, but they exhibit different timing and noticeable signs.

1.2 Driver State Measures

Driving performance measures are commonly used to assess a driver's state. Key indicators include average speed, speed variability, the standard deviation of lane position (SDLP), and the rate of steering wheel reversals. Previous studies have shown that increased cognitive load, fatigue, or drowsiness can affect these measures, often leading to greater lane variability or more frequent steering corrections. High workload can overwhelm drivers, while extended periods of low-demand driving can lead to fatigue and drowsiness [1,15].

In automated and assisted driving, these effects are more critical because drivers may be disengaged for long periods and still be expected to take back control when automation fails, which depends strongly on the driver's mental model, their understanding of the system and its limits [11]. Studies show that takeover performance improves when drivers are asked to prepare before taking control. Wu et al. demonstrated that a two-stage takeover procedure increased drivers' monitoring behaviour and improved post-takeover driving performance during planned transitions [20], highlighting the need to continuously monitor the driver's state to support the human collaboration of the vehicle.

Physiological Measures. Physiological sensing provides more direct insight into the driver's internal state. Heart rate (HR) is commonly used as an indicator of general arousal and tends to increase under high mental workload or stress. However, the relationship between HR and fatigue is inconsistent. Heart rate variability (HRV) reflects autonomic nervous system activity and is more informative for detecting fatigue and drowsiness, especially over longer time windows [7]. EEG provides rapid and accurate measurements of brain activity. It can detect quick changes in our thoughts and emotions. Increases in theta and alpha brainwave activity often signify that a person is feeling tired or drowsy. [10]. Despite its sensitivity, the EEG is more intrusive and more affected by motion artefacts, which limit its standalone use in realistic driving environments.

Behavioural and Postural Indicators. The driver state is also reflected in observable behaviour. Changes in posture, movement patterns and control strategies can indicate behavioural adaptation to increased workload or fatigue [19]. Vision-based posture and movement tracking provides a non-contact way to capture these cues and complements physiological and performance-based measures, especially when eye tracking is unreliable due to lighting conditions or occlusion.

1.3 Multimodal and Event-Aligned Driver Monitoring

Each sensing modality captures only part of the driver state. Performance measures are affected by road geometry and automation levels. Physiological signals vary in sensitivity and robustness, while behavioural indicators depend on context. As a result, single-modality approaches often lack reliability across drivers and scenarios [17]. A key challenge is the temporal mismatch between signals. EEG and posture can respond rapidly to driving events, heart rate responds more gradually, and HRV and fatigue-related changes develop over longer time scales [7, 10]. Consequently, assuming that all signals are identical over time may limit the identification of important relationships.

To address these limitations, recent work increasingly adopts multimodal driver monitoring approaches that combine performance, physiological, and behavioural signals. Aligning these signals to driving events enables the short-term workload effects to be analysed alongside longer-term fatigue trends [4].

This highlights the need for frameworks that integrate multiple sensing modalities while accounting for their distinct temporal characteristics. While some studies focus on individual sensing modalities, most concentrate on isolated signals or offline analysis, with limited attention given to synchronising heterogeneous data streams or incorporating human-state estimates into vehicle software architectures. From the perspectives of digital health and SDV, this gap hinders the translation of sensing data into actionable adaptations. This highlights the need for integrated multimodal frameworks, such as HiLAS, that enable human-centred interactions within vehicle systems.

2 Materials and Methods

2.1 Proposed System Overview

HiLAS is a multimodal driver-state monitoring framework that integrates the driver into software-defined vehicle architectures [13]. As illustrated in Fig. 1, human-state estimates are fed to vehicle software layers to support adaptive warnings, improved HMI behaviour, and safer navigation assistance. The framework combines multiple sensors to assess the driver's state, including drowsiness, mental workload, and fatigue. It gathers physiological signals from EEG and wearable devices to provide insights into mental workload and heart functions. Furthermore, it incorporates visual inputs to examine the driver's posture, enabling the monitoring of behavioural changes over time. To better interpret these signals, HiLAS integrates driving-related information from Controller Area Network (CAN) signals and data from a forward-facing dash camera. This enables the identification of external driving events such as intersections, braking, and lane changes.

Extracted features from all sensor streams are aligned in a central synchronisation node using a window-based timeline. This design reflects the fact that driver state is inherently dependent on driving context and task demands, rather than being an isolated internal condition. Unlike prior approaches that estimate driver state independently of external events, HiLAS explicitly couples internal human-state signals with vehicle and environment context.

Following synchronisation, a data fusion and machine learning pipeline estimates driver states using both sensor-derived features and identified driving

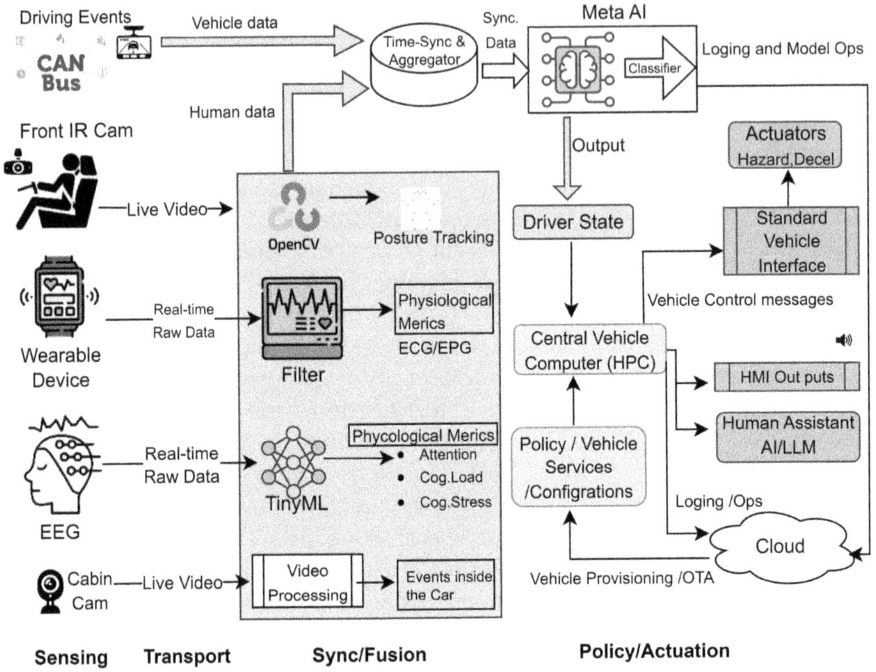

Fig. 1. Conceptual HiLAS architecture illustrating multimodal sensing and integration with software-defined vehicle software layers.

events, and the resulting outputs are fed into the vehicle's data and control pipeline by utilising the COVESA Vehicle Signal Specification (VSS), ROS 2 middleware, and other industry-relevant standards and platforms. This allows vehicle-level policies to determine how different driver states should influence HMI behaviour and safe navigation assistance strategies within the SDV paradigm.

The design of HiLAS is guided by the following principles:

- **Complementarity of modalities:** No single sensor can robustly capture driver state across all conditions. HiLAS combines EEG, wearable physiology, posture, and contextual data to exploit their complementary strengths and mitigate individual limitations.
- **Context-aware interpretation:** Driver state is interpreted relative to driving events and environmental demands, rather than as an absolute or context-free signal.
- **Temporal alignment and interpretability:** Window-based synchronisation ensures that heterogeneous signals can be analysed and interpreted at the level of session and task-relevant events.
- **Human-in-the-loop integration:** Human-state estimates are not treated as standalone outputs, but as first-class signals within the SDV software stack that can influence interaction and assistance behaviour.

– **Scalability toward real vehicles:** The framework is designed using industry-relevant standards (VSS, ROS 2) to facilitate future deployment in real-world SDV platforms.

2.2 Experimental Setup

This work reports a preliminary, simulator-based pilot study designed to evaluate the feasibility of multimodal driver-state sensing under controlled conditions. The experimental setup, shown in Fig. 2, and the Table 1 reflect sensing modalities that will be plausibly mapped to future in-vehicle implementations.

Table 1. Simulator Components and Real-Vehicle Equivalents

Component	Pilot Setup	Real Vehicle
EEG	5-channel dry electrodes	Workload/vigilance (future 2-channel ear-EEG)
Wearable	Heart-rate and stress watch	ECG/PPG via SDK
Posture	OpenCV keypoint tracking	IR camera–posture monitoring
360° Camera	Cabin view	Occupant/cabin monitoring
Simulation	ETS2 + CAVE setup	Varied real-road driving

The pilot study was conducted in a Cave Automatic Virtual Environment (CAVE) providing a horizontal field of view of approximately 200°, achieved using three WUXGA projectors with corrected projection profiles. The driving setup consisted of a Logitech G923 steering wheel with automatic transmission and a race-style seat, positioned at the centre of the CAVE. The simulated environment included road networks with navigation guidance, traffic signs, and structural elements such as bridges. Participants were instructed to drive naturally in order to encourage realistic driving behaviour.

Each participant completed a goal-directed driving task using Euro Truck Simulator 2, which was selected as a close approximation of real-world driving rather than a purely game-like environment. The simulator provides realistic vehicle behaviour, traffic flow, road layouts, and traffic rules, supporting natural driving behaviour.

Driver behaviour was recorded using an in-cabin camera setup. A front-facing Logitech HD1080p webcam (30 fps) captured upper-body posture and head movement, while a wide-angle cabin view was recorded using an Insta360 X4 camera. Camera placement aimed to maximise visibility while minimising intrusion, while acknowledging practical limitations such as occlusion and lighting variability. The primary front-facing camera was positioned approximately 90 cm in front of the participant, slightly to the right, and angled downward by 15–20° to mimic a typical in-truck monitoring perspective. The wide-angle camera was included to capture the full cabin view and to support future in-vehicle use cases, such as monitoring passenger movement.

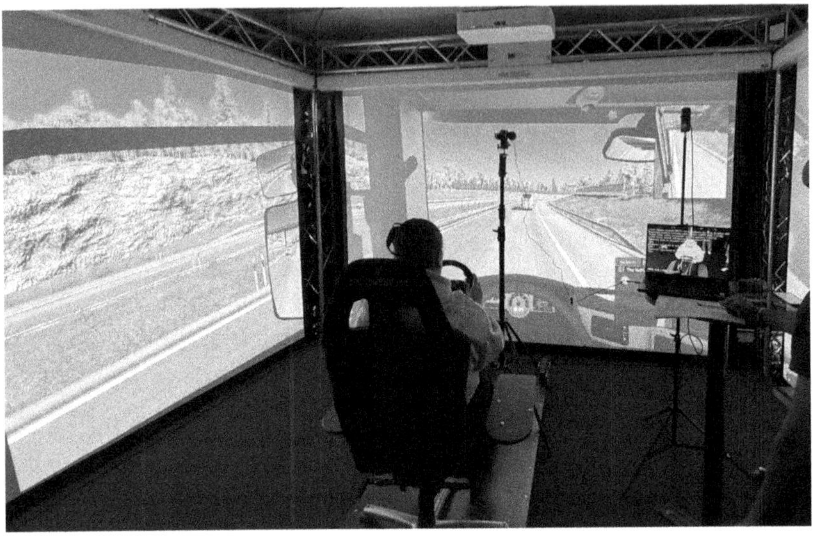

Fig. 2. Truck-driving simulator used in the pilot study, including steering wheel, pedals, and immersive visual display.

The front camera in HiLAS focuses on robust upper-body posture and gross behavioural movement rather than eye tracking. Extracted posture features included hand, trunk, and neck angles, postural stability over time windows, and posture-change intensity as a proxy for behavioural adaptation during demanding driving events. Eye-based gaze estimation was not prioritised due to reduced reliability under realistic in-vehicle conditions, including lighting variation and the use of sunglasses. An OpenCV-based pose estimation pipeline was used to compute posture metrics, and ergonomic compliance was assessed descriptively using ISO 11226 guidelines for static working postures [2].

Physiological data were collected using two sensing modalities. EEG signals were recorded using a 5-channel dry-electrode headset (EMOTIV Insight) positioned over frontal and central regions to capture neural correlates of cognitive workload and attention. In parallel, a wearable smartwatch (Samsung Galaxy Watch6 Classic) recorded heart rate and stress-related metrics derived from photoplethysmography, providing cardiovascular indicators linked to workload and fatigue.

2.3 Data Collection and Analysis

Five participants (three female, two male), all in their mid-twenties to mid-thirties, took part in the study after providing informed consent. Three participants held valid driving licences and were experienced drivers, while two participants were less experienced but had basic driving proficiency. For further studies, a more versatile and larger group of drivers will be hired.

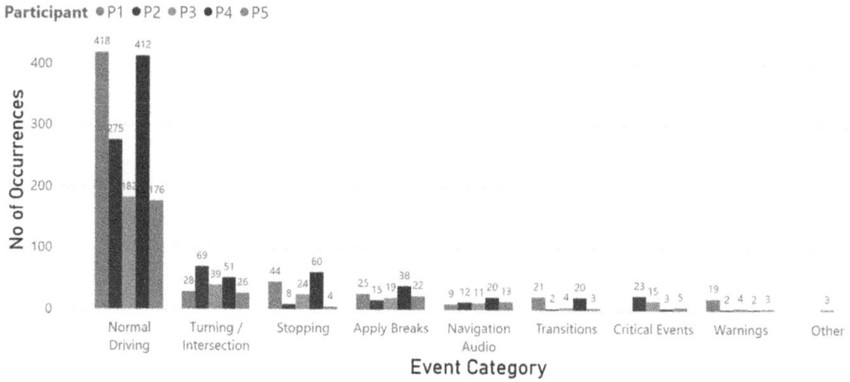

Fig. 3. Frequency of annotated driving event categories across participants used in the event-aligned analysis.

Participants were instructed to drive a truck from a predefined start location to a target destination. During the drive, they performed common driving tasks, including lane keeping, lane changes, overtaking, obeying speed limits, responding to traffic lights, road signs, navigating intersections, and parking at the final destination. Voice-based navigation instructions were provided in the simulator at key points along the route.

Figure 3 shows the distribution of annotated driving event categories across participants. Normal driving accounted for the largest portion of the sessions, while task-relevant events such as intersections, stopping, braking, navigation prompts, and critical events occurred less frequently and varied across participants.

Session durations ranged from approximately five to fifteen minutes. During each session, multimodal data streams were recorded, including simulated driving video, EEG signals, wearable physiological data, in-cabin video, and time-stamped posture metrics. All recorded streams were stored as participant-specific, time-stamped files and organised by sensing modality to support offline synchronisation, traceability, and subsequent analysis. All data were processed offline and aligned using timestamp-based synchronisation.

Stress metrics were derived from the wearable smartwatch using heart-rate variability patterns from photoplethysmography signals, while posture features were extracted using an OpenCV-based pipeline. Driving events, including navigation cues, lane changes, braking, and crashes, were identified from simulator logs and annotated with timestamps and task labels, as illustrated in Fig. 3. Analysis focused on aligning these events with multimodal sensor data to examine short-term, event-related changes in driver state rather than relying on whole-session averages.

Mental workload was defined as an event-dependent increase in cognitive effort required for perception, decision-making, and vehicle control. Fatigue was treated as a gradual, cumulative cognitive-physiological state associated with time-on-task and posture stability, while stress reflected physiological arousal. Although these states may overlap in natural driving, they were treated as analytically distinct for this study.

2.4 Feature Extraction and Modelling Pipeline

Multimodal data were segmented into overlapping, temporally aligned time windows across modalities. Windows of 10 s duration with a 5 s step were used, providing sufficient temporal context to capture physiological and behavioural responses while preserving short driving events. EEG was treated as a sensitive modality for relative workload changes rather than as a standalone or deployable predictor.

For each 10 s window, posture and behavioural features were extracted using summary statistics including mean, variance, slope, and range, while categorical driving-context variables were represented by the most frequent value within the window. For the EEG-based pipeline, additional window-level features were computed from the available channels, including band-power measures (theta, alpha, beta, and gamma), relative band power, signal variance, RMS, spectral entropy, and peak absolute z-score. Two datasets were then formed: one using posture and behavioural features only, and another combining posture and EEG features.

Supervised machine learning models were trained separately to estimate mental workload (three-class classification) and fatigue (binary classification) using a Random Forest classifier, as it is known to be simple and effective for such classification tasks and to provide preliminary results.

The model was trained using a fixed hyperparameter configuration rather than automated hyperparameter tuning. The number of trees was set to 450 to reduce variance and stabilise predictions, and class imbalance was addressed using `class_weight = "balanced"`. All remaining hyperparameters were kept at their default values, including unlimited tree depth, square-root feature sampling at each split, a minimum of two samples is required to split a node, and a minimum of one sample per leaf. These defaults were retained to allow flexible tree growth, while regularisation was primarily achieved through bootstrap aggregation, feature sub-sampling, and ensemble averaging rather than explicit constraints on individual trees. Hyperparameters were applied during model fitting within the training folds, while participant-wise `GroupKFold` cross-validation was used to evaluate performance in a subject-independent manner and prevent data leakage across participants.

Given the exploratory nature of the pilot study and limited sample size, the modelling pipeline was used to assess feasibility and the comparative contribution of sensing modalities rather than to optimise predictive performance. In selected analyses, cognitive load was normalised by posture-change intensity to capture sustained demand and reduce movement-related EEG noise, while fatigue was treated as a cumulative cognitive-physiological state. Labels were derived from driving context and time-on-task, with EEG included as an input feature but not used to define the labels.

3 Results

Pilot data were analysed by aligning key driving events with multimodal sensor streams, enabling event-based examination of changes in driver state across EEG, wearable physiological signals, and posture metrics.

3.1 Vision-Based Posture and Behaviour

Vision-based posture analysis revealed systematic changes in driver movement during demanding driving situations. Increased upper-body and hand movement was observed during navigation decisions, sharp steering actions, and other task-intensive events, indicating higher behavioural engagement.

Posture-tracking reliability was affected by practical conditions, such as low lighting and dark clothing. While posture sensing provided useful behavioural context, these observations confirm that vision-based measures alone are insufficient for robust driver-state estimation and benefit from integration with physiological sensing modalities.

3.2 Wearable Physiological Measures

Physiological signals from wearables exhibited substantial inter-individual variability. Average heart rate showed no consistent association with task completion or driving phase, highlighting the importance of individual baselines, consistent with previous findings [7]. In contrast, stress-related metrics showed a modest increase during driving relative to baseline. Participants who completed the driving task tended to exhibit higher average stress values than those who crashed, suggesting that elevated physiological arousal in the simulator may reflect task engagement rather than degraded performance. This observation is preliminary and requires validation in larger-scale studies.

3.3 EEG-Derived Mental Workload

EEG-based workload estimation was feasible in the simulator environment. Predicted workload exhibited clear event-aligned peaks, with higher values consistently observed during critical and decision-intensive situations such as crashes, loss of control, complex turning manoeuvres, and stopping at traffic lights or gates. Figure 4 summarises the driving events associated with the highest EEG-derived workload values across all recorded sessions.

EEG signal quality was sensitive to head movement and headset instability, leading to occasional noise during posture adjustments and steering actions. These limitations are expected in realistic driving-like behaviour and motivate improved noise handling and less intrusive EEG designs for longer-term and in-vehicle deployment.

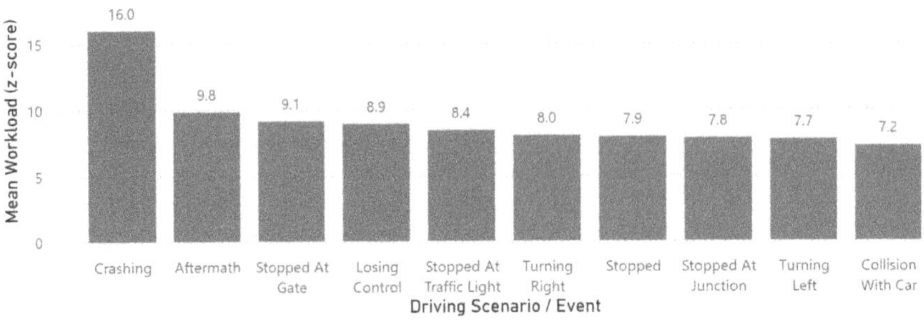

Fig. 4. Driving events associated with the highest EEG-derived mental workload, shown as mean normalised workload scores across all sessions.

3.4 Multimodal Modelling Outcomes

Supervised models were trained to estimate mental workload and fatigue using windowed multimodal features from all sensors combined, with and without EEG. Including EEG substantially improved mental workload estimation: the model achieved an accuracy of 0.966, compared to 0.878 without EEG. These window-level results indicate feasibility under participant-wise validation rather than generalisable performance. This confirms that EEG provides complementary information for capturing short-term cognitive demand beyond posture and behavioural features alone. Mental workload is reported using discrete class predictions or normalised EEG-derived workload scores, whereas fatigue is visualised probabilistically to reflect its cumulative nature.

In contrast, fatigue-prediction performance with EEG achieved an accuracy of approximately 0.72. Compared with similar recent studies [4], the achieved accuracy is comparable under realistic driving conditions. This supports the view that fatigue is a gradual, cumulative state without a clear temporal onset and is therefore better captured by longer-term physiological and behavioural trends than by brief, event-aligned EEG changes. Higher reported accuracies typically rely on large-scale datasets, deep transfer-learning architectures, and multimodal fusion strategies [3,4].

3.5 Event-Aligned Multimodal Patterns

Figure 5 presents an event-aligned multimodal segment from an intersection scenario for a representative participant. The right y-axis shows the model-predicted probability of cumulative fatigue, while the left y-axis represents a posture-normalised cognitive load indicator, defined as estimated cognitive load divided by positive posture-change intensity. This representation distinguishes cognitive demand during active movement from demand under relatively static posture. High cognitive load with little movement may indicate sustained mental effort, whereas posture changes may reflect adaptive behaviour.

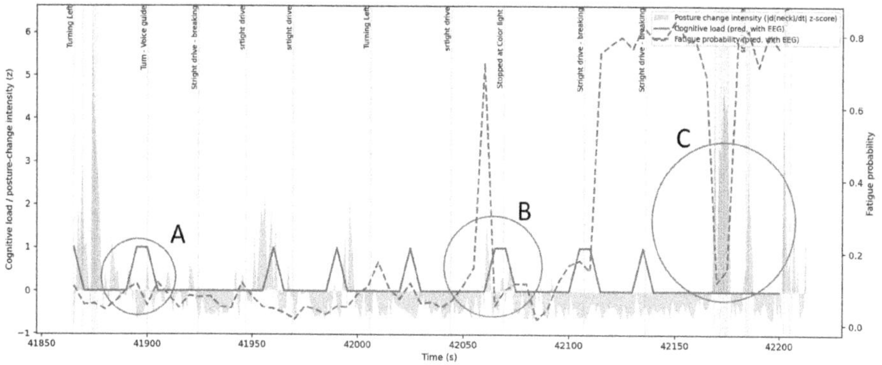

Fig. 5. Event-aligned time series showing posture change intensity, estimated cognitive load, and fatigue probability for selected driving events during a representative intersection scenario.

Normalising cognitive load by posture-change intensity also reduces movement-related EEG artefacts, thereby emphasising periods when increased EEG activity is more likely to reflect mental processing. Selected events illustrate these effects: (A) navigation cues coincide with increased posture-normalised cognitive load, indicating added cognitive demand from voice-based navigation guidance; (B) during an intersection manoeuvre, reduced posture change combined with increased cognitive load and fatigue probability reflects elevated task demand; and (C) large posture adjustments are followed by reduced fatigue probability despite low cognitive load, suggesting relief following prolonged static posture.

In this work, the driver's state is not treated as a single fixed label, but as a combination of posture intensity, cognitive load, fatigue probability, and the driving event occurring in each time window. This state evolves over time and changes with both driver behaviour and driving context.

3.6 Participant Feedback

Following recent studies on driving-simulator validation, we collected short post-task feedback on three key aspects: perceived simulator realism, sensor comfort (intrusiveness), and perceived workload [21]. A semi-structured questionnaire was used to capture participants' perceptions of simulator realism and authenticity, as well as comfort and any simulator-related discomfort, providing contextual information for interpreting the multimodal measurements.

Most participants described the simulator environment as realistic and sensitive to driving inputs, even without prior truck-driving experience. One participant stated:

> "very realistic, very sensitive. I haven't driven a truck, but a car."

Crash events were often perceived as serious rather than purely game-like. However, one participant still described elements of the setup as resembling a game, particularly due to visual presentation and speed perception.

> "I feel more like a game, especially with the front screening. You don't see how fast you are going."

Perceived immersion was also discussed. While participants acknowledged that the simulator was not as demanding as real driving, several reported a strong sense of presence created by the immersive display. One participant commented:

> "I don't think it's as intensive as real driving, but it definitely feels like you are there, especially with all the immersion going on with all the screens."

Control sensitivity was highlighted as an important factor influencing workload and simulator realism

> "The steering and the accelerator were very sensitive."

Wearable sensing and camera-based monitoring were generally perceived as unobtrusive. However, several participants reported mild discomfort from the EEG headset, particularly during longer sessions, highlighting the need for less intrusive neural-sensing solutions in future studies.

4 Discussion

This study demonstrates the feasibility of multimodal driver-state monitoring by integrating EEG, wearable physiological sensing, and vision-based posture analysis within a software-defined vehicle context. Rather than aiming to maximise prediction accuracy, HiLAS focuses on synchronising and interpreting heterogeneous human-state signals in an event-aligned manner, showing that mental workload and behavioural responses vary dynamically with driving context and task demands.

Event-based analysis indicated that demanding situations such as navigation decisions, loss of control, crashes, and voice-based guidance were associated with increased EEG-derived mental workload. These responses were often accompanied by posture changes and increased movement, suggesting that task demand is reflected across both neural and behavioural channels. Wearable stress measures differed widely between participants, making individual baselines more meaningful than fixed thresholds. The findings further suggest that auditory navigation cues are not cognitively neutral. Voice-based guidance introduced additional processing demands, particularly during already challenging driving moments, highlighting the importance of timing and personalisation in human-machine interaction.

Multimodal integration proved essential for interpreting these effects. EEG, wearable, and posture signals captured complementary aspects of driver state:

EEG was sensitive to short-term cognitive demand, wearables reflected gradual physiological fatigue and stress, and posture captured behavioural adaptation and movement-based regulation. EEG, posture, and wearable signals each exhibited distinct limitations when used in isolation, but their combination enabled more interpretable event-level analysis. In particular, posture-normalised workload representations highlighted sustained cognitive effort despite limited behavioural adaptation while mitigating movement-related EEG noise.

Several limitations should be acknowledged. The study was conducted as a small-scale, simulator-based pilot with a limited number of participants, and the results should therefore be interpreted as exploratory rather than generalisable. EEG measurements were sensitive to movement-related noise, posture tracking was affected by lighting and occlusion, and wearable metrics showed strong individual variability. In addition, modelling and analysis were performed offline and were not optimised for real-time deployment. While the study does not target clinical diagnosis, the monitored states' workload, fatigue-related trends, and physiological responses are relevant to preventive digital health and everyday well-being.

The present evaluation should be interpreted as a feasibility-oriented pilot rather than a performance benchmark. The sample size was small ($n = 5$), session durations were relatively short, and the event distribution was imbalanced, with normal driving windows substantially outnumbering critical events. These factors increase the likelihood that the reported window-level performance estimates are unstable and may not generalise to broader driver populations or real-world conditions. Accordingly, the reported classification results are intended to illustrate the comparative value of multimodal sensing, rather than to claim robust deployable accuracy.

To support future benchmarking of HiLAS, evaluation will include system-level metrics beyond classification accuracy, such as multi-stream synchronisation drift, end-to-end processing latency, real-time throughput under onboard constraints, and robustness to signal dropout and sensing noise. Together, these measures help assess whether a multimodal pipeline is not only predictive but also stable and reliable in real-world SDV settings. This work establishes an empirical foundation for multimodal, human-in-the-loop driver monitoring, highlighting key challenges and opportunities for health-aware vehicle systems.

Future work will extend HiLAS from simulator-based evaluation to real-vehicle studies. Planned in-vehicle experiments will deploy the sensing framework in a Toyota RAV4, with onboard processing performed on an NVIDIA Jetson Orin Nano Super Developer Kit. The system will integrate Emotiv MN8 2-channel EEG earphones, infrared in-cabin cameras, and an Android-based wearable sensor into a compact, real-time sensing and fusion pipeline built on ROS2. These multimodal streams will support a driver-state model coupled with a lightweight, onboard LLM that serves as a driving companion rather than a conventional assistant. The LLM will reason over driver state and driving context to provide adaptive, voice-based guidance without cloud connectivity. This paper focuses on multimodal sensing and event-aligned analysis; the LLM component is planned for future work and is not evaluated here. Future validation will include more participants, longer driving sessions, and testing in a real car under real driving conditions to assess how well the system generalises beyond this pilot study. In addition, future work will incorporate explicit driver drowsiness estimation using established observer-based drowsiness levels, as adopted in wearable-based driver monitoring studies [5]. Further evaluations will focus on driver experience, perceived control during assistance, robustness to noisy or missing data, and the stability of driver-state estimates.

5 Conclusion

This paper presents HiLAS, a multimodal human-in-the-loop sensing framework for driver-state monitoring in software-defined vehicles. Through a simulator-based pilot study, we demonstrated the feasibility of synchronising EEG, wearable physiological sensing, and vision-based posture analysis to capture event-driven changes in driver mental workload and behaviour. The results highlighted the complementary roles of different sensing modalities. These findings demonstrate the feasibility of multimodal integration in a pilot setting.

EEG was sensitive to short-term cognitive effort, posture metrics captured behavioural adaptation, and wearable signals reflected longer-term physiological responses, together enabling a more interpretable representation of driver state than any single modality alone.

Beyond technical feasibility, this work highlights the relevance of multimodal driver monitoring for digital wellness and adaptive automotive systems. While the present study is exploratory, it outlines a clear pathway toward real-vehicle deployment and more human-aware software-defined vehicles that not only perceive their environment but also better understand and collaborate with their drivers.

Acknowledgments. We thank the Advanced Intelligence Centre (AIC) Smart Campus Lab Lounge at the University of Oulu for providing the facilities used in this study. This research infrastructure has been partially supported by the European Union NextGenerationEU instrument funded by the Research Council of Finland (grant number 352726). We also acknowledge Chamika Karunarathne for support with data collection, and we thank all participants for their valuable contributions.

This work was supported by the EU HORIZON projects CHIPS-JU CIA FEDERATE (grant number 101139749), CHIPS-JU RIA HAL4SDV (grant number 101139789), and CHIPS-JU IA SHIFT2SDV (grant number 101194245), as well as the Business Finland projects 6G Visible (grant number 10743/31/2022), HAL4SDV national funding (grant number 7655/31/2023), and SHIFT2SDV national funding (grant number 5972/31/2024).

Disclosure of Interests. The authors declare that they have no competing interests relevant to the content of this article.

References

1. Ayas, S., He, D., Donmez, B.: Driver state classification: identifying high cognitive load and drowsiness through driver performance and physiology. IEEE Trans. Intell. Transp. Syst. (2025)
2. Delleman, N., Dul, J.: International standards on working postures and movements iso 11226 and en 1005–4. Ergonomics **50**(11), 1809–1819 (2007)
3. Dello Iacono, F., et al.: Analysis of neurophysiological correlates of mental fatigue in both monotonous and demanding driving conditions. Brain Sci. **15**(9) (2025). https://doi.org/10.3390/brainsci15091001, https://www.mdpi.com/2076-3425/15/9/1001
4. Kakhi, K., Asgharnezhad, H., Khosravi, A., Alizadehsani, R., Acharya, U.R.: Fatigue detection with multimodal physiological signals via uncertainty-aware deep transfer learning. J. Bionic Eng. 1–16 (2026)
5. Kundinger, T., Sofra, N., Riener, A.: Assessment of the potential of wrist-worn wearable sensors for driver drowsiness detection. Sensors **20**(4), 1029 (2020)
6. LAL, S., Craig, A.: Driver fatigue: electroencephalography and psychological assessment. Psychophysiology **39**, 313–21 (2002). https://doi.org/10.1017/S0048577201393095
7. Lu, K., Dahlman, A.S., Karlsson, J., Candefjord, S.: Detecting driver fatigue using heart rate variability: a systematic review. Accid. Anal. Prev. **178**, 106830 (2022)
8. Lu, S., Shi, W.: Vehicle Computing: From Traditional Transportation to Computing on Wheels. Springer, Cham (2024). https://doi.org/10.1007/978-3-031-59963-7
9. Muralidhar, A., Bindroo, R., Panimohzi, K.: Analysis of real-time cognitive fatigue detection systems for driver safety. In: 2024 International Conference on Emerging Technologies in Computer Science for Interdisciplinary Applications (ICETCS), pp. 1–6. IEEE (2024)
10. Naseri, N., Parastesh, F., Ghassemi, F., Jafari, S., Perc, M., Završnik, J.: Synchronization levels in eeg connectivity during cognitive workloads while driving. Nonlinear Dyn. **113**(7), 7243–7258 (2025)
11. Nasser, G., Morrison, B.W., Wiggins, M.W.: Mental models and driver takeover in automated vehicles: a systematic review. Ergonomics 1–14 (2025)
12. Pan, H., et al.: Exploring the effect of driver drowsiness on takeover performance during automated driving: an updated literature review. Accid. Anal. Prev. **216**, 108023 (2025)
13. Peltonen, E., Basnayake, V., Elgendy, N., Kämä, B., Seppänen, P., Päivärinta, T.: Towards data-centric and context-aware decision making in software-defined vehicles. In: 2025 IEEE 22nd International Conference on Software Architecture Companion (ICSA-C), pp. 574–577. IEEE (2025)
14. RoSPA: Driver fatigue and road collisions (2024). https://www.rospa.com/siteassets/pages/health-and-safety/health-and-safety-news/driver-fatigue-and-road-collisions/driver-fatigue-factsheet-0324.pdf, driver fatigue may contribute to up to 20% of road collisions
15. Saccomanno, F.F., Yu, M., Shortreed, J.: Effect of driver fatigue on truck accident rates. WIT Trans. Built Environ. **18** (2025)
16. Slater, J.D.: A definition of drowsiness: One purpose for sleep? Med. Hypotheses **71**(5), 641–644 (2008)

17. Visconti, P., Rausa, G., Del-Valle-Soto, C., Velázquez, R., Cafagna, D., De Fazio, R.: Innovative driver monitoring systems and on-board-vehicle devices in a smart-road scenario based on the internet of vehicle paradigm: a literature and commercial solutions overview. Sensors **25**(2), 562 (2025)
18. World Health Organization: Global Status Report on Road Safety 2023. World Health Organization (2023)
19. Wu, J., et al.: Research on driver posture recognition and prediction in vehicle. Proc. Inst. Mech. Eng. Part D: J. Automob. Eng. **239**(2–3), 796–808 (2025)
20. Wu, Y., Hasegawa, K., Kihara, K.: How to request drivers to prepare for takeovers during automated driving. Transport. Res. F: Traffic Psychol. Behav. **109**, 938–950 (2025)
21. Zhang, S., Zhao, C., Zhang, Z., Lv, Y.: Driving simulator validation studies: a systematic review. Simul. Model. Pract. Theory **138**, 103020 (2025). https://doi.org/10.1016/j.simpat.2024.103020, https://www.sciencedirect.com/science/article/pii/S1569190X24001345

Multiparametric MRI Analysis in Glioma Grading: Added Value of ADC Maps

Nourhan Ibrahim[1(✉)], Egor Panfilov[1], Niina Salokorpi[2,3,4], and Tuija Keinänen[2,3,4]

[1] Research Unit of Health Sciences and Technology, University of Oulu, Oulu, Finland
nourhan.ibrahim.ml@gmail.com
[2] Research Unit of Clinical Medicine, Faculty of Medicine, Oulu University Hospital and University of Oulu, Oulu, Finland
[3] Medical Research Center Oulu, Oulu University Hospital and University of Oulu, Oulu, Finland
[4] Neurocenter, Oulu University Hospital, Oulu, Finland

Abstract. The current standard in glioma diagnosis and grading relies on histopathological analysis of tumor tissue obtained through biopsy or surgical resection. These invasive procedures may expose patients to increased risk of complications. In this study, we investigated the potential of using multi-sequence MRI as a noninvasive method for glioma grading. The analysis was conducted on a dataset of 36 glioma patients with contrast-enhanced T1 (T1c) images, Apparent Diffusion Coefficient (ADC) maps, tumor annotations, and patient demographics. The imaging data was preprocessed using intra-subject registration, brain extraction, and resampling. A subset of 19 T1c and 14 ADC radiomics was selected for further analysis. After dimensionality reduction, bias-corrected and accelerated bootstrapping was utilized alongside Firth logistic regression for developing a T1c-based model, and a multi-sequence model. The two models were compared using the likelihood ratio test and the Akaike information criterion. The inclusion of ADC parameters significantly improved the model in terms of the quality of fit to the data. The results further implied that increased tumor texture heterogeneity and decreased ADC values could be associated with higher glioma grade. These findings highlight the potential utility of multi-sequence MRI for digital biopsy in glioma grading, although validation in a larger patient cohort is required.

Keywords: Magnetic Resonance Imaging · Radiomics · Glioma Grading

1 Introduction

Aggressiveness and malignancy of gliomas are reflected in their histopathological grade, with low-grade (LG) gliomas typically showing slower progression and

M. Särestöniemi et al. (Eds.): NCDHWS 2026, CCIS 3010, pp. 297–304, 2026.
https://doi.org/10.1007/978-3-032-28819-6_19

a better prognosis compared to high-grade (HG) gliomas [1]. Conventionally, glioma grading is determined through histopathological analysis of tumor tissue obtained by stereotactic biopsy, open biopsy, or surgical resection. Although stereotactic biopsy could be considered less invasive than the other two methods, it still involves a direct interaction with brain tissue, which poses a risk of complications of varying severity. Moreover, conventional tissue-based grading is subject to inter-observer variability which may affect diagnostic reliability [2]. In addition, biopsy samples may not adequately represent the spatial heterogeneity of the tumor and may fail to capture the most aggressive regions, potentially leading to underestimation of the tumor grade [3]. These limitations underscore the need for accurate and reliable non-invasive methods for glioma grading.

Radiomics is a set of quantitative imaging-based features that can convey information that is not visible to the naked eye [4,5]. These features can be used for analyzing the structure, shape, and texture of the whole tumor unlike traditional biopsy. Radiomics was used in previous studies for developing machine learning models for automatic glioma grading using either a specific MRI sequence or a combination of structural sequences. Although the use of diffusion-weighted imaging (DWI) was recommended, the number of studies that actually used DWI in general, ADC maps specifically, or combined structural and DWI sequences is much less than those using structural sequences [6–8]. Furthermore, most of the previous studies were more focused on model development rather than the associations between radiomics and glioma grades.

In this study, the main objective was to assess the value of ADC radiomics in addition to T1c radiomics in classification of LG and HG glioma grades. Additionally, we studied the associations between radiomics and glioma grades as well as the quality of fit of the models to the data.

2 Materials and Methods

The study included 36 glioma patients aged 20–79 years. Of these, 25 patients (69.4%) were male and 11 patients (30.6%) were female. A total of 22 patients (61.1%) were diagnosed with high-grade glioma (grade III–IV), while 14 patients (38.9%) were diagnosed with low-grade glioma (grade I–II). The dataset comprised preoperative imaging, demographic data, and histopathological diagnoses. The imaging data consisted of two sequences, namely contrast-enhanced T1 (T1c) and apparent diffusion coefficient (ADC) maps-together with reference annotations of the tumor for each patient.

Image preprocessing was performed by applying rigid intra-subject registration, brain extraction, re-orientation to the right-anterior-posterior (RAS) coordinate system, resampling to the standard (1.0, 1.0, 1.0) mm voxel spacing, and global normalization. The tumor masks were resampled to their corresponding source images used by the expert for the original annotation. The resampled masks were further processed by warping using the transformation produced during the image preprocessing, brain extraction, reorientation and resampling to the standard spacing to match the images.

Radiomic features were extracted from the preprocessed images after outlier intensity truncation and global min-max normalization. Absolute gray level discretization using a fixed bin width of 0.05 was utilized for better reproducibility, and the texture features were computed over the distances of 1, 2, and 3 pixels to capture both local and global texture characteristics of the tumor. A subset of the features was selected following the recommendations of previous studies to avoid selection bias [9–12]. Dimensionality reduction using principal component analysis (PCA) was then applied, with the first two principal components for each sequence selected for modeling. It should be noted that PCA was applied to the selected features only to avoid noise corrupting the principal components.

Finally, two models were fitted using Firth logistic regression [13,14] and bias-corrected and accelerated (BCa) bootstrapping [15]. These methods were specifically chosen to correct the confidence intervals for systematic bias and skewness as well as to penalize extreme estimations. The first model was parametrized by the T1c-derived components only, while the second model consisted of components from both T1c and ADC sequences. The two models were then compared in terms of the quality of fit and model complexity using the likelihood ratio test (LRT) [16,17] and the Akaike information criterion (AIC) [18]. An overview of the processing pipeline is shown in Fig. 1

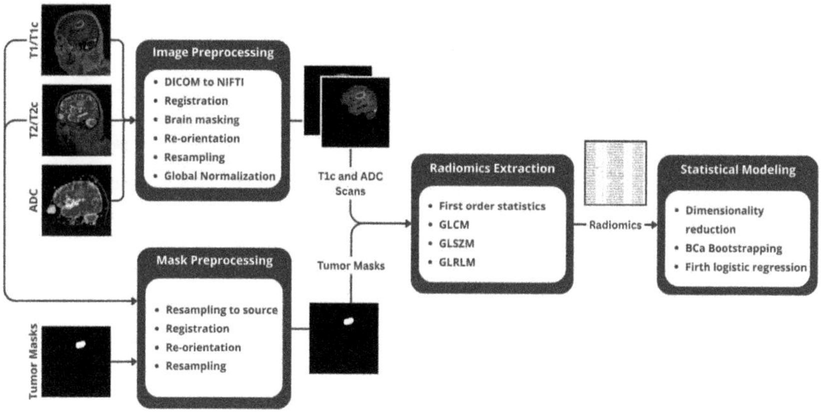

Fig. 1. An overview of the modeling pipeline. T1c = contrast-enhanced T1-weighted image; T2c = contrast-enhanced T2-weighted image; ADC = apparent diffusion coefficient map

3 Results

The selected radiomics from the T1c sequence consisted of 7 first order statistics, 9 gray level co-occurrence matrix (GLCM) features, and 3 gray level size zone matrix (GLSZM) features. From the ADC sequence, the selected radiomics consisted of 7 first order statistics and 7 GLCM features. Figure 2a shows the weights of each feature in each principal component. The cumulative variances were 0.433 and 0.797 for the first and second T1c components respectively. The results show that some features were more dominant in one feature than the other. Similarly, the weights of the ADC features are indicated in Fig. 2b, and the cumulative variances were 0.356 and 0.617 for the first and second ADC components respectively.

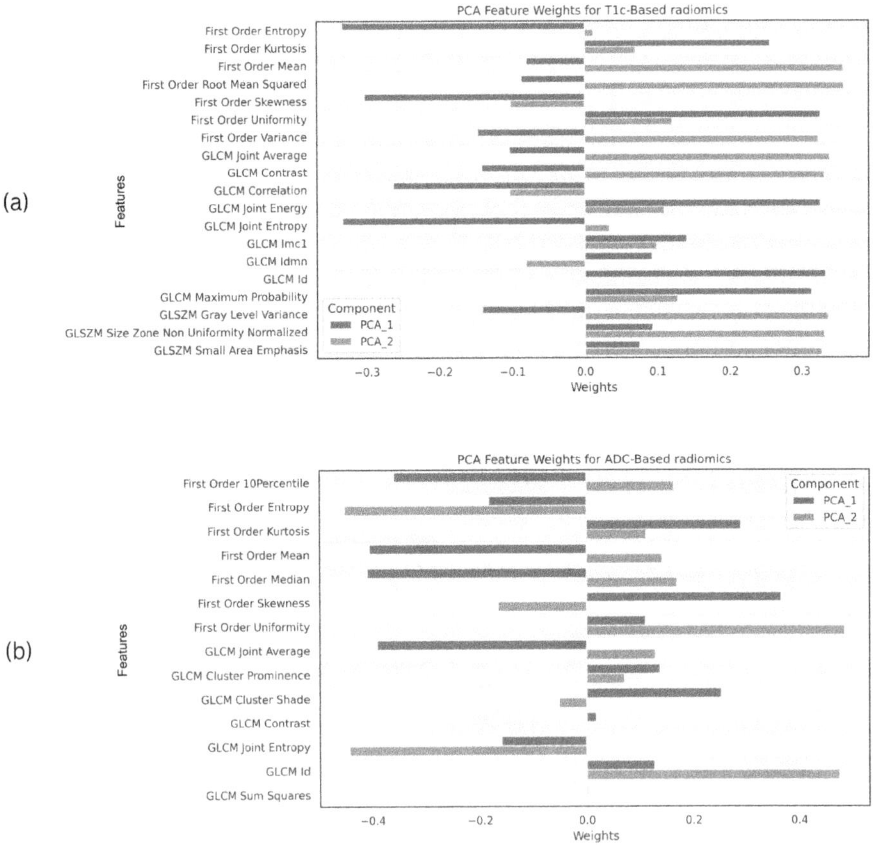

Fig. 2. Contributions of the T1c-based (top) and ADC-based (bottom) radiomics in the principal components; PCA_1 and PCA_2 are the first and the second principal components, respectively.

The forest plot in Fig. 3a indicates the associations between the T1c-based model parameters and the increase in the glioma grade; and it suggests that the first T1c component (OR: 1.005, 95% CI: [0.963, 1.021]) could be less relevant to the model compared to the second T1c component (OR: 1.247, 95% CI: [1.206, 1.268]), and that the positive association between the second component and high-grade glioma in this model was statistically significant. Figure 3b on the other hand suggests that all the parameters in the combined T1c and ADC model were significantly associated with the glioma grade. More specifically, the association was negative for the first T1c (OR: 0.960, 95% CI: [0.923, 0.974]) and the second ADC (OR: 0.884, 95% CI: [0.855, 0.916]) components, and positive for the second T1c (OR: 1.218, 95% CI: [1.157, 1.243]) and the first ADC (OR: 1.375, 95% CI: [1.321, 1.412]) components.

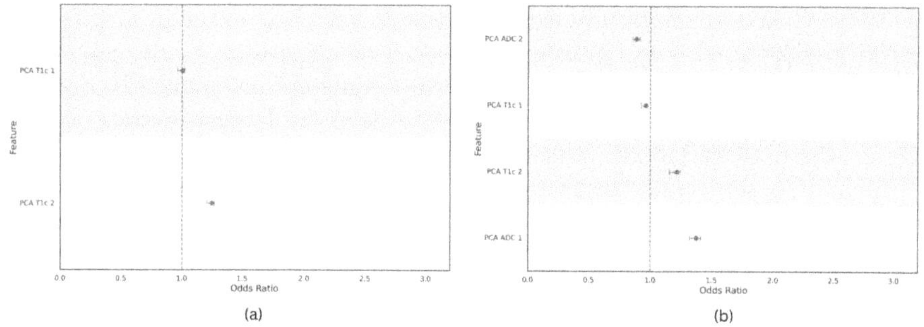

Fig. 3. Odds ratios and 95% confidence intervals of the parameters in the T1c-only model (left) and the T1c and ADC model (right). Null value is indicated by the dotted red line. (Color figure online)

When the two models were compared using the likelihood ratio test, the resulting p-value was 0.003, which was below the significance limit of 0.05. The AIC for the T1c-only model was 41.184, and for the T1c and ADC model was 33.547, with a ΔAIC of 7.637. Consequently, the multi-sequence model was better in terms of the fit to the data and the model complexity than the T1c model.

4 Discussion

According to the LRT, the p-value suggests that the ADC parameters improved the fit of the regression model to the data, and hence the improved discriminatory power of the multi-sequence model. The trends in the radiomics contributions to the model parameters indicate that the increase in the heterogeneity and coarse texture of the tumor as well as the decrease in the ADC values in the tumor region could be significantly associated with the increase in the glioma grades.

The two most significant parameters were the first ADC component and the second T1c component respectively with the former's negative correlation with the first order mean, median, and 10th percentile indicating a tendency towards low water diffusion in high grade glioma tumors. This finding is further supported by the component's negative correlation with GLCM joint average, and positive correlation with GLCM cluster shade. The result aligns with prior observations that lower ADC values in high-grade gliomas reflect restricted water diffusion caused by increased cellular density [19]. The second T1c component's positive correlation with the first order mean and variance, as well as the GLCM contrast, GLSZM size zone non-uniformity normalized, and GLSZM small area emphasis highlights the hyper-intensity in the tumor and its complex pronounced texture.

Despite the existence of previous studies that investigated the classification of glioma grades using radiomics, this work is one of few that is more concerned with inferential analysis and the interactions between the model parameters than predictive modeling. However, the small sample size imposed some constraints on the design choices in this study including the dependence on the prior literature for feature selection instead of using a data-driven algorithms. Model complexity also had to be restricted, allowing only two parameters per sequence to ensure convergence. These constraints highlight the need for larger datasets to fully leverage the potential of radiomics.

Expanding the cohort further would enable more robust feature selection methods and support the development of more complex models that better capture interactions across individual MRI sequences. Incorporating additional MRI contrasts—such as perfusion, magnetic resonance spectroscopy, or blood oxygen level dependent imaging—could further enhance grading accuracy by reflecting the tumor biological characteristics [20]. As datasets grow, machine learning–based fusion of multiparametric MRI and radiomic features may allow more reliable, clinically useful prediction of glioma grade.

5 Conclusion

Combining multiparametric MRI data represents a positive development towards non-invasive digital biopsy. Integrating ADC with T1c radiomic components improved the model's fit and discriminatory power compared to using T1c alone. The combined model benefited from the significant contributions of all components, reflecting both structural heterogeneity and diffusivity patterns associated with higher tumor grades. These findings demonstrate that leveraging information from multiple MRI-derived feature sets enhances robustness in glioma grade prediction.

References

1. Weller, M., et al.: Glioma. Nat. Rev. Dis. Primers **10**(1) (2024). https://doi.org/10.1038/s41572-024-00516-y
2. van den Bent, M.J.: Interobserver variation of the histopathological diagnosis in clinical trials on glioma: a clinician's perspective. Acta Neuropathol. **120**(3), 297–304 (2010). https://doi.org/10.1007/s00401-010-0725-7
3. Gatto, L., Franceschi, E., Di Nunno, V., Tosoni, A., Lodi, R., Brandes, A.A.: Liquid biopsy in glioblastoma management: from current research to future perspectives. Oncologist **26**(10), 865–878 (2021). https://doi.org/10.1002/onco.13858

4. van Timmeren, J.E., Cester, D., Tanadini-Lang, S., Alkadhi, H., Baessler, B.: Radiomics in medical imaging - "how-to" guide and critical reflection. Insights Imaging **11**(1) (2020). https://doi.org/10.1186/s13244-020-00887-2
5. Mayerhoefer, M.E., et al.: Introduction to radiomics. J. Nucl. Med. **61**(4), 488–495 (2020). https://doi.org/10.2967/jnumed.118.222893
6. Dequidt, P., et al.: Exploring radiologic criteria for glioma grade classification on the BRATS dataset. IRBM **42**(6), 407–414 (2021). https://doi.org/10.1016/j.irbm.2021.04.003
7. Sun, P., Wang, D., Mok, V.C., Shi, L.: Comparison of feature selection methods and machine learning classifiers for radiomics analysis in glioma grading. IEEE Access **7**, 102010–102020 (2019). https://doi.org/10.1109/access.2019.2928975
8. Foltyn-Dumitru, M., et al.: Advancing noninvasive glioma classification with diffusion radiomics: exploring the impact of signal intensity normalization. Neuro-Oncol. Adv. **6**(1) (2024). https://doi.org/10.1093/noajnl/vdae043
9. Ubaldi, L., Saponaro, S., Giuliano, A., Talamonti, C., Retico, A.: Deriving quantitative information from multiparametric MRI via radiomics: evaluation of the robustness and predictive value of radiomic features in the discrimination of low-grade versus high-grade gliomas with machine learning. Physica Med. **107**, 102538 (2023). https://doi.org/10.1016/j.ejmp.2023.102538
10. Moodi, F., et al.: Glioma tumor grading using radiomics on conventional MRI: a comparative study of WHO 2021 and WHO 2016 classification of central nervous tumors. J. Magn. Reson. Imaging **60**(3), 923–938 (2023). https://doi.org/10.1002/jmri.29146
11. Vijithananda, S.M., et al.: Texture feature analysis of MRI-ADC images to differentiate glioma grades using machine learning techniques. Sci. Rep. **13**(1) (2023). https://doi.org/10.1038/s41598-023-41353-5
12. De Maria, L., et al.: The current diagnostic performance of MRI-based radiomics for glioma grading: a meta-analysis. J. Integr. Neurosci. **23**(5) (2024). https://doi.org/10.31083/j.jin2305100
13. Firth, D.: Bias reduction of maximum likelihood estimates. Biometrika **80**(1), 27 (1993). https://doi.org/10.2307/2336755
14. Heinze, G., Schemper, M.: A solution to the problem of separation in logistic regression. Stat. Med. **21**(16), 2409–2419 (2002). https://doi.org/10.1002/sim.1047
15. Efron, B., Narasimhan, B.: The automatic construction of bootstrap confidence intervals. J. Comput. Graph. Stat. **29**(3), 608–619 (2020). https://doi.org/10.1080/10618600.2020.1714633
16. Neyman, J., Pearson, E.S.: On the use and interpretation of certain test criteria for purposes of statistical inference part I. Biometrika **20A**(1–2), 175–240 (1928). https://doi.org/10.1093/biomet/20a.1-2.175
17. Wilks, S.S.: The large-sample distribution of the likelihood ratio for testing composite hypotheses. Ann. Math. Stat. **9**(1), 60–62 (1938). https://doi.org/10.1214/aoms/1177732360
18. Cavanaugh, J.E., Neath, A.A.: The Akaike information criterion: background, derivation, properties, application, interpretation, and refinements. WIREs Comput. Stat. **11**(3) (2019). https://doi.org/10.1002/wics.1460
19. Momeni, F., et al.: Differentiating between low- and high-grade glioma tumors measuring apparent diffusion coefficient values in various regions of the brain. Oman Med. J. **36**(2) (2021). https://doi.org/10.5001/omj.2021.59
20. Lohela, J., Lehtiö, K., et al.: Improved brain tumor diagnostics and follow-up with novel magnetic resonance imaging methods: a single center study protocol. PLOS One **20**(11) (2025). https://doi.org/10.1371/journal.pone.0336387

A Modular Approach for Multi-scale Whole-Brain Simulation: Integrating a Neuron-Astrocyte-Vascular Model into the Virtual Brain

Rok Virant(✉) and Marja-Leena Linne

Faculty of Medicine and Health Technology, Computational Neuroscience Group, Tampere University, Tampere, Finland
{rok.virant,marja-leena.linne}@tuni.fi

Abstract. Whole-brain simulation frameworks have become important tools for studying large-scale brain dynamics, disease mechanisms, and personalized neuroimaging signals such as BOLD fMRI. As these platforms move toward increased biological realism and multi-scale integration, their underlying architecture becomes a critical factor for ensuring scalability, extensibility, and long-term usability. Integrating heterogeneous biophysical processes across neuronal, glial, and vascular domains poses significant architectural challenges. Here, we demonstrate that a modular design is not only compatible with, but fundamentally necessary for, incorporating complex multi-compartment physiological cascades into whole-brain simulation frameworks without modifying their core computational infrastructure. Using The Virtual Brain (TVB) as a reference platform, we present a case study in which a Neuron-Astrocyte-Vascular (NAV) extension is integrated as a set of modular components. In this implementation, astrocytic calcium dynamics and neurovascular coupling mechanisms are incorporated alongside existing neuronal models while preserving core system properties such as computational efficiency, scalability, and personalization. Our results show that neuronal, astrocytic, and vascular subsystems can be implemented as independent yet interoperable layers within the simulation framework, maintaining the integrity of connectivity, coupling, and solver structures. This integration blueprint provides a generalizable template for extending whole-brain models toward richer multi-scale representations. To our knowledge, this work represents the first demonstration of integrating a biologically detailed Neuron-Astrocyte-Vascular cascade into a modular whole-brain simulation framework without altering its core architecture. Beyond its immediate application, this approach facilitates more flexible and scalable neuroscientific modeling and opens new opportunities for brain-inspired neuromorphic systems and energy-aware computing.

Keywords: Whole-brain-simulation · Architectural-modularity · Scalability · Neuron-Astrocyte-Vascular model · BOLD-fMRI

M. Säreströniemi et al. (Eds.): NCDHWS 2026, CCIS 3010, pp. 305–313, 2026.
https://doi.org/10.1007/978-3-032-28819-6_20

1 Introduction

Whole-brain simulation frameworks and platforms allow the study of local and global brain states. These large-scale computational platforms are particularly designed to model and predict large-scale brain dynamics. Simplified neuronal population models are coupled through structural connectivity of network interactions, alongside the effects of structural organization on functional dynamics. One such whole-brain simulation framework is The Virtual Brain (TVB) simulator [2]. The research done using the TVB platform has demonstrated that connectome-based simulations can reproduce empirically observed large-scale brain activity patterns [8] and support personalized modeling of healthy and pathological brain states [3].

Current whole-brain simulators are progressing toward richer biological detail and broader data integration, highlighting the importance of architectural strategies that support scalability, interpretability, and traceability [5, 6]. In monolithic architectures, where model components are tightly interdependent rather than modular, changes must be implemented across the entire system, which restricts extensibility and complicates adaptation to new scientific questions. Recent architectural extensions of TVB further demonstrate how modular designs enable large-scale parameter exploration and systematic model evaluation without requiring modifications to the simulation core [4]. Additionally, modular approaches allow individual components to be developed, validated, and scaled independently, while maintaining coherent system-level dynamics. This flexibility supports reproducibility, facilitates integration of novel biophysical and biochemical models, and enables simulators to evolve alongside emerging neuroscientific discoveries. As a concrete example, we showcase our work integrating the Neuron-Astrocyte-Vascular (NAV) model, previously developed to better understand the origin of BOLD fMRI signal [9], into the TVB framework.

In this study, we show how a modular design enables biophysical extensions to coexist and interact seamlessly with large-scale brain simulations. Modularity is framed here not merely as a choice of software engineering, but rather a scientific driver, a foundational principle for the future generation of whole-brain modeling. Here, we demonstrate, for the first time, the integration of a biologically detailed Neuron-Astrocyte-Vascular (NAV) model into the modular architecture of The Virtual Brain, establishing a scalable framework for incorporating multiscale physiological mechanisms into whole-brain simulations. While this study primarily focuses on the architectural demonstration and its feasibility, the quantitative validation is seen as an additional, essential future step.

2 Architectural Design Principles of the Virtual Brain Simulator

The foundation of The Virtual Brain simulator is defined by its modular architecture. Rather than a single biological model, its modular structure is based on interoperable and interchangeable components [1–3]. TVB's architectural core is defined by several well-defined components. Structural connectivity represents the large-scale network topology of the brain. This is typically produced from diffusion-weighted magnetic resonance imaging (dMRI) using tractography methods. The resulting connections are specified by connection weights and transmission delays between regions or nodes.

Dynamical models of the activity of local populations of neuronal cells are typically presented as neural mass models or neural field models, providing a representation of population-level activity across spatial and temporal dimension [4–6]. What defines these models is the intrinsic activity of each individual brain region. The coupling function determines how neuronal activity propagates across the network. Numerical Integration schemes orchestrate and govern the evolution of the system, in other words, how the signal is computed from a temporal perspective. Finally, observation (forward) models map the simulated neuronal activity to empirically measurable signals, enabling direct comparison with experimental data. These signals include, but are not limited to, electroencephalography (EEG), magnetoencephalography (MEG), and blood-oxygen-level-dependent (BOLD) functional magnetic resonance imaging (fMRI) which can be recorded non-invasively in humans [2, 3].

From a conceptual perspective, the above-mentioned components are intentionally separated, allowing each component to be modified and specified independently. The structural data do not constrain the choice of local dynamics, and the observational model remains independent of both the network topology and the underlying neuronal mechanisms. This clear division forms the foundation of modularity in the whole-brain simulator that we have selected to use, the TVB, allowing the system to be flexible, extendable, and modular [2, 3].

From a technical standpoint, TVB is organized in a way that well defines layers, each implemented as a free-standing module with a transparent interface. Neuronal models, coupling functions, and forwards models can be shaped and extended independently, without touching the core simulation engine. In a controlled and systematic approach, this structure makes it easier to compare different models with each other, extending the architecture if needed.

In summary, the components and the design principles used in TVB define the simulator as a modular modeling framework. On this architecture, we have integrated an auxiliary biophysical module into one simulator, illustrating how a modular design can enable structured and interpretable extensions of whole-brain simulators.

3 Methods

The Neuron-Astrocyte-Vascular (NAV) model (see Fig. 1) describes a biophysical cascade that links neuronal activity to vascular responses through astrocytic signaling pathways. In this framework, synaptic activity modulates astrocytic metabotropic glutamate receptor activation, leading to intracellular inositol 1,4,5-trisphosphate (IP_3) production and Ca^{2+} dynamics. Astrocytic calcium activity modulates downstream vascular signaling pathways, including arachidonic acid metabolites and prostaglandins, which in turn modulate local blood flow and volume, giving rise to BOLD/fMRI signals. This cascade provides a link between the neuronal population activity and the macroscopic hemodynamic observations, as introduced by Tesler et al. (2023) [9].

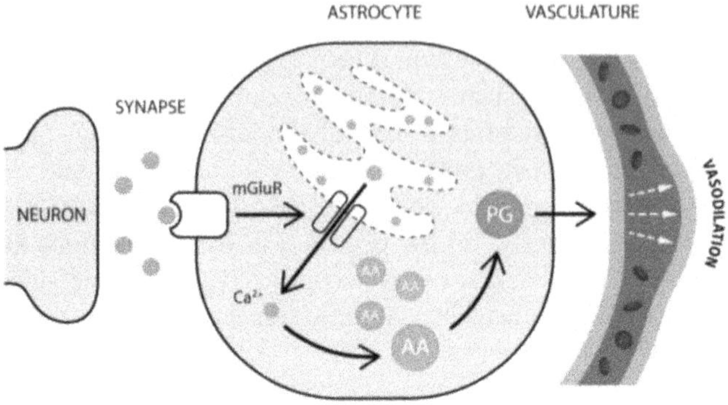

Fig. 1. Signaling pathway mediated through a Neuron-Astrocyte-Vascular system. Synaptic glutamate activates metabotropic glutamate receptors (mGluRs) in the astrocyte. This triggers intracellular inositol 1,4,5-trisphosphate (IP_3) production and Ca^{2+} dynamics, further regulating the production and the release of vasoactive substances (including arachidonic acid (AA) metabolites and prostaglandins (PG)), resulting in vascular dilation. The schematic illustration follows the biophysical NAV model described in Tesler et al. [9].

At the level of local brain dynamics, astrocytic and vascular processes are incorporated as additional state variables within the brain area model. Neuronal population activity is generated using a mean-field model of Adaptive Exponential integrate-and-fire (AdEx) excitatory and inhibitory neurons, each described by differential equations for membrane voltage and adaptation current. The activity of the excitatory population serves as the driving input to the astrocytic layer. Astrocytic calcium dynamics are governed by dedicated subsystems that evolve in parallel with neuronal activity. Driven by synaptic input from neurons, the layers remain separated from the neuronal model. This separation further confirms that biologically detailed glial dynamics can be incorporated as independent layer within an existing neuronal model, without the need to modify the mean-field formulation. Similar biophysically grounded mean-field approaches have been used to bridge cellular mechanisms and whole-brain dynamics, supporting the integration of additional physiological subsystems within TVB [6, 7].

At the coupling level, the NAV does not change the large-scale structural connectivity either. Instead, the Neuron-Astrocyte-Vascular interactions are executed locally within the selected or given nodes. This further maintains the original network topology and the definition of inter-regional coupling. This kind of structure ensures that global dynamics remain governed by the exact same connectome-based interactions, whereas additional biophysiological mechanisms focus on modulating local responses. This confirms that the addition of the NAV cascade is isolated from connectivity and inter-regional coupling. At the observational level, vascular variables are linked to the hemodynamic forward model to generate a BOLD signal. These observation models are separated from the neuronal modules and the astrocytic module. This makes it possible to study and test different neurovascular formulations alongside their hypotheses without changing the core of the system.

In summary, the described modular framework enables the NAV cascade to be simulated independently, driven by external inputs such as synaptic activity or neuromodulator signals. Each component can be modified or replaced without affecting the overall system, underscoring the flexibility and modularity of the TVB architecture [11]. The reproduced dynamics are consistent with those reported in Tesler et al. (2023) [9], while detailed quantitative validation against empirical BOLD fMRI data is beyond the scope of the present study.

4 Results from the Use Case Study

The modular integration of the NAV cascade into TVB is demonstrated using a stimulation experiment (see Fig. 2). An external pulse-train stimulus drives excitatory neuronal populations, producing transient increases in neuronal firing rate accompanied by adaptation dynamics. These neuronal responses serve as inputs to the astrocytic module, where activity-dependent signaling triggers IP_3 production and intracellular calcium dynamics in each astrocytic unit. Astrocytic calcium signals subsequently drive the vascular subsystem via the arachidonic acid and prostaglandin pathways, resulting in a delayed and temporally smoothed BOLD-like response. The temporal separation between neuronal firing rate, astrocytic calcium activity, and vascular output reflects the hierarchical organization of the NAV cascade, highlighting the functional modularity and multi-scale interactions within the system (see Fig. 3). While the reproduced dynamics are consistent with the ones present in Tesler et al. (2023) [9], the quantitative validation against empirical fMRI is beyond the scope of the current study.

These results demonstrate that additional physiological and biophysiological processes can be incorporated locally within TVB nodes without affecting large-scale connectivity, coupling mechanisms, or numerical solvers. The NAV-TVB use case illustrates how a modular architectural design enables multi-stage physiological and signaling cascades to be simulated coherently within a whole-brain framework.

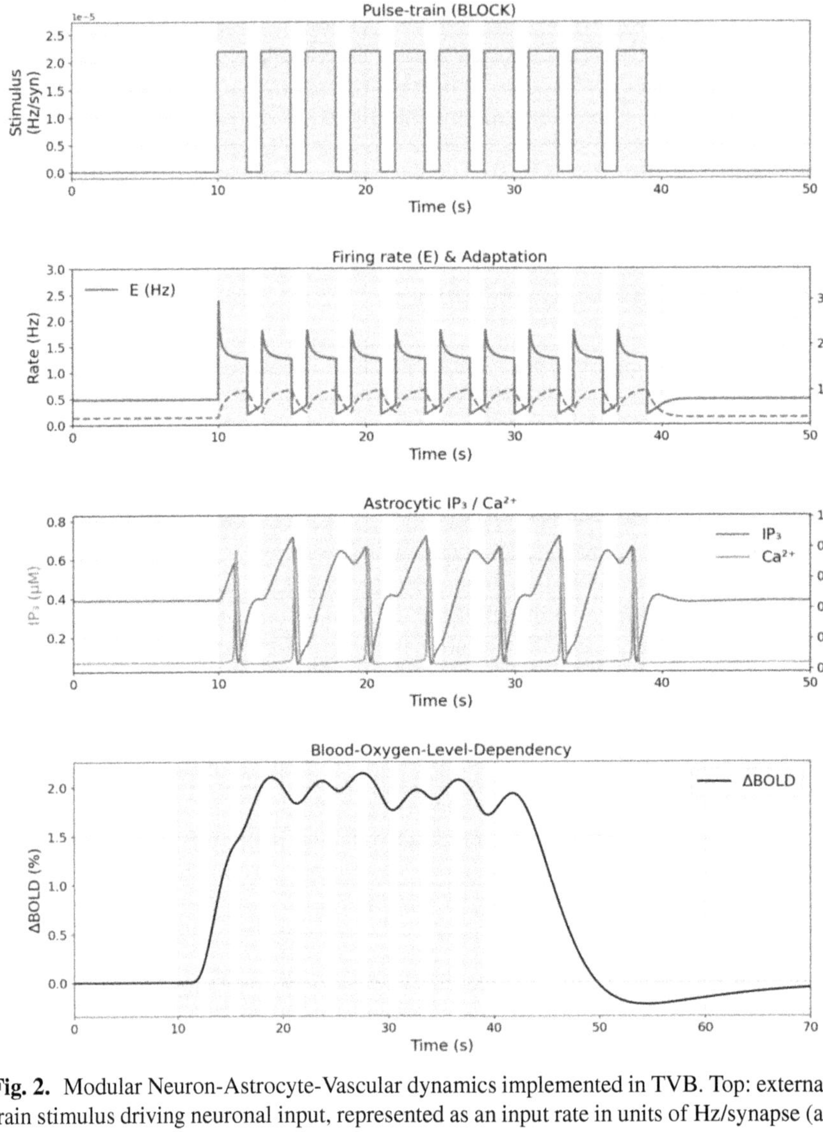

Fig. 2. Modular Neuron-Astrocyte-Vascular dynamics implemented in TVB. Top: external pulse train stimulus driving neuronal input, represented as an input rate in units of Hz/synapse (average presynaptic firing rate per synapse). Second panel: the resulting excitatory firing rate with spike-frequency adaptation, illustrating transient neuronal responses to repeated stimulation; the dashed red curve represents the mean adaptation variable, while the blue curve represents the mean neuronal activity. Third panel: astrocytic signaling dynamics, showing IP_3 accumulation and Ca^{2+} transients triggered by neuronal activity. Bottom: vascular response is presented as a BOLD signal generated via the astrocyte-mediated pathway. The figure illustrates the temporal propagation of activity across neuronal, astrocytic, and vascular modules, highlighting their modular coupling within the TVB framework.

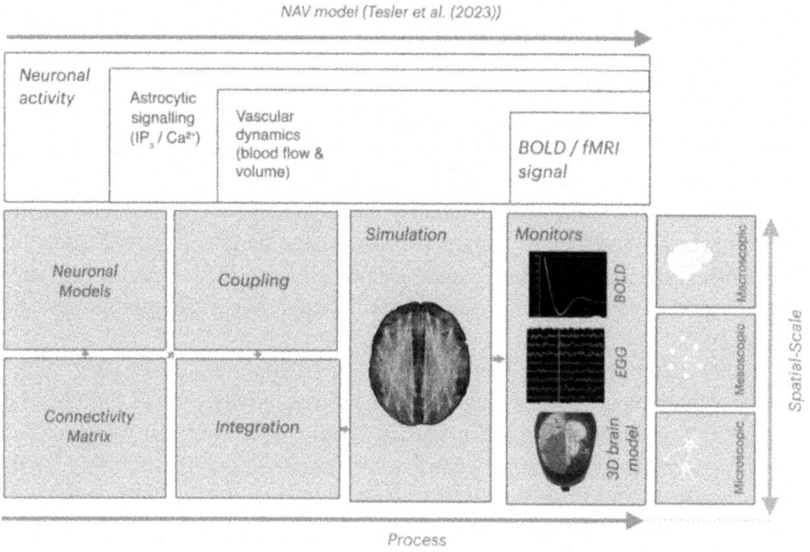

Fig. 3. Modular workflow of the TVB architecture extended with a Neuron-Astrocyte-Vascular (NAV) cascade. Neuronal models combined with the connectivity matrix define local neuronal activity, which is propagated through coupling and numerical integration to generate whole-brain simulations. Neuronal outputs drive astrocytic signaling (IP_3/Ca^{2+}) and subsequent vascular dynamics (blood flow and volume), which are mapped to macroscopic observables (e.g., BOLD/fMRI, EEG) via monitor modules. The workflow illustrates a structured process spanning microscopic, mesoscopic, and macroscopic spatial scales, following the NAV modeling concept of Tesler et al. [9].

5 Discussion

In this study, we demonstrate, for the first time, the integration of a full Neuron-Astrocyte-Vascular cascade into The Virtual Brain. This provides further evidence that TVB's modular architecture can support low-level biophysical and biochemical interactions as independent layers, without requiring modifications to its core computational infrastructure. By maintaining a clear separation between neuronal, astrocytic, and vascular processes, each component can be simulated, modified, or replaced independently [2, 3]. This use case illustrates how detailed local physiological mechanisms can be incorporated while preserving the integrity of connectivity, coupling schemes, and numerical solvers [5, 11].

While a modular architectural approach provides flexibility and extensibility it introduces tradeoffs between biological realism and computational efficiency. Specifically, separating neuronal, astrocytic, and vascular components may simplify their interactions, and the overall system behavior depends on the assumptions and parameterization of each module. Additionally, integrating processes across different scales could face challenges for the consistency and validation of parameters. These tradeoffs are acknowledged as possible directions of future validation work.

Our work primarily focuses on demonstrating architectural feasibility rather than introducing new biological validation. Importantly, the implemented NAV model builds upon the previously validated framework by Tesler et al. (2023) [9], where the model was already evaluated against BOLD fMRI data, providing strong support for its biological relevance. The reproduced dynamics in our implementation are consistent with those reported in the original study, further confirming the correctness of the integration. While this work does not aim to re-establish biological validity, it provides a crucial step in extending a validated cellular-level model into a whole-brain simulation framework. Future work will focus on further validation using increasingly detailed experimental data, including in vivo astrocytic calcium recordings and human neurovascular coupling measurements. Systematic comparisons between NAV-derived signals and empirical data will be essential to assess and refine the biological realism of the model in a whole-brain context.

A modular structure enables whole-brain simulators to be extended in a controlled and scalable manner, reducing architectural complexity even as biological detail increases [4, 5]. Such modularity is also consistent with neuromorphic design principles, which rely on distributed, component-level computation, allowing different physiological processes to be modeled as interacting but independent units. In this context, the NAV module provides a pathway for incorporating energy-related constraints into large-scale brain simulations [9, 10].

From a digital health perspective, this modular whole-brain framework supports the development of personalized brain digital twins [12] by enabling the integration of multimodal data and providing mechanistic, model-based insights into disease mechanisms and potential therapeutic interventions. Together, these features position modular architectures as a key enabler for the next generation of whole-brain simulation frameworks, supporting both flexibility and increased physiological realism [13].

In conclusion, modular whole-brain simulation frameworks provide a strong foundation for the next generation of computational neuroscience. The integration blueprint presented here offers a concrete example of how increasingly detailed and complex physiological mechanisms can be incorporated into whole-brain simulations.

Funding. This research has received funding from the European Union's Horizon Europe Programme (https://commission.europa.eu/index_en) under Specific Grant Agreement No. 101147319 (EBRAINS 2.0 Project) and from Research Council of Finland (https://www.aka.fi/en/), decision No. 373683, to M-LL. The project also received funding from the strategic profiling of Tampere University in health data science (Academy of Finland, 2021–2026).

References

1. Jirsa, V.K., Sporns, O., Breakspear, M., Deco, G., McIntosh, A.R.: Towards the virtual brain: network modeling of the intact and the damaged brain. Arch. Ital. Biol. **148**(3), 189–205 (2010)
2. Sanz Leon, P., et al.: The Virtual Brain: a simulator of primate brain network dynamics. Front. Neuroinform. **7**, 10 (2013)
3. Sanz-Leon, P., Wang, Y., Cabral, J., Knock, S.A., McIntosh, A.R., Jirsa, V.K.: The virtual brain: a computational framework for large-scale brain network modeling. Neuroimage **111**, 385–430 (2015)

4. van der Vlag, M., Kusch, L., Destexhe, A., Jirsa, V.K., Diaz-Pier, S., Goldman, J.S.: Vast parameter space exploration of the virtual brain: a modular framework for accelerating the multi-scale simulation of human brain dynamics. Appl. Sci. **14**(5), 2211 (2024)
5. Kusch, L., et al.: Multiscale co-simulation design pattern for neuroscience applications. Front. Neuroinform. **18**, 1156683 (2024)
6. Sacha, M., Tesler, F., Cofré, R., Destexhe, A.: A computational approach to evaluate how molecular mechanisms impact large-scale brain activity. Nat. Comput. Sci. **5**(5), 405–417 (2025)
7. Tesler, F., et al.: Multiscale modeling of neuronal dynamics in hippocampus CA1. Front. Comput. Neurosci. **18**, 1432593 (2024)
8. Stenroos, P., et al.: EEG-fMRI in awake rat and whole-brain simulations show decreased brain responsiveness to sensory stimulations during absence seizures. eLife **13**, RP90318 (2024)
9. Tesler, F., Linne, M.-L., Destexhe, A.: Modeling the relationship between neuronal activity and the BOLD signal: contributions from astrocyte calcium dynamics. Sci. Rep. **13**, 6451 (2023)
10. Jiang, H.-J., et al.: Modeling neuron-astrocyte interactions in neural networks using distributed simulation. PLoS Comput. Biol. **21**(9), e1013503 (2025)
11. Palesi, F., et al.: The importance of cerebellar connectivity on simulated brain dynamics. Front. Cell. Neurosci. **14**, 240 (2020)
12. Schirner, M., Domide, L., Perdikis, D., Triebkorn, P., Stefanovski, L., Pai, R., et al.: Brain simulation as a cloud service: the virtual brain on EBRAINS. Neuroimage **251**, 118973 (2022)
13. Linne, M.-L.: Computational modeling of neuron-glia signaling interactions to unravel cellular and neural circuit functioning. Curr. Opin. Neurobiol. **85**, 102838 (2024)

A Safety-Constrained Architecture for Adaptive Clinical Decision Support

Kavishwa Wendakoon(✉) and Nirnaya Tripathi

University of Oulu, P.O. Box 123, 90014 Oulu, Northern Ostrobothnia, Finland
{Kavishwa.WendakoonMudiyanselage,Nirnaya.Tripathi}@oulu.fi

Abstract. AI-assisted clinical decision support systems (CDSS) increasingly incorporate adaptive and generative components to personalize recommendations and improve workflow efficiency. However, runtime adaptation in safety-critical clinical settings introduces significant governance challenges, including loss of predictability, unclear accountability, and limited auditability of system behavior over time. Existing CDSS architectures largely focus on model performance or explainability, while providing insufficient support for governing how and when adaptive changes are permitted in practice.

This paper presents a safety-constrained self-adaptive software architecture for AI-assisted CDSS that enables bounded personalization while preserving clinician authority, patient safety, and regulatory accountability. Following a Design Science Research methodology, we design and iteratively refine an architecture based on a MAPE-K control loop augmented with an explicit Constraint Layer. The constraint layer enforces an adaptation boundary through bounded parameter updates, multi-clinician validation gates, evidence anchoring with contradiction checks, and auditable change records with versioning and rollback.

We instantiate the architecture in a nurse-led triage-to-disposition workflow, modeling escalation paths and safety gates as an explicit state machine, and demonstrate interoperability via SMART on FHIR-style interfaces that exchange clinical context while keeping adaptation logic and governance mechanisms internal to the system. A formative stakeholder evaluation with clinicians indicates that the proposed approach improves perceived predictability, trust calibration, and confidence in oversight compared to unconstrained adaptive CDSS.

The results suggest that governing adaptation, rather than restricting AI capability, is a key design strategy for deploying trustworthy, adaptive decision support in regulated digital health environments.

Keywords: Clinical Decision Support Systems · Adaptive AI · Self-Adaptive Systems · Safety-Constrained Architecture · AI Governance · Digital Health · Auditability · Design Science Research

1 Introduction

Clinical decision support systems (CDSS) are widely regarded as a core digital health capability for improving the safety, consistency, and efficiency of care.

M. Säreströniemi et al. (Eds.): NCDHWS 2026, CCIS 3010, pp. 314–338, 2026.
https://doi.org/10.1007/978-3-032-28819-6_21

Their real-world impact, however, is often limited less by algorithmic performance than by persistent socio-technical failure modes. Prior work has documented recurring problems such as workflow misalignment, high override rates, and alert fatigue, where repeated or poorly timed alerts reduce adherence to otherwise useful guidance [1]. More broadly, CDSS benefits and harms are tightly coupled: the same mechanisms that scale clinical knowledge can also increase cognitive burden, introduce new safety risks, and erode trust when system behavior is poorly integrated into clinical work or cannot be meaningfully scrutinized [2].

These concerns become more acute with the increasing use of machine learning (ML) and generative AI in decision support. ML-enabled systems may offer greater personalization and context sensitivity, but they can also behave in ways that are harder for clinicians and organizations to anticipate, interpret, and govern [3]. In practice, clinicians may place undue confidence in AI-generated advice even when it is incorrect, thereby shifting both judgment and confidence calibration [4]. Transparency alone is not a sufficient safeguard. Explainable AI (XAI) may improve interpretability, but it does not automatically provide accountability, provenance, or enforceable operational limits [5]. Clinical users often need more than an explanation of a single output; they need structured information about intended use, limitations, data provenance, and monitoring expectations in order to support safe use [6].

A more difficult challenge arises when AI-assisted CDSS are *adaptive*, that is, when they modify aspects of their behavior over time in response to feedback, environmental change, or newly incorporated knowledge. Self-adaptation is well established in software-intensive systems as a means of managing uncertainty and dynamic operating conditions [7,8]. In clinical settings, however, adaptation is not merely a technical optimization mechanism. It can introduce silent behavioral drift: small changes in thresholds, prompting strategies, knowledge sources, or interface presentation may alter clinician attention, reliance, and downstream action without being sufficiently visible, validated, or auditable. In regulated and trust-sensitive healthcare environments, such drift complicates accountability and weakens organizational oversight.

This tension is particularly visible in systems that generate textual recommendations. Retrieval-augmented generation (RAG) has been proposed to ground outputs in external evidence by coupling language models with document retrieval [9]. While such approaches can improve provenance and updateability relative to purely parametric generation, they do not by themselves guarantee safe adaptation. A system may still change its retrieval sources, prompting logic, decision thresholds, or presentation strategies in ways that materially affect clinical action. Evidence grounding therefore addresses only part of the problem; it does not determine what is allowed to change, under what constraints, with what validation process, or with what rollback guarantees.

Existing research addresses important parts of this challenge, but largely in separate streams. Prior work covers workflow fit and alert fatigue in CDSS [1,10,11], trust calibration and transparency in clinician-AI interaction [4,5,12], and governance expectations for adaptive CDS and regulated clinical AI [13–

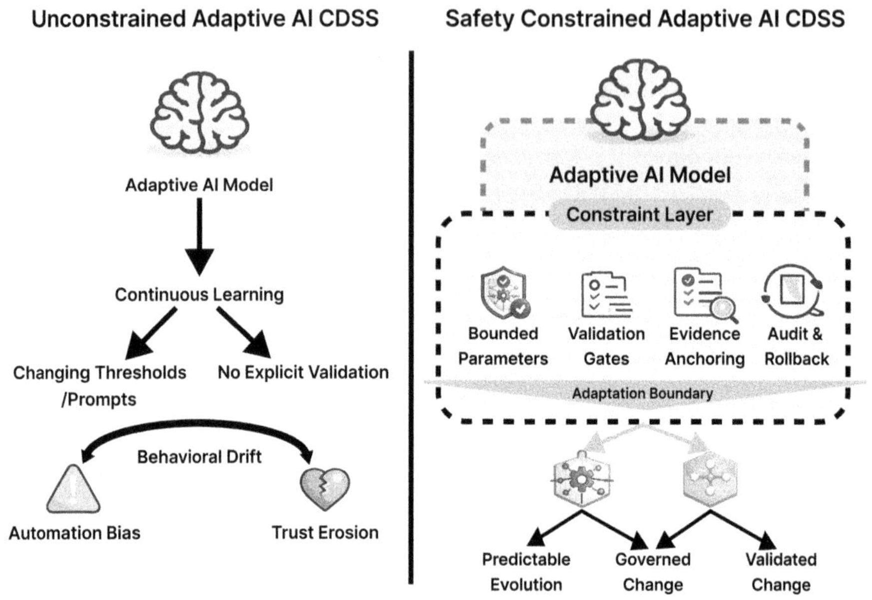

Fig. 1. Conceptual contrast between unconstrained adaptive AI-assisted clinical decision support and the proposed safety-constrained adaptive architecture.

15]. Related work also addresses high-risk regulatory accountability under the EU AI Act, evidence grounding for generative models, and self-adaptive software mechanisms for runtime change [9,16,17] [7,8,18]. What remains insufficiently addressed is the *architectural synthesis* of these concerns into a single runtime governance approach. The novelty of this paper lies not in proposing adaptation, explainability, or evidence grounding in isolation, but in combining explicit adaptation boundaries, validation states, evidence checks, and rollback-oriented accountability into one safety-constrained architecture for adaptive clinical decision support (Fig. 1).

We therefore argue that adaptation itself should be treated as a safety-critical capability to be explicitly governed. Rather than viewing adaptive behavior as an implementation detail, we frame it as a digital health governance problem: which aspects of the system may change, within what limits, under whose validation, and with what forms of auditability and reversibility. To address this problem, we propose a safety-constrained adaptive architecture for AI-assisted CDSS that embeds governance directly into the architectural design. The architecture introduces an explicit adaptation boundary, restricts change to bounded system parameters, requires multi-clinician validation before learned patterns influence future recommendations, anchors recommendations to retrievable evidence where applicable, and supports audit logging with rollback.

The study follows a Design Science Research (DSR) approach aimed at producing and evaluating an artifact that addresses a practically relevant socio-technical problem [19,20]. To align claims with artifact maturity, the evaluation strategy is grounded in established DSR guidance [21]. We instantiate the proposed architecture in a nurse-to-physician referral workflow representative of primary care decision-making and conduct a formative stakeholder evaluation with clinicians to examine perceived safety, trust calibration, transparency requirements, and governance alignment [12].

This paper makes three contributions. First, it offers a governance-first framing of adaptive AI in CDSS as a safety-critical socio-technical problem rather than a purely technical optimization problem. Second, it presents a safety-constrained adaptive architecture that operationalizes explicit adaptation boundaries, validation gates, evidence anchoring, and auditability. Third, it provides an instantiation and formative stakeholder evaluation that surfaces practical requirements for trustworthy adaptive decision support in clinical workflows. We do not claim clinical effectiveness or diagnostic superiority. Rather, the contribution is design knowledge: an architectural foundation for governing adaptive AI decision support more safely in healthcare and other regulated domains.

2 Background Work

This section situates the paper within six strands of prior work: (i) CDSS adoption and socio-technical failure modes, (ii) trust calibration in clinician-AI interaction, (iii) adaptive CDS governance and regulatory accountability, (iv) evidence-grounded language models, (v) self-adaptive software engineering foundations, and (vi) the positioning of the present study. Taken together, these strands show that the challenge in adaptive clinical AI is not only how to improve model output, but how to govern changes in system behavior over time.

2.1 Clinical Decision Support: Effectiveness Depends on Workflow Fit

CDSS effectiveness depends as much on workflow fit as on technical capability. Successful systems are typically integrated into clinician workflow, delivered at the point of decision-making, and framed as actionable support rather than interruption [10,11]. Conversely, poor integration can increase cognitive burden, provoke overrides, and erode trust, with alert fatigue remaining the canonical example of socio-technical failure [1,2]. These lessons matter directly for adaptive CDSS: if alerting behavior, recommendation cadence, or interface prominence change over time without governance, adaptive components may intensify the very failure modes that have historically limited CDSS impact.

2.2 Trust Calibration and Clinician Behavior with AI Decision Aids

Clinician interaction with AI decision aids raises risks of miscalibrated trust and overreliance. Trust is a major determinant of adoption, yet clinicians may shift both decisions and confidence toward AI advice even when that advice is incorrect [4,12]. This makes calibrated reliance, rather than maximal trust, the relevant design objective. Explainable AI may improve interpretability, but explanation alone does not provide accountability or deployment governance [5]. Related work therefore emphasizes structured communication of intended use, limitations, and evaluation evidence, for example through "model facts"-style artifacts [6]. For adaptive CDSS, trustworthy use requires not only explanation, but system-level controls over how AI behavior may change and influence clinical action.

2.3 Adaptive CDS Governance, Regulation, and Evaluation Expectations

Adaptive CDS has increasingly been framed as a governance problem rather than a purely technical one. The AMIA position paper on adaptive CDS argues that systems that learn and change over time require explicit lifecycle oversight, monitoring, and coordinated change management [13]. More recent work on dynamic deployment similarly highlights that evolving medical AI challenges conventional assumptions about what is being evaluated and when [22]. In parallel, regulatory frameworks reinforce that adaptive change must remain accountable: the MDR places continuing conformity and risk-management responsibilities on manufacturers [14]; FDA PCCP guidance frames adaptive change as pre-specified and lifecycle-governed [15]; and the EU AI Act adds obligations for high-risk medical AI, further strengthening provider accountability [16,17]. Although CONSORT-AI remains relevant as a reporting guideline for clinical trials, the broader implication here is that adaptive clinical AI must be designed for transparent evaluation, controlled change, and clear accountability rather than informal local evolution [23].

2.4 Evidence Grounding for Language Models in Clinical Settings

Generative AI introduces additional safety concerns because language models can produce fluent but incorrect outputs. Retrieval-augmented generation (RAG) addresses part of this problem by coupling generation with external retrieval, thereby improving provenance and factual grounding [9]. In clinical settings, retrieval-augmented language models have shown promise in grounding outputs in curated medical resources and improving perceived safety relative to purely parametric generation [18]. However, evidence grounding is not equivalent to governance. A system may retrieve evidence and still adapt its prompting, thresholds, source selection, or presentation logic in ways that materially affect clinical work. RAG therefore supports provenance, but does not by itself determine what may change, who validates change, or how changes are audited and reversed.

2.5 Self-adaptive Systems: Bounding and Assuring Runtime Change

Self-adaptive and autonomic systems provide an important technical foundation for reasoning about runtime change under uncertainty [7,8]. These traditions contribute concepts such as feedback control, uncertainty management, and runtime assurance. In clinical AI, however, adaptation cannot be treated as an unconstrained optimization mechanism. Even small changes may affect clinician attention, escalation behavior, or downstream patient management. For that reason, adaptation must be bounded by design, validated against explicit rules, and made auditable through traceable change artifacts such as provenance trails, version histories, and rollback points. The self-adaptive systems literature supplies the architectural basis for this, but not the clinical governance rules needed to determine what counts as acceptable change in regulated settings.

2.6 Positioning of This Work

The literature reviewed above points to a clear gap at the intersection of clinical AI, adaptive CDS, regulation, and software architecture. Prior CDSS research has established that workflow integration, timing, and alert management are decisive for real-world effectiveness [1,10,11]. AI-specific studies further show that clinically consequential systems must address miscalibrated trust, overreliance, and insufficiently actionable transparency [4,5,12]. At the same time, adaptive CDS governance work, including the AMIA position paper, makes clear that systems that learn and change over time require explicit lifecycle oversight, monitoring, and change-management processes rather than informal local evolution [13].

This need for governance is reinforced by emerging regulatory frameworks. In regulated medical-device contexts, adaptive change cannot be treated as a purely local technical matter. The MDR places continuing responsibility for conformity, risk management, and lifecycle control on the manufacturer [14]. FDA guidance on Predetermined Change Control Plans similarly frames adaptive change as something that must be pre-specified, validated, and governed within an approved lifecycle process [15]. The EU AI Act adds further accountability obligations for high-risk AI systems, including many clinically consequential medical AI applications [16,17]. Together, these developments indicate that adaptive clinical AI must be designed not only for performance and usability, but also for bounded change, accountability, and controlled evolution.

Evidence-grounded language-model approaches such as RAG improve provenance and factual support, while self-adaptive systems research provides general mechanisms for runtime monitoring and change [7,9,18] [8]. However, neither stream by itself resolves the central problem addressed in this paper: how adaptive AI behavior should be explicitly bounded, validated, audited, and aligned with clinical accountability in safety-critical workflows. In other words, existing work addresses important parts of the problem, but largely in separate streams.

Relative to this field, the contribution of the present work is an architectural synthesis. It does not propose adaptation as unrestricted local learning, nor does it treat explanation, evidence grounding, or regulatory awareness as sufficient safeguards in isolation. Instead, it brings together explicit adaptation boundaries, differentiated validation states, evidence checks, and rollback-oriented accountability within a single safety-constrained architecture for adaptive clinical decision support. In this sense, the contribution is not a claim of clinical effectiveness or regulatory compliance, but design knowledge: a structured architectural response to the problem of governing adaptive AI behavior in clinical decision support.

3 Research Method and Context (Design Science Research)

3.1 Methodological Rationale, Research Question, and Design Objectives

This study follows a Design Science Research (DSR) approach because its primary outcome is a design artifact: a safety-constrained adaptive software architecture for AI-assisted CDSS. DSR is appropriate when the contribution is prescriptive, for example, an architecture, method, or model and should be evaluated for utility, coherence, and rigor rather than explained only through observational inference [19,24]. We operationalize the study through the Design Science Research Methodology (DSRM), which structures the work from problem identification through artifact design, demonstration, and evaluation [20]. Consistent with established DSR guidance, the study is intended to generate design knowledge rather than claims of clinical effectiveness or diagnostic benefit [25].

The research question is therefore framed to elicit architectural knowledge:

RQ: How can self-adaptive software architectures be designed to support AI-assisted clinical decision support while preserving patient-safety constraints?

From the literature on CDSS adoption barriers, trust calibration, adaptive-system assurance, and clinical governance (Sect. 2), we derived four design objectives:

- **DO1: Bounded runtime adaptation.** Enable adaptation to evolving workflows and evidence while limiting unsafe behavioral drift.
- **DO2: Preserved clinician authority.** Ensure that AI remains advisory, with explicit override and bounded influence on clinical action.
- **DO3: Validation gates for learning.** Prevent promotion of patterns derived from noisy, isolated, or weakly supported feedback.
- **DO4: Auditability and rollback.** Provide traceability, accountability, and reversibility appropriate to clinical governance.

These objectives guide both artifact construction (Sect. 4) and evaluation (Sect. 6), thereby maintaining traceability between the problem, the design choices, and the resulting claims [19,25].

Table 1. Summary of design cycles and their main outcomes.

Cycle	Focus	Main outcome
1	Baseline adaptive CDSS architecture and risk elicitation	Refined problem framing: adaptation in clinical decision support must be treated as a safety-critical capability requiring explicit governance.
2	Governance mechanisms as architectural constraints	Consolidated constraint layer including adaptation boundaries, bounded parameter updates, validation gates, evidence anchoring, and audit/rollback mechanisms.
3	Refinement for clinical plausibility and usability	Clearer enforcement points, tighter control of recommendation prominence, more reviewable provenance, and stronger differentiation of governance levels for change.

3.2 DSR Process and Iterations

We followed the standard DSRM activities of problem identification, objective definition, design and development, demonstration, evaluation, and communication [20]. The work was conducted iteratively across three design cycles so that the architecture could be progressively refined through build-evaluate loops rather than through a single-pass design process [19] (Table 1).

3.3 Context, Stakeholder Relevance, and Evaluation Strategy

The architecture is demonstrated through a nurse-to-physician referral workflow representative of primary care and triage contexts. In this scenario, nurses capture initial case information and create a referral, while physicians review the referral, inspect supporting evidence, and determine the next clinical action. Within DSR, this serves the purpose of *demonstration*: it instantiates the artifact in a realistic workflow so that its governance properties can be examined concretely rather than only abstractly [20,24]. At the same time, the scenario is not intended to represent all Nordic primary-care settings or organizational cultures; it is used as a plausible and clinically meaningful instantiation.

Stakeholder involvement was used to ensure practical relevance and to test whether the proposed governance mechanisms align with clinical expectations of safety, accountability, and trust. Participants contributed to requirements elicitation, design critique, and evaluation sessions, enabling the study to surface how different professional backgrounds interpret bounded adaptation, evidence visibility, override authority, and reviewability. Because this is a formative DSR study, the role of participants is to provide expert critique of the artifact rather than representative evidence about clinical practice [19].

The evaluation therefore focuses on formative design validation rather than summative clinical effectiveness. We structure the evaluation using the Framework for Evaluation in Design Science (FEDS), which distinguishes formative evaluation for plausibility and alignment from summative evaluation for real-world effectiveness [21]. Accordingly, the evaluation targets four questions: the perceived safety of bounded adaptation, preservation of clinician authority and calibrated reliance, transparency and evidence-provenance requirements at the point of care, and governance fit with respect to auditability, accountability, and rollback. This positioning deliberately avoids over-claiming: it does not test diagnostic superiority, patient outcomes, workflow efficiency, or cross-regional generalizability [21,25].

3.4 Scope and Claim Boundaries

This study evaluates architectural mechanisms and stakeholder perceptions rather than patient outcomes. No claims are made about diagnostic accuracy, treatment efficacy, clinical effectiveness, or regulatory compliance in practice; such claims would require controlled clinical studies, broader multi-site evaluation, and appropriate ethical and organizational governance. The contribution is therefore limited to architectural claims supported by formative design validation, while questions of summative effectiveness and real-world deployment remain future work [19,21].

4 Safety-Constrained Adaptive Architecture

This section presents the core artifact of the study: a safety-constrained adaptive architecture for AI-assisted clinical decision support. The design objective is not to maximize adaptivity, but to govern it. We build on established self-adaptive systems principles, in which a managed system is supervised by an adaptation manager organized as a feedback control loop [7,8,26]. In clinically consequential settings, however, adaptive behavior must remain bounded, reviewable, and attributable. Accordingly, the architecture is presented as a governance-oriented design concept for controlled adaptation rather than as a claim that runtime adaptation can occur outside formal oversight structures [14–16].

4.1 Architectural Overview

Self-adaptive systems are commonly structured around a feedback loop in which the system monitors its operation, analyzes conditions, plans adaptation, and executes changes [7]. In our setting, this loop is implemented as a Monitor-Analyze-Plan-Execute over a shared Knowledge base (MAPE-K) architecture supervising a managed clinical workflow system. The central challenge is that naive adaptation can introduce silent behavioral drift: recommendations, thresholds, evidence presentation, or interface prominence may change over time in

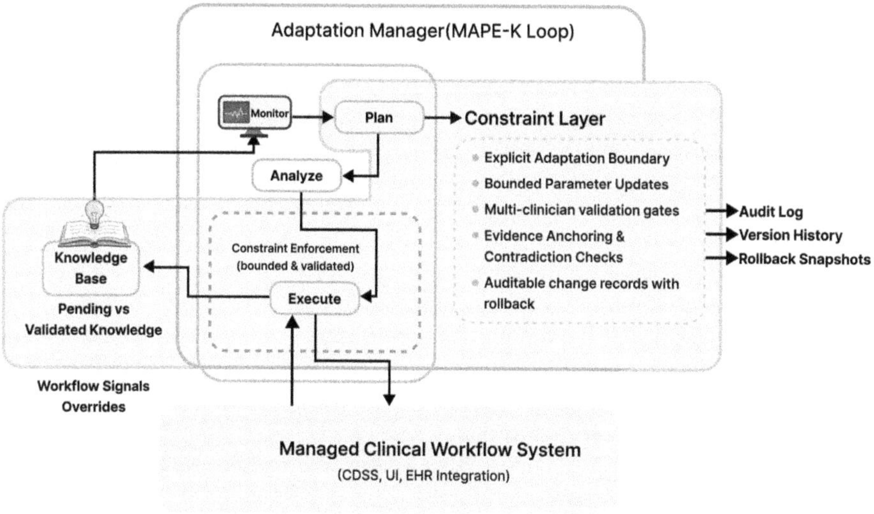

Fig. 2. Safety-constrained adaptive architecture for AI-assisted clinical decision support systems (CDSS).

ways that clinicians do not immediately notice, even though such changes may influence decision-making.

Figure 2 shows two major subsystems: (i) the **Managed System**, namely the clinical workflow application, and (ii) the **Adaptation Manager**, which implements the MAPE-K loop over a shared knowledge base [7,26]. A dedicated **Constraint Layer** governs this loop by enforcing explicit adaptation boundaries, bounded parameter updates, validation gates for learned patterns, evidence anchoring with contradiction checks, and auditable change records with rollback support. The knowledge base further distinguishes *pending* from *validated* knowledge so that interaction-derived patterns do not silently become active behavior without review.

4.2 Explicit Adaptation Boundary

A frequent cause of unsafe adaptation is an ill-defined adaptation space. We therefore define an **adaptation boundary** that partitions system properties into four classes:

- **Non-adaptive invariants**: properties that must not change at runtime without offline governance (e.g., clinician override, triage priority definitions, and safety-critical hard rules).
- **Adaptive parameters**: bounded parameters that may change under explicit constraints (e.g., confidence thresholds, suggestion density, and user-interface prominence).

- **Adaptive knowledge candidates**: reusable patterns derived from interaction feedback that may be considered for promotion only after validation and safety checks.
- **Governance escalation classes**: a distinction between lower-impact changes that may remain within the approved adaptation envelope and higher-impact changes that require designated governance review or external change control.

The first three classes define *what* may change, while the fourth defines *how change is governed.* This distinction is important because not all technically feasible changes are acceptable candidates for local runtime adaptation. Some changes may require review by a clinical quality lead, a designated safety officer, or a manufacturer-led change-control process, particularly where the change could materially affect clinical risk or intended use [13–15]. The adaptation boundary therefore constrains runtime change by design and makes explicit that consequential adaptation must remain embedded within stronger organizational and regulatory oversight [8,26].

4.3 Constraint Layer: Governing the Adaptation Loop

The main architectural novelty is the **Constraint Layer**, embedded across the analysis, planning, and execution stages of the adaptation loop. It performs three functions: it prevents unsafe plans by checking proposed changes against approved bounds and governance classes; it gates learning so that candidate knowledge cannot influence future recommendations without satisfying predefined review criteria; and it ensures accountability by producing structured change artifacts, including audit records, provenance links, and rollback snapshots. In this way, the architecture extends self-adaptive systems assurance from general runtime control toward explicitly governed change in safety-critical clinical settings [8,27].

4.4 Safety Constraint Mechanisms

We implement four model-agnostic constraint mechanisms that govern how the system changes and how those changes become operational.

C1. Bounded Adaptation of Influence and Presentation. In clinical decision support, seemingly minor shifts in presentation can materially affect clinician reliance. The architecture therefore bounds changes to influence-bearing parameters such as confidence thresholds, alerting cadence, and interface prominence by requiring all updates to remain within an approved envelope. This mechanism limits abrupt or weakly reviewed behavioral shifts and makes the intensity of AI influence itself subject to governance [8,26].

C2. Validation Gates for Learning and Promotion. Learning from clinician interaction may improve workflow fit, but it can also amplify individual error or local bias. Candidate knowledge items are therefore stored as *pending* and promoted only after explicit validation. Lower-impact candidates require repeated support across time, validation by multiple distinct clinicians, and no contradiction with active evidence constraints; higher-impact candidates additionally require designated governance review. The rationale is not that agreement guarantees correctness, but that promotion criteria must be predefined, role-aware, and proportionate to the impact of the change [13,15].

C3. Evidence Anchoring as a Constraint. Evidence grounding is treated as a governance constraint rather than only an interface feature. AI suggestions must attach references to retrieved evidence items, and candidate learned patterns are blocked from promotion if they conflict with currently retrieved evidence. Although retrieval-augmented generation can improve provenance and factual grounding, it does not by itself govern adaptive change; here, provenance is used to constrain what may become persistent system behavior [9,18].

C4. Audit Logging and Rollback for Accountable Adaptation. Each executed adaptation must generate an auditable change record that captures the triggering signals, proposed plan, affected parameters or knowledge items, relevant provenance links, the reviewing actor or role, and resulting version identifiers. Every change is also associated with a restorable configuration or knowledge snapshot. This mechanism supports post-hoc review, incident analysis, and recovery to known-safe states, thereby extending familiar documentation practices into runtime governance [27].

4.5 Constraint Enforcement Points

Constraints are enforced at multiple stages of the adaptation loop. At the analysis and planning stages, unsafe parameter updates are rejected and learning proposals are checked against validation and provenance requirements. At execution, changes are applied only if the required review conditions have been met and audit and rollback artifacts can be created. Within the knowledge base, the system preserves the distinction between pending and validated knowledge, together with parameter version histories and immutable audit trails.

Table 2 summarizes the mechanisms and their governance role. Together, these constraints operationalize the central architectural claim of the paper: adaptation is permitted only within an explicitly governed envelope, and only when the resulting behavior remains reviewable, attributable, and reversible.

4.6 What this Architecture Claims, and does not Claim

To avoid over-claiming, we distinguish architectural claims from clinical, organizational, and regulatory claims. The architecture claims: (i) bounded runtime

Table 2. Constraint mechanisms and their primary governance purpose.

Constraint	What it governs	Safety/governance rationale
C1: Bounds	Influence-bearing parameters (thresholds, cadence, prominence)	Prevent silent drift and sudden shifts that could induce unsafe reliance
C2: Validation gates	Promotion of learned patterns	Reduce amplification of isolated errors and local bias in adaptive learning; require role-appropriate review for higher-impact changes
C3: Evidence anchoring	Provenance + contradiction blocking	Prevent ungrounded or conflicting suggestions from becoming persistent behavior
C4: Audit & rollback	Traceable change history and reversibility	Enable accountability, post-hoc review, and recovery to known-safe versions

change through explicit adaptation boundaries and parameter envelopes; (ii) gated learning through validation and evidence anchoring; and (iii) accountable evolution through audit logging and rollback. It does *not* claim improved diagnostic accuracy, improved patient outcomes, automatic regulatory compliance, or immediate deployability in real clinical settings. Those would require separate clinical validation, human-factors evaluation, organizational integration, manufacturer-led quality management, and prospective regulatory assessment [14–16]. The contribution is therefore design knowledge: a governance-first architectural pattern for making adaptive AI behavior more inspectable and controllable within clinical workflows.

5 Instantiation in Clinical Workflow

This section demonstrates how the proposed safety-constrained adaptive architecture can be instantiated in a Nordic primary-care workflow in which nurse-led triage and telephone counselling are common, and escalation to a physician is available when uncertainty or risk warrants it. The purpose is *demonstration* in the Design Science Research sense: to make the architecture concrete in a realistic workflow and to show how its governance mechanisms may operate in practice. It is not intended to claim that the resulting workflow represents all Nordic primary-care settings or organizational cultures. Rather, it provides a plausible and clinically meaningful instantiation through which the architecture can be examined and refined.

Prior work from Sweden suggests that structured triage combined with a "Nurse on Call" model can improve teamwork and perceived quality of care, while also surfacing organizational and competence-related barriers that must be managed during adoption [28]. Evidence from Norway similarly shows that nurse-led telephone triage can vary in urgency grading and that systematic evaluation and training are important for safety in out-of-hours settings [29]. These observations motivate two design choices in our instantiation: first, escalation and "second-check" pathways are treated as first-class workflow elements rather than exceptional cases; second, auditability is treated as part of the safety case rather than as optional operational telemetry.

5.1 Clinical Setting and Roles

We assume a primary-care center or out-of-hours cooperative in which patient entry occurs through phone or portal contact, and in some cases walk-in assessment. The instantiated workflow includes four core roles: a triage nurse responsible for intake, symptom characterization, and escalation initiation; an on-call physician responsible for adjudication of escalated cases and justified override; a medical secretary or coordinator responsible for scheduling and logistics; and a system safety officer or quality lead responsible for monitoring incidents and approving configuration changes under formal change control. This role structure separates clinical care from governance oversight and reflects the reviewer concern that responsibility for adaptive system safety cannot be assumed to rest solely with frontline clinicians. Access control is therefore structured around role-based separation of duties consistent with RBAC principles [30].

5.2 Workflow Fit: Triage-to-Escalation as a Safety Pattern

Nordic primary care frequently uses nurse-led triage supported by decision aids and explicit escalation to a physician when required [28,29]. We instantiate this as an explicit state machine with built-in safety gates. The workflow begins with intake and red-flag screening, followed by structured nurse-led risk stratification. The system then produces a bounded recommendation, for example self-care advice, same-day nurse assessment, same-day physician assessment, or emergency escalation. If red flags or high-risk patterns are detected, the adaptive layer is not permitted to down-triage; instead, the workflow enforces escalation or an emergency pathway. For uncertain or high-risk cases, the physician reviews the case summary, rationale, and evidence trace before authorizing the next action. The workflow concludes with disposition, follow-up, and documented safety-netting advice.

This state machine is shown in Fig. 3. It should be understood as an *instantiation pattern*, not as a universal model of Nordic care. Local protocols, staffing models, and escalation rules vary across settings; any real-world implementation would therefore require local tailoring and, in regulated settings, alignment with approved change-control and safety-governance processes.

5.3 Interoperability Layer

The instantiation assumes integration with an electronic health record (EHR) ecosystem through standards-based APIs so that adaptive decision support can be embedded into clinical work rather than operate as a disconnected parallel tool. SMART on FHIR provides a practical approach for interoperable clinical applications using standardized authorization and data access patterns [31]. We therefore model patient context and key clinical objects including encounter summaries, observations, medications, and conditions as normalized resources exchanged through a FHIR-compatible interface, while keeping the safety-constrained adaptation logic inside the architecture boundary. This preserves interoperability without externalizing governance.

5.4 Auditability in the Live Workflow

Figure 3 also illustrates how auditability is embedded into the workflow. The instantiation assumes a structured event stream that records who performed which action, in what patient context, what recommendation was shown, which constraints were active, whether escalation or override occurred, and what downstream actions followed. Such records are essential because they provide the evidentiary basis for inspecting whether constraints were activated appropriately, whether overrides cluster in specific contexts, and whether adaptive changes remain aligned with intended governance boundaries [32,33]. For the present paper, auditability is included to demonstrate how the architecture can be made inspectable and reviewable in practice; it does not by itself establish clinical benefit or regulatory sufficiency. A fuller event taxonomy can be provided in supplementary material or an appendix if needed.

6 Stakeholder Evaluation

Because the contribution of this paper is an architectural artifact, namely, a governance-first, safety-constrained adaptive CDSS architecture rather than a clinically validated intervention, the evaluation is intentionally formative. Its purpose is to assess design plausibility, surface safety-relevant requirements, and examine whether the proposed governance mechanisms align with clinical expectations of trust, accountability, and reviewability. This positioning follows Design Science Research guidance that evaluation strategies should match both artifact maturity and the type of claim being made [19,21]. Accordingly, the evaluation does not test clinical effectiveness, diagnostic superiority, or regional representativeness; rather, it examines whether the artifact is sufficiently coherent and practically grounded to justify further refinement and future summative study.

6.1 Evaluation Goals

The evaluation addressed four system-level questions: whether the proposed adaptation boundaries and constraints plausibly reduce unsafe behavioral drift; whether the governance mechanisms support calibrated reliance and preserve clinician authority; whether evidence anchoring and contradiction checks are

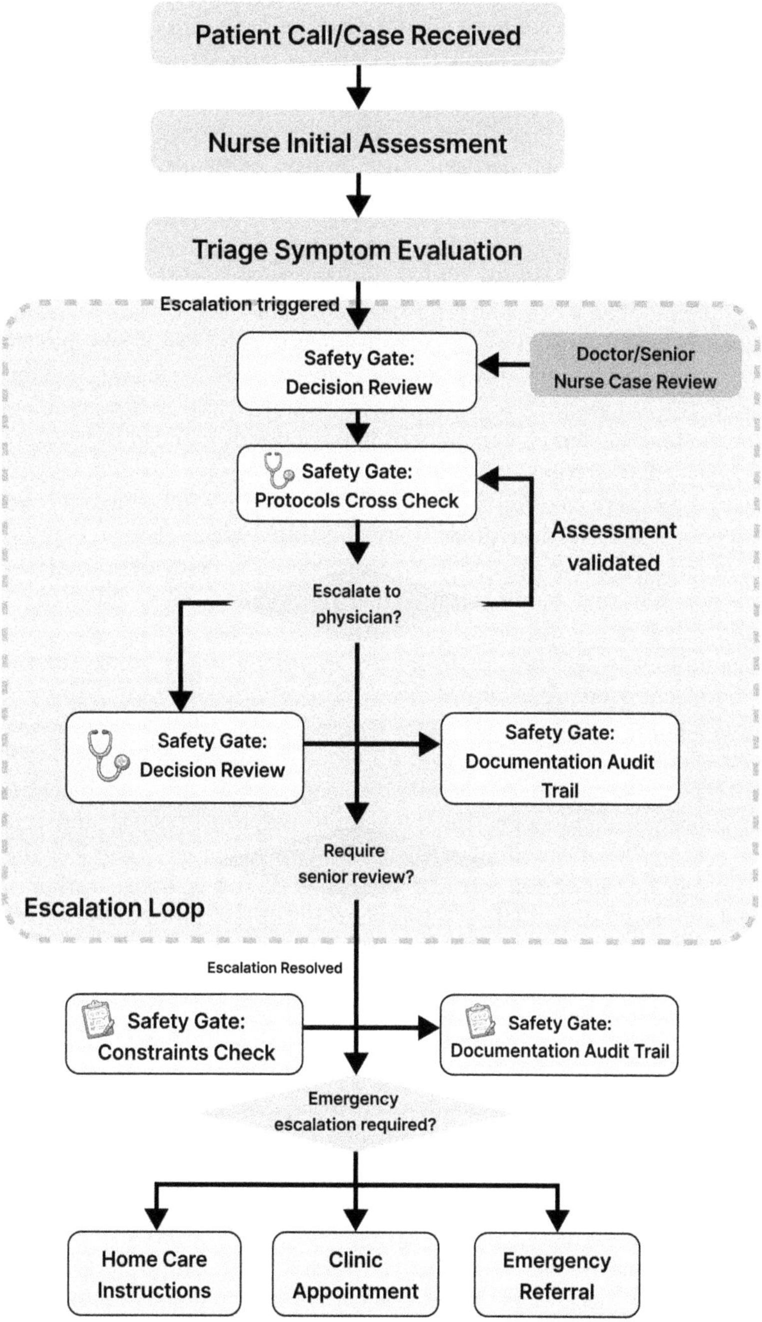

Fig. 3. Nordic triage-to-disposition workflow modeled as a state machine for nurse-led triage and "Nurse on Call" services.

practical for credibility assessment at the point of care; and whether audit, roll-back, and validation mechanisms align with expectations for accountability and incident response. These questions focus on how adaptive behavior is bounded and governed, rather than on predictive performance or patient outcomes.

6.2 Participants, Recruitment, and Scope of Sample

We conducted formative evaluation sessions with seven clinical stakeholders: five physicians and two triage nurses. The physicians represented multiple specialties, namely General Practice (6 years of experience), Neurology (8 years), Cardiology (15 years), Orthopedics (4 years), and Internal Medicine (12 years). The inclusion of multiple specialties was intentional, as it allowed us to probe whether the same adaptive mechanism might raise different concerns across clinical domains, such as different tolerances for risk, escalation thresholds, and acceptable degrees of automation. The two nurses contributed perspectives grounded in triage practice and workflow coordination.

Participants were recruited purposively through professional networks in order to obtain informed critique from clinicians with relevant experience in decision-making, escalation, and care workflow. The aim of recruitment was therefore not demographic or institutional representativeness, but relevance to the architectural and governance questions under study.

The sample was selected for formative expert critique rather than for statistical representation. A group of seven clinical stakeholders is not sufficient to support claims of representativeness across Nordic primary-care settings, nor to establish clinical consensus across different organizational cultures. Rather, the goal was to elicit expert perspectives capable of surfacing recurring governance concerns, challenging the plausibility of the artifact, and informing iterative refinement. Consistent with qualitative and DSR practice, the value of this sample lies in the depth and relevance of the feedback rather than in numerical coverage alone [34]. We therefore interpret the findings as recurrent expert concerns within a formative design study rather than as evidence of broad population-level saturation.

6.3 Protocol and Analysis

Each session followed a structured walkthrough of the instantiated workflow (Sect. 5) and the proposed architectural controls (Sect. 4). Participants reviewed intake summaries and triage recommendations, examined evidence links, escalation cues, validation logic, and override pathways, and were encouraged to think aloud while interacting with these workflow and governance features. Sessions concluded with a semi-structured interview focused on perceived risks of adaptive behavior, acceptable boundaries of change, evidence visibility, and the audit information required for accountability. This protocol was motivated by prior findings that clinicians may shift both decisions and confidence toward AI advice even when that advice is incorrect, making calibrated reliance and visible clinician authority central concerns [4,12,35].

We collected audio-recorded interview responses and walkthrough commentary, structured notes documenting concerns and suggested refinements, and artifact-linked observations identifying which architectural feature triggered specific feedback. The material was analyzed using reflexive thematic analysis following Braun and Clarke, with two researchers independently coding an initial subset to establish a shared coding frame and then refining themes through iterative discussion [36]. To support transparency and credibility, the evaluation design and reporting were aligned with COREQ recommendations, investigator triangulation was used during initial coding, and participants were given a brief summary of the high-level interpretations for comment [36,37].

6.4 Findings

Across sessions, four themes recurred consistently. These themes should be interpreted as formative findings about perceived governance fit and artifact plausibility, not as evidence of clinical effectiveness.

F1: Predictability is preferred over apparent "smartness." Participants consistently preferred a system that behaved predictably and changed slowly over one that appeared more adaptive but less stable. Even small, unannounced shifts for example in recommendation prominence or display behavior were seen as capable of altering clinician attention and inducing inappropriate reliance. This finding supports the decision to bound influence-bearing parameters and to separate pending knowledge from validated knowledge (C1-C2).

F2: Evidence links are necessary, but must be cognitively lightweight. Stakeholders regarded evidence anchoring as important for credibility, especially when recommendations could change over time. At the same time, they emphasized that evidence presentation must remain concise and actionable at the point of care, for example through short guideline snippets and clear source references rather than long documents. This indicates that provenance is necessary, but must not impose cognitive burden beyond what is feasible during triage and escalation.

F3: Validation gates must reflect clinical accountability, not only technical logic. Participants supported the principle that learned patterns should not be promoted from isolated feedback alone. However, they also stressed that *who* validates matters: higher-impact changes were seen as requiring review aligned with clinical responsibility, such as sign-off by a senior clinician or designated quality lead. This finding supports treating validation gates as socio-technical governance mechanisms rather than as purely statistical thresholds.

F4: Auditability and rollback are prerequisites for acceptable adaptive CDSS. Participants consistently emphasized the need to answer basic accountability questions: what changed, when it changed, why it changed, and how prior behavior could be restored if needed. Auditability and rollback were therefore viewed not as optional enhancements, but as prerequisites for acceptable adaptive decision support in clinical pathways. This finding reinforces the architecture's emphasis on versioned change records, provenance-aware audit trails, and rollback capability.

6.5 Implications for Artifact Refinement

The evaluation directly informed refinement of both the instantiation and the architectural controls. Specifically, it led to tighter bounds on user-interface prominence changes (C1), clearer differentiation between low-impact and high-impact knowledge candidates (C2), concise point-of-care evidence summaries with retained provenance trails (C3), and more standardized audit records to support clinical review and incident response (C4). In line with FEDS, these results support formative conclusions about plausibility, coherence, and governance alignment, but they do not establish clinical effectiveness, workflow superiority, or safety benefit in deployment [21]. Broader multi-site studies and prospective evaluation would still be required to assess clinical outcomes and real-world workflow effects.

7 Discussion and Implications

This paper addressed a recurring problem in digital health: how adaptive AI behavior in clinical decision support systems (CDSS) can be governed safely when system behavior may evolve over time. Rather than treating adaptation as an implementation detail or a purely technical optimization mechanism, we argued that it should be engineered as a safety-critical and governable property of the system. The proposed architecture therefore shifts the focus from maximizing adaptivity to bounding, validating, and making adaptation accountable.

7.1 Governance and Clinician Authority

A central implication of this work is that adaptation in AI-assisted CDSS should be framed primarily as a governance challenge rather than as an optimization challenge. Prior CDSS research shows that even static systems can introduce harms through alert fatigue, workflow disruption, and erosion of trust [1,2]. Our findings suggest that adaptive behavior can amplify these risks if changes occur without explicit boundaries, validation, and traceability. From this perspective, the key question is not simply whether an adaptive model can improve recommendations, but whether the resulting changes remain visible, reviewable, and acceptable in safety-critical work [3,4].

This point is closely tied to clinician authority. Human-AI collaboration research consistently emphasizes that trust should be calibrated rather than maximized [12]. Our formative evaluation reinforces this: participants valued predictability, inspectability, and the ability to override system behavior more than aggressive or opaque adaptivity. The architecture responds by bounding influence-bearing parameters, making learning contingent on validation, and ensuring that changes remain reviewable and reversible. In doing so, it supports controlled evolution while preserving visible clinician authority and reducing the risk of silent deference to AI output.

The same logic applies to explainability. Prior work shows that explanations alone do not guarantee safety, accountability, or appropriate use [5]. Our contribution is therefore not to treat evidence grounding as a sufficient safeguard in itself, but to recast provenance and contradiction checks as constraints on adaptive change. By linking evidence, validation, and rollback, the architecture moves from static explanation toward accountable change control and offers a more operational view of governance for evolving clinical AI [27].

7.2 Regulatory Accountability and Translational Feasibility

A major implication of this work concerns regulatory accountability. In real-world medical-device settings, responsibility for device safety and conformity does not rest solely with clinicians or local practitioners. AI-assisted CDSS used in clinically consequential contexts may fall within software-as-a-medical-device or related regulated product categories, where responsibility for risk management, technical documentation, post-market control, and conformity remains centered on the manufacturer and formal governance structures around the device [14–16]. This places an important practical boundary around how any adaptive architecture can be interpreted.

For that reason, the architecture proposed here should not be read as enabling unconstrained local adaptation by clinical users or healthcare organizations outside broader accountability frameworks. Rather, it should be understood as a governance-oriented architectural concept whose key mechanisms, including adaptation boundaries, validation gates, evidence anchoring, and auditability, would need to be instantiated within stronger organizational and regulatory control structures. In practice, higher-impact forms of adaptive change would likely require designated governance review and, in regulated deployments, consistency with manufacturer-led quality management and formally approved change-control processes [13, 15].

This qualification narrows and strengthens the contribution of the paper. The work does not claim to solve the legal allocation of responsibility for adaptive medical AI, nor does it claim that the proposed architecture is by itself sufficient for regulatory approval or operational deployment. Instead, it contributes a structured architectural response to a problem that regulatory and organizational frameworks must also address: how adaptive behavior can be bounded and made inspectable enough to support accountability. In that sense, the architecture is best understood as a translationally aware design concept rather than a complete deployment model.

7.3 Design-Science Contribution and Future Work

From a Design Science Research perspective, the main contribution of this study is design knowledge: a reusable architectural pattern for governing adaptive behavior in safety-critical, human-facing systems. Following established DSR typologies, this contribution takes the form of a design artifact and associated design principles rather than a predictive or explanatory theory [25]. The formative evaluation supports claims of plausibility, relevance, and governance fit, but it does not establish clinical effectiveness, regional representativeness, or implementation readiness.

Although the instantiation focuses on a primary-care triage workflow, the architectural principles are relevant beyond this specific setting. Similar governance challenges arise wherever adaptive AI influences consequential human decision-making. What generalizes is the need to define explicit adaptation boundaries, distinguish lower-impact from higher-impact change, preserve human authority, and make runtime evolution reviewable. What does not automatically generalize are the specific validation thresholds, workflow states, escalation rules, or accountability structures, all of which remain context-dependent.

Future work should therefore proceed in three directions. First, the architecture should be examined in richer empirical settings, including broader clinical roles, multi-site deployments, and organizationally heterogeneous contexts. Second, its effects on workflow, safety, and user behavior should be studied through prospective and summative evaluation. Third, research should explicitly address how runtime governance architectures such as the one proposed here can be aligned with quality management, post-market surveillance, and regulated change-control models for adaptive medical AI [23]. Without such alignment, technically strong adaptive systems may remain translationally weak because the mechanisms of responsibility, authorization, and review are insufficiently specified. More broadly, the paper suggests that an architectural theory of governed change is not a substitute for clinical validation, but a prerequisite for making later validation meaningful.

8 Limitations and Conclusion

8.1 Limitations

This study has four main limitations.

First, the evaluation is formative and qualitative, consistent with Design Science Research (DSR) guidance for early-stage architectural artifacts [19,21]. It supports claims of plausibility, design relevance, and perceived governance fit, but does not establish clinical effectiveness, safety improvement, cognitive-burden reduction, or workflow efficiency. Demonstrating such outcomes would require prospective deployment, controlled study designs, and appropriate ethical and organizational oversight [23].

Second, the stakeholder sample was intentionally small and designed for formative expert critique rather than representativeness. The inclusion of five physicians and two nurses was sufficient to surface recurring high-level concerns, but not to support claims of saturation across primary-care settings or across the full range of clinical roles involved in triage workflows. Broader participation would be needed to assess variation in usability, workflow impact, and governance expectations across settings [34,37].

Third, the architecture is demonstrated through a nurse-to-physician triage and referral workflow intended as a plausible primary-care instantiation, not as a universal model of practice. Although the architectural principles are designed to be reusable, implementation details including governance processes, validation thresholds, role responsibilities, and audit practices would need to be adapted to local clinical, legal, and organizational realities [2].

Fourth, the paper does not resolve the legal and regulatory distribution of accountability for adaptive behavior in clinically consequential systems. In regulated medical-device contexts, responsibility for conformity, risk management, and post-market change control cannot be assumed to rest with clinicians or local practitioners alone. The proposed architecture should therefore be understood as a governance-oriented design concept, not as a complete deployment model for adaptive software as a medical device [13–15]. In addition, the proposed constraints reduce but do not eliminate residual risk: incomplete, outdated, or incorrectly interpreted knowledge may still influence recommendations, and ongoing monitoring, training, and human oversight remain necessary [3].

8.2 Conclusion

Adaptive and generative AI are increasingly entering clinical decision support, but in safety-critical settings adaptation can itself become a source of silent behavioral drift, blurred accountability, and erosion of clinician trust. This paper argued that these challenges are fundamentally architectural and governance-related rather than purely algorithmic.

To address this problem, we presented a safety-constrained adaptive architecture for AI-assisted CDSS that treats adaptation as a capability to be explicitly bounded, validated, and audited. Using a Design Science Research approach, we instantiated the architecture in a primary-care triage workflow and conducted a formative stakeholder evaluation focused on perceived safety, trust calibration, transparency requirements, and governance fit.

The contribution of this work is design knowledge: a governance-first architectural pattern for making adaptive AI behavior more inspectable, reviewable, and controllable in safety-critical, human-facing systems. We deliberately do not claim clinical effectiveness, diagnostic superiority, or regulatory readiness. Instead, the paper provides a structured foundation on which later clinical, organizational, and regulatory evaluation can be more meaningfully built. Future work should examine the architecture in broader empirical settings, evaluate its effects through prospective studies, and explore how runtime governance mechanisms can be aligned with formal accountability and regulated change-control models for adaptive medical AI.

Acknowledgments. This research is supported by FAST (Finnish Software Engineering Doctoral Research Network), funded by the Finnish Ministry of Education and Culture, and conducted as part of the doctoral program at the University of Oulu in close collaboration with academic and industrial partners.

Disclosure of Interests. The author has no competing interests to declare that are relevant to the content of this article.

References

1. Ancker, J.S., et al.: Effects of workload, work complexity, and repeated alerts on alert fatigue in a clinical decision support system. BMC Med. Inform. Decis. Mak. **17**(1), 36 (2017)
2. Sutton, R.T., Pincock, D., Baumgart, D.C., Sadowski, D.C., Fedorak, R.N., Kroeker, K.I.: An overview of clinical decision support systems: benefits, risks, and strategies for success. NPJ Digit. Med. **3**(1), 17 (2020)
3. Rajkomar, A., Dean, J., Kohane, I.: Machine learning in medicine. N. Engl. J. Med. **380**(14), 1347–1358 (2019)
4. Gaube, S., et al.: Do as AI say: susceptibility in deployment of clinical decision-aids. NPJ Digit. Med. **4**(1), 31 (2021)
5. Tjoa, E., Guan, C.: A survey on explainable artificial intelligence (XAI): toward medical XAI. IEEE Trans. Neural Netw. Learn. Syst. **32**(11), 4793–4813 (2021)
6. Sendak, M.P., Gao, M., Brajer, N., Balu, S.: Presenting machine learning model information to clinical end users with model facts labels. NPJ Digit. Med. **3**(1), 41 (2020)
7. Kephart, J.O., Chess, D.M.: The vision of autonomic computing. Computer **36**(1), 41–50 (2003)
8. de Lemos, R., et al.: Software engineering for self-adaptive systems: a second research roadmap. In: de Lemos, R., Giese, H., Müller, H.A., Shaw, M. (eds.) Software Engineering for Self-Adaptive Systems II. LNCS, vol. 7475, pp. 1–32. Springer, Heidelberg (2013). https://doi.org/10.1007/978-3-642-35813-5_1
9. Lewis, P., et al.: Retrieval-augmented generation for knowledge-intensive NLP tasks. In: Advances in Neural Information Processing Systems (NeurIPS) (2020)
10. Kawamoto, K., Houlihan, C.A., Balas, E.A., Lobach, D.F.: Improving clinical practice using clinical decision support systems: a systematic review of trials to identify features critical to success. BMJ **330**(7494), 765 (2005)
11. Bates, D.W., et al.: Ten commandments for effective clinical decision support: making the practice of evidence-based medicine a reality. J. Am. Med. Inform. Assoc. **10**(6), 523–530 (2003)
12. Asan, O., Bayrak, A.E., Choudhury, A.: Artificial intelligence and human trust in healthcare: focus on clinicians. J. Med. Internet Res. **22**(6), e15154 (2020)
13. Petersen, C., et al.: Recommendations for the safe, effective use of adaptive CDS in the us healthcare system: an AMIA position paper. J. Am. Med. Inform. Assoc. **28**(4), 677–684 (2021). https://academic.oup.com/jamia/article/28/4/677/6100038
14. European Parliament and Council of the European Union: Regulation (EU) 2017/745 of the European parliament and of the council of 5 April 2017 on medical devices, amending directive 2001/83/EC, regulation (EC) no 178/2002 and regulation (EC) no 1223/2009 and repealing council directives 90/385/EEC and

93/42/EEC, Official Journal of the European Union, L 117, 5 May 2017, pp. 1–175 (2017). https://eur-lex.europa.eu/eli/reg/2017/745/oj?locale=en
15. U.S. Food and Drug Administration: Marketing submission recommendations for a predetermined change control plan for artificial intelligence-enabled device software functions, final guidance (2025). https://www.fda.gov/regulatory-information/search-fda-guidance-documents/marketing-submission-recommendations-predetermined-change-control-plan-artificial-intelligence
16. European Parliament and Council of the European Union: Regulation (EU) 2024/1689 of the European parliament and of the council of 13 June 2024 laying down harmonised rules on artificial intelligence (Artificial Intelligence Act), Official Journal of the European Union, L, 2024/1689, 12 July 2024 (2024). https://eur-lex.europa.eu/eli/reg/2024/1689/oj
17. Aboy, M., Minssen, T., Vayena, E.: Navigating the EU AI act: implications for regulated digital medical products. NPJ Digit. Med. **7**, 237 (2024). https://www.nature.com/articles/s41746-024-01232-3
18. Zakka, C., et al.: Almanac - retrieval-augmented language models for clinical medicine. NEJM AI **1**(2) (2024)
19. Hevner, A.R., March, S.T., Park, J., Ram, S.: Design science in information systems research. MIS Q. **28**(1), 75–105 (2004)
20. Peffers, K., Tuunanen, T., Rothenberger, M.A., Chatterjee, S.: A design science research methodology for information systems research. J. Manag. Inf. Syst. **24**(3), 45–77 (2007)
21. Venable, J., Pries-Heje, J., Baskerville, R.: FEDS: a framework for evaluation in design science research. Eur. J. Inf. Syst. **25**(1), 77–89 (2016)
22. Rosenthal, J.T., Beecy, A., Sabuncu, M.R.: Rethinking clinical trials for medical AI with dynamic deployments of adaptive systems. NPJ Digit. Med. **8**, 252 (2025). https://www.nature.com/articles/s41746-025-01674-3
23. Liu, X., et al.: Reporting guidelines for clinical trial reports for interventions involving artificial intelligence: the CONSORT-AI extension. BMJ **370**, m3164 (2020)
24. March, S.T., Smith, G.F.: Design and natural science research on information technology. Decis. Support Syst. **15**(4), 251–266 (1995)
25. Gregor, S., Hevner, A.R.: Positioning and presenting design science research for maximum impact. MIS Q. **37**(2), 337–355 (2013)
26. de Lemos, R., et al.: Software engineering for self-adaptive systems: a second research roadmap. In: de Lemos, R., Giese, H., Müller, H.A., Shaw, M. (eds.) Software Engineering for Self-Adaptive Systems II. LNCS, vol. 7475, pp. 1–32. Springer, Heidelberg (2013). https://doi.org/10.1007/978-3-642-35813-5_1
27. Mitchell, M., et al.: Model cards for model reporting. In: Proceedings of the Conference on Fairness, Accountability, and Transparency (FAT*/FAccT), pp. 220–229 (2019)
28. Gelin, M., Gesar, B., Källberg, A.-S., Ehrenberg, A., Gustavsson, C., et al.: Introducing a triage and nurse on call model in primary health care, a focus group study of health care staff's experiences. BMC Health Serv. Res. **23**(1), 1299 (2023)
29. Hansen, E.H., Hunskaar, S.: Telephone triage by nurses in primary care out-of-hours services in Norway: an evaluation study based on written case scenarios. BMJ Qual. Saf. **20**(5), 390–396 (2011)
30. Sandhu, R.S., Coyne, E.J., Feinstein, H.L., Youman, C.E.: Role-based access control models. Computer **29**(2), 38–47 (1996)
31. Mandel, J.C., Kreda, D.A., Mandl, K.D., Kohane, I.S., Ramoni, R.B.: SMART on FHIR: a standards-based, interoperable apps platform for electronic health records. J. Am. Med. Inform. Assoc. **23**(5), 899–908 (2016)

32. Kannampallil, T., Adler-Milstein, J.: Using electronic health record audit log data for research: insights from early efforts. J. Am. Med. Inform. Assoc. **30**(1), 167–171 (2023)
33. Adler-Milstein, J., Adelman, J.S., Tai-Seale, M., Patel, V.L., Dymek, C.: EHR audit logs: a new goldmine for health services research? J. Biomed. Inform. **101**, 103343 (2020)
34. Guest, G., Bunce, A., Johnson, L.: How many interviews are enough? An experiment with data saturation and variability. Field Methods **18**(1), 59–82 (2006)
35. van den Haak, M.J., de Jong, M.D.T., Schellens, P.J.: Retrospective vs. concurrent think-aloud protocols: testing the usability of an online library catalogue. Behav. Inf. Technol. **22**(5), 339–351 (2003)
36. Braun, V., Clarke, V.: Using thematic analysis in psychology. Qual. Res. Psychol. **3**(2), 77–101 (2006)
37. Tong, A., Sainsbury, P., Craig, J.: Consolidated criteria for reporting qualitative research (COREQ): a 32-item checklist for interviews and focus groups. Int. J. Qual. Health Care **19**(6), 349–357 (2007)

AI and LLMs in Healthcare: Tools for Professionals, Support for Citizens

Prognostic Risk Stratification of Hypertrophic Cardiomyopathy

Linking Sarcomere Gene Variants with Multimodal Phenotypes via Unsupervised Clustering

Long Dang[1](✉), Felix Agakov[2], Jari Hyttinen[1], Iacopo Olivotto[3], and Mark van Gils[1]

[1] Faculty of Medicine and Health Technology, Tampere University, Tampere, Finland
long.dang@tuni.fi
[2] Pharmatics Limited, Edinburgh, UK
[3] University of Florence, Florence, Italy

Abstract. Hypertrophic Cardiomyopathy (HCM) is an inherited disorder that provokes pathological cardiac changes across molecular-to-tissue scales, clinically presenting as enlarged heart. HCM causes severe health problems and unexpected deaths. Driven by sarcomeric variants, the genotype-phenotype relationship in HCM is highly heterogeneous. Unsupervised clustering reveals hidden genotype-phenotype associations without prior labels. However, conventional algorithms often overlook subgroup patterns, due to potential biases in feature selection and prior algorithm assumptions. This study outlines a clustering-based approach for HCM risk stratification based on clinical data where unsupervised methods with optimized parameters benchmarked across genetic cohorts.

Multimodal dataset from over 2,600 individuals, including clinical, physiological, imaging data were aggregated, standardized, transformed, reduced in dimensionality using PCA guided by reconstruction-error threshold. Three algorithms: K-Means, DBSCAN, GMM were applied separately to each group. Optimal parameters were selected by a custom framework that employed metrics: Davies-Bouldin, Calinski-Harabasz Index, Silhouette Score.

Two clusters consistently revealed in each cohort. K-Means outperformed others. Regardless of genotype, one cluster was linked with higher rates of stroke, heart failure, and sudden death, particularly in pathogenic sarcomeric variant carriers. Members in this cluster exhibited an 11.75-fold higher fatality rate, earlier disease onset, and reduced lifespan. Factor loadings suggest that CMR, Echocardiography were the main contributors to shape clusters and enhance separation.

The identification of high-mortality clusters highlights the value of integrating phenotype-genotype data for risk stratification. The study proposes an approach for monitoring disease progression by observing cluster shifts using recent clinical data. Result validation with external dataset is still required in future work.

Keywords: hypertrophic cardiomyopathy · unsupervised clustering · multimodal data analysis · clinical decision support

M. Särestöniemi et al. (Eds.): NCDHWS 2026, CCIS 3010, pp. 341–361, 2026.
https://doi.org/10.1007/978-3-032-28819-6_22

1 Introduction

1.1 Background of Hypertrophic Cardiomyopathy

The human heart is a muscular organ responsible for the continuous circulation of blood throughout the body. Most of the time, this system operates normally, but certain asymptomatic disorders may develop silently, leading to severe complications, and unexpected deaths. One such condition is Hypertrophic Cardiomyopathy (HCM), a disease that is characterized by abnormal thickening of the myocardial tissue in the heart [1], commonly in the left ventricle (LV) [2, 3]. HCM provokes pathological changes that span from molecular alterations to cellular and tissue morphology, resulting in heart enlargement as clinical evident. In adults, HCM is diagnosed by an LV wall thickness $\geq$15 mm on echocardiography or cardiovascular magnetic resonance (CMR), in the absence of other causes of hypertrophy such as athletic remodelling [4, 5]. The estimated prevalence of HCM in the adult population lies between 0.16% and 0.29%, corresponding to roughly one case per 300–600 individuals [6–9]. While there is no clear mapping between HCM and specific geographic, ethnic, or sex factors [1], the presence of HCM shows a positive correlation with adverse clinical outcomes, including sudden cardiac death (SCD) and heart failure (HF) [10, 11], particularly among adolescents and athletes [12, 13]. Although HCM is commonly associated with signs such as exertional dyspnoea, fatigue, palpitations, and chest pain [10, 14, 15], its manifestation and progression can vary considerably or, in some cases, remain entirely asymptomatic until discovered by chance [2].

HCM is commonly caused by changes in genes (variants) encoding proteins that control heart muscle contraction, known as sarcomere genes. This genetic alteration can be inherited from either parent [1, 16], affects cardiac muscle cells [10], and gradually causes thickening of the heart wall, leading to hypertrophy [17]. The most common sarcomere genes in HCM [18–21] are *MYBPC3* [22], *MYH7* [23], *TNNT2* [24], *TNNI3* [25], *TPM1* [26], *MYL2* [27], *MYL3* [27], and *ACTC* [28]. Sarcomere gene variants account for 30–60% HCM cases [4, 29, 30], however, considerable variability in the clinical presentation of HCM, regardless of genetic background, and likewise a comparable diversity of phenotypic expression of variants within known genes has been observed in recent studies [3, 30–33]. Thus, while the genetic profile can inform clinical management [34], the presence of inconsistencies and uncertainties calls for further investigation to elucidate genotype-phenotype associations and uncover additional genetic or non-genetic modifiers influencing disease expression.

In response, data analytic approaches and clinical decision support models based on different types of healthcare data have been developed over the years. The adoption of machine learning (ML) techniques combined with data from multiple clinical modalities not only enables clinicians to gain a comprehensive view of HCM progression from various perspectives but also uncovers complex, nonlinear patterns within heterogeneous datasets [35–39]. In settings with limited annotated data, as is typical healthcare data analysis research, including in HCM research, unsupervised clustering may show advantages by revealing the latent genotype-phenotype associations without reliance on exact prior labels. Most of the prior research using cluster-based techniques has relied on single-source data, though the role of multimodality in HCM research is gradually being recognized, particularly by using imaging and clinical data [37, 40, 41]. Although unsupervised learning holds promise for prognostic stratification using multimodal data, attention needs to be paid to the interpretability and clinical relevance of clusters, which are highly sensitive to feature and algorithm selection, potentially leading to inconsistent results [37].

1.2 Research Objectives and Strategies

This research aims to advance clinical decision support models by revealing hidden phenotypic substructures from commonly accessible medical data of individuals with HCM, thereby potentially enabling patient stratification, continuous risk monitoring, and, eventually, individualized and adaptive care across diverse genetic backgrounds. Specifically, to address the gap in current research regarding multi-modal approaches, this study introduces an interpretable clustering-based approach for stratifying HCM phenotypes using approximately 20 modalities of data obtained from a specialized HCM centre in Florence, Italy [42], applied independently to each of the three sarcomere cohorts. Additionally, it proposes a methodological framework for monitoring changes in patients at risk through the continued analysis of evolving clinical data.

The work is carried out in the EU-funded project SMASH-HCM (Stratification, Management, and Guidance of Hypertrophic Cardiomyopathy Patients using Hybrid Digital Twin Solutions), which aims to develop next-generation diagnostic, prognostic, and therapeutic approaches [43]. It will deliver a hybrid digital twin platform that combines biophysical and data-driven approaches through a multimodal framework to enable precision medicine in HCM [44]. The work reported in this paper forms part of a broader research effort to develop clinically interpretable referral models using routinely collected clinical data to achieve more precise risk stratification.

This research uses both multimodal clinical data, gene variant profiles together with an aggregated statistical approach to summarize longitudinal records. Segregating sarcomere gene categories facilitates precise genotype-phenotype characterization across carriers of pathogenic/likely pathogenic (P/LP) variants, individuals with variants of uncertain significance (VUS), and those without variants in the common sarcomere genes. In addition, by using a shared assessment framework and testing various algorithms across genetic cohorts, this work minimizes selection bias to ensure robust and reproducible outcomes. Furthermore, the results were interpreted to promote clinical relevance and suggest actionable insights.

The paper continues with Sect. 2 that details the methodology, Sect. 3 that reports the results, and Sect. 4 in which the findings, implications, strengths and limitations are discussed. Section 5 draws the conclusions of the study.

2 Methods

2.1 Overview of Methodology

This study presents a systematic methodology to analyse and interpret complex patterns in multimodal repositories related to HCM, as illustrated by the workflow in Fig. 1.

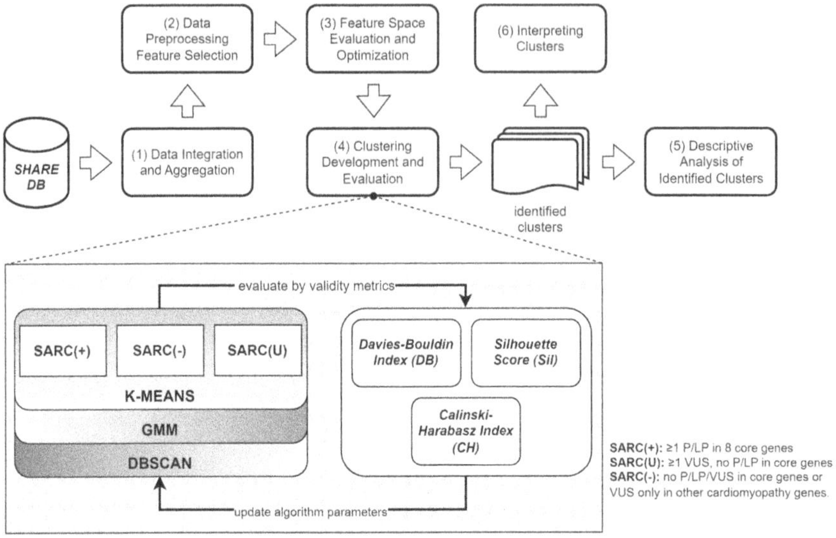

Fig. 1. Overview of the study workflow: From aggregated data, dimensionality reduction to independent clustering and descriptive analysis.

The workflow starts with selecting the appropriate data source, followed by integrating and preprocessing diverse data modalities into a comprehensive analytical dataset. To address the high dimensionality of the data, Principal Component Analysis (PCA) guided by reconstruction-error threshold are implemented. Eight core genes: *ACTC1*, *MYBPC3*, *MYH7*, *MYL2*, *MYL3*, *TNNI3*, *TNNT2*, and *TPM1* were examined. Individuals were classified into three cohorts: SARC(+) with any P/LP variant in core genes, SARC(U), with VUS in core genes and SARC(−) with no variant in core genes or only VUS in other cardiac genes. Following this, three unsupervised algorithms: K-Means, DBSCAN, and Gaussian Mixture Models (GMM) were benchmarked to evaluate performance across varied data distributions, cluster shapes in the heterogeneous data [45–47]. They were independently applied to each of the three sarcomere cohorts, thereby enabling the classification of phenotypic data in respect to their genetic profiles.

Parameter optimization for each algorithm was carried out via a custom evaluation framework, utilizing normalized clustering validity metrics including the Davies-Bouldin Index (DB) [48], Calinski-Harabasz Index (CH) [49], and Silhouette Score (Sil) [50]. The resulting clusters were subsequently analysed descriptively and comparatively, both within and across genetic subsets, to reveal underlying patterns, and risk characteristics based on phenotypic profiles. Finally, to enhance the clinical utility of the results, cluster interpretation was performed by evaluating the contribution of the top three principal components (PCs) from the PCA results, observing the contribution of medical features to cluster formation within sarcomere cohorts.

2.2 Dataset

In this study, a dataset of over 2600 patients and their relatives was obtained from the Sarcomeric Human Cardiomyopathy Registry (SHaRe) database [42], provided by Careggi University Hospital in Florence, Italy. SHaRe is the result of an international collaboration among cardiovascular centres, maintaining standardized genetic and longitudinal clinical data on individuals affected by cardiopathies, including HCM [42, 51].

Genetic testing results were available for 56% of the study cohort. Individuals without genetic testing were excluded from further analysis. Among those tested, 59.2% carried variants in eight sarcomere gene associated with HCM (HCM core genes): *ACTC1*, *MYBPC3*, *MYH7*, *MYL2*, *MYL3*, *TNNI3*, *TNNT2*, and *TPM1*, 5.6% had variants in other cardiac disorder genes, and 35.2% had no detectable variants in either the HCM core genes or other inherited cardiac disorder genes. Within the detected variants, 96% were located in the HCM core genes, with only a small proportion arising from other genes implicated in other aetiologies such as metabolic and storage diseases. Variants in *MYBPC3* and *MYH7* represented the greatest proportion of all analysed variants, and they also showed the greatest classification diversity, spanning P/LP to VUS and Likely Benign (LB). P/LP variants were prominently represented in 5/8 HCM core genes, in which the proportion of P/LP variants ranged from 73.1% to 87.2% per gene. Additionally, VUS had the highest proportion in 3/8 core genes, with the largest shares being 58.3% in *TPM1*, 87.5% in *MYL3*, and occurring exclusively in *ACTC1*. Within those core genes, LB variants were uncommon, even in the gene with the highest proportion, the LB category accounted for only 4.9% of variants.

Alongside genetic information, this study utilizes multimodal health records in a tabular format encompassing demographic background, behavioural factors, longitudinal physiological measurements, ambulatory monitoring, stress test outcomes, and medication profiles, along with imaging derived features from echocardiography, CMR, ECG, and cardiac catheterization. Additionally, familial cardiac history and observed cardiovascular events, such as Premature Ventricular Contraction (PVC), Atrial Fibrillation, Premature Atrial Contraction (PAC), and syncope were also incorporated. Mortality-related variables were intentionally excluded from the learning dataset to enable subsequent stages of the study and avoid leakage of possible outcome information into the training data.

Summary statistics of demographic and contextual variables used in the comparative analysis between cohorts are presented in Supplementary Table 1. The majority of participants were the first affected family members (probands), whereas relatives of affected individuals represented 16.33% of the total. The dataset exhibited a skewed gender distribution with a ratio of approximately 60:40 males: females. In terms of racial composition, White individuals represented the majority (97.84%), while participants from Asian and Black racial groups were also included. Whereas the reported use of harmful substances such as alcohol or drugs was low, at under 1%, up to 31.7% participants identified themselves as smokers. While patients with diabetes represented 7.4% of the cohort, hypertension was present in approximately 40% of the population.

Within a follow-up period averaging roughly 18–20 years, the mean age at primary diagnosis was 44.60 years, and the 1st cardiac event occurred at a mean age of 46.44 years. Individuals carrying P/LP variants in one of the eight sarcomere cores genes presented younger mean ages at primary diagnosis and 1st cardiac event, whereas those without such variants and VUS variants, revealed later onset compared to the cohort average. The prevalence of arrhythmic events such as PVC, Atrial Fibrillation, PAC, and syncope was higher among individuals carrying P/LP variants in the core genes compared to those without P/LP/VUS variants within these genes. Similarly, echocardiographic indicators of systolic dysfunction, including Left Ventricular Ejection Fraction (LVEF) $\leq$50% and LVEF $\leq$35%, occurred nearly twice as frequently in the P/LP carrier group. However, while stroke rates were comparable across groups, compared to carriers of P/LP variants, the prevalence of obstruction was roughly 1.5 times higher among individuals carrying only VUS in core genes, and 2 time higher among those without any variants. These findings shed light on risk stratification and highlight the need to categorize variant subsets to better explain genotype- phenotype correlations.

2.3 Integration and Preprocessing of Multimodal Data

To facilitate understanding of phenotypic variation within each sarcomere group, a patient grouping approach based on genetic profiles was introduced (Fig. 2). The Sarcomere Plus, or SARC(+), refers to individuals carrying a P/LP variant in at least one of the eight HCM core genes. The Sarcomere Uncertain or SARC(U) group represents an ambiguous category, comprising individuals who do not carry any P/LP variants, but have at least one VUS in one of those core genes. The Sarcomere Negative or SARC(−) refers to individuals without variants in the HCM core genes, though a VUS may appear in other cardiac disorder genes outside the core set.

By this criterion, the sarcomere cohorts were established, comprising 701 cases in SARC(+), 596 cases in SARC(−), and 173 cases in SARC(U).

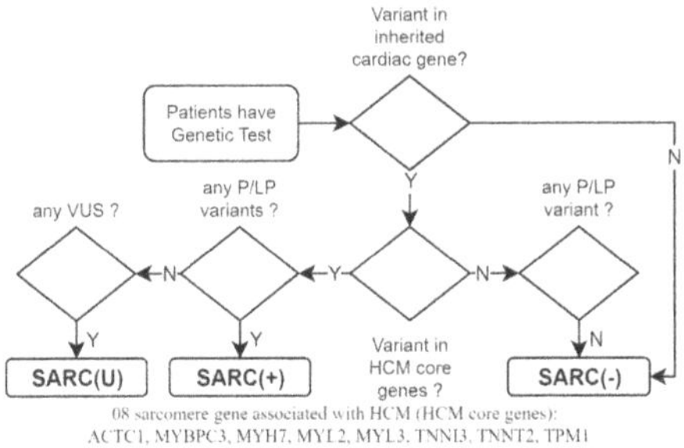

Fig. 2. Workflow outlines the stepwise classification of participants into three sarcomere cohorts based on their genetic background.

Longitudinally recorded clinical variables were summarized using statistical descriptors selected according to the characteristics of each data modality (Table 1). For instance, cardiac event variables were captured by type and age at the first and the most recent occurrence to reflect current clinical relevance, while initial and final ECG values were highlighted to show disease progression over time. Boolean indicator variables were subsequently introduced to indicate the presence of missing values in selected features, reflecting data unavailability specific to certain modalities. Approximately 20% of aggregated variables showing no variation or notable modality inconsistency were excluded, resulting in 1,032 retained variables in the final dataset. Aggregated features were standardized and transformed to address inconsistent value ranges across modalities and ensure compatibility with downstream algorithms.

A dimensionality reduction step using PCA was applied to address the residual high dimensionality in the retained data. The Variance of the Reconstruction Error (VRE) criterion was used to quantitatively determine the optimal number of PCs while simultaneously evaluating the cumulative variance retained [52, 53]. The reconstruction error varied across the sarcomeric subsets, with a peak value of approximately 0.06 Using a reconstruction error threshold of 0.02 (corresponding to the third quartile, Q3), we selected 32, 29, 24 PCs in SARC(+), SARC(−), and SARC(U), respectively, which preserves approximately 74% of the cumulative variance. The retained PCs were used as inputs for subsequent analyses.

Table 1. Summary How Statistics Methods Applied Across Modalities CMR: Cardiovascular Magnetic Resonance, ECG: Electrocardiography, Amb: Ambulatory x: means Yes, blank: means No and - means not Applicable.

Modalities	First Age	Last Age	Mode	Mean	Count	Min Value	Max Value	First Value	Last Value
Genetic data					x				
Event History	x	x	x		x				
Echocardiogram						x	x	x	x
CMR						x	x	x	x
Medication	x	x		x					
Physiology data						x	x	x	x
Stress Test						x	x	x	x
Implant / Explant	x	x			x				
ECG	x	x			x	x	x	x	x
Laboratory Test						x	x	x	x
Amb. Monitoring						x	x	x	x
Familial History					x				
Risk Score						x	x	x	x
Clinical History	x	x		x		x	x	x	x
Measurements						x	x	x	x
Demographic	–	–	–	–	–	–	–	–	–
Behaviour	–	–	–	–	–	–	–	–	–
Catheterization	–	–	–	–	–	–	–	–	–

2.4 Cluster Discovery Using Unsupervised Learning

Due to the heterogeneous nature of the dataset, three clustering algorithms: K-Means, Gaussian Mixture Models (GMM), and DBSCAN, reflecting different assumptions regarding cluster shape, distribution, and density [45–47], were applied to each predefined sarcomere subset to assess clustering performance from diverse perspectives. Clustering algorithm selection was guided by two key criteria: inter-cluster separation and intra-cluster compactness.

Clustering parameters were optimized using a custom evaluation framework and consistently applied for each subset. It was constructed by incorporating three clustering validity metrics: Davies-Bouldin (DB) [48], Silhouette (SH) [50], and Calinski-Harabasz (CH) [49]. For each algorithm, let θ represent a specific parameter configuration within the candidate set Θ ($\theta \in \Theta$), and DB(θ), Sil(θ), CH(θ) corresponding to normalized clustering validity metrics of θ. The composite score (CS) associated with θ, represents the equally weighted average of those metric values, and is formulated as:

$$\overline{\mathrm{CS}}(\theta) = \frac{[1 - DB(\theta)] + Sil(\theta) + CH(\theta)}{3} \tag{1}$$

The parameter set corresponding to the highest composite score was identified as the optimal configuration for the algorithm [54, 55]. Thus, the optimal parameter configuration θ^* is defined as:

$$\theta^* = \underset{\theta \in \Theta}{\mathrm{argmax}} \overline{CS}(\theta) \tag{2}$$

While in K-Means and GMM, the construction of the candidate set Θ focused on the potential number of clusters, which was varied from 2 to 10, candidate set Θ of DBSCAN involved both neighbourhood radius (eps) set within the 10th - 90th percentile range of pairwise distances and the minimum number of neighbours required to define a dense region, spanning from 2 to 40.

2.5 Interpretation Clusters

Given the first three PCs capture about 40% of the total variance, the study focuses on analysing the factor loadings of those PCs to examine the influence of individual variables and their modalities in interpreting segmentation outcomes. Furthermore, to assess the contribution of variables to cluster differentiation, the study analysed the absolute coefficients of each variable on the first PC (PC1), second PC (PC2) and third PC (PC3), with higher values indicating a greater influence on separation of cluster.

2.6 Characterization of Identified Clusters

To elucidate the distinguishing phenotypic characteristics of the identified clusters, the study employed various descriptive analyses to examine and compare the obtained cluster profiles within and across sarcomeric variant cohorts. Initially, the patterns of mortality causes were assessed to reveal trends associated with each cluster. With respect to each genetic profile, death rates within the observed follow-up period were subsequently compared across clusters to evaluate variation in both overall and cardiomyopathy-specific mortality. Kaplan-Meier curve analyses were then performed to reveal pathological progression and survival probability among the stratified clusters.

3 Results

3.1 Outcome of Cluster Identification

Application of K-Means, DBSCAN, and GMM to stratify sarcomere cohorts revealed remarkable variability in optimal parameter settings and resulting outputs. While K-Means and GMM achieved the highest composite scores consistently at the optimal number of clusters k = 2 across all sarcomere subsets (Fig. 3), DBSCAN presented variability in the selection of optimal parameters, with both the neighbourhood radius and density threshold differing between genetic cohorts.

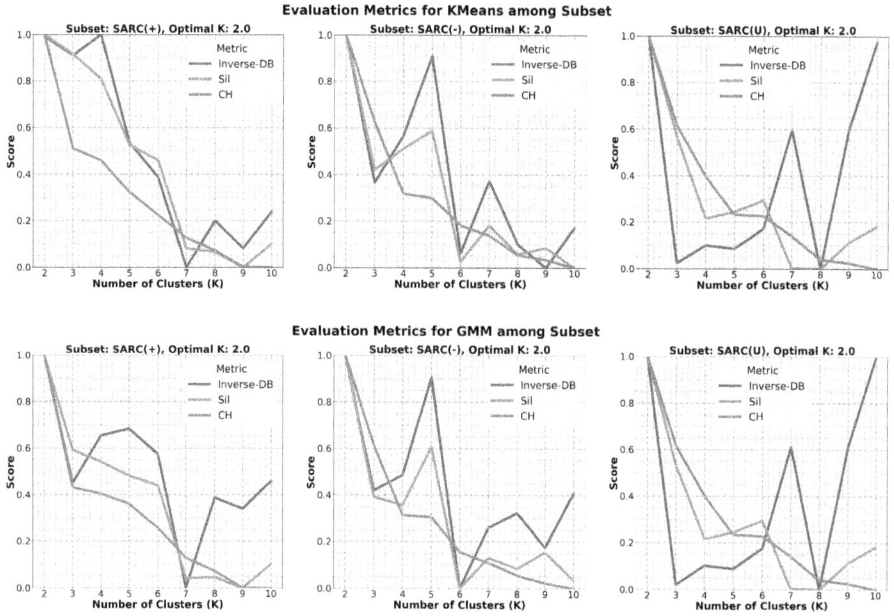

Fig. 3. Evaluation metrics for K-Means, GMM showing variability in clustering validity metrics across different cluster options., with the highest composite scores achieved at the optimal cluster number k = 2 for both algorithms in all genetic groups.

Although consensus was achieved between 3 algorithms in identifying two clusters under optimal parameter settings, DBSCAN failed to produce a relatively balanced distribution among clusters in all genetic groups. Meanwhile, similarity in cluster structures was found between K-means and GMM across all subgroups when visualized using t-SNE and UMAP (Fig. 4). However, K-Means outperformed others by demonstrating better inter-cluster separation and intra-cluster compactness, therefore, it was adopted as the model for subsequent studies.

Cluster membership varied across the subsets. Given the inherent arbitrariness of clustering annotations, numerical labels are used solely for reference and identification, without implying any ordering, hierarchy, or semantic meaning. They are interpreted based on their characteristic patterns rather than on the label assignment.

In SARC(+), clusters 1 and 2 comprised 358 (51.1%) and 343 (48.9%) individuals, respectively. In SARC(−), 336 (56.4%) persons were assigned to cluster 1 and 260 persons (43.6%) to cluster 2. For SARC(U), 89 (51.4%) people belonged to cluster 1 and 84 (48.6%) to cluster 2.

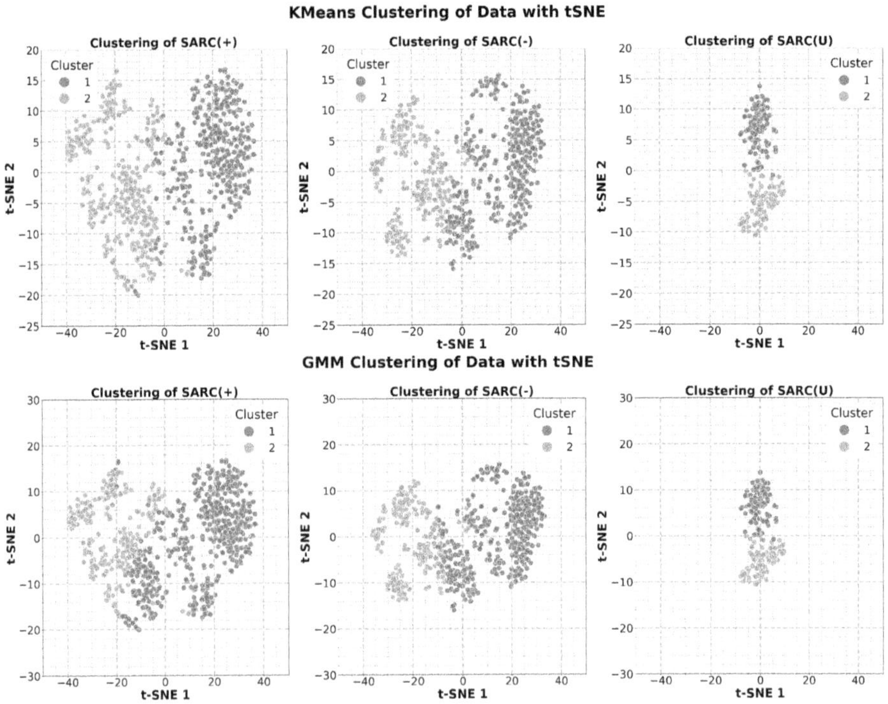

Fig. 4. Visualization of two identified clusters in 2D space using t-SNE with K-Means and GMM. Results indicate a relative similarity between the two algorithms; however, K-Means demonstrates superior performance by producing more compact clusters and clearer separation.

3.2 Characterization of Identified Clusters

The follow-up duration or the study period was evaluated separately for each sarcomere cohort and showed variability, with a median of 14.76 years, 16.23 years, and 18.39 years in SARC(−), SARC(U), and SARC(+), respectively.

Mortality and Causes of Death Assessment

Mortality analysis and cause-of-death assessment revealed noticeable differences across genetic cohorts (Fig. 5). Findings indicated that stroke occurred exclusively in one cluster (cluster 2), which also exhibited abnormally elevated mortality associated with HF and SCD across three genetic cohorts. The most notable rise was seen in the SARC(+), where 26 deaths with HF (96.3%) and 15 with SCD (83.3%) belonged to cluster 2. A similarity was observed in the SARC(−), in which 5 deaths with HF (71.4%) and 5 with SCD (62.5%) were found in the same cluster 2. Although this cluster 2 showed a pronounced increase in HCM fatalities including deaths due to HF, SCD, and stroke, the proportion of mortality resulting from these causes in each cohort remained relatively limited: 42.20% in SARC(+), 22.72% in SARC(−), and 33.33% in SARC(U).

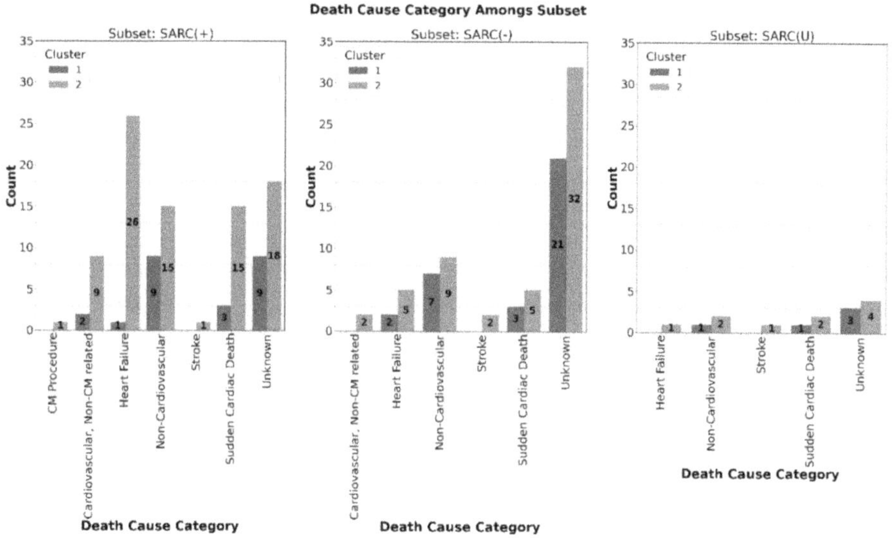

Fig. 5. Distribution Of Causes of Death by Cluster and Genetic Cohorts. The figure highlights elevated rates of HF, SCD, as well as stroke occurring exclusively in cluster 2. It also shows that unknown causes of death account for a substantial proportion across all genetic cohorts.

Throughout the follow-up period, cumulative all-cause mortality remained consistently higher in one cluster (cluster 2) across all subgroups (Fig. 6). Notably, within the SARC(+), death rates reached 24.8% in cluster 2 compared to 6.7% in cluster 1, while in SARC(−), they were 21.2% in cluster 2 and 9.8% in cluster 1. In SARC(U), death rates were the lowest, at 11.9% and 5.6% for clusters 2 and 1, respectively.

When restricting the examination to cardiomyopathy-related fatalities and excluding cases of unknown, non-cardiovascular, or cardiovascular but non-cardiomyopathy causes, the disparity between the two clusters became even more pronounced across all cohorts. Interestingly, mortality due to cardiomyopathic complications in cluster 2 among SARC(+) individuals was found to be roughly 11.75 times greater than in cluster 1 and about 3.4–4.3 times higher compared to other sarcomere groups. Given the pronounced elevated fatality rate in cluster 2, which peaked at 14.3%, in comparison with the cohort average ranging from 3.1%-7.4%, these findings suggest the potential promise for identifying individuals at elevated risk for cardiomyopathy-related deaths.

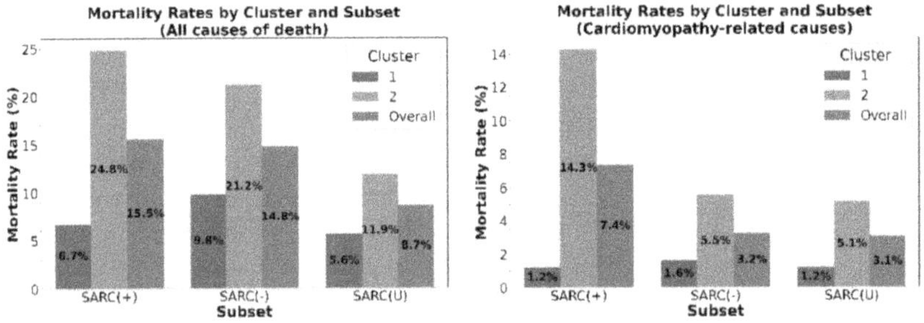

Fig. 6. All-Cause And Cardiomyopathy Fatalities Across Clusters and Genetic Cohorts. The figure shows a higher mortality rate in cluster 2 regardless of genotype profile. A difference becomes even more pronounced when considering cardiomyopathy-related fatalities alone.

Survival Analysis Using the Kaplan-Meier Estimator

Assessment of outcomes revealed a consistent pattern across the different variant categories, indicating that one cluster (cluster 2) is associated with an earlier onset of mortality (Fig. 7). Specifically, in the SARC(−) group, cluster 2 exhibited a reduction in survival probability beginning in the fourth decade of life, whereas the SARC(+) and SARC(U) groups demonstrated an accelerated deterioration, with a marked decline evident starting at age 20. This observation reflects more severe disease progression at an earlier stage of life among patients classified to cluster 2, particularly among carriers of sarcomeric variants, thus suggesting potential value for timely risk assessment.

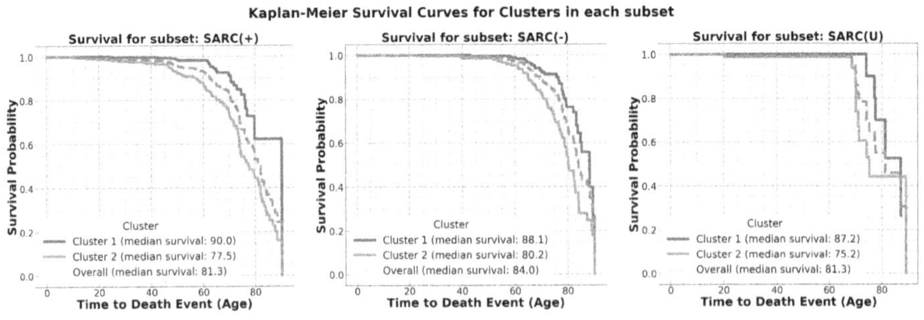

Fig. 7. Kaplan-Meier Survival Curves Stratified by Cluster Within Each Genetic Cohort.

Figures illustrate earlier onset of mortality in cluster 2, with survival probability declines at age 20 among sarcomeric variants carriers, compared to age 40 in those without these variants.

Moreover, Cluster 2 is also distinguished by comparatively reduced life expectancy, with the maximum recorded ages being 80.2 years in SARC(−), 77.5 years in SARC(+) and only 75.2 years in SARC(U). The observed range falls considerably short of the projected mean lifespans across all variant groups, which range from 81.3 to 84.0 years. Furthermore, participants within cluster 1 generally demonstrated a median survival exceeding that of the entire genetic cohort. Notably, individuals in cluster 1 with P/LP sarcomeric variants achieved the greatest longevity, attaining 90 years of age.

3.3 Interpreting Clusters via Component Loadings

The comparative analysis reveals consistent fluctuations in absolute coefficients across components across variant groups, predominantly within the 0–0.10 range. Among these groups, the third quartiles (Q3) of absolute coefficient values in the first 3 PCs are approximately 0.020, serving as the threshold for identifying high-loading variables that may shape cluster structure and increase cluster separation.

In SARC(+), CMR variables account for the largest share of absolute coefficients across all three PCs, contributing 52%, whereas in SARC(−), SARC(U), their influence is limited to PC1, PC2. Within these CMR variables, those related to ventricular ejection fractions, and end-systolic, end-diastolic volumes showed as the most influential contributors. Additionally, stress test variables with blood pressure indices are also distinguished as major contributors, accounting for over 20% of high-loading features and primarily linked to PC2 and PC3.

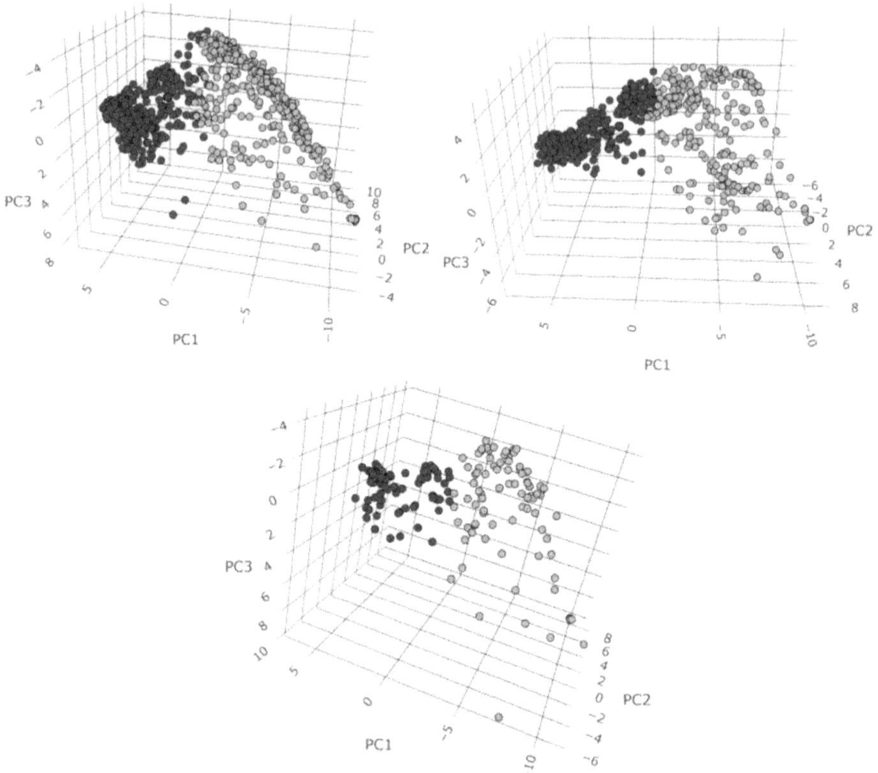

Fig. 8. Visualization of K-Means Clusters Across Genetic Cohorts in 3D SARC(+): top-left, SARC(−): top-right, SARC(U): below, Cluster 1: blue, Cluster 2: orange. While cluster 1 tends to condense around similar values, cluster 2 exhibits substantial variability across three dimensions.

Alongside the 42% contribution of CMR variables, the SARC(−) subset also showed the inclusion of roughly 33% echocardiographic features in PC1 and PC3. Additionally, the analysis highlights the emergence of body index-related features, such as Body Mass Index (BMI) and Body Surface Area (BSA), which contributed approximately 11.3% of the high-loading variables, ranking just behind CMR and echocardiographic variables. Within the SARC(U) subset, CMR features represented the largest share, contributing 47% of the high-loading variables, followed by a 39% proportion of stress test features, observed solely in PC3. As a result, only a small proportion was left for other variables, such as cardiac event, comprised less than 14% of the total.

Furthermore, the interpreted clustering outcomes consistently highlighted critical variables that play a major role in separating clusters and shaping their structural formation. In the 3D space, identified clusters are separated along the axes by PC1, PC2 and PC3, reflecting the influence of CMR and echocardiographic variables in promoting inter-cluster separation and intra-cluster compactness.

4 Discussion

4.1 Key Observations and Their Significance

The emergence of one cluster (cluster 2) suggests potential clinical relevance, as individuals within this subgroup demonstrate considerably elevated mortality rates, diminished projected life expectancy, and an increased likelihood of adverse complications, including SCD, HF, and stroke. These risks are particularly amplified in the SARC(+) subgroup, comprising carriers of P/LP sarcomeric variants, reinforcing the importance of genetic stratification within the diagnostic framework for HCM. Additionally, this observation indicates that relying solely on genetic variant status as a prognostic marker may be insufficient, given the comparable risk profiles observed among individuals belonging to the same cluster. This evidence provides additional justification for adopting an integrated, multimodal approach to HCM management, rather than depending exclusively on individual markers such as genotype or clinical traits.

The failure of DBSCAN to identify phenotypic patterns suggests that that although DBSCAN effectively detects dense clusters, its application to datasets with heterogeneous structures requires more precise parameter tuning than solely relying on basic calculations. Meanwhile, K-means and GMM showed comparable cluster structures across sarcomere cohort under t-SNE and UMAP visualization, indicating a relatively compact distribution with roughly spherical or elliptical shapes, aligning well with the assumptions of those algorithms.

While cluster 2 is characterized by substantial variability, cluster 1 is more tightly distributed along PC3, driven mainly by body index factors in SARC(−) and stress test metrics in other variant categories. This observation highlights that individuals at lower risk, especially those lacking sarcomeric variants, share relatively consistent body characteristics, whereas higher risk individuals demonstrate broader variation in cardiac performance under stress, regardless of genetic background. Additionally, the prominence of body index-related features among high-loading variables in those without sarcomeric genetic variants suggests that metabolic and body size may act as additional modifiers of HCM phenotypic expression, contributing to variability in HCM beyond genetic factors alone.

Furthermore, in 3D projection (Fig. 8), the separation of clusters along the horizontal and vertical axes by PC1 and PC3, where CMR and echocardiographic variables dominate, indicates a notable divergence in disease expression and progression among clusters, confirming the essential role of imaging features in stratifying phenotypic distinctions. Besides that, imaging-derived parameters are often subject to criticism regarding rotational variability, which can introduce inconsistencies in measurement outcomes and affect the accuracy of the derived results [56]. In this study, this concern was mitigated as imaging data were collected under standardized protocols at specialized HCM centres, ensuring that variability in measurements was controlled and minimized.

4.2 Novelty of the Study

This work outlines an interpretable clustering-based approach that may stratify HCM risk using variant profiles. It highlights a distinct patient cohort that exhibits unfavourable risk characteristics, associated with elevated mortality and shortened survival. Additionally, this research suggests a potential direction for developing a new classification model by utilizing prior cluster centroids. In this approach, cluster membership for patient is determined by identifying the nearest centroid using Euclidean distance, given the clinical and imaging data. Complementing risk stratification for new admissions, the proposed approach enables continuous monitoring disease progression through cluster membership transition among follow-up patients by detecting temporal risk patterns through ongoing integration of recent clinical data.

Furthermore, the study presents a conceptual framework that integrates genotype and phenotype data to explore their joint contribution to understanding disease mechanisms and improving diagnostic precision. The study proposes an approach of using multiple clustering methods for benchmarking, since relying solely on parameter tuning does not ensure optimal results, as illustrated by DBSCAN's limitations. The consistent detection of two stable cluster structures across algorithms suggests that the custom evaluation framework provides a reliable basis for parameter selection, although external validation was not performed, which limits the certainty of the identified insights.

This work introduces a tailored extension of traditional clustering methods, offering partial mitigation of common limitations in unsupervised learning. Specifically, to mitigate the challenge of excessive sensitivity to feature selection, this research proposes a systematic framework for harmonizing multimodality data by reorganizing longitudinal datasets into aggregated and synthesized variables to effectively capture disease progression throughout the follow-up period. To address potential biases arising from data heterogeneity, we benchmarked three clustering methods, each with tailored parameter optimization, to inform our evaluation before drawing final conclusions.

4.3 Limitations and Future Direction

Most modalities employed in this study rely on manual measurements, which may introduce variability to the recorded data. Such variability is particularly concerning when used in aggregated indicators, such as minimum or maximum values, and subsequently incorporated into clustering algorithm. Additionally, most essential features for cluster formation and subgroup differentiation, extracted from imaging data such as CMR and echocardiography, are vulnerable to rotational variability, which may introduce additional inconsistencies in data acquisition.

Furthermore, because only a relatively small proportion of deaths are attributed to HF, SCD, and stroke, events considered directly related to HCM, accurately estimating the true burden of HCM in each cluster remains challenging. HCM may contribute to secondary causes of death, undocumented fatalities, or deaths with unknown classification [4, 5, 57], as observed in 60% of death cases in the SARC(−) group. Therefore, these observations underscore the need for comprehensive mortality assessments in data to accurately capture the full impact of HCM on patient outcomes.

Although the dominant factors demonstrate the clinical relevance of the findings by confirming features routinely used in HCM risk stratification, the interpretation remains primarily theoretical, conceptual and at a general analytical level. Instead, applying predictive modelling approaches, such as LASSO-penalized logistic regression or SHAP-based feature importance analysis of a richer predictive model, could be used in future work to identify variables most strongly associated with cluster memberships. Additionally, comprehensive comparative assessments and significance tests for high-loading features among clusters and across variant subsets are needed in subsequent study to make the interpretability of the findings more robust and formally verified.

In addition, the exclusive reliance on a single dataset introduces uncertainty regarding the generalizability of the research. Addressing this limitation requires supplementary validation sets and retrospective analyses to confirm the applicability of the proposed model in broader contexts. Moreover, the potential strategy of utilizing cluster centroids to construct a novel classification framework is still at a conceptual stage, indicating the need for subsequent refinement, validation, and benchmarking against independent datasets to assess its generalizability and practical utility.

In this work, we have only focused on comparing and analysing unsupervised clustering methods, which ignore any information about HCM endpoints during learning. In the future we plan to extend this work by considering semi-parametric discriminative mixtures (mixtures-of-experts), where cluster memberships will be learned simultaneously with cluster-specific predictive mappings to improve predictions of endpoints at follow-up, with validations in independent samples within and across cohorts.

5 Conclusions

This study presents a clustering approach that may offer potential value for prognostic risk assessment in HCM. The findings confirm that individuals grouped within a specific cluster are at an elevated mortality risk, diminished lifespan, and greater vulnerability to adverse cardiovascular events, including SCD, HF, and stroke. This contrast becomes even more pronounced among carriers of P/LP sarcomeric variants, reinforcing the contribution of genetic factors HCM risk stratification. Nonetheless, relying solely on sarcomeric variant type for outcome estimation may be insufficient, given the consistent risk patterns observed among individuals within the same cluster, irrespective of genotype. This underscores the need to implement a multimodal approach in HCM research, particularly for elucidating the interaction between genetic determinants and phenotypic expressions, and for addressing the inherent complexity and heterogeneity of HCM development.

Furthermore, the study highlights the relevance and translational potential of the findings by revealing contributions of certain clinical features to cluster structures and separation through interpretation using factor loading analysis. Although not yet validated within this study, our research outcomes may facilitate the development of a stratified approach to prognostic assessment and disease progression management.

Lastly, while the research provides a solid methodological framework for data preparation and analysis, which contributes to greater reproducibility and reliability, it also simultaneously acknowledges existing constraints and highlights prospects for further refinement and advancement as outlined.

Acknowledgments. This study was funded by the European Union under GA #101137115.

Disclosure of Interests. This research was funded by the European Union under GA #101137115. Views and opinions expressed are however those of the author(s) only and do not necessarily reflect those of the European Union or HADEA. Neither the European Union nor the granting authority can be held responsible for them.

References

1. Marian, A.J., Braunwald, E.: Hypertrophic cardiomyopathy: genetics, pathogenesis, clinical manifestations, diagnosis, and therapy. Circ. Res. **121**, 749–770 (2017). https://doi.org/10.1161/CIRCRESAHA.117.311059
2. Suboc, T.: Hypertrophic cardiomyopathy - cardiovascular disorders - MSD manual professional edition. In: MD, Rush University (2024). https://www.msdmanuals.com/professional/cardiovascular-disorders/cardiomyopathies/hypertrophic-cardiomyopathy. Accessed 13 May 2025
3. Yiu, K.H., Atsma, D.E., Delgado, V., et al.: Myocardial structural alteration and systolic dysfunction in preclinical hypertrophic cardiomyopathy mutation carriers. PLoS One **7** (2012). https://doi.org/10.1371/journal.pone.0036115
4. Ommen, S.R., Ho, C.Y., Asif, I.M., et al.: 2024 AHA/ACC/AMSSM/HRS/PACES/SCMR guideline for the management of hypertrophic cardiomyopathy: a report of the American heart Association/American college of cardiology joint committee on clinical practice guidelines. Circulation **149**, e1239–e1311 (2024). https://doi.org/10.1161/CIR.0000000000001250
5. Arbelo, E., Protonotarios, A., Gimeno, J.R., et al.: 2023 ESC Guidelines for the management of cardiomyopathies: developed by the task force on the management of cardiomyopathies of the European Society of Cardiology (ESC). Eur. Heart J. **44**, 3503–3626 (2023). https://doi.org/10.1093/eurheartj/ehad194
6. Maron, B.J., Gardin, J.M., Flack, J.M., et al.: Prevalence of hypertrophic cardiomyopathy in a general population of young adults: echocardiographic analysis of 4111 subjects in the CARDIA study. Circulation **92**, 785–789 (1995). https://doi.org/10.1161/01.CIR.92.4.785
7. Maron, B.J., Mathenge, R., Casey, S.A., et al.: Clinical profile of hypertrophic cardiomyopathy identified de novo in rural communities. J. Am. Coll. Cardiol. **33**, 1590–1595 (1999). https://doi.org/10.1016/S0735-1097(99)00039-X
8. Hada, Y., Sakamoto, T., Amano, K., et al.: Prevalence of hypertrophic cardiomyopathy in a population of adult Japanese workers as detected by echocardiographic screening. Am. J. Cardiol. **59**, 183–184 (1987). https://doi.org/10.1016/S0002-9149(87)80107-8
9. Zou, Y., Song, L., Wang, Z., et al.: Prevalence of idiopathic hypertrophic cardiomyopathy in China: a population-based echocardiographic analysis of 8080 adults. Am. J. Med. **116**, 14–18 (2004). https://doi.org/10.1016/j.amjmed.2003.05.009
10. Basit, H., Alahmadi, M.H., Rout, P., Sharma, S.: Hypertrophic cardiomyopathy. In: StatPearls Treasure Island (FL) (2024). https://www.ncbi.nlm.nih.gov/books/NBK430788/. Accessed 13 May 2025
11. Maron, B.J., Desai, M.Y., Nishimura, R.A., et al.: Management of hypertrophic cardiomyopathy: JACC state-of-the-art review. J. Am. Coll. Cardiol. **79**, 390–414 (2022). https://doi.org/10.1016/j.jacc.2021.11.021
12. Maron, B.J., Haas, T.S., Ahluwalia, A., et al.: Demographics and epidemiology of sudden deaths in young competitive athletes: from the United States national registry. Am. J. Med. **129**, 1170–1177 (2016). https://doi.org/10.1016/j.amjmed.2016.02.031
13. Santos E de, S., Castro, P.H.G., Lima, L.P.S., et al.: Mortality from hypertrophic cardiomyopathy in Brazil—historical series. Int. J. Environ. Res. Public Health **21** (2024). https://doi.org/10.3390/IJERPH21111498
14. Van Driel, B., Nijenkamp, L., Huurman, R., et al.: Sex differences in hypertrophic cardiomyopathy: new insights. Curr. Opin. Cardiol. **34**, 254–259 (2019). https://doi.org/10.1097/HCO.0000000000000612

15. Kraft, T., Montag, J.: Altered force generation and cell-to-cell contractile imbalance in hypertrophic cardiomyopathy. Pflugers Arch. **471**, 719–733 (2019). https://doi.org/10.1007/s00424-019-02260-9
16. Autosomal Dominant Disorder. https://www.genome.gov/genetics-glossary/Autosomal-Dominant-Disorder. Accessed 13 May 2025
17. Mattsson, G., Magnusson, P., Mattsson, G., Magnusson, P.: Cardiomyopathy - disease of the heart muscle (2021). https://doi.org/10.5772/INTECHOPEN.91489
18. Carrier, L., Hengstenberg, C., Beckmann, J.S., et al.: Mapping of a novel gene for familial hypertrophic cardiomyopathy to chromosome 11. Nat. Genet. **4**, 311–313 (1993). https://doi.org/10.1038/NG0793-311
19. Thierfelder, L., MacRae, C., Watkins, H., et al.: A familial hypertrophic cardiomyopathy locus maps to chromosome 15q2. Proc Natl Acad Sci U S A **90**, 6270–6274 (1993). https://doi.org/10.1073/pnas.90.13.6270
20. Watkins, H., Macrae, C., Thierfelder, L., et al.: A disease locus for familial hypertrophic cardiomyopathy maps to chromosome 1q3. Nat. Genet. **3**, 333–337 (1993). https://doi.org/10.1038/ng0493-333
21. Jarcho, J.A., McKenna, W., Pare, J.A.P., et al.: Mapping a gene for familial hypertrophic cardiomyopathy to chromosome 14q1. N. Engl. J. Med. **321**, 1372–1378 (1989). https://doi.org/10.1056/nejm198911163212005
22. Gautel, M., Zuffardi, O., Freiburg, A., Labeit, S.: Phosphorylation switches specific for the cardiac isoform of myosin binding protein-C: a modulator of cardiac contraction? EMBO J. **14**, 1952–1960 (1995). https://doi.org/10.1002/j.1460-2075.1995.tb07187.x
23. Seidman, J.G., Seidman, C.: The genetic basis for cardiomyopathy: from mutation identification to mechanistic paradigms. Cell **104**, 557–567 (2001). https://doi.org/10.1016/S0092-8674(01)00242-2
24. Thierfelder, L., Watkins, H., MacRae, C., et al.: α-tropomyosin and cardiac troponin T mutations cause familial hypertrophic cardiomyopathy: a disease of the sarcomere. Cell **77**, 701–712 (1994). https://doi.org/10.1016/0092-8674(94)90054-X
25. Kimura, A., Harada, H., Park, J.E., et al.: Mutations in the cardiac troponin I gene associated with hypertrophic cardiomyopathy. Nat. Genet. **16**, 379–382 (1997). https://doi.org/10.1038/ng0897-379
26. Schleef, M., Werner, K., Satzger, U., et al.: Chromosomal localization and genomic cloning of the mouse α-tropomyosin gene TPM-1. Genomics **17**, 519–521 (1993). https://doi.org/10.1006/geno.1993.1361
27. Poetter, K., Jiang, H., Hassanzadeh, S., et al.: Mutations in either the essential or regulatory light chains of myosin are associated with a rare myopathy in human heart and skeletal muscle. Nat. Genet. **13**, 63–69 (1996). https://doi.org/10.1038/ng0596-63
28. Olson, T.M., Doan, T.P., Kishimoto, N.Y., et al.: Inherited and de novo mutations in the cardiac actin gene cause hypertrophic cardiomyopathy. J. Mol. Cell. Cardiol. **32**, 1687–1694 (2000). https://doi.org/10.1006/jmcc.2000.1204
29. Burke, M.A., Cook, S.A., Seidman, J.G., Seidman, C.E.: Clinical and mechanistic insights into the genetics of cardiomyopathy. J. Am. Coll. Cardiol. **68**, 2871–2886 (2016). https://doi.org/10.1016/j.jacc.2016.08.079
30. Topriceanu, C.-C., Pereira, A.C., Moon, J.C., et al.: Meta-analysis of penetrance and systematic review on transition to disease in genetic hypertrophic cardiomyopathy. Circulation **149**, 107–123 (2024). https://doi.org/10.1161/CIRCULATIONAHA.123.065987
31. Maron, B.J., Seidman, J.G., Seidman, C.E.: Proposal for contemporary screening strategies in families with hypertrophic cardiomyopathy. J. Am. Coll. Cardiol. **44**, 2125–2132 (2004). https://doi.org/10.1016/j.jacc.2004.08.052

32. Popa-Fotea, N.M., Micheu, M.M., Bataila, V., et al.: Exploring the continuum of hypertrophic cardiomyopathy—from DNA to clinical expression. Medicina (Lithuania) **55** (2019). https://doi.org/10.3390/medicina55060299
33. Alexa, I.D., Cozma, L.G., Constantinescu, G., et al.: Early diagnosis in hypertrophic cardiomyopathy–case report. Rev. Med. Chir. Soc. Med. Nat. Iasi. **108**, 361–365 (2004)
34. Ashraf, M., Jan, M.F., Jahangir, A., et al.: Abstract 14514: hypertrophic cardiomyopathy - genotype distribution and genotype-phenotype correlations - a unique perspective from a single center study. Circulation **148** (2023). https://doi.org/10.1161/CIRC.148.SUPPL_1.14514
35. Cardim, N., Galderisi, M., Edvardsen, T., et al.: Role of multimodality cardiac imaging in the management of patients with hypertrophic cardiomyopathy: an expert consensus of the European association of cardiovascular imaging endorsed by the Saudi Heart Association. Eur. Heart J. Cardiovasc. Imaging **16**, 280–280hh (2015). https://doi.org/10.1093/ehjci/jeu291
36. Karamarkou, C., Babady, M., Maltsinioti, C., Bruder, O.: Update on imaging in hypertrophic cardiomyopathy. Echocardiography **42**, e70146 (2025). https://doi.org/10.1111/echo.70146
37. Loncaric, F., Marti Castellote, P.M., Gonzalez Lopez, E., et al.: Exploring phenotypes in hypertrophic cardiomyopathy with machine learning data integration. a multicentric, multimodality pilot study. Eur. Heart J. **42** (2021). https://doi.org/10.1093/EURHEARTJ/EHAB724.3072
38. Amano, Y., Kitamura, M., Takano, H., et al.: Cardiac MR imaging of hypertrophic cardiomyopathy: techniques, findings, and clinical relevance. Magn. Reson. Med. Sci., 120–131 (2018). https://doi.org/10.2463/mrms.rev.2017-0145
39. Ashiwaju, B.I., Orikpete, O.F., Uzougbo, C.G.: The intersection of artificial intelligence and big data in drug discovery: a review of current trends and future implications. Matrix Sci. Pharma **7**, 36–42 (2023). https://doi.org/10.4103/MTSP.MTSP_14_23
40. Wengrofsky, P., Akivis, Y., Bukharovich, I.: Cardiac multimodality imaging in hypertrophic cardiomyopathy: what to look for and when to image. Curr. Cardiol. Rev. **19**, E160323214676 (2023). https://doi.org/10.2174/1573403X19666230316103117
41. Hourqueig, M., Bouzille, G., Mirabel, M., et al.: Hypertrophic cardiomyopathies requiring more monitoring for less atrial fibrillation-related complications: a clustering analysis based on the French registry on hypertrophic cardiomyopathy (REMY) for the REMY working group of the French Society of Cardiology **111**, 163–174 (2022). https://doi.org/10.1007/s00392-020-01797-5
42. SHaRe – SHaRe Project. https://www.thehareregistry.org/. Accessed 3 Jul 2025
43. SMASH-HCM. https://smash-hcm.eu/. Accessed 8 Jul 2025
44. Värri, A.O., Van Gils, M., Hyttinen, J.: Multilevel modelling for decision support in hypertrophic cardiomyopathy in the SMASH-HCM project. Finnish J. eHealth eWelfare **16** (2024). https://doi.org/10.23996/FJHW.143516
45. Fabianpedregosa, F.P., Michel, V., Oliviergrisel, O.G., et al.: Scikit-learn: machine learning in Python Gaël Varoquaux Bertrand Thirion Vincent Dubourg Alexandre Passos PEDREGOSA, VAROQUAUX, GRAMFORT ET AL. Matthieu Perrot. J. Mach. Learn. Res. **12**, 2825–2830 (2011)
46. Arthur, D., Vassilvitskii, S.: How slow is the k-means method? In: Proceedings of the Annual Symposium on Computational Geometry, vol. 2006, pp. 144–153 (2006). https://doi.org/10.1145/1137856.1137880
47. Schubert, E., Sander, J., Ester, M., et al.: DBSCAN revisited, revisited: why and how you should (still) use DBSCAN. ACM Trans. Database Syst. **42** (2017). https://doi.org/10.1145/3068335
48. Davies, D.L., Bouldin, D.W.: A cluster separation measure. IEEE Trans. Pattern Anal. Mach. Intell. PAMI-**1**, 224–227 (1979). https://doi.org/10.1109/TPAMI.1979.4766909

49. Caliñski, T., Harabasz, J.: A dendrite method foe cluster analysis. Commun. Stat. **3**, 1–27 (1974). https://doi.org/10.1080/03610927408827101
50. Shahapure, K.R., Nicholas, C.: Cluster quality analysis using silhouette score. In: Proceedings - 2020 IEEE 7th International Conference on Data Science and Advanced Analytics, DSAA 2020, pp. 747–748 (2020). https://doi.org/10.1109/DSAA49011.2020.00096
51. Ho, C.Y., Day, S.M., Ashley, E.A., et al.: Genotype and lifetime burden of disease in hypertrophic cardiomyopathy: insights from the Sarcomeric human cardiomyopathy registry (SHaRe). Circulation **138**, 1387 (2018). https://doi.org/10.1161/CIRCULATIONAHA.117.033200
52. Valle, S., Li, W., Qin, S.J.: Selection of the number of principal components: the variance of the reconstruction error criterion with a comparison to other methods. Ind. Eng. Chem. Res. **38**, 4389–4401 (1999). https://doi.org/10.1021/IE990110I. ISSUE:ISSUE: https://doi.org/10.1021/IECRED.1999.38. ISSUE-11;PAGEGROUP:STRING:PUBLICATION
53. Joe Qin, S., Dunia, R.: Determining the number of principal components for best reconstruction. IFAC Proc. Volumes **31**, 357–362 (1998). https://doi.org/10.1016/S1474-6670(17)44953-6
54. Sowan, B., Hong, T.P., Al-Qerem, A., et al.: Ensembling validation indices to estimate the optimal number of clusters. Appl. Intell. **53**, 9933–9957 (2023). https://doi.org/10.1007/S10489-022-03939-W
55. Shi, C., Wei, B., Wei, S., et al.: A quantitative discriminant method of elbow point for the optimal number of clusters in clustering algorithm. EURASIP J. Wirel. Commun. Netw. **2021** (2021). https://doi.org/10.1186/S13638-021-01910-W
56. Van Dalen, B.M., Soliman, O.I.I., Vletter, W.B., et al.: Feasibility and reproducibility of left ventricular rotation parameters measured by speckle tracking echocardiography. Eur. J. Echocardiogr. **10**, 669–676 (2009). https://doi.org/10.1093/ejechocard/jep036
57. Mielczarek, S., Syska, P., Lewandowski, M., et al.: P990Assessment of clinical risk factors for all-cause mortality among hypertrophic cardiomyopathy patients with ICDs. Eur. Heart J. **40** (2019). https://doi.org/10.1093/EURHEARTJ/EHZ747.0583

Trustworthy Federated Machine Learning in Healthcare: A Sociotechnical and Risk-Based Evaluation Using the Z-Inspection® Method

Pedro Kringen[1], Antti P. Happonen[2], Petra Ekman[1], Charles Vesteghem[5], Benjamin Barlous[5], Antonios Danelakis[6], Mark van Gils[2(✉)], Pedro A. Moreno-Sánchez[2,3], and Magnus Westerlund[1,4]

[1] Laboratory of Trustworthy AI, Arcada, 00560 Helsingfors, Finland
[2] Faculty of Medicine and Health Technology, Tampere University, 33100 Tampere, Finland
mark.vangils@tuni.fi
[3] Tecnalia, Basque Research & Technology Alliance (BRTA), 48160 Derio, Spain
[4] Faculty of Human and Social Sciences, Abo Akademi University, Turku, Finland
[5] Research Unit in General Practice, Aalborg University, Aalborg, Denmark
[6] NorHead, Norwegian University of Science and Technology, Trondheim, Norway

Abstract. Clinical use of AI requires verifiable trust in governance, fairness, privacy, and robustness. Federated machine learning (FML) changes how models are trained and audited and must be assessed in clinical settings. This work presents a sociotechnical governance study of FML on unstructured clinical notes across two Nordic healthcare sites. Using the Z-Inspection® methodology, we assess an AI system for predicting migraine and headache treatment, where data remain local and only model updates are shared.

Through co-design sessions with software developers and the assessment team, claims, issues, tensions, resolutions, and monitorable risks were identified and linked via sociotechnical scenarios that reveal improvement paths. Findings were mapped to the European Commission's High-Level Expert Group on AI requirements and the MIT AI Risk Repository, showing how trustworthiness requirements and risks can be operationalized in line with legislation such as the GDPR and the EU AI Act.

The study suggests that cross-jurisdictional governance can support the integration of FML into clinical practice. To our knowledge, this is the first Z-Inspection® review of a federated clinical application mapped end-to-end to the EU AI HLEG requirements. We show that a governance model aligned with technology readiness levels, using coordinated assessment tracks with shared minimum controls and explicit deployment gates, can manage uneven readiness across sites. This work demonstrates cross-border learning over heterogeneous health records by combining structured primary-care data with unstructured neurology notes without transferring raw data. It also provides a practical barrier assessment template for evaluating and improving the trustworthiness of federated clinical AI systems.

Keywords: AI assessment · Z-Inspection® · headache and migraine treatment · federated machine learning · research product development · trustworthy AI · artificial intelligence

M. Särestöniemi et al. (Eds.): NCDHWS 2026, CCIS 3010, pp. 362–378, 2026.
https://doi.org/10.1007/978-3-032-28819-6_23

1 Introduction

Electronic Health Records (EHRs) support coordinated care and must ensure patient safety and confidentiality in the digital society. A common practice in the use of healthcare data for research purposes, e.g., to perform statistical analyses or develop decision-support methods, is to centralize records from various EHRs into a single location. Combining data from different sources typically increases the number of cases, improving the power of analyses, the performance of algorithms, and the accuracy of performance estimates. It also provides datasets with broader population coverage (e.g., across different demographic groups or geographic locations). However, combining data sources requires transferring data across multiple locations, potentially raising concerns about patient privacy, compliance with national regulations, and data governance, especially when dealing with non-anonymized health records. While fully anonymized data can be in principle transferred easily and is not subject to the GDPR, full data anonymization almost systematically leads to a significant loss of information leaving little usable information for scientific research or development.

Federated learning (FL) was proposed by Google [1] as an alternative option. The idea is intuitively clear: keep the data where it was collected, move the model computation pipeline to the data, perform the needed computations locally at the different sites, transfer only the output of computations (that do not contain personal information), and finally combine the outputs from the various sites into a single model. This way, clinical organizations can learn from one another without transferring their patients' files, thereby facilitating the secondary use of clinical data. From a European Union perspective, FML is well-suited for healthcare data as it aligns with the digital strategy and regulations like the General Data Protection Regulation (GDPR), national data-sovereignty requirements, and yet allows for cross-institution collaboration [2, 3]. Theoretically, this approach reduces the risk of cross-site data breaches, simplifies compliance with ethics reviews and regulations, and most importantly, in the age of AI, facilitates the pooling of multi-institutional data sources that promote data diversity and allow for obtaining sufficiently large data sets to develop AI methods in the first place.

The federated learning is a technical concept, and thus, 'disease agnostic' by nature. In this study we have been focusing on headache disorders. Headache disorders, including migraine, are common and debilitating [4, 5], and their treatment is challenging as patients require both acute pain relief and preventive treatment, and it is highly personalized: what helps one person may fail for another [6, 7]. In the Nordic context, extensive EHR coverage across both primary care and neurology is available, potentially enabling the development of machine learning predictive models to improve treatment personalization of headache disorders, notably through an FML approach.

As a proof-of-concept, the project has been focusing on a common drug used for headache disorders, amitriptyline, to ensure clinical relevance. This was deemed as an appropriate real-world use case for testing whether federated AI can help clinicians make better, privacy-respecting decisions.

Healthcare is built on trust; patients believe that clinicians will act in their best interests, even in the absence of certainty. Bringing AI-based healthcare decision support systems into this context raises new questions, not just whether such systems work as intended, but whether their use is ethical, transparent, and in line with clinical guidelines and responsibilities [8]. A new understanding that can arise from examining such questions is whether established guidelines and best practices in the clinical domain overlap with those derived from AI solutions, or whether they are orthogonal, given the absence of human intuition vs. the data-driven nature of ML. Trust is an attitude, but trustworthiness is a property (set of achieved requirements) of a system, and an AI-driven tool may or may not deserve the trust placed in it. In the past couple of years, the "black box" nature of AI, as well as of federated systems [9–11], has brought the need for mechanisms to assure reliability, explainability, and fairness in the entire lifecycle of an AI-based system to the fore [12]. There is a growing body of work that calls for calibrated trust, so that clinicians do not over- nor under-trust what an AI-based system does [13]. Thus, any decision support solution that uses AI must be proven to be accurate and robust, ensure privacy, and be accounted for according to transparent ethical and accountability governance, or it risks introducing harm to the clinical field and patients, and, in the long term, diluting the quality of clinical judgment [8].

The European Commission's HLEG work [14] led to tools such as ALTAI (the Assessment List for Trustworthy AI) [15], and has been translated directly into the EU's Artificial Intelligence Act, adopted in 2024 [16], defining Europe's preference for *trustworthy AI by design.* The HLEG Ethics Guidelines translate broad and abstract principles (respect for human autonomy, non-maleficence, justice, and explicability) into seven requirements: human agency and oversight, robustness and safety, privacy and data governance, transparency, fairness, the well-being of society, and accountability. Concurrently, there have been attempts by independent initiatives to translate these ideas into practice [17, 18]. Of these, Z-Inspection® presents a structured, interdisciplinary approach to evaluating the trustworthiness of specific and environmentally contextualized AI-based systems over their lifecycle [19–21]. In integrating legal, technical, and ethical considerations, these frameworks provide a governance context within which federated AI for healthcare may be studied and developed responsibly [22].

A Z-Inspection® assessment is an expert-led qualitative methodology designed to discover issues and dilemmas with AI systems. Rather than producing quantitative metrics, it systematically elicits claims and evidence, which are then interpreted in light of Trustworthy AI requirements and qualitative frameworks such as the MIT AI Risk Repository. The results presented in this paper should therefore be read as a structured sociotechnical mapping of issues, tensions, and resolutions, not as a quantitative performance evaluation of the federated learning system itself.

The Z-Inspection® method [21] was applied in the assessments of the artefacts produced in the FEHLS project. After completing the Z-Inspection® assessment (set-up, assessment, and resolution phases), the key issues and tensions were extracted and mapped with respect to the EU HLEG requirements for Trustworthy AI [14]. Following this, as part of the process, we interrogated what this means for clinical relevance, bias, privacy, and explainability [23, 24]. The approach is more practice-oriented than theoretical, to demonstrate how a structured ethical review can translate high-level principles into specific design choices and governance measures for real-world clinical AI [18].

As a novel extension to the process, we applied a structured risk taxonomy that enables socio-technical hazards to be specified, compared, and audited. Accordingly, this work applies the *MIT AI Risk Repository* (Table S1) to code plausible harmful pathways in federated clinical AI, using its numbered, domain-spanning sub-domains to ensure consistent coding, traceability, and cross-study comparability while aligning with emerging governance [25].

The primary contribution of this work is the structured governance assessment of a federated clinical AI system, not the machine learning technique itself. Gradient boosting was selected as a suitable classifier for the available data, but the novelty lies in the independent, end-to-end trustworthiness evaluation using Z-Inspection® mapped to both the EU HLEG requirements and the MIT AI Risk Repository.

The paper is organized as follows. First, we describe the study setup, the federated datasets, learning architecture, and ethical evaluation framework, including the Z-Inspection® procedure and the risk-mapping method. Next, the quantitative results of the performance and fairness analyses and the risk-mapping outcomes are presented. The following section discusses these findings in the context of technology readiness, model transparency, and ethical principles, highlighting the interplay between the HLEG and MIT perspectives and deriving practical implications and limitations. Finally, the paper concludes by underscoring the main contributions and offering recommendations for future research and implementation.

To frame the results presented in this paper, it is essential to distinguish between the quality of the technical work and the maturity level the project was designed and funded to reach. Both national teams developed their contributions with solid engineering practice, yet the overall system operated at an early technology readiness level (TRL 3–4). The limitations identified in the assessment, therefore, reflect the scope, data constraints, and developmental stage of the prototype rather than shortcomings in the technical work itself. The analysis aims to clarify what an early-stage federated learning system reveals about the requirements for advancing to higher TRL levels, not to critique individual contributors. This distinction should guide the interpretation of the claims, evidence, and recommendations presented in the main text and appendices.

2 Materials and Methods

2.1 Study Design

The FEHLS project was established as a cross-national research collaboration among Denmark, Norway, and Finland. The AI-driven decision-support solution for migraine interventions integrated the technical development of two coordinated machine learning pipelines to ensure the compatibility of their outputs, with a separate trustworthiness assessment. ML models were trained on patient data to predict the efficacy of amitriptyline, a treatment for headache disorders, using an FML strategy. The trained models take as input a set of patient-specific features extracted from the initial data and output a continuous score ranging from 0 to 1 that represents the risk of treatment failure within 3 months.

The technical teams (Aalborg University/RUGP in Denmark and NTNU/St. Olav's Hospital in Norway) developed the predictive models, while an independent assessment team (Arcada University of Applied Sciences and Tampere University) applied the Z-Inspection® methodology. The project's dual-track approach facilitated technical flexibility and ethical reflection in parallel.

By keeping patient records on-site in Denmark and Norway and sharing only parameters for the locally trained models, the project allowed teams to independently build the pipelines and train models, test them in their respective countries, without moving personal data across borders. Further, teams could collectively consolidate models and test each other's datasets to assess generalization performance and improve data representativeness in the final federated solution. The goal was to accomplish two things: 1) to test the viability of the federated setup in practice and 2) to verify trustworthiness in a prototype in a clinical cross-national sandbox environment.

The Danish data originated from general practice electronic patient records (EG Clinea and CGM XMO) assembled in the RUGP database. They included data from more than 64,000 patients with chronic conditions over roughly two decades. From this source, a neurology-referred subset of 5,971 patients was identified, and 106 individuals with a headache disorder diagnosis, an amitriptyline prescription, and at least 2 neurology visits formed the analytic cohort. Using Python scripts, diagnostic, medication, and sociodemographic variables were extracted into structured tables. ICPC-2 and SKS-D codes were approximately mapped to ICD-10 at the three-character level, and medications were coded using ATC, so that the core features after harmonization included age, sex, the 25 most frequent ICD-10 diagnoses, and the 24 most commonly prescribed ATC medications shared across the Danish and Norwegian cohorts.

The Norwegian dataset (NorHead) contained neurology outpatient documentation, combining unstructured notes from neurology departments and specialists with standard clinical variables. For the FEHLS use case, the modelling cohort comprised 454 patients (115 males (25.33%), 273 females (60.13%), and 66 (14.54%) with unknown sex) aged 16–90 years. Coded entries for demographic descriptors, diagnoses, medications, and procedures were extracted using Python scripts and stored to structured tables. ICPC-2, ATC, and SKS-D were mapped to ICD-10 for analysis, with the mappings treated as approximate where granularity differs between systems. In both countries, the datasets were in the respective national languages, Danish and Norwegian, and the metadata followed distinct national guidelines, which differed but shared specific medical codes; core features after processing included sex, age, high-frequency diagnoses, and regularly prescribed medications.

Data Processing. Both sites implemented a standardized pipeline to transform raw clinical data into harmonized modelling variables. At the Danish node, Python scripts using *regex* and *pandas* were applied to extract three classes of data from general-practice records: (1) sociodemographic variables (age, sex), (2) diagnostic codes (ICD-10, SKS-D, ICPC-2, and free-text matches), and (3) medication data (ATC-coded prescriptions or free-text pattern matches). At the Norwegian node, custom scripts similarly extracted coded entries for diagnoses, medications, and procedures from unstructured neurology notes. For both datasets, ICPC-2 and SKS-D codes were mapped approximately to ICD-10 at the three-character level to enable cross-country comparability, with recognition that some granularity was lost in the process. Following harmonization, the common feature set comprised age, sex, the 25 most frequent ICD-10 diagnoses, and the 24 most frequently prescribed ATC medications shared across the Danish and Norwegian cohorts.

To avoid data leakage, the target drug amitriptyline (ATC N06AA09) was excluded from the predictor feature set. The processed outputs were stored as structured tables of demographics, diagnoses, medications, procedures, and treatment variables, forming the aligned input space for federated training.

Model Development. Given the limited data sets, which may raise concerns about representativeness, and the presence of missing data, a gradient boosting classifier, a model predicting response to migraine treatment, was chosen [26, 27]. For both local datasets, the data was split 70:20:10 into training, testing sets, and validation, and hyperparameters were optimized using randomized cross-validation on the training folds.

Model performance was compared to a baseline (logistic regression) using average precision and confusion-matrix summaries. In the federated setup, only model updates, not raw patient records, were shared among sites. Testing was performed locally and independently, by both teams, on each other's models and the FL model.

Assessment Design. The assessment of the FEHLS federated learning system followed the Z-Inspection® methodology [21]. This process was applied in parallel with the technical developments to initiate a first ethical, socio-legal, and technical reflection on the trustworthiness of the federated AI tool.

Z-Inspection®. The methodology consists of three phases (Fig. 1). During the setup phase, the team verified the legal and ethical preconditions. It assembled an independent, multidisciplinary assessment group at Arcada University of Applied Sciences and Tampere University, distinct from the developers at Aalborg University and NORHead at NTNU/St Olav's Hospital. This twofold operation led to the decoupling of technical development from the independent evaluation and ensured the review was conducted without any conflicts of interest. In the *assessment phase*, co-design sessions with the Danish and Norwegian technical teams generated socio-technical scenarios capturing the context (e.g., technical implementation, data handling, and compliance aims), actors, and evaluation criteria. Structured analysis of the socio-technical scenarios, using the Claims-Arguments-Evidence (CAE) framework, identified developer claims and arguments that, in the absence of evidence, led to the identification of issues and tensions. A consensus process then mapped these observations to the seven AI HLEG requirements for Trustworthy AI using an "open-to-closed vocabulary" for governance measures and monitoring of emerging harms [28] (Audit Algorithms, 2020). This three-phase process decoupled ethical evaluation from model development and aligned the assessment with European governance instruments [16, 18, 29]. The specific sub-requirements applied in the mapping are described in [14].

The results section summarizes the assessment results in an integrated table that reports the issues and tensions identified, maps them to the selected HLEG requirement they affect, and suggests succinct, actionable mitigation actions. Together, these steps constitute a barrier assessment, in which identified risks are linked to preventive detectability, and mitigable controls with defined recommendations.

Assessment Extensions - Risk Mapping to the MIT AI Risk Repository. Identified issues were systematically mapped to the MIT AI Risk Repository to provide a consistent, auditable risk lens appropriate for the federated clinical setting [25]. The inputs

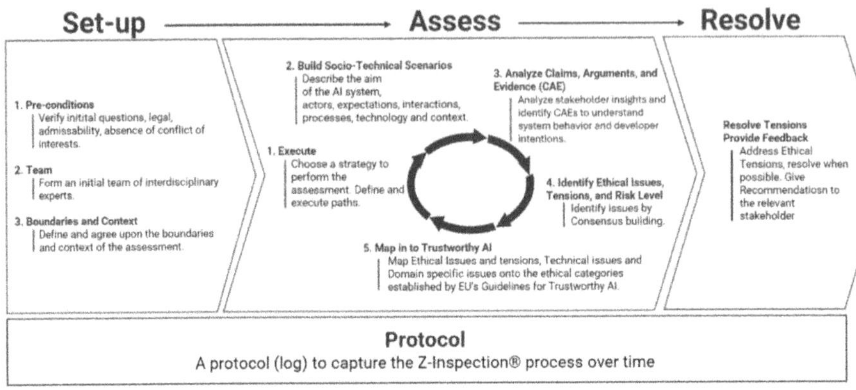

Fig. 1. Overview of the Z-Inspection® process. The process is divided into three phases: Set-Up, Assess, and Resolve – covering pre-condition verification, socio-technical scenario analysis, ethical mapping, and tension resolution to provide actionable recommendations for stakeholders. The Z-Inspection® process in a nutshell. Adapted after Zicari et al., 2021.

comprised the finalized issue and tension set derived from Claim-Argument-Evidence sessions and from the mapping to the EU AI HLEG requirements. For each issue, a one-sentence statement specified the risk mode, MIT AI Risk Repository locus, and clinical relevance. Independent assessors then selected primary risks from the repository that best characterized the plausible harm pathways. Disagreements were adjudicated by seeking consensus. The resulting table serves as the prespecified method for risk categorization used throughout the manuscript. This risk mapping, in combination with the issue–tension–resolution synthesis, operationalizes a barrier assessment by identifying missing barriers and proposing ways to reinforce them.

3 Results and Discussion

3.1 Technical Result Background

Technical teams in Denmark and Norway successfully developed federated learning pipelines using local datasets. The Gradient Boosting Tree model [30] from the python lightgbm library [26, 31] was utilized. This model consecutively generates a series of tree classifiers with each tree having a weighting relative to the error rate present when a given tree is generated. It is appropriate for a federated learning pipeline, because it can be further trained multiple times over different datasets and has demonstrated exemplary performance on predicting structured medical data [27, 32].

The model was jointly trained on the individual datasets and hyperparameters such as the learning rate, the number of trees, max tree depth, and minimum data per leaf hyperparameters have been optimized. Missing values are handled using the default implementation in lightgbm. Linear models with elastic net regularization (eta = 0.001) have been trained on the training datasets to act as a baseline metric of the predictive model.

The jointly trained model outperformed linear baselines in expected tests, and performance was assessed using area under the curve of the precision recall curve (average precision in Scikit-Learn). Other shown metrics include F1, ROC-AUC, precision, and accuracy.

Some crucial limitations still appeared to exist, such as a small use-case cohort, incomplete demographic fields (gender is missing in approximately 15% of records), and a need for more complete integration with Norwegian data to assess generalizability. These limitations require further investigation, which is beyond the scope of this study, as we emphasize the holistic results of the federated system's trustworthy assessment described below.

3.2 Priority Actions

To surface practical issues and tensions around trustworthiness, we used the Claims, Arguments, Evidence framework. The federated approach promises to maintain data privacy. However, several specific risks still exist with a federated architecture. By framing the CAE resulting issues, tensions, and suggested resolutions as part of a barrier assessment, we demonstrate how technical and ethical shortcomings translate into actionable barriers that need strengthening before the system can be considered trustworthy (Table S3).

Priority actions that were identified were to a) make explicit what "similarity-based" predictions mean in clinical terms, b) produce explanations clinicians can actually use in practice, c) design traceability versus audit mechanisms that only allow patient identification retrospectively when medically needed, and d) put in place a lightweight but formalized ethics/governance onboarding process that follows the system from development into clinical operation. A synthesis of the identified issues mapped to HLEG requirements, potential tensions, and proposed resolutions is presented in Table S4 in the Appendices. Each issue in the assessment report has a descriptive column, the technical implication, and the recommended ethical/organizational action (Table S4), with a more detailed issue-level overview provided in Appendix Table S5.

3.3 Identified Core Assessment Issues

Below, we describe selected issues identified during the assessment (see also Table 1). These are highlighted to emphasize their general nature in the federated machine learning (FML) system design.

Technology Readiness Level (TRL) Discrepancy and Uneven Readiness Across Sites. An initial difference in TRL aim was identified between the Danish and the Norwegian cases. This distinction influenced each partner's technical capacity to deliver

Table 1. Summary of key issues identified in the Z-Inspection® assessment, with primary HLEG requirements and MIT AI Risk Repository domains. Full details are provided in Tables 4 and 5 (Appendices).

Issue	HLEG Requirement	MIT Risk Domain	Key Resolution
TRL discrepancy across sites	Reliability, Traceability	5.1 Overreliance, 6.5 Governance failure	TRL-aware staged gates with shared minimum controls
Cohort bias and missing demographics	Fairness, Human Agency	1.1 Discrimination, 1.3 Unequal performance	Fairness constraints, document cohort bias, exclude incomplete records
SHAP plots unsuitable for clinical use	Explainability, Communication	5.1 Overreliance, 7.4 Lack of interpretability	Dual-layer XAI, clinician micro-training, user testing
Transparency and audit trails not defined	Traceability, Privacy	6.5 Governance failure, 7.4 Lack of transparency	Privacy-preserving model cards and audit logs
No adversarial or edge-case testing	Accuracy, Reliability	2.2 Security vulnerabilities, 7.3 Lack of robustness	Add edge-case test sets, present results to stakeholders

a framed evaluation (e.g., DK focused on demonstration outputs, whereas NO remained at formative evaluation). Technically, the mismatch makes direct benchmarking and federated aggregation difficult because nodes have distinct model maturity, data pipelines, and testing regimes. Governance-wise, this was raised and discussed with partners during the self-assessment to align the technical partners on project aims.

Bias and Cohort Composition (Fairness). The result analysis identified demographic bias (overrepresentation of female patients), missing data (missing sex), and the type of cohort as the main factors contributing to algorithmic bias. From an ML perspective, class imbalance and missing values reduce statistical power and increase uncertainty in predictions for the subgroup. Clinically, this could lead to incorrect generalizations about underrepresented patients. We advocate for explicit fairness testing (subgroup metrics), pre-processing techniques such as re-weighting or calibration, and model cards documenting cohort limitations so that clinicians know the extent of applicability bounds (see Table S4 in Appendices for specific mitigations).

Explainability and Clinical Usability of Explanations. Although SHAP and probability scores were generated for the NorHead/NTNU solution, clinicians could find it challenging to understand their interpretability [33]. This is a usability issue rather than an issue of algorithm accuracy; an explanation can be technically valid yet clinically inadequate. This should be treated as a translator problem, suggesting an explainable artificial intelligence (XAI) workflow (summary for the clinician and detail for the expert) with user testing and training to balance trust and avoid over-reliance.

Transparency, Traceability, and Auditability vs. Privacy. The assessment concluded that the transparency techniques (logs, model cards) were not sufficiently specified. Traceability in federated settings is a trade-off; more extensive logs facilitate audits but heighten the exposure risk. The assessment suggests using privacy-preserving designs, such as pseudonymized IDs, minimal audit fields, strict role-based access, and short, documented retention periods, as a balanced solution.

Interoperability and Engineering constraints in a Federated Architecture. In this study, an FML system was built using Python and different electronic health record (EHR) descriptions (ICPC/SKS $\rightarrow$ ICD-10). Heterogeneous EHR representations and APIs introduced friction into federated processes by increasing preprocessing load, potentially limiting the scalability of the FML system. We recommend implementing a common data dictionary, keeping the shared variable set small, and connecting separate sites with a lightweight technical integration layer. Our other findings from the ICPC-2/SKS-D and ICD-10 descriptions, along with related alignment choices, support this observation and the suggested alignment.

EHR Data Quality and "Garbage-In" Risks. Algorithms trained on EHR data can reproduce recording errors and human errors from the source records. This suggests that continuous monitoring, such as clinician review of (physical) outliers before their removal, and transparency about what the model can and cannot correct in noisy or corrupted EHR data, should be discussed during the development phase of the FML system.

Robustness, Edge-Case Testing, and Validation Scope. The assessment identified limitations in hostile-attack testing, rare-event testing, and robustness. The undetected insertion of malicious data or systematic erroneous data into local datasets may have severe consequences for the resulting FML model. These issues may indicate blind spots in the implementation, potentially enabling malicious actions that will be hard to detect at an aggregated level later. A phased cross-site validation plan, including synthetic edge cases, latency stress tests, and possible local pilot projects, can provide tools to address these issues. These considerations should also be taken into account when justifying the developer's opinions on the TRL of the FML system and when evaluating a system's TRL progression. In a federated system design process, these challenges become pronounced and demand specific attention.

Absence of Legal Experts and Limits of Ethical Review. Clinical/medical leads covered ethics in our project. Legal expertise was not part of the assessment team. Thus, e.g., GDPR questions were technical (identifying roles, reasoning & purposes, cross-border, DPIA content). Adherence to the EU AI sandbox provisions for research was considered a basis for the project (including considerations for the perceived risk class, documentation, human oversight obligations, post-market surveillance, and incident reporting). The implementation of traceability/audit logs did not account for proportionality, and storage limitations and access rights were deemed out of scope for the sandbox verification. The issues of the research-to-clinical boundary (intended use, triggers of conformity assessment) and of secondary data use/purpose limitations were not considered.

Comparative Benchmarking and Reproducibility. The assessment found that the algorithm choice in the study (gradient boosting) lacked a full comparative justification.

This demonstrates why model choice matters (transparency vs. predictive performance), and these reasons recommend using multi-criteria decision analysis (MCDA) or systematic benchmarking to select a suitable algorithm that meets FML standards. If the environment in use has some code-sharing restrictions, auditor access based on trusted relationships can provide a pragmatic path to reproducibility of FML system results.

3.4 Overall Interpretation

The path to developing trusted federated machine learning in healthcare is both challenging and promising. The study shows that technical advances and ethical reflection must be developed hand in hand. The federated design enabled cross-border privacy-preserving training, but constraints on cohort size, data completeness, and model interpretability show that innovation is not everything. Trustworthiness requires continuous integration of technical robustness, interpretability, and fairness. The Z-Inspection® process provides a structured means to operationalize these requirements and to connect technical progress with ethical accountability.

Interpretation of Technical and Ethical Findings. Federated pipelines were set up in both Denmark and Norway, spanning structured general-practice data and unstructured neurology notes. Gradient-boosting models outperformed linear baselines, indicating that predicting migraine treatment response is feasible [27, 32].

At the same time, missing sex information and a strongly female-skewed cohort limit generalizability and raise fairness concerns. Some other crucial limitations appeared to exist, such as a small use-case cohort, incomplete demographic fields (gender is missing in approximately 15% of records), and a need for more complete integration with Norwegian data to assess generalizability. These limitations require further investigation, which was beyond the scope of this study.

The Z-Inspection® assessment flagged the same points as potential sources of bias. And while SHAP plots and probability-readouts count as technical "interpretability," clinicians struggle to use them in practice. In effect, the technical limitations and the ethical issues line up; they are two angles on the same underlying problem.

Interpreting Key Issues Through the MIT AI Risk Repository. To place our findings in a broader AI-risk context, we compared the issues identified in Table S4 with those in the MIT AI Risk Repository. This living database aggregates more than 1600 AI-related risks drawn from 64 taxonomies as of 27th October 2025 and was designed to help both newcomers and experts see how existing frameworks overlap and where gaps remain [25, 34]. By cataloguing risks, the repository encourages organizations to address vulnerabilities proactively and shows that most frameworks cover only a fraction of the risk landscape [34]. Our comparison highlights four domains that are particularly relevant to the Norwegian and Danish pilots. First, the systems' low technology readiness levels (TRL 3 and ~4) relate to the *AI system safety, failures & limitations* domain, limited validation, and immature infrastructure, which increase the likelihood of unexpected behavior and therefore demand cautious deployment. Second, *model choice and explainability* intersect the *human–computer interaction* and *discrimination & toxicity* domains. The Danish team used a logistic regression baseline, which offers greater transparency but still requires bias mitigation and careful calibration. The Norwegian team used only a gradient boosting model, which poses additional interpretability challenges and may require post-hoc explanation methods to understand predictions in relation to the data. Third, our findings on *transparency* and *privacy & security*, insufficient documentation, unclear contestability mechanisms, and potential data-protection issues align with repository risks such as unequal performance across groups. Finally, questions about governance and organizational readiness hint at socio-economic implications. Integrating such predictive tools into clinical workflows could influence resource allocation and trust in healthcare institutions, even if those impacts are not yet visible at this early stage.

Notably, *misinformation* and *malicious misuse* domains do not feature prominently in our analysis because the pilots are not yet widely deployed or exposed to adversarial actors. However, the repository's emphasis on these domains serves as a reminder that responsible scaling must anticipate them. Overall, framing our discussion through the MIT taxonomy underscores where current efforts meet international best practice and where blind spots persist. Seen through this lens, the MIT mapping functions as a barrier assessment, transforming abstract risks into preventive, detective, and mitigative barriers that guide the co-creation process.

Comparison with Other Federated Healthcare AI studies. The results are consistent with those observed in other federated learning-based health care projects. Radiology groups have trained imaging models across hospitals without needing to share raw scans [35, 36], and genomics teams have employed federated setups to find markers across wide, distributed cohorts [37, 38]. These cases demonstrate that federation is possible in a clinical situation and further delivers actual clinical value. They also reverberate with the same points of friction as is observed here, interoperability frictions, questions of fairness, and explainability gaps recur across domains, not only in migraine care [2, 39, 40]. As [41] discussed, EHR-based models may encode the inconsistencies and cognitive errors found in the records. In line with this, it is shown here that the performance of models is limited to how well and consistently clinical documentation is captured [41].

3.5 Study Strengths and Challenges

An obvious strength is the hands-on proof of the concept that federated machine learning can work in a Nordic setting, within the technical constraints of GDPR, and with respect for national data sovereignty. It was demonstrated that international collaborations can take place even in sensitive areas such as migraine care.

Several constraints remain. The use-case cohort was small, and essential demographics were incomplete; matching structured fields to free-text notes was challenging. Variance in technology-readiness between the Danish demonstration and the Norwegian proof-of-concept indicates that governance should be harmonized and that sites should share milestones. Inadequacy of available legal and philosophical expertise to contribute to the assessment constrained the ethical and social examination that could be done. National guidelines for treatment and medical innovations are developed with new research. That calls for regular retraining of the system to keep the recommendations up to date.

3.6 Role of Z-Inspection® as a Complement to Regulatory Frameworks

The assessment made one point clear, federated learning, as well as its variants, is not a hack to fairness, transparency, or accountability. Z-Inspection® played a role in bringing these gaps to the surface and proactively transforming them to practical solutions-monitoring for social impacts, privacy-preserving audit logs [28]. These actions are complementary to the EU AI Act, which builds reflection and oversight into daily development, not just at the end. As a combined effort, the two-track process of technical work with focused ethical review can move systems from mere compliance to earned trust [8]. Similar approaches to operationalizing ethics in practice have also been proposed outside healthcare [17].

3.7 Future Work

Several steps are needed for the future. The broader participation of legal scholars, ethicists, and patient representatives will help to refine the analysis and ensure that it remains inclusive. Security and traceability of federated infrastructures may be enhanced by the consideration of emerging technologies such as distributed ledgers (blockchain), wherever suitable [42, 43].

As international cooperations progress, diverse and multidisciplinary teams drive not only technical advancement but also more adaptive and transparent governance [44, 45]. As a space where innovation and patient-centered care overlap, the true value of federated learning will depend on how this capability develops alongside integrity. As treatment processes can be complicated, it is essential to keep in mind that a data-driven AI is a tool to support decision-making, but the clinician needs to consider the variables that vary within the patients, such as comorbidities, sex, age, and family planning [46].

The Z-Inspection® assessment produces a structured set of issues, tensions, and resolutions as its primary output. Each resolution (Table S4) specifies concrete actions that the development teams can implement to address the identified concerns. In FEHLS, this assessment was performed post-hoc on a TRL 3–4 prototype, and a formalized mechanism for tracking the implementation of resolutions was not part of the project scope. However, ongoing parallel work is developing dedicated follow-up tooling that enables iterative monitoring and reassessment of identified issues across the AI system lifecycle.

4 Conclusions

The FEHLS project shows that privacy-preserving federated learning for cross-border headache research is technically feasible but constrained by small, heterogeneous datasets and explicability limits identified in the independent Z-Inspection® assessment. Together, the pipeline evaluation and trustworthy AI review indicate that federated models alone cannot resolve biases or opacity; progress in model performance must be coupled with governance that explicitly addresses safety, fairness, and transparency in clinical use.

By mapping issues to both the EU HLEG Trustworthy AI requirements and the MIT AI Risk Repository, co-creation teams can systematically prioritize risk domains such as

AI system safety, discrimination, human–computer interaction, and privacy and security, and target them with concrete controls. In this setting, federated headache AI becomes not just a technical choice but an ethical one: integrating robust validation, risk-aware design, and patient and expert feedback is essential if federated AI innovations are to improve care without eroding trust in clinical practice.

Given the findings presented across the technical evaluation and the Z-Inspection® assessment, the limitations highlighted in this study should be understood as properties of an early-stage TRL 3–4 research prototype operating under defined project constraints, rather than an indication of insufficient technical work. The Z-Inspection® assessment was performed post-hoc on the project outcomes and does not cover the deployment phase. Detailed pseudocode and code for the federated pipeline are outside the scope of this governance-focused paper and will be reported in a dedicated technical publication. Similarly, iterative follow-up procedures for monitoring and resolving identified issues over time are being developed in parallel work and were not part of the FEHLS project design.

Acknowledgments. This work was conducted within the FEHLS project, funded by the Nordic Ministerial Council for Digitalization through Nordic Innovation (Case No. 407-7003-P22027). Norwegian clinical data were approved by REK (application no. 696721). The Danish component used data approved by the Danish Health Authorities (ref. 2021-043721) under the Danish Health Act §46, with no research ethics committee approval required. The authors thank the clinical and technical teams at Aalborg University, NTNU/St. Olav's Hospital, Arcada University of Applied Sciences, and Tampere University. AI-assisted tools were used for language editing of this manuscript.

Disclosure of Interests. The authors have no competing interests to declare that are relevant to the content of this article.

References

1. Konečný, J., McMahan, H.B., Yu, F.X., et al.: Federated learning: strategies for improving communication efficiency (2016). https://doi.org/10.48550/ARXIV.1610.05492
2. Rahman, A., Hossain, Md.S., Muhammad, G., et al.: Federated learning-based AI approaches in smart healthcare: concepts, taxonomies, challenges and open issues. Clust. Comput. **26**, 2271–2311 (2023). https://doi.org/10.1007/s10586-022-03658-4
3. Tariq, A., Serhani, M.A., Sallabi, F.M., et al.: Trustworthy federated learning: a comprehensive review, architecture, key challenges, and future research prospects. IEEE Open J. Commun. Soc. **5**, 4920–4998 (2024). https://doi.org/10.1109/OJCOMS.2024.3438264
4. Steiner, T.J., Jensen, R., Uluduz, D., et al.: Migraine remains second among the world's causes of disability, and first among young women: findings from GBD2019. J. Headache Pain **21**, 137 (2020). https://doi.org/10.1186/s10194-020-01208-0
5. Stovner, L.J., Nichols, E., Steiner, T.J., et al.: Global, regional, and national burden of migraine and tension-type headache, 1990–2016: a systematic analysis for the global burden of disease study 2016. Lancet Neurol. **17**, 954–976 (2018). https://doi.org/10.1016/S1474-4422(18)30322-3
6. Eigenbrodt, A.K., Ashina, H., Khan, S., et al.: Diagnosis and management of migraine in ten steps. Nat. Rev. Neurol. **17**, 501–514 (2021). https://doi.org/10.1038/s41582-021-00509-5

7. Puledda, F., Sacco, S., Diener, H.-C., et al.: International Headache Society global practice recommendations for the acute pharmacological treatment of migraine. Cephalalgia **44**, 03331024241252666 (2024). https://doi.org/10.1177/03331024241252666
8. Bærøe, K., Miyata-Sturm, A., Henden, E.: How to achieve trustworthy artificial intelligence for health. Bull. World Health Organ. **98**, 257–262 (2020). https://doi.org/10.2471/BLT.19.237289
9. Guidotti, R., Monreale, A., Ruggieri, S., et al.: A survey of methods for explaining black box models. ACM Comput. Surv. **51**, 1–42 (2019). https://doi.org/10.1145/3236009
10. Li, B., Qi, P., Liu, B., et al.: Trustworthy AI: from principles to practices. ACM Comput. Surv. **55**, 1–46 (2023). https://doi.org/10.1145/3555803
11. Zhao, J., Bagchi, S., Avestimehr, S., et al.: The federation strikes back: a survey of federated learning privacy attacks, defenses, applications, and policy landscape. ACM Comput. Surv. **57**, 1–37 (2025). https://doi.org/10.1145/3724113
12. Albahri, A.S., Duhaim, A.M., Fadhel, M.A., et al.: A systematic review of trustworthy and explainable artificial intelligence in healthcare: assessment of quality, bias risk, and data fusion. Inf. Fusion. **96**, 156–191 (2023). https://doi.org/10.1016/j.inffus.2023.03.008
13. Schlicker, N., Baum, K., Uhde, A., et al.: How do we assess the trustworthiness of AI? Introducing the trustworthiness assessment model (TrAM). Comput. Hum. Behav. **170**, 108671 (2025). https://doi.org/10.1016/j.chb.2025.108671
14. European Commission: Ethics guidelines for trustworthy AI. Publications Office of the European Union (2019)
15. European Commission. Directorate General for Communications Networks, Content and Technology.: The Assessment List for Trustworthy Artificial Intelligence (ALTAI) for self assessment. Publications Office, LU (2020)
16. European Commission: Shaping Europe's digital future: AI Act. European Commission (2024)
17. Charton, J.E., Lucas, S., Vogd, W., et al.: Operationalising digital ethics: establishment of an ethics evaluation tool for data analytics. AI Soc. (2025). https://doi.org/10.1007/s00146-025-02621-2
18. Radclyffe, C., Ribeiro, M., Wortham, R.H.: The assessment list for trustworthy artificial intelligence: a review and recommendations. Front. Artif. Intell. **6**, 1020592 (2023). https://doi.org/10.3389/frai.2023.1020592
19. Düdder, B., Möslein, F., Stürtz, N., et al.: Ethical maintenance of artificial intelligence systems. In: Pagani, M. and Champion, R. (eds.) Artificial Intelligence for Sustainable Value Creation. Edward Elgar Publishing (2021). https://doi.org/10.4337/9781839104398.00018
20. Stahl, B.C., Antoniou, J., Bhalla, N., et al.: A systematic review of artificial intelligence impact assessments. Artif. Intell. Rev. **56**, 12799–12831 (2023). https://doi.org/10.1007/s10462-023-10420-8
21. Zicari, R.V., Brodersen, J., Brusseau, J., et al.: Z-Inspection®: a process to assess trustworthy AI. IEEE Trans. Technol. Soc. **2**, 83–97 (2021). https://doi.org/10.1109/TTS.2021.3066209
22. IEEE guide for framework for trustworthy federated machine learning (2024). https://doi.org/10.1109/IEEESTD.2024.10807155
23. Vetter, D., Amann, J., Bruneault, F., et al.: Lessons learned from assessing trustworthy AI in practice. Digit. Soc. **2**, 35 (2023). https://doi.org/10.1007/s44206-023-00063-1
24. Zicari, R.V., Amann, J., Bruneault, F., et al.: How to assess trustworthy AI in practice. Digit. Soc. **2**, 35 (2023). https://arxiv.org/abs/2206.09887
25. Slattery, P., Saeri, A.K., Grundy, E.A.C., et al.: The AI risk repository: a comprehensive meta-review, database, and taxonomy of risks from artificial intelligence (2024). https://doi.org/10.48550/ARXIV.2408.12622
26. Pedregosa, F., Varoquaux, G., Gramfort, A., et al.: Scikit-learn: machine learning in Python. J. Mach. Learn. Res. **12** (2011)

27. Vesteghem, C., Szejniuk, W.M., Brøndum, R.F., et al.: Dynamic risk prediction of 30-day mortality in patients with advanced lung cancer: comparing five machine learning approaches. JCO Clin. Cancer Inform. e2200054 (2022). https://doi.org/10.1200/CCI.22.00054
28. Supreme Audit Institutions of Finland, Germany, the Netherlands, Norway and the UK: auditing machine learning algorithms. A white paper for public auditors (2023)
29. Ala-Pietilä, P., Bonnet, Y., Bergmann, U., et al.: Assessment list for trustworthy artificial intelligence (ALTAI) for self-assessment. Shaping Europe's digital future (2020)
30. Friedman, J.H.: Greedy function approximation: a gradient boosting machine. Ann. Stat. **29** (2001). https://doi.org/10.1214/aos/1013203451
31. Ke, G., Meng, Q., Finley, T., et al.: LightGBM: a highly efficient gradient boosting decision tree. In: Proceedings of the 31st International Conference on Neural Information Processing Systems, pp. 3149–3157. Curran Associates Inc., Red Hook (2017)
32. Shwartz-Ziv, R., Armon, A.: Tabular data: deep learning is not all you need. Inf. Fusion. **81**, 84–90 (2022). https://doi.org/10.1016/j.inffus.2021.11.011
33. Markus, A.F., Kors, J.A., Rijnbeek, P.R.: The role of explainability in creating trustworthy artificial intelligence for health care: a comprehensive survey of the terminology, design choices, and evaluation strategies. J. Biomed. Inform. **113**, 103655 (2021). https://doi.org/10.1016/j.jbi.2020.103655
34. MIT Initiative: MIT Researchers Create an AI Risk Repository. https://ide.mit.edu/insights/mit-researchers-create-an-open-ai-risk-repository/. Accessed 23 Sep 2025
35. Linardos, A., Kushibar, K., Walsh, S., et al.: Federated learning for multi-center imaging diagnostics: a simulation study in cardiovascular disease. Sci. Rep. **12**, 3551 (2022). https://doi.org/10.1038/s41598-022-07186-4
36. Ng, D., Lan, X., Yao, M.M.-S., et al.: Federated learning: a collaborative effort to achieve better medical imaging models for individual sites that have small labelled datasets. Quant. Imaging Med. Surg. **11**, 852–857 (2021). https://doi.org/10.21037/qims-20-595
37. Montalvo, N., Requena, F., Capriotti, E., et al.: Federated learning for the pathogenicity annotation of genetic variants in multi-site clinical settings. Bioinformatics **41**, btaf523 (2025). https://doi.org/10.1093/bioinformatics/btaf523
38. Raimondi, D., Chizari, H., Verplaetse, N., et al.: Genome interpretation in a federated learning context allows the multi-center exome-based risk prediction of Crohn's disease patients. Sci. Rep. **13**, 19449 (2023). https://doi.org/10.1038/s41598-023-46887-2
39. Ducange, P., Marcelloni, F., Renda, A., et al.: Federated Learning of XAI models in healthcare: a case study on Parkinson's Disease. Cogn. Comput. **16**, 3051–3076 (2024). https://doi.org/10.1007/s12559-024-10332-x
40. Zhang, Y., Zeng, D., Luo, J., et al.: A survey of trustworthy federated learning: issues, solutions, and challenges. ACM Trans. Intell. Syst. Technol. **15**, 1–47 (2024). https://doi.org/10.1145/3678181
41. Alzubaidi, L., Al-Sabaawi, A., Bai, J., et al.: Towards risk-free trustworthy artificial intelligence: significance and requirements. Int. J. Intell. Syst. **2023**, 4459198 (2023). https://doi.org/10.1155/2023/4459198
42. Chen, C., Liu, J., Tan, H., et al.: Trustworthy federated learning: privacy, security, and beyond. Knowl. Inf. Syst. **67**, 2321–2356 (2025). https://doi.org/10.1007/s10115-024-02285-2
43. Guo, J., Pietzuch, P., Paverd, A., et al.: Trustworthy AI using confidential federated learning: federated learning and confidential computing are not competing technologies. Queue. **22**, 87–107 (2024). https://doi.org/10.1145/3665220
44. Fehr, J., Citro, B., Malpani, R., et al.: A trustworthy AI reality-check: the lack of transparency of artificial intelligence products in healthcare. Front. Digit. Health. **6**, 1267290 (2024). https://doi.org/10.3389/fdgth.2024.1267290

45. Moreno-Sánchez, P.A., Del Ser, J., Van Gils, M., et al.: A design framework for operationalizing trustworthy artificial intelligence in healthcare: requirements, tradeoffs and challenges for its clinical adoption. Inf. Fusion. **127**, 103812 (2025). https://doi.org/10.1016/j.inffus.2025.103812
46. Silberstein, S.D.: Preventive migraine treatment. Continuum **21**, 973–989 (2015). https://doi.org/10.1212/CON.0000000000000199

Pre-treatment Chemotherapy Resistance Prediction in Endometrial Cancer: A Machine Learning Approach

Salma Niny[1(✉)], Chaïmaâ Kissi[1], Pradeep Reddy Challa[2], and Mohamed Nabil Srifi[1]

[1] Advanced Systems Engineering Laboratory, National School of Applied Sciences, Ibn Tofail University, Kenitra, Morocco
{salma.niny,chaimaa.kissi,srifimn}@uit.ac.ma
[2] School of Engineering and Technology, CGC University, Mohali, Punjab, India
pradeep@cgcuniversity.in

Abstract. Chemotherapy resistance reduces treatment success in endometrial cancer and limits patient survival. Many predictive models depend on genomic or imaging data that are expensive and difficult to use in everyday care. This work introduces a machine learning framework that predicts chemotherapy resistance using only data collected before treatment. Two feature sets were evaluated. The first used four core variables: age, tumor stage, grade, and site of resection or biopsy. The second added race, and ethnicity.

This study used data from the TCGA-UCEC cohort and applied Random Forest, XGBoost, logistic regression, and support vector machines. Disease progression was used as the target outcome to reflect resistance more accurately than treatment response. Models were tested with stratified validation and cross-dataset evaluation on CPTAC-UCEC cohort.

The best models achieved an accuracy of 0.98, precision of 0.98, recall of 1.00, and F1-score of 0.998. Results showed that the four-feature model performed nearly the same as the six-feature model, supporting the value of simple inputs. SHAP analysis explained the influence of each variable on model output. An interactive decision-support module allows clinicians to input patient data and receive real-time risk estimates.

This approach helps clinicians/pathologists/oncologists predict resistance early, improve treatment planning, and avoid unnecessary toxicity. The framework provides a clear, interpretable path toward personalized chemotherapy selection using routine clinical datas.

Furthermore, a proof-of-concept study based on an extension analysis of transcriptomic data (RNA-seq) derived from TCGA-UCEC was performed to assess if the addition of only using molecular biomarkers could increase the prediction of resistance. Even with careful feature selection and rigorous cross validation, the RNA-based models had poor and unstable performance given the high dimensionality, class imbalance, as well as limited sample size. These observations underline that in realistic data situation simple and interpretable clinical models might well offer more robust and deployable predictions as high-dimensional molecular strategies.

M. Säreströniemi et al. (Eds.): NCDHWS 2026, CCIS 3010, pp. 379–399, 2026.
https://doi.org/10.1007/978-3-032-28819-6_24

Keywords: Endometrial cancer · chemotherapy resistance · machine learning · deep learning · clinical decision support · precision oncology

1 Introduction

In developed nations, endometrial cancer is the most prevalent gynaecologic cancer. Due to obesity and ageing populations, its incidence is still increasing [1]. Chemotherapy is still a crucial component of treatment for many women, particularly those with advanced or recurrent disease. However, a sizable percentage of patients do not improve with these treatments. Disease progression, increased relapse rates, and decreased overall survival are all consequences of chemotherapy resistance. Oncologists could customise treatment and steer clear of ineffective medications by anticipating resistance before treatment starts [2].

Present clinical methods lack dependable instruments for early detection of resistant cases. Physicians that focus on cancer employ broad clinical markers, such as disease stage, tumor grade, and histological characteristics, to choose therapies. These elements give restricted forecast precision. Molecular diagnostics and imaging markers have demonstrated potential, yet they remain expensive and frequently unattainable in standard practice. Consequently, numerous therapy choices still hinge on personal interpretation, leading to inconsistency in patient results [3].

Computational techniques like machine learning and deep learning present new ways for enhancing therapy prediction. They analyse complex connections within medical, genetic, or radiographic information that conventional analytical techniques commonly ignore. ML algorithms identify nonlinear trends in basic measures, whereas DL frameworks derive abstract attributes from multidimensional data like MRI scans or tissue slides [4]. Both strategies have yielded promising findings in forecasting treatment effectiveness across various malignancies. However, Most of the models in use today work, as opaque systems giving little insight into how they make predictions. This deficiency in clarity hinders confidence and utilization in medical environments.

Despite advances in oncology-focused AI, several key gaps remain. Many studies depend on high-dimensional genomic or radiomic inputs that require costly resources and specialized infrastructure. Some models rely only on clinical information collected before treatment, which is the most common and useful data available when a diagnosis is made [5]. In addition, most previous work defines the prediction target as treatment response recorded after therapy. This definition is confounded by treatment heterogeneity, physician bias, and incomplete follow-up [6]. Another limitation is that feature minimality, the smallest set of clinical variables needed for reliable prediction, has rarely been evaluated. Finally, few systems provide explainability or interactive functionality that clinicians can use directly [7].

These limitations motivate the need for a simpler and more interpretable approach. Using only pre-treatment clinical features would make predictive models faster, transparent, and easier to integrate into standard oncology workflows. We propose that a minimal subset of clinical data can predict chemotherapy resistance with accuracy comparable to larger feature sets. To make this prediction clinically meaningful, resistance is redefined as disease progression during or after chemotherapy, which better reflects biological nonresponse.

This work presents a machine learning framework that uses pre-treatment clinical data to predict chemotherapy resistance in endometrial cancer. A limited set containing four crucial variables and an expanded set of six variables with extra pathologic information are the two feature configurations that are contrasted. The framework offers an interactive decision-support interface that calculates each patient's risk and integrates model explainability using SHAP-based feature importance. The TCGA-UCEC dataset is used to assess model performance [8], and CPTAC-UCEC is used for external validation [9].

This study focused on three core questions. First, how well can pre-treatment clinical data be used to predict chemotherapy resistance in endometrial cancer? Second, does expanding the number of clinical variables lead to a significant improvement in predictive performance or clinical usefulness? Third, how can clinical workflows incorporate interpretable machine learning models to help oncologists make customized treatment decisions? The answers aim to guide future data-efficient and transparent AI tools in gynecologic oncology.

The rest of this paper is organized as follows. Section 2 covers materials and methods, including dataset selection and preprocessing, feature importance analysis, model development, and an interactive prediction system. Section 3 presents experimental results with model performance comparisons, visual interpretations, and external cross-validation with an independent dataset, highlighting the discussion on clinical interpretability, limitations, and practical implications. Section 4 concludes the study and suggests recommendations for future research and clinical integration.

2 Materials and Methods/Study Scenario

In this study we designed this study to build an interpretable machine learning framework that predicts chemotherapy resistance in endometrial cancer using only information available before treatment. Our goal was to see how well simple, interpretable models perform compared with deep learning approaches when we limit the input to basic clinical variables.

We worked with two feature sets. The first one used only four core clinical features. The second included six variables to test whether adding more data improved results in a meaningful way. Our workflow included data extraction, cleaning, model training, validation, and interpretation. Figure 1 summarizes how we structured the entire process from data selection to interpretation.

2.1 Data Source and Study Population

We based our study on the TCGA-UCEC (The Cancer Genome Atlas Uterine Corpus Endometrial Carcinoma) dataset, one of the most comprehensive and publicly accessible resources for endometrial cancer research. The clinical data represented spans several institutions and contains clinical, demographic, pathological and treatment information for patients with endometrial carcinoma. It serves as a curated and normalized starting point for model building and validation in cancer outcome prediction. The table that was utilized is the clinical data table found on the GDC data portal.

Our analysis focused solely on individuals undergoing chemotherapy. We retained records with full pre-treatment details: age, tumor grade, FIGO stage, histology type, lymphovascular invasion status. Commonly gathered in most clinics before therapy starts.

Dropped cases with incomplete outcomes or vague follow-up data. Ensuring only subjects with clear chemo response or disease progression remained. Post filtering, our cohort displayed diverse tumor stages and histologic varieties.

No external data blending or adjustments. Every preprocessing step—filtering, cleaning—occurred inside the TCGA dataset. For reproducibility. The refined collection enabled testing machine learning models' ability to forecast chemo resistance. Using just baseline diagnostic info. A streamlined approach.

2.2 Data Preprocessing

TCGA-UCEC was downloaded from Genomic Data Commons (GDC) portal as five files with following extensions: clinical.tsv, exposure.tsv, family_history.tsv, follow_up.tsv and pathology_detail.tsv which had clinical and pathology informations collected from patients with endometrial cancer.

Among these files, clinical.tsv had patient-level demographics and diagnostic informations (age, stage etc.), follow_up.tsv had outcome informations such as disease progression and recurrence information. pathology_detail.tsv had tumor-level information (pathological grade, histological subtype, lymphovascular invasion etc.). Follow_up.tsv and pathology_detail.tsv were merged with clinical.tsv files using caseID. All three files had caseID common to each patient. After merging the three files, duplicates were observed and checked. Since all three files had the information from before any treatment, only one row per patient was sufficient. So only unique patientIDs were taken into account.

The merged dataset was filtered to select only patients that received chemotherapy. Patients with unclear follow-up details were excluded from the dataset after removing NaN values from necessary pre-treatment variables like stage and grade. This would be our target variable whether the patient was chemotherapy resistant or not.

2.3 Feature Selection and Importance Analysis

Feature importance analysis was performed to identify which pre-treatment clinical variables contributed most to predicting chemotherapy resistance. After merging and cleaning the dataset, an XGBoost-based approach was used to rank the variables according to their predictive power.

The merged dataset contained 71,034 entries and 492 columns before filtering. After selecting only the relevant patients who had a clear chemotherapy outcome, 5,579 samples remained, including 4,721 chemotherapy-sensitive cases and 858 resistant cases. This distribution reflects the clinical imbalance observed in real patient cohorts, where complete response is more common than progression.

The analysis considered eight candidate clinical features that were commonly available in the TCGA-UCEC records. Only six of these variables were present in the merged dataset and used for the importance ranking. These included age at diagnosis, FIGO stage, tumor grade, site of resection or biopsy, race, and ethnicity.

Each categorical feature was label-encoded, and numerical variables were standardized. An XGBoost classifier was trained using 300 estimators, a maximum depth of four, and a learning rate of 0.05. The model was evaluated using log loss as the performance metric.

The top six most important features identified by the XGBoost model are shown in Table 1:

Table 1. Top Six Most Important Pre-Treatment Clinical Features.

Rank	Feature	Importance Score
1	diagnoses.tumor_grade	0.2712
2	diagnoses.figo_stage	0.2530
3	diagnoses.site_of_resection_or_biopsy	0.2185
4	diagnoses.age_at_diagnosis	0.1763
5	demographic.race	0.0487
6	demographic.ethnicity	0.0324

These results indicate that tumor grade, FIGO stage, and site of resection or biopsy were the strongest predictors of chemotherapy resistance, followed by age at diagnosis, race, and ethnicity.

This six-feature subset was used in all subsequent modeling steps, representing the most informative pre-treatment clinical variables available in the dataset. The outcome confirmed that interpretable models can rely on a few of routinely collected clinical features while maintaining predictive strength.

The six clinical variables identified as most informative are summarized in Table 2, along with their TCGA references and inclusion in each model configuration.

Table 2. Selected pre-treatment clinical features used in the machine learning models.

Feature Name	TCGA Column Reference	Description	Included in Model
Age at Diagnosis	diagnoses.age_at_diagnosis	Patient age in years at the time of diagnosis, converted from days	4F/6F
Tumor Grade	diagnoses.tumor_grade	Histologic grade of the tumor (G1–G3, High Grade)	4F/6F

(*continued*)

Table 2. (*continued*)

Feature Name	TCGA Column Reference	Description	Included in Model
FIGO Stage	diagnoses.figo_stage	Clinical tumor stage based on FIGO classification	4F/6F
Site of Resection or Biopsy	diagnoses.site_of_resection_or_biopsy	Anatomical site of the biopsy or tumor resection	4F/6F
Race	demographic.race	Self-reported race of the patient	6F only
Ethnicity	demographic.ethnicity	Self-reported ethnicity (Hispanic or Latino, Not Hispanic or Latino)	6F only

2.4 Model Development and Training Protocol

Two supervised classification models were developed to predict chemotherapy resistance in patients with endometrial cancer. The first model used six pre-treatment features identified through XGBoost feature importance ranking, while the second used four top-ranked features determined from the same importance analysis. The goal was to compare how feature reduction affected model performance and interpretability.

The workflow was implemented in Python 3.10 using the pandas, scikit-learn, and xgboost libraries. The analysis was executed locally on a workstation equipped with a 12th Gen Intel Core i7-1270P (2.20 GHz) processor, 16 GB RAM, and a 64-bit Windows operating system. There is no GPU acceleration that was used, and all the simulations has been completed within a few minutes, which confirms the computational efficiency of the framework.

Due to the dataset containing labeled outcomes, specifically Complete Response and Progressive Disease, which clearly distinguished chemotherapy-sensitive and resistant patients, supervised learning was selected for this study. These defined targets allowed models to learn direct mappings between pre-treatment clinical features and known outcomes. Unsupervised methods were not appropriate in this context because of their focus on clustering or pattern discovery without predefined labels [10]. The availability of explicit clinical outcomes made supervised classification the most suitable approach for this predictive task [11].

Four algorithms were compared to determine the most effective predictor: Random Forest Classifier, XGBoost Classifier, Logistic Regression, Support Vector Machine (SVM).

Data were divided into 80% training and 20% testing subsets using stratified sampling to maintain balanced class proportions. For SVM and Logistic Regression models, data were standardized using StandardScaler to ensure numerical stability and faster convergence.

Each model was trained on the training subset and then evaluated on the testing subset using four standard performance metrics:

- Accuracy to measure overall correctness
- Precision to assess the reliability of positive predictions
- Recall to evaluate the ability to identify resistant cases
- F1-score as a balance between precision and recall

After evaluation, the model with the highest predictive performance was selected to serve as the basis for the interactive prediction component developed later in the study. The same selection process was applied to both the six-feature and four-feature configurations, ensuring that each interactive module relied on the most reliable supervised algorithm identified during testing.

2.5 Study Scenario: Interactive Clinical Prediction System

The second phase of this study has focused on creating a simple and practical interactive system to replicate how the predictive model might be used in a real clinical setting. The system acted as a model for combining machine learning predictions with the decision-making processes that oncologists use when treating endometrial cancer.

An interactive console was created after the best-performing supervised model for each configuration (four-feature and six-feature models) was determined. This console allowed for the real-time input of patient data and generated instantaneous predictions regarding chemotherapy resistance. The design focused a lot on making things easy to use and clear, with straightforward inputs, quick results, and easy-to-understand information for clinicians.

Each patient case was entered using the same clinical variables that had been used during model training. For the six-feature configuration, the system required tumor grade, FIGO stage, site of resection or biopsy, age, race, and ethnicity. For the four-feature model, only tumor stage, tumor grade, site of resection or biopsy, and age were needed. These variables represented information that is routinely available at diagnosis, making the system directly applicable in a real clinical context.

Based on the actual values found in the TCGA-UCEC dataset, the system presented a list of options for each categorical variable to make the interaction easier for users. For instance, users could choose from options like Stage IA, Stage IB, Stage II, Stage IIIC1, or Stage IVB when entering the tumour stage. Likewise, G1, G2, G3, and High Grade were the options that could be used to specify the tumour grade. This reduced the possibility of inaccurate or unreliable inputs and guaranteed that each input complied with legitimate data categories used during training.

After all the inputs had been selected, the system automatically encoded the categorical choices, combined them with the numerical features, and used the trained model to make a prediction. The output included both a binary classification (Resistant or Not Resistant) and a probability score that showed how likely it was that the person would be immune to chemotherapy.

To make sure the comparison was fair, the same patient profiles were put into both models. This made it possible to directly test whether adding two more features to the six-feature configuration changed the outcome or the probability level of the prediction. Since both models used the same patient data, any differences in the results could only be due to the feature set and not to changes in the data.

After testing them internally, both models were ready for external cross-validation with a dataset that was not linked to either model. The goal of this phase was to see if they could generalise beyond the TCGA-UCEC data and to make sure they could still predict resistance in new patients. If the outcomes were the same across all datasets, it would make a stronger case for clinical integration.

In general, this interactive system showed how a trained machine learning model could be turned into a simple, clear, and easy-to-use tool for doctors. By guiding users through structured input options based on real data, it connected the dots between creating models and making decisions in real life about how to treat endometrial cancer.

2.6 RNA-seq–Based Biomarker Analysis: A Feasibility Study

a) **Introduction**

Since treatment failure is frequently caused by underlying molecular mechanisms that are not captured by traditional clinical assessment, accurately predicting chemotherapy response and resistance remains a crucial challenge in oncology. To enhance response prediction and treatment stratification across various cancer types, a variety of quantitative biomarkers derived from medical imaging, radiomics, and multi-omics data have been studied in recent years.

In breast cancer, imaging-based biomarkers have been thoroughly investigated, especially in the context of neoadjuvant chemotherapy. By capturing tumour perfusion, cellularity, and diffusion characteristics, multiparametric MRI has been demonstrated to offer predictive value. In locally advanced breast cancer, Lu et al. [12] showed that combining diffusion-weighted imaging with DCE-MRI features could predict the pathological response to neoadjuvant chemotherapy. However, because of scanner variability, imaging protocols, and cohort-specific feature selection, these methods may have limited generalisability and rely on indirect imaging surrogates of tumour biology. Moreover, the molecular mechanisms underlying chemoresistance are not directly reflected in imaging features.

Similarly, Jahani et al. [13] reported better treatment response prediction after investigating early changes in tumour heterogeneity derived from longitudinal DCE-MRI registration. Although this work emphasises the significance of temporal heterogeneity, the extracted features are still phenotypic rather than mechanistic, and its reliance on serial imaging restricts its applicability in standard clinical workflows. Beyond imaging, efforts have been made to incorporate molecular information through multi-omics integration.

Ran et al. [14] proposed an artificial intelligence framework that integrates genomic, transcriptomic, and other omics data for precision stratification and drug resistance prediction in breast cancer. While this approach acknowledges the molecular basis of resistance, it requires large, well-annotated multi-omics datasets that are not always available in clinical practice, and its focus is not specific to chemotherapy resistance mechanisms in endometrial cancer.

Quantitative diffusion-based imaging biomarkers have also been explored in other tumor types. Zhao et al. [13] reported that apparent diffusion coefficient (ADC) values derived from diffusion-weighted MRI were predictive of response to neoadjuvant chemoradiotherapy in locally advanced rectal cancer. However, ADC values are influenced by multiple physiological factors and provide limited insight into the gene-level regulatory processes that drive resistance.

Histopathological features derived from pre-treatment biopsies have likewise been investigated for response prediction. While these features provide direct cellular-level information, they are inherently limited by sampling bias and fail to capture intratumoral heterogeneity at the molecular scale, particularly in cancers with complex genomic landscapes such as endometrial cancer.

Collectively, existing studies demonstrate that imaging-based and radiomics-derived biomarkers can capture phenotypic manifestations of treatment response and tumor heterogeneity. However, their predictive performance is often inconsistent, their biological interpretability is limited, and most are not designed to directly identify the molecular mechanisms of chemotherapy resistance. In contrast, RNA sequencing (RNA-seq) offers a direct and comprehensive view of gene expression programs associated with drug response and resistance. Despite the growing clinical relevance of chemotherapy resistance in endometrial cancer, transcriptomic biomarkers remain underexplored in this context. This gap motivates the present work, which investigates, in a proof-of-concept setting, the feasibility of leveraging RNA-seq profiles for chemotherapy resistance prediction in endometrial cancer and for comparing the practical utility of molecular biomarkers with that of simple clinical variables.

In contrast to breast and colorectal cancers, the application of quantitative biomarkers and machine learning for chemotherapy response prediction in endometrial cancer remains comparatively underexplored, despite the growing incidence and clinical importance of this disease. Most existing studies focus either on prognostic modeling or on general molecular characterization, rather than on pre-treatment prediction of chemotherapy resistance. This lack of dedicated, clinically oriented predictive models motivates the present work and underlines the need for both simple, deployable clinical predictors and exploratory investigations into molecular biomarkers in this specific cancer type.

b) **RNA-seq Dataset and Preprocessing**

RNA sequencing (RNA-seq) gene expression data for uterine corpus endometrial carcinoma (UCEC) were obtained from The Cancer Genome Atlas (TCGA) project [15]. The dataset comprises genome-wide expression profiles measured for more than 20,000 genes per tumor sample. In order to construct a cohort suitable for supervised prediction of chemotherapy response, transcriptomic profiles were were integrated with clinical and follow-up records containing treatment outcome information from the TCGA dataset [8].

Only patients with both RNA-seq data and reliable chemotherapy response information were included. After matching and filtering, 67 patients made up the final group. This group included 56 cases that responded to chemotherapy and 11 cases that did not.

This significant class imbalance shows the natural distribution of outcomes in the data and makes the learning task even more challenging. The initial gene expression matrix had over 20,000 features, creating a situation with high dimensions and few samples. To maintain data quality and numerical stability, all gene expression values were changed to numeric format. Genes with only missing values in all samples were eliminated. For the remaining genes, missing values were filled in using the median expression value calculated from the patients.

Where necessary, a logarithmic transformation was performed to homogenize variance and decrease the impact on extreme expression values. Due to the extremely high dimensionality of the feature space with respect to the available number of samples, a multi-level reduction approach was followed. First, genes with low variance (near-zero) across patients were discarded as they contain little discriminatory information. Then a univariate feature selection procedure using ANOVA F-statistics was used to select only the best genes.In this proof-of-concept study, the number of selected genes was limited to a small subset (e.g., 200) to reduce the risk of overfitting and to improve model stability.

Importantly, all preprocessing, filtering, and feature selection operations were embedded within the cross-validation pipeline, ensuring that no information from the test folds was leaked into the training process. This design choice provides an unbiased estimation of generalization performance and is particularly critical in small-sample, high-dimensional transcriptomic prediction settings.

Given the limited cohort size, the extreme dimensionality of the transcriptomic data, and the strong class imbalance, this RNA-seq analysis is not intended to produce a clinically deployable molecular predictor. Instead, it should be interpreted as a proof-of-concept exploration of the feasibility of transcriptomic biomarkers in this setting.

c) **Models and Evaluation Protocol**

The same models of supervised learning, employed in the clinical-feature analysis, were tested to determine whether transcriptomic profiles offer valuable information for predicting chemotherapy resistance. This choice ensures a fair and consistent comparison of clinical and molecular predictors. XGBoost, Random Forest, Support Vector Machine (SVM), and Logistic Regression are four widely used classifiers that were examined. These models reflect complementary modeling philosophies and range from simple linear decision functions to more flexible, non-linear ensemble techniques.

One significant issue with this dataset is the stark disparity between chemotherapy-sensitive and chemotherapy-resistant cases. Rather than using synthetic oversampling techniques, which can introduce artificial patterns in very small cohorts, we adopted a cost-sensitive learning strategy. For Logistic Regression, SVM, and Random Forest, class imbalance was handled by assigning higher weights to the minority (resistant) class. The scale_pos_weight parameter for XGBoost was used to correct the imbalance; it was set based on the ratio of negative to positive samples. This approach encourages the models to pay more attention to resistant cases without altering the original data distribution.

All models were trained within a unified preprocessing and feature selection pipeline. This pipeline includes logarithmic transformation (when required), variance-based filtering, and univariate feature selection. Embedding these steps directly into the learning pipeline ensures that feature selection is performed using only the training data of each fold, thereby preventing information leakage and overly optimistic performance estimates.

The performance of the different classifiers evaluated on the RNA-seq dataset is summarized in Table 3, where results are reported as mean and standard deviation across repeated stratified cross-validation runs. Overall, the transcriptomic models exhibit modest and, in some cases, unstable predictive performance, which reflects the intrinsic difficulty of the problem in this small and highly imbalanced cohort.

Table 3. Performance of RNA-seq–based models.

Model	Accuracy	Precision	Recall	F1-score
XGBoost	0.812 ± 0.063	0.128 ± 0.304	0.078 ± 0.176	0.094 ± 0.211
Random Forest	0.835 ± 0.026	0.000 ± 0.000	0.000 ± 0.000	0.000 ± 0.000
SVM (linear)	0.783 ± 0.064	0.000 ± 0.000	0.000 ± 0.000	0.000 ± 0.000
Logistic Regression	0.629 ± 0.127	0.213 ± 0.195	0.442 ± 0.334	0.270 ± 0.204

Table 3 reports the standard classification metrics for the four evaluated models. At first glance, several methods achieve relatively high accuracy values. However, this metric is misleading in the present setting, as the dataset contains a large majority of chemotherapy-sensitive patients. A model that predicts almost all patients as sensitive can therefore achieve high accuracy while completely failing to identify resistant cases. This behavior is clearly observed for the Random Forest and SVM models, which reach high accuracy but exhibit zero recall and zero F1-score, indicating that they fail to detect resistant patients in most cross-validation splits.

Logistic Regression shows a different behavior. It achieves the highest recall and F1-score among all models, meaning that it is able to identify a larger fraction of resistant patients. However, this comes at the cost of low precision and high variability across folds, indicating that its predictions are unstable and often include many false positives. XGBoost achieves a more balanced behavior, with slightly better overall trade-offs between precision and recall, but its F1-score and recall remain low, showing that only a small proportion of resistant patients are correctly identified.

Figures 1 and 2 provide a complementary view of the behavior of the RNA-based model, showing both its classification errors and its overall ranking ability.

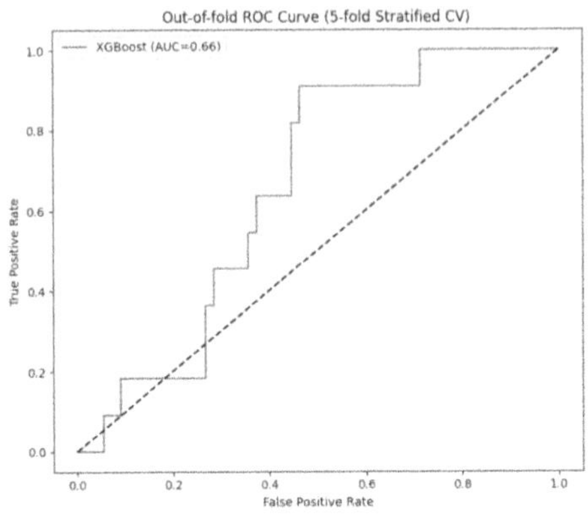

Fig. 1. ROC curves for four-feature XGBoost models.

Figure 1 shows the corresponding out-of-fold ROC curve. The curve lies only moderately above the diagonal, with an area under the curve of approximately 0.66. This indicates that the model has a limited ability to rank resistant patients ahead of sensitive ones, but that this ranking signal remains weak and insufficient for reliable clinical use. In practice, this means that while some information related to resistance may be present in the transcriptomic data, it is not strong or stable enough to support accurate decision-making in this cohort.

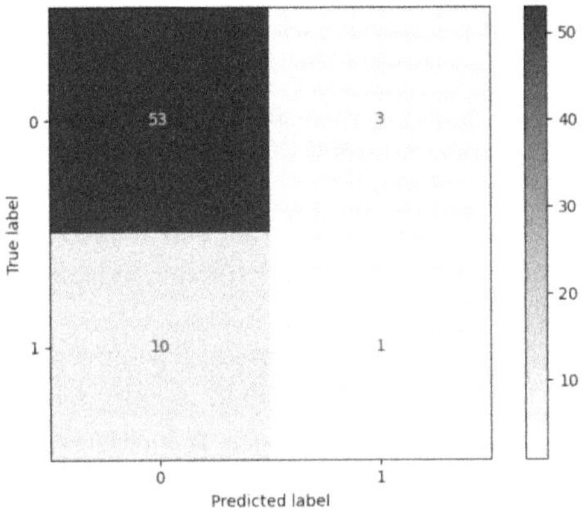

Fig. 2. Confusion matrix for four-feature XGBoost models.

To further illustrate the behavior of the RNA-based models, Fig. 2 presents the out-of-fold confusion matrix obtained with the best-performing model according to cross-validation ranking (XGBoost). This matrix shows that the model correctly classifies most sensitive patients, but misses the majority of resistant cases. In particular, only one resistant patient is correctly identified, while ten resistant patients are misclassified as sensitive. This confirms that the model is very biased toward the majority class and struggles to capture the molecular signal associated with resistance.

When combined, the findings in Table 1 and Figs. 1 and 2 demonstrate how severely limited RNA-seq-based prediction is in this situation. Strong class imbalance, small sample size, and extremely high dimensionality result in unstable models that either collapse to predicting only the majority class or yield highly variable results across splits. This demonstrates that transcriptomic biomarkers by themselves do not offer the same degree of robustness and reliability as the previously presented clinical-feature-based models in the current data regime.

3 Results and Discussion

The experimental evaluation aimed to assess how well supervised learning models could predict chemotherapy resistance in patients with endometrial cancer using only pre-treatment clinical data.

Two experimental configurations were tested: one using a minimal set of four clinical features and another using six features identified through prior feature importance analysis.

In this section, we present and discuss the performance results, visual analyses, and clinical implications of both models. The main goal is to find out if using fewer input features improves clarity or if it lowers the accuracy, which is very important for using the model in a real medical setting.

3.1 Model Performance Comparison

The assessment examined the impact of feature reduction on clinical interpretability and classification accuracy by comparing two predictive configurations. Only the four most predictive features were included in the second configuration, whereas six pre-treatment variables determined by feature importance ranking were used in the first. The same supervised algorithms and evaluation parameters already mentioned were used to test both.

The performance of the four algorithms on both feature sets is shown in Tables 4 and 5.

Overall, both models did well, obtaining high recall and accuracy in every assessment. While Logistic Regression and SVM performed mediocrely, XGBoost and Random Forest consistently generated the most accurate predictions.

Table 4. Performance of supervised models using four pre-treatment clinical features.

Model	Accuracy	Precision	Recall	F1-score	ROC-AUC
Random Forest	0.957	0.785	1.000	0.880	0.994
XGBoost	0.965	0.845	0.953	0.896	0.994
Logistic Regression	0.730	0.327	0.680	0.442	0.809
Support Vector Machine (SVM)	0.788	0.409	0.779	0.536	0.902

Table 4 summarizes the performance of the supervised models trained using only four pre-treatment clinical features: age, tumor grade, FIGO stage, and site of resection or biopsy. Among the evaluated algorithms, tree-based models clearly outperformed linear approaches. XGBoost achieves the best balance between sensitivity and precision (F1-score = 0.896), followed by Random Forest, which has perfect sensitivity (1.000). These results shows that all chemotherapy-resistant samples were detected. This is crucial in the real world because false negatives can lead to suboptimal treatment decisions. Logistic Regression and SVM performed poorly in terms of discrimination ability, as shown by their lower precision and F1-scores.

These results indicate that nonlinear models are more suited to capture the complex relationships between the clinical variables. Despite the feature selection, the feature combination of the four features demonstrated exceptional discriminative ability (ROC-AUC = 0.994), highlighting that only a few clinical variables are needed to provide outstanding predictive performance.

Table 5. Performance of supervised models using six pre-treatment clinical features.

Model	Accuracy	Precision	Recall	F1-score	ROC-AUC
Random Forest	0.969	0.809	1.000	0.894	0.998
XGBoost	0.982	0.920	0.945	0.933	0.998
Logistic Regression	0.743	0.305	0.745	0.433	0.862
Support Vector Machine (SVM)	0.839	0.444	0.900	0.595	0.912

Table 5 presents the performance of the same algorithms when two additional demographic variables—race and ethnicity—were incorporated into the model. Overall, performance metrics improved slightly for the best-performing models. XGBoost achieved the highest overall performance (F1-score = 0.933, ROC-AUC = 0.998), indicating a marginal gain in classification accuracy when additional features were included. Random Forest similarly maintained perfect recall while achieving higher precision compared to the four-feature configuration.

However, the performance gains associated with the six-feature model were modest. The recall of XGBoost decreased slightly compared to the four-feature model (0.945 vs. 0.953), and improvements in F1-score came at the cost of increased model complexity. Logistic Regression and SVM again showed only moderate performance, reinforcing the advantage of ensemble-based methods for this task. These findings suggest that while demographic variables may contribute incremental information, the core clinical features remain the dominant predictors of chemotherapy resistance.

3.2 Model Interpretation

We did visual analyses to better understand how the models worked and to confirm that their predictions were reliable. The receiver operating characteristic (ROC) curves in Figs. 3 and 4 show that both the four-feature and six-feature XGBoost models were almost perfect at telling the difference between chemotherapy-resistant and sensitive patients, with ROC-AUC values above 0.99. The curves were almost the same, which means that the minimal feature set kept most of the predictive signal.

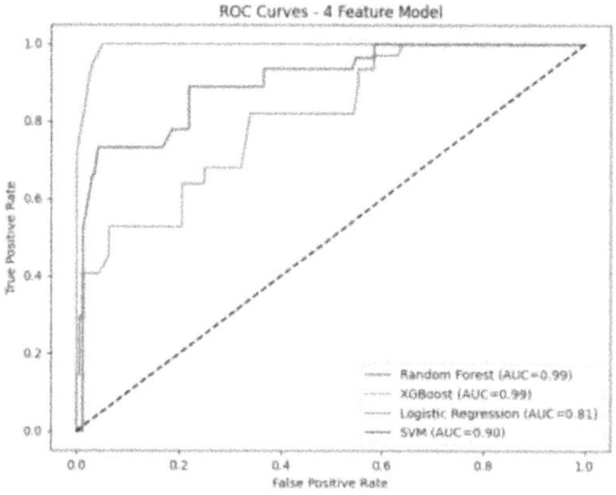

Fig. 3. ROC curves for four-feature XGBoost models.

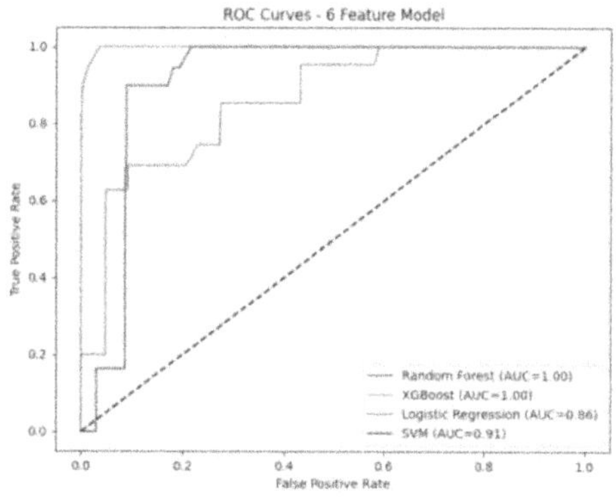

Fig. 4. ROC curves for six-feature XGBoost models.

Figure 5 illustrates the confusion matrix of the six-feature XGBoost model. The model correctly classified the majority of chemotherapy-sensitive patients (719 true negatives) and successfully identified most resistant cases (104 true positives). Only six resistant patients were misclassified as sensitive, resulting in a low false-negative rate and a high recall of 0.945. This is a critical property in a clinical context, as false negatives correspond to patients who may receive ineffective chemotherapy. Although a small number of false positives were observed (nine cases), this trade-off is clinically acceptable, as overestimating resistance is generally safer than failing to detect it. In general, the confusion matrix shows that the six-feature XGBoost model offers a good balance between sensitivity and specificity, which makes it appropriate for decision-support situations where reducing the number of resistant cases that are missed is crucial.

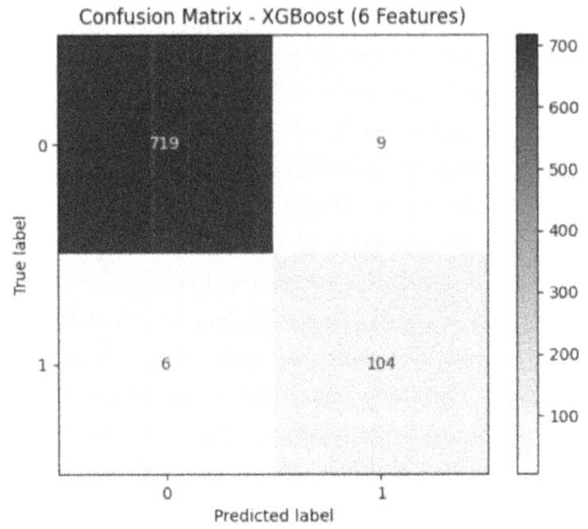

Fig. 5. Confusion matrix of the six-feature XGBoost model.

Tumour grade and stage were the most significant predictors, followed by biopsy site and age, according to feature importance analysis (Fig. 6). The conclusion that demographic variables add little predictive value beyond core clinical features is supported by the minor contributions of race and ethnicity.

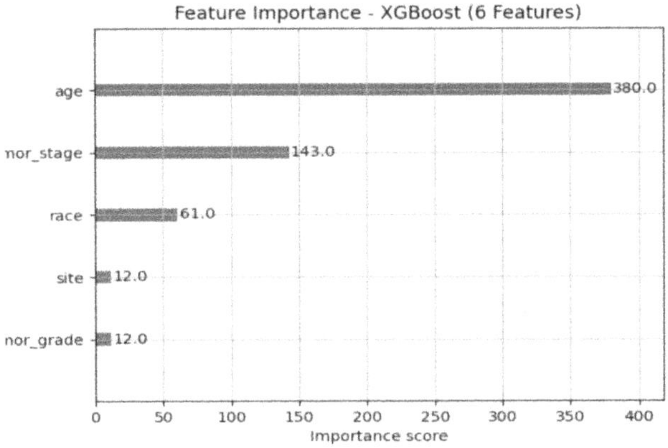

Fig. 6. Feature importance ranking for six-feature model.

3.3 Interactive Model Evaluation

An interactive prediction component was incorporated into the study to assess the usefulness of the developed models. This part functioned as a clinical decision support prototype as well as a validation tool. It gave users the ability to manually enter patient characteristics and get chemotherapy resistance predictions in real time.

The system was created to mimic a situation involving a clinical consultation. The user was prompted to enter pre-treatment characteristics, including age, tumour stage, tumour grade, and the location of the resection or biopsy. The system showed a list of acceptable choices for categorical variables that were taken straight from the dataset, such as G1 to High Grade for tumour grade and Stage IA to Stage IVB for FIGO stage.

After obtaining all of the responses, the system automatically encoded the variables, applied any necessary scaling, and generated a prediction. The output included a probability score that indicated the risk of chemotherapy resistance as well as a binary classification (Resistant or Sensitive). The predictions that were produced right after the final input verified that the model could operate in real time on a standard workstation without GPU acceleration.

To verify the system's validity, the same patient case was tested on both configurations: the four-feature and six-feature models. The goal was to observe if adding the two variables (race and ethnicity) influenced the prediction outcome. Nearly similar classifications were produced by both models, with only minor variation in probability values. This confirmed that the four-feature configuration maintained comparable performance while being simpler to use in a clinical environment.

An external dataset from the Clinical Proteomic Tumour Analysis Consortium (CPTAC-UCEC) was used to confirm the models' dependability and generalisability. This dataset is a good benchmark for independent testing because of its clinical and pathological records from patients with endometrial cancer. Two representative cases were chosen to assess model behaviour across disparate clinical profiles.

The first case had a low-risk profile with Stage IA and Grade 1 disease, which is clinically linked to a favorable response to treatment. Both models correctly identified the patient as sensitive, with resistance probabilities of 0.00% and 0.01%. This alignment with clinical expectations validated the model's ability to find beneficial treatment profiles and effectively generalize across datasets.

The second external validation case was chosen from the CPTAC-UCEC dataset. The patient was 74 years old at diagnosis, and had Grade 3 disease and FIGO Stage IVB. Both characteristics are associated with unfavorable chemotherapy response patterns. Given a 97.33% probability of resistance, the four-feature model classified this case as resistant using both interactive model inputs when including the patient's pretreatment characteristics. Using a resistance probability of 1.07%, the six-feature model predicted this case to be sensitive. This difference showed that instead of enhancing the precision of the model, the inclusion of demographic features such as race and ethnicity actually impaired it. The four-feature model were more in accordance with what was expected clinically since it only included features such as tumour stage, grade, site, and age. The results demonstrate that small and clinically-informed models can offer more accurate and interpretable predictions than their more feature-rich counterpartsespecially when tested on external patient data.

3.4 Discussion

The study results indicate that clinical machine learning needs to balance the trade-off between interpretability and model complexity. It is true that highly sophisticated algorithms and deep learning methods have the ability to model complex nonlinear relationships, but unfortunately, they are often less reliable and less transparent in medical applications [16]. On the other hand, our work demonstrates that even a very limited number of some traditional clinical variables can yield reliable predictions which can be easily understood by doctors.

The four features model in real life offers a very good middle ground between simplicity and good performance. The inputs needed are accessible at the time of diagnosis with minimal effort for preprocessing. Such models with little computational requirements can be integrated quickly in clinical environments including those with limited resources.

The consistency and applicability of the method were demonstrated through external testing with the CPTAC-UCEC dataset. The stable results of the four features model on different datasets suggest that a few basic clinical variables like tumor grade, stage, site, and age carry most of the essential information related to chemotherapy response. At the same time, the six features model that also incorporated race and ethnicity brought slight discrepancies without raising the accuracy thus, by adding unnecessary complexity, it became less stable and less interpretable, as pointed out by the results.

These findings highlight an important point: simply adding more variables does not always lead to a better predictive performance. In clinical settings where data are often heterogeneous or incomplete, it is usually more practical to have compact and transparent models rather than complex ones. Hence, the four features method is a good deal in terms of computational efficiency and clinical relevance for its early integration into clinical decision support systems.

We tried to see if molecular biomarkers could lead to better prediction performance and we did an additional proof-of-concept experiment with RNA-seq transcriptomic data of the same patients. We tried various ways to improve the performance of RNA based models through extensive feature selection, preprocessing, and cost-sensitive learning, yet the models showed poor and highly variable performance. The reason for such behavior was the very small number of samples, very high dimensionality, and severe imbalance of classes in the data. In some cases, the models just predicted the majority class and, in others, they showed high variability in the results of cross, validation runs. While this does not diminish the biological relevance of transcriptomic data, it highlights an important methodological reality: in small clinical cohorts, high-dimensional molecular data does not necessarily produce more reliable predictors than simple clinical variables.

This informative result strengthens the main conclusion of this work, suggesting that routinely available clinical variables currently offer a more robust and deployable basis for chemotherapy resistance prediction than genome-wide molecular profiles used alone. The RNA-seq experiment should therefore be interpreted as an exploratory extension illustrating both the potential and current limitations of molecular biomarkers.

Despite these encouraging findings, certain limitations must be acknowledged. The study relies on retrospective data from TCGA and CPTAC, which may not reflect global variations in clinical practice or patient populations. In addition, the binary definition of chemotherapy response simplifies real clinical outcomes. Future work should consider multi-class response modeling and the integration of treatment-specific or molecular features.

Integration evaluation in clinical software settings and real-world validation utilising institutional datasets should be included in future development [17]. The system's performance when integrated into oncologists' workflows, where time restrictions and data variability are more noticeable, might be evaluated through prospective studies [18]. A balanced approach that improves accuracy without sacrificing explainability could be achieved by combining interpretable machine learning with limited deep feature extraction.

4 Conclusion

Our proposed model with four features was not only simple, interpretable, and clinically actionable but also provided high predictive performance by focusing on commonly-available variables: grade, FIGO stage, biopsy_site, and age. The smaller model performed comparably or better than a larger six-feature counterpart that included demographic features such as colour and ethnicity, particularly when applied to an external dataset (CPTAC-UCEC) for validation. This finding highlights the value of smaller, curated sets of features to improve model interpretability and robustness, two important facets for clinical utility. We also demonstrated how intuitive AI could be integrated into cancer decision support workflows during the interactive prediction step by allowing users to input patient data and receive real-time, probability-based predictions.

In addition to clinical factors, we also carried out a proof-of-concept extension based on RNA-seq transcriptomic data, as we believe there may still be potential in using molecular biomarkers to predict chemotherapy resistance. However, even with significant preprocessing and feature selection efforts, we found that predictive performance of RNA-based models was fairly limited and unstable. We attribute this to compounding effects of small sample size, high dimensionality, severe class imbalance, as a notable lesson for the field, we did not find that high-dimensional molecular data was capable of outperforming simple, clinically-grounded predictors in realistic clinical data regimes when used as a standalone predictor.

In general, we have shown that lightweight, clinically-grounded supervised models can produce reliable, reproducible, and interpretable predictions that behave reasonably in real-world settings. Moving forward, we encourage prospective validation in heterogeneous patient populations, integration with clinical information systems, and exploration of hybrid methods that utilize robust clinical prediction with tightly-constrained molecular biomarkers or deep representations in to augment performance.

Acknowledgments. The authors acknowledge their university for providing the hardware and software resources to conduct the simulations presented in this work.

Disclosure of Interests. The authors have no competing interests to declare that are relevant to the content of this article.

References

1. Berek, J.S., et al.: FIGO staging of endometrial cancer: 2023. Int. J. Gynecol. Obstet. (2023)

2. Lloyd, K., Cree, I.A., Savage, R.S.: Prediction of resistance to chemotherapy in ovarian cancer: a systematic review. BMC Cancer **15**, 117 (2015). https://doi.org/10.1186/s12885-015-1101-8
3. Tiwari, A., Mishra, S.N., Kuo, T.-R.: Current AI technologies in cancer diagnostics and treatment. Mol. Cancer (2025). https://doi.org/10.1186/s12943-025-02369-9
4. Tran, K., et al.: Deep learning in cancer diagnosis, prognosis and treatment selection. Genome Med. **13**, 152 (2021). https://doi.org/10.1186/s13073-021-00968-x
5. Yeh, A.C., et al.: Radiogenomics of breast cancer using dynamic contrast-enhanced MRI and gene expression profiling. Cancer Imaging **19**, 48 (2019). https://doi.org/10.1186/s40644-019-0233-5
6. Chekroud, A.M., et al.: Illusory generalizability of clinical prediction models. Science **384**, eadg8538 (2024). https://doi.org/10.1126/science.adg8538
7. Sporsem, T., et al.: What does explainable AI mean in practice? Evaluative requirements from a longitudinal clinical case study (2025). arXiv. https://doi.org/10.48550/arxiv.2501.09592
8. The Cancer Genome Atlas Program: TCGA-UCEC: Uterine Corpus Endometrial Carcinoma. https://portal.gdc.cancer.gov/projects/TCGA-UCEC
9. Clinical Proteomic Tumor Analysis Consortium (CPTAC): CPTAC-UCEC dataset. https://www.linkedomics.org/data_download/CPTAC-UCEC/
10. Lopez, C., Tucker, S., Salameh, T., Tucker, C.: An unsupervised machine learning method for discovering patient clusters based on genetic signatures. J. Biomed. Inform. **85**, 30–39 (2018). https://doi.org/10.1016/j.jbi.2018.07.004
11. Calster, B., et al.: Performance evaluation of predictive AI models to support medical decisions: overview and guidance (2024). https://doi.org/10.48550/arxiv.2412.10288
12. Lu, N., Dong, J., Fang, X., et al.: Predicting pathologic response to neoadjuvant chemotherapy in patients with locally advanced breast cancer using multiparametric MRI. BMC Med. Imaging **21**, 155 (2021)
13. Zhao, M., Zhao, L., Yang, H., et al.: Apparent diffusion coefficient for the prediction of tumor response to neoadjuvant chemo-radiotherapy in locally advanced rectal cancer. Radiat. Oncol. **16**, 17 (2021)
14. Ran, D., Li, J., Zhao, M., Du, L., Zhang, Y., Zhu, J.: Artificial intelligence integrates multi-omics data for precision stratification and drug resistance prediction in breast cancer. Front. Oncol. **15**, 1612474 (2025)
15. UCSC Xena Browser: TCGA-UCEC HiSeqV2 gene expression dataset. https://xenabrowser.net/datapages/?dataset=TCGA.UCEC.sampleMap%2FHiSeqV2&host=https%3A%2F%2Ftcga.xenahubs.net&removeHub=https%3A%2F%2Fxena.treehouse.gi.ucsc.edu%3A443
16. Abdullah, T.A.A., Zahid, M.S.M., Ali, W.: A review of interpretable ml in healthcare: taxonomy, applications, challenges, and future directions. Symmetry. **13**(12), 2439 (2021). https://doi.org/10.3390/sym13122439
17. Manktelow, M., et al.: Clinical and operational insights from data-driven care pathway mapping: a systematic review. BMC Med. Inform. Decis. Mak. **22**, 93 (2022). https://doi.org/10.1186/s12911-022-01756-2
18. Santos, C.F.D., Amorim-Lopes, M.: Externally validated and clinically useful machine learning algorithms to support patient-related decision-making in oncology: a scoping review. BMC Med. Res. Methodol. (2025). https://doi.org/10.1186/s12874-025-02463-y

EEG-Based Mental Workload Classification Using Machine Learning in Software Engineering Tasks: A Methodological Approach

Sameera Gamage(✉), Pantea Keikhosrokiani, and Minna Isomursu

Empirical Software Engineering in Software, Systems and Services (M3S), University of Oulu, 90014 Oulu, Finland
{sameera.gamage,Pantea.Keikhosrokiani,Minna.Isomursu}@oulu.fi

Abstract. Mental workload affects the performance and well-being of software engineers, yet most existing assessment methods rely on self-reports and do not support continuous or objective monitoring. Electroencephalography (EEG) provides a direct measure of brain activity related to cognitive effort, but reliable workload classification requires careful signal processing and well-designed learning models.

This paper presents an EEG-based methodological framework for mental workload classification during software engineering tasks. We describe a complete and reproducible pipeline, including digital filtering, artifact reduction using Independent Component Analysis (ICA), and Power Spectral Density (PSD), which represents the distribution of signal power across EEG frequency bands. PSD representations are used to train both a deep learning model (ResNet-34) and a classical machine learning model (SVM). To improve classification reliability, a stacking-based meta-learning approach combines the outputs of the two models. Unlike prior EEG workload studies, this paper presents a fully reproducible pipeline grounded in software engineering tasks.

Experimental results show that EEG-based models can reliably distinguish between workload levels, while the meta-learning model reduces model-specific errors, particularly between neighboring workload classes. This work focuses on methodological foundations for EEG-based workload monitoring and does not make clinical claims.

Keywords: Mental workload · EEG-based workload estimation · Signal processing pipeline · Power spectral density · Meta-learning · Software engineering

1 Introduction

Software engineering tasks require sustained attention, problem solving, and context switching. These demands increase mental workload and can reduce

M. Säreströniemi et al. (Eds.): NCDHWS 2026, CCIS 3010, pp. 400–417, 2026.
https://doi.org/10.1007/978-3-032-28819-6_25

productivity, code quality, and well-being. Measuring mental workload can help to understand cognitive demands and support better work design.

Traditional methods such as questionnaires are subjective and can be biased. They also do not support continuous monitoring. EEG offers an objective signal source with high temporal resolution and has been used for workload estimation in many cognitive domains [1,2]. However, building a reliable EEG-based classification system requires (i) clear signal processing steps and (ii) models that can learn workload patterns robustly.

Software engineering tasks create a type of mental workload that is different from generic cognitive tasks often used in workload research [3]. Unlike controlled laboratory tasks such as N-back or simple memory tests, software engineering involves abstract reasoning, problem solving, and continuous decision making [4]. Developers frequently switch between understanding requirements, writing code, debugging errors, and evaluating solutions. These activities require maintaining complex mental models and handling uncertainty, which causes mental workload to change dynamically during the task rather than remain constant.

Many EEG-based mental workload studies focus on domains such as driving and aviation [5], where tasks are highly structured and environmental stimuli are clearly defined. In such domains, mental workload is often dominated by sustained attention, visual processing, and motor coordination. In contrast, software engineering workload is mainly driven by internal cognitive processes such as logical reasoning, memory retrieval, and problem solving. Because of these differences, workload patterns identified in driving or aviation tasks cannot be directly assumed to generalize to software engineering work.

This paper focuses on EEG signal processing and machine learning methods to classify the mental workload of software engineers. We present a full pipeline from raw EEG to workload classification and show how deep learning and classical learning can be combined. Our key contribution is not only the model accuracy but also the reproducible steps from filtering and artifact handling to PSD generation and training. We also add a simple stacking-based meta-learning step to reduce misclassifications between neighboring workload levels, which is a common challenge in EEG-based mental workload estimation due to overlapping cognitive states [1,2,6].

In this research, mental workload is analyzed using EEG data collected during realistic software engineering tasks rather than abstract cognitive benchmarks. The dataset reflects workload variations that arise from real development activities, such as code comprehension, problem solving, and task switching [3]. By grounding EEG analysis in a software engineering context, this work aims to improve the relevance and ecological validity of mental workload classification for knowledge-intensive work environments.

Despite many studies on EEG-based workload estimation, there is still a lack of clear and reproducible methodological guidance, especially for software engineering tasks. Existing work often reports final accuracy without clearly describing the full signal processing and learning pipeline, which limits reproducibility and practical adoption [7,21–23]. To address this gap, this study focuses on a method-driven investigation of EEG-based mental workload classification. Unlike many existing studies that focus on single models and lack detailed pipeline descriptions, this work presents a unified and reproducible framework.

This study makes three main contributions. First, we provide a complete end-to-end EEG processing pipeline, including filtering, artifact removal, and PSD-based representation. Second, we combine a deep learning model (ResNet-34) with a feature-based SVM to use both learned and manually extracted features. Third, we introduce a stacking-based meta-learning approach that improves classification performance, especially when workload levels overlap.

1.1 Research Question

How can EEG signal processing and machine learning be used to reliably estimate mental workload during software engineering tasks?

1.2 Contributions

The main contributions of this paper are described in more detail as follows. First, we provide a detailed implementation of an end-to-end EEG-based workload classification pipeline, including filtering, ICA-based artifact reduction, and PSD estimation. Second, we demonstrate how PSD representations can be used to train a deep learning workload classifier based on ResNet-34. Third, we implement an SVM-based classifier using both EEG-derived numerical features and task-related behavioral features, including task performance accuracy and completion time, to provide a complementary workload estimation approach. Fourth, we introduce a simple stacking-based meta-learning approach that combines deep learning and classical machine learning models to improve classification reliability. Finally, we provide a gap-driven related work analysis that highlights current limitations in EEG-based workload estimation for software engineering tasks.

2 Related Work

Mental workload is usually measured using self-reports and task performance metrics [2]. Self-report tools are easy to use and cheap, but they are subjective. People may overestimate or underestimate their workload, and their answers can change based on mood, stress, or how they remember the task. Task performance measures (such as accuracy and time) are also useful, but they do not always reflect the real cognitive effort. For example, a highly skilled person can perform well even under high workload, and a beginner can perform poorly even under moderate workload. Because of these issues, many studies use physiological signals to measure workload in a more objective way [1].

Among physiological signals, EEG is widely used for workload estimation because it captures brain activity directly and has high time resolution [1]. Many studies report that changes in theta, alpha, and beta activity are linked with attention and cognitive effort. Still, EEG signals are very sensitive to noise.

Eye blinks, muscle movements, electrode shifts, and environmental interference can easily distort the signal. Because of this, careful preprocessing and artifact handling are needed before workload classification [7,21].

To classify workload from EEG, machine learning is commonly used. Classical methods such as Support Vector Machines (SVM) are popular because they can work well with high-dimensional data and smaller datasets [6,8]. More recent studies use deep learning to learn complex patterns directly from EEG representations, reducing the need for manual feature engineering [9]. Transfer learning is also used when datasets are limited, because pre-trained models can provide strong feature extraction and reduce training time [12].

In software engineering contexts, only a limited number of studies have examined mental workload using EEG during realistic programming tasks. Existing work has shown that combining EEG with other physiological measures can capture changes in cognitive state during software development activities, indicating that EEG features reflect variations in mental effort during real programming tasks [3]. Studies on cognitive load detection using EEG have also demonstrated that time–frequency representations of EEG signals can effectively identify different cognitive load levels [10]. More recent studies have investigated EEG-based cognitive workload detection using machine learning techniques on benchmark workload datasets, demonstrating that EEG features are effective for workload classification [11]. However, compared to generic cognitive experiments, EEG-based workload studies that focus specifically on software engineering tasks remain relatively limited.

Even with these advances, there are still important gaps. First, many papers focus mainly on final accuracy and do not explain the complete EEG processing steps clearly (such as filtering, ICA, PSD computation, and segmentation). This makes it hard to reproduce the results and compare methods fairly [7,21]. Second, EEG workload studies are often tested in aviation, driving, or general cognitive experiments, and fewer studies focus on software engineering tasks, even though software work is a clear example of high cognitive demand. Third, single-model systems can be unstable because workload classes may overlap in EEG patterns, especially between neighboring levels. In many studies, model disagreement is not handled well, and meta-learning style combination is still limited in this context. Finally, PSD is a well-established representation in EEG analysis. However, in many studies, the process of converting PSD features into learning-ready inputs is not always clearly described, which can affect transparency and reproducibility.

In this paper, we address these gaps by presenting a clear EEG signal processing pipeline, using PSD-based deep learning together with an SVM baseline, and introducing a meta-learning step to improve classification reliability.

3 Methodology

3.1 Research Method

To answer the research question, this study follows the Design Science Research (DSR) methodology, which is suitable for developing and evaluating technical artifacts that address identified research problems [14,15]. DSR methodology enables structured artifact development through iterative cycles of relevance, rigor, and evaluation. Figure 1 outlines the six DSRM stages used in this research.

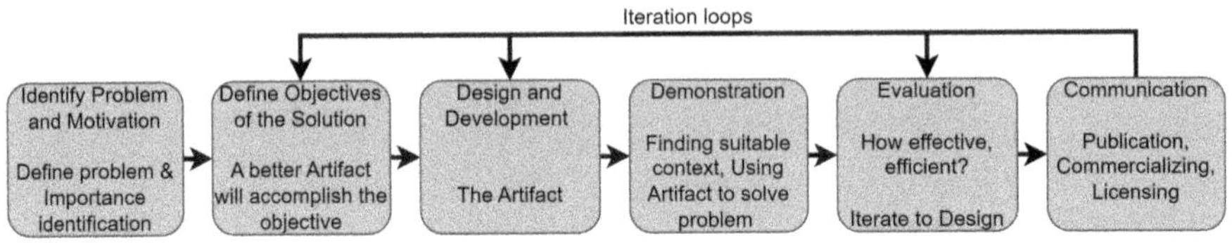

Fig. 1. Design Science Research Steps.

In this work, the designed artifact is an EEG-based mental workload classification pipeline, consisting of signal preprocessing, feature representation, machine learning models, and a meta-learning integration step. The artifact is evaluated through experimental analysis using real EEG data collected during software engineering tasks. Figure 2 shows the overall DSR iterations for the development of the artifacts.

3.2 EEG Data Acquisition

EEG signals were collected using a wearable EEG headset while participants performed cognitively demanding software engineering tasks. The headset records multi-channel brain activity with a sampling frequency of $f_s = 256$ Hz. Data were saved as CSV files for preprocessing. The dataset consists of EEG recordings collected from multiple participants performing software-related tasks, with mental workload labeled into discrete levels to support supervised learning. The participants were graduate-level students and early-career researchers in computer science with prior experience in software development. Participants were recruited through university mailing lists and voluntary participation. The inclusion criteria considered normal or corrected-to-normal vision and no known neurological disorders that could affect EEG recordings. All participants provided informed consent prior to participation.

EEG data used in this study were continuously collected during software-related task execution in a controlled experimental setting. EEG was recorded from 12 participants using an Emotiv headset with 14 EEG channels at a sampling rate of 256 Hz. The continuous EEG signals were segmented into non-overlapping 8 s windows. Each EEG segment represents a short time window (8 s) of brain activity, while the assigned workload label reflects the overall perceived workload of the corresponding task. This allows task-level self-reported workload to be used for supervised learning at the window level. For each window, power spectral density (PSD) features were computed separately for all 14 channels and converted into labeled PSD images. Mental workload labels were obtained using NASA-TLX self-reports [19], collected immediately after each software

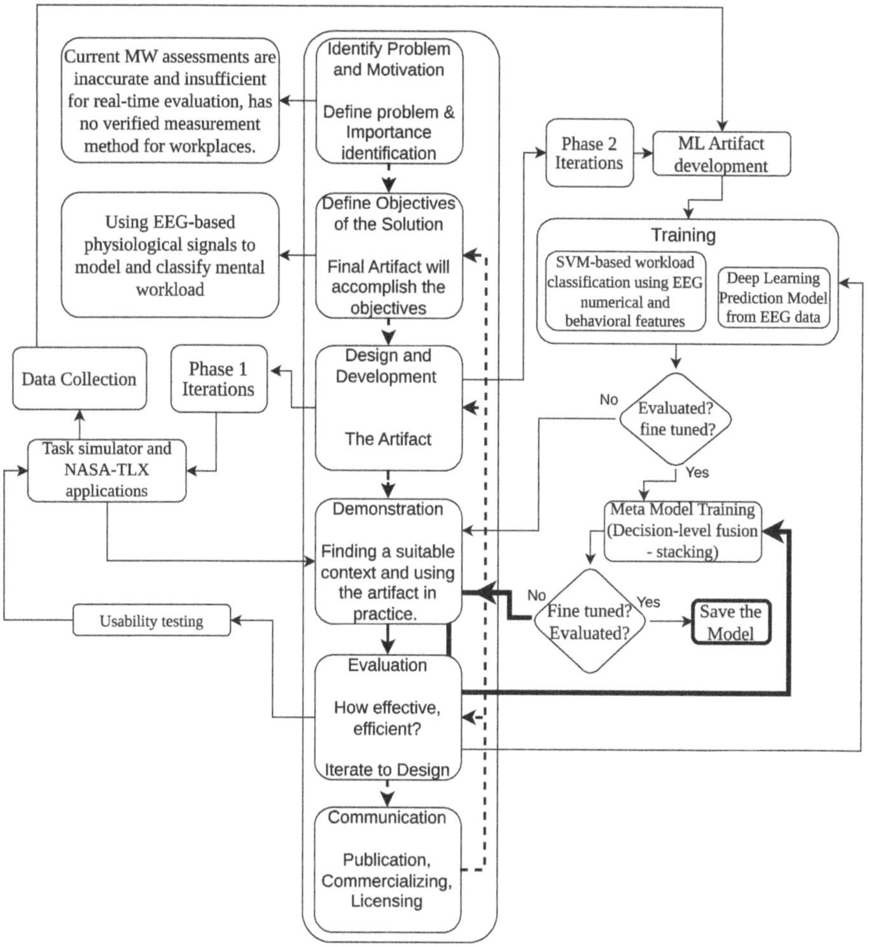

Fig. 2. Overall DSR steps for artifact development.

engineering sub-task. A single workload value was calculated by averaging the six NASA-TLX dimensions. The scores were normalized across participants and divided into six ordered workload levels (L1–L6), where L1 represents the lowest workload and L6 represents the highest workload. Equal-width binning was used to preserve gradual changes in workload across tasks.

During data collection, self-reported workload values were recorded along with timestamps. EEG signals and task-related behavioral data, including task performance accuracy and task completion time, were also recorded with corresponding timestamps. Using timestamp alignment, each NASA-TLX score was mapped to the EEG segments, PSD images, and behavioral features belonging to the same sub-task interval. Since NASA-TLX scores were collected at the sub-task level, the same workload label was assigned to all EEG segments and PSD images within that interval. This assumes that mental workload remains relatively stable during each sub-task. For deep learning, PSD values were converted into fixed-size 2D images (224×224), where frequency information is represented spatially, and color intensity reflects spectral power. In addition, numerical feature vectors were constructed by extracting average power values from four frequency bands (delta, theta, alpha, and beta) for each channel, resulting in 56 features per EEG segment (14 channels $\times$ 4 bands). After preprocessing, artifact removal, and labeling, a total of 1,368 PSD images were generated for model training and evaluation.

Six workload levels were used to preserve fine-grained variations during model training. For meta-learning evaluation, these levels were grouped into three categories: low (L1–L2), medium (L3–L4), and high (L5–L6). This grouping reduces label noise and improves classification stability, as adjacent workload levels often show similar EEG patterns. While the number of participants is limited, the goal of this study is to validate the EEG processing and learning pipeline rather than achieve population-level generalization.

3.3 Signal Preprocessing Pipeline

Raw EEG signals usually include slow baseline drift, power-line noise, and physiological artifacts (e.g., eye blinks and muscle activity). We applied a standard preprocessing pipeline based on filtering and ICA, which is commonly used in EEG studies [21–23].

Digital Filtering. First, low-frequency drift was removed using a high-pass filter ($f_c = 0.5$ Hz). A simple discrete-time representation of a first-order high-pass IIR filter [21,28] can be written as:

$$y[n] = a_0 x[n] + a_1 x[n-1] - b_1 y[n-1], \tag{1}$$

where the coefficients $\{a_0, a_1, b_1\}$ are selected based on f_c and the sampling rate f_s using standard digital filter design.

Power-line interference was attenuated with a notch filter at 50 Hz (nominal grid frequency in Europe) [21,28]. The notch transfer function is:

$$H(z) = \frac{1 - 2\cos(\omega_0)z^{-1} + z^{-2}}{1 - 2r\cos(\omega_0)z^{-1} + r^2 z^{-2}}, \qquad \omega_0 = \frac{2\pi f_0}{f_s}, \tag{2}$$

where r controls the notch bandwidth.

Finally, we applied a band-pass filter (1–40 Hz) to keep the main EEG frequency content used in workload analysis and suppress out-of-band noise [21,22]. A compact FIR representation is:

$$y[n] = \sum_{k=0}^{N} b_k\, x[n-k], \tag{3}$$

The filter length can be selected using minimum-length FIR estimation approaches [13]. In practice, the filter coefficients were obtained using standard FIR design methods rather than manual coefficient selection.

ICA-Based Artifact Reduction. After filtering, ICA was used to separate independent sources and reduce artifacts such as eye blinks and muscle activity [24,25]. The observed EEG X is modeled as a linear mixture of independent sources S:

$$X = AS, \qquad S = WX, \tag{4}$$

where A is the mixing matrix and W is the unmixing matrix.

Before estimating W, the EEG data were centered and whitened to remove second-order correlations. Using the eigen-decomposition of the covariance matrix, a common whitening formulation was applied, following standard ICA preprocessing procedures [24,26].

$$X_{\text{white}} = D^{-\frac{1}{2}} E^T (X - \mu), \tag{5}$$

where E and D are the eigenvectors and eigenvalues, and μ is the channel-wise mean. Independent components were then estimated using FastICA, and artifact-related components were removed before reconstructing the cleaned signal [24,26]. The quality of artifact removal was checked by visually comparing EEG signals before and after ICA processing. Common artifacts such as eye blinks and muscle noise were reduced while preserving the main EEG signal patterns. This whitening step ensures unit variance and removes second-order correlations before ICA estimation.

PSD Estimation. Power spectral density (PSD) features were computed from the cleaned EEG using Welch's method, which improves spectral stability by averaging modified periodograms across windowed segments [21,27]. A compact Welch PSD expression is:

$$\hat{P}[m] = \frac{1}{K} \sum_{k=1}^{K} \frac{1}{U} \left| X_k[m] \right|^2, \qquad PSD_{\text{dB}}[m] = 10 \log_{10} \big(\hat{P}[m] \big). \tag{6}$$

where K is the number of segments, U is the window-energy normalization, and $X_k[m]$ is the DFT of the k-th windowed segment. The PSD representations highlight workload-related spectral changes and can be used directly as learning inputs (e.g., numerical PSD features or PSD-based images).

After filtering, PSD curves for all the channels were obtained. Workload differences often appear as changes in spectral power across frequency ranges.

PSD plots were converted into image-like inputs for deep learning. They were placed upon their corresponding power spectral density range using a color intensity distribution. Figure 3 shows a sample PSD image that was used as a model input. The deep learning model learns frequency patterns related to different workload levels.

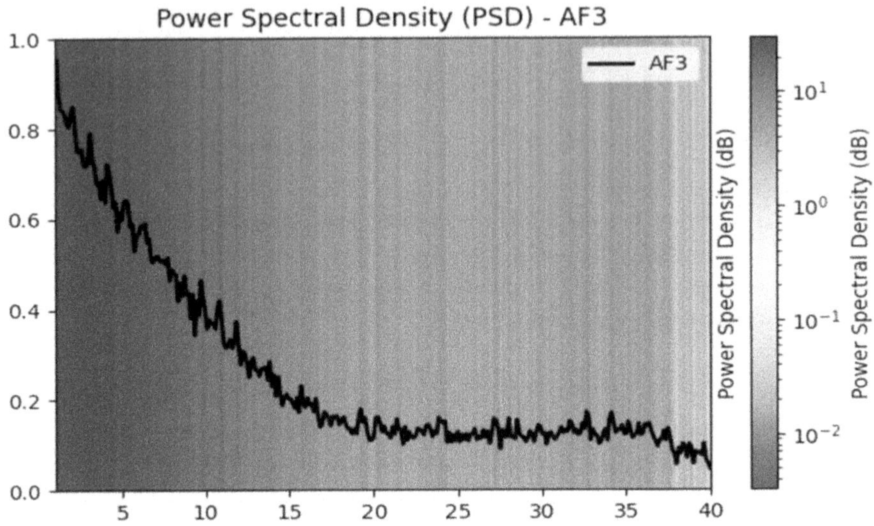

Fig. 3. PSD image example for one EEG channel.

3.4 Model Training

Deep Learning Model (ResNet-34). A ResNet-34 model was trained on PSD images. Transfer learning was applied to adapt a pre-trained model to the workload classification task [9,12]. We fine-tuned the final layers and trained with standard optimization settings. This helps reduce overfitting when the dataset size is limited. Figure 4 shows the overall model development method used.

SVM Model. In addition to the deep learning model, we trained a Support Vector Machine (SVM) as a feature-based classifier. The SVM model was trained using a combination of EEG-derived numerical features and task-related behavioral features. EEG numerical features were extracted from power spectral density (PSD) representations by computing average spectral power values across standard frequency bands (delta, theta, alpha, and beta) for each EEG channel. These features capture workload-related frequency changes in the EEG signal.

In addition to EEG features, task performance accuracy and task completion time were included as behavioral features. These features were aligned with EEG segments using timestamps, ensuring that all features correspond to the same task interval. The SVM model, therefore combines physiological and behavioral information, providing a complementary representation of mental workload. Unlike the deep learning model, which learns spatial patterns from PSD images, the SVM relies on explicit numerical features, making it suitable for use in the meta-learning stage. NASA-TLX values were used only for workload label generation and were not included as input features to the SVM model.

SVM was selected because it performs well with high-dimensional data and limited sample sizes, which is common in EEG studies. Unlike the deep learn-

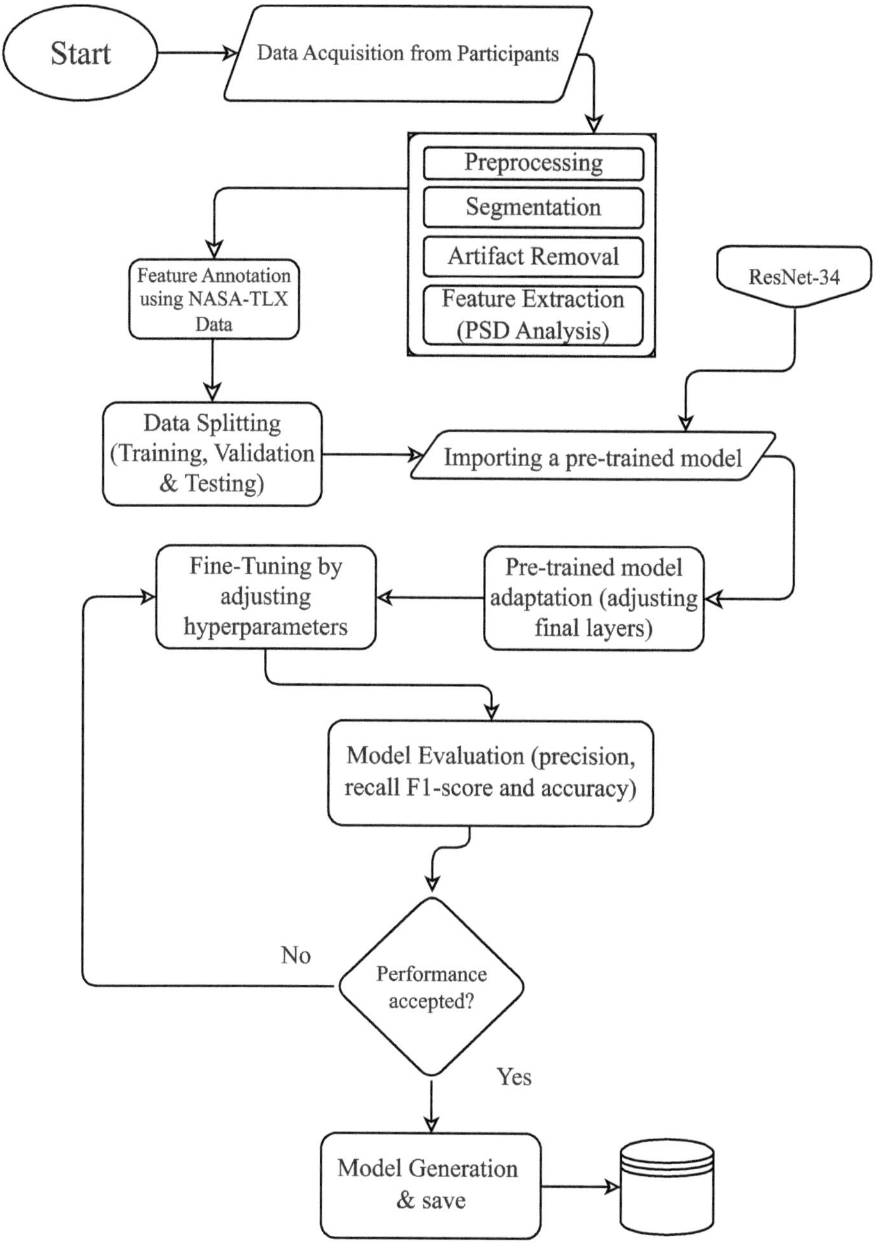

Fig. 4. Overall system architecture for the proposed deep learning-based EEG workload classification pipeline.

ing model, which learns spatial patterns from PSD images, the SVM relies on explicit frequency-domain features. This difference makes the SVM complementary to the deep model and suitable for use in the meta-learning stage. SVM is a strong baseline for high-dimensional classification and can work well with limited data [6,8]. **Meta-Learning** To reduce disagreement between models, a stacking-based meta-learning approach was used. The base models (ResNet-34 and SVM) first produce class probability outputs for each EEG segment. These probability values are used as input features for a lightweight meta-classifier, which produces the final workload classification. This approach helps improve classification when workload levels overlap in EEG patterns.

The meta-classifier was trained using validation-fold classifications to avoid information leakage. This stacking strategy improves classification stability by combining the strengths of the deep learning model and the feature-based model. The base models were trained using six workload levels to preserve fine-grained variations in mental workload. However, due to overlap between adjacent workload levels and subjectivity in self-reported data, the meta-learning model was evaluated using three grouped categories (low, medium, high) to improve classification stability. This evaluation strategy reduces label noise and supports more robust cross-model validation.

The meta-classifier was implemented using an SVM (`SVC`) and trained on the model output features after standardization using `StandardScaler`. We used an 80/20 train–test split with a fixed random seed (`random_state=42`). Hyperparameters were selected using grid search with 5-fold cross-validation (`GridSearchCV, cv=5`) by tuning the regularization parameter C, the kernel parameter γ, and the kernel type. The best configuration was selected based on cross-validation accuracy. The final meta-model used an RBF kernel with $C = 1$ and $\gamma = 1$. This approach improves classification stability, particularly for overlapping workload levels, without increasing model complexity. All implementation scripts were developed in Python and are publicly available for reproducibility[1]. Thus, the two base models operate on different representations of the data. The deep learning model uses PSD images derived from EEG signals, while the SVM uses combined EEG numerical and behavioral features. This enables a multi-perspective representation of mental workload.

3.5 Example of the Meta-learning Process

For a given EEG segment, the ResNet-34 model outputs workload class probabilities (0.20,0.55,0.25) for low, medium, and high workload, respectively, while the SVM outputs (0.10,0.40,0.50). These six probability values are concatenated and used as input to the meta-classifier. Based on learned validation patterns, the meta-model produces a final workload classification (e.g., medium), resolving disagreements between the base models and improving classification stability.

[1] Code and materials are available at https://github.com/Sameera-G/Mental_Workload_Analysis_Meta_Model_Approach.

4 Results

The deep learning model achieved stable learning and was able to classify mental workload levels from PSD images. Figure 5(a) shows the variation of training accuracy over epochs, and Fig. 5(b) shows the classification performance.

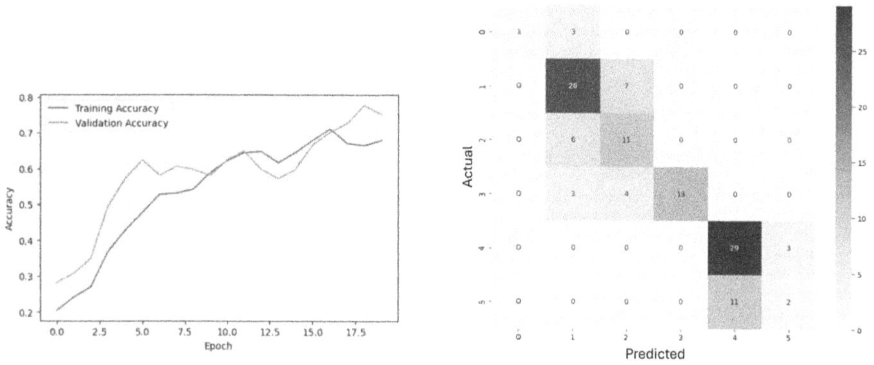

(a) Training accuracy variation

(b) Confusion matrix of Deep Learning ResNet-34 (Labels correspond to workload levels (1–6), where 1 = very low and 6 = very high.)

Fig. 5. Deep learning model results using PSD-based EEG input.

The meta-learning model outperforms individual models. The ResNet-34 model achieved 63% accuracy, while the SVM model achieved 50%. The meta-learning model improved the accuracy to 83%. This indicates that combining both models helps reduce errors and improve classification performance. Final model results are summarized using the confusion matrix. Figure 6 shows that the final model has improved stability compared to the individual models. In addition, Fig. 6(a) presents the confusion matrix of the SVM model, which was developed using both EEG-derived numerical features and task-related behavioral features, including task performance accuracy and completion time. While Fig. 6(b) shows the confusion matrix of the meta-learning model. The SVM model shows reasonable classification performance, achieving an accuracy of 50%, but it produces noticeable misclassifications between neighboring workload levels. In contrast, the meta-learning model reduces these errors and achieves an improved accuracy of 83%, providing more consistent classifications across classes. Due to the limited sample size, statistical significance testing was not applied, and the results are intended to demonstrate methodological feasibility rather than statistically generalizable conclusions. Most mistakes occur between closely related workload classes due to overlapping EEG patterns. This shows that similar workload levels are harder to separate, and the meta-learning approach helps improve classification in these cases. While the deep learning model demonstrates strong standalone performance, the meta-learning model combines classifications from the ResNet-34 and SVM models to improve classification stability and produce a more stable final workload classification, especially between neighboring workload levels.

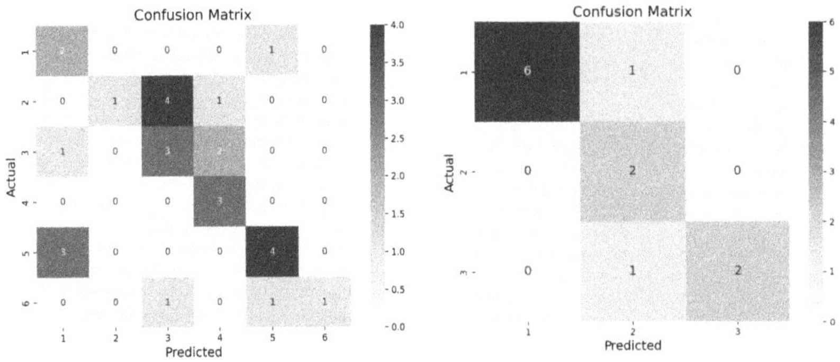

(a) SVM model confusion matrix (b) Meta-model confusion matrix

Fig. 6. Confusion matrices comparing the SVM model and the meta-learning model, which uses collapsed workload categories (1 = low, 2 = medium, 3 = high).

Table 1 summarizes precision, recall, F1-score, and accuracy for the final model. Precision, recall, and F1-score are reported as weighted averages to account for class imbalance in the dataset. High precision indicates strong reliability when classifying workload.

Table 1. Final model performance metrics

Precision	Recall	F1-Score	Accuracy
0.92	0.83	0.85	0.83

The performance of individual models and the proposed meta-learning approach were evaluated using the test dataset. As seen in the Table 2, the Deep learning ResNet-34 model achieved an accuracy of 63%, while the SVM model achieved 50%. The stacking-based meta-learning model improved the performance to 83% accuracy. This shows that combining deep learning and feature-based models helps improve classification reliability and reduces errors between similar workload levels.

Table 2. Model Performance Comparison

Model	Accuracy
ResNet-34	63%
SVM	50%
Meta-model	83%

5 Discussion

This study demonstrates that EEG-based machine learning can be used to estimate mental workload during software engineering tasks when signal processing is carefully designed. Power Spectral Density (PSD) is an effective representation because it captures workload-related frequency changes in EEG signals. The deep learning model trained on PSD images learns complex patterns, while the SVM provides a complementary and interpretable feature-based model. Due to the limited dataset size, the results indicate performance trends rather than statistically generalizable outcomes. Nevertheless, the findings directly address the research question by showing that a structured EEG processing pipeline combined with meta-learning can improve the reliability of workload estimation in software engineering contexts.

5.1 Effect of Meta-learning on Workload Classification Reliability

The stacking-based meta-learning model improves mental workload classification by combining complementary information from the deep learning and classical models. Instead of relying on a single classifier, the meta-model learns to balance the confidence scores produced by the ResNet-34 and the SVM. For each EEG segment, both base models output class probability distributions, which are used as input features for the meta-classifier. This allows the final classification to be based on agreement patterns between models rather than a single decision boundary.

From a statistical perspective, the meta-model functions as a lightweight decision-level fusion mechanism. When both base models assign high probability to the same workload class, the decision is reinforced. When disagreement occurs, the meta-classifier learns which model is more reliable for specific workload ranges using validation data. This reduces model-specific bias and random fluctuations, particularly between neighboring workload levels where EEG patterns tend to overlap. The effectiveness of this approach is reflected in improved classification stability and reduced misclassification between adjacent workload categories. Individual models may confuse nearby workload levels due to subjective variability in NASA-TLX self-reports, whereas the meta-model produces more consistent outputs by evaluating collapsed workload groups (low, medium, and high). This strategy reduces label noise without introducing additional features or increasing model complexity.

The meta-learning approach is also suitable for future deployment in mobile or wearable systems due to its low computational cost. The base models can operate independently, while the meta-model requires only probability-level inputs to generate stable workload estimates. This design supports real-time workload monitoring and provides a practical foundation for interpretable workload visualization in applied software engineering environments.

5.2 Implications for Software Engineering Practice

The proposed EEG-based workload classification pipeline can support future research on mental workload in software engineering environments. By providing objective and continuous workload estimates, such methods could help study adaptive work environments where task difficulty, interruptions, or support tools are adjusted based on cognitive load. In addition, workload monitoring approaches may support research on developer well-being by identifying periods of sustained high mental effort. While this work does not propose a deployable system, the methodological framework can inform the design of future tools for analyzing mental workload in software engineering tasks.

5.3 Limitations

Dataset size and class balance can affect model reliability. The workload labels are based on NASA-TLX self-reports, which may introduce subjectivity across participants. In addition, wearing EEG devices with multiple electrodes may affect user comfort and could influence cognitive state during task execution. Since workload labels are derived from NASA-TLX self-reports collected at the task level, the same label is assigned to multiple EEG segments within a task. This assumes that workload remains relatively stable during the task and may not capture short-term fluctuations in cognitive state. Wearable EEG devices can include noise, so preprocessing is essential [7,21]. Future work should use larger datasets and more diverse software engineering tasks. As this work focuses on methodological development, future studies with larger and more diverse participant groups are needed to evaluate generalizability.

6 Conclusion

We presented a complete EEG-based pipeline for mental workload classification in software engineering tasks. The pipeline includes filtering, ICA, PSD estimation, and machine learning model training. ResNet-34 and SVM were used as workload classifiers, and a meta-learning step improved reliability. The proposed approach achieved an accuracy of 83%, showing that combining deep learning and machine learning models using meta-learning improves workload classification performance.

This work provides a methodological foundation for objective workload monitoring in knowledge work domains. Future work will focus on larger datasets, handling class imbalance, and evaluation in more natural workplace settings. This study provides a reproducible methodological baseline for future EEG-based workload monitoring in knowledge-intensive work environments.

Acknowledgments. This research is supported by FAST (Finnish Software Engineering Doctoral Research Network), funded by the Finnish Ministry of Education and Culture, and conducted as part of the doctoral program at the University of Oulu in close collaboration with academic and industrial partners.

Disclosure of Interests. The authors have no competing interests to declare that are relevant to the content of this article.

References

1. Holm, A., Lukander, K., Korpela, J., Sallinen, M., Müller, K.M.: Estimating brain load from the EEG. Sci. World J. **9**, 639–651 (2009)
2. Longo, L., Wickens, C.D., Hancock, G., Hancock, P.A.: Human mental workload: a survey and a novel inclusive definition. Front. Psychol. **13**, 883321 (2022)
3. Medeiros, J., et al.: EEG as a potential ground truth for the assessment of cognitive state in software development activities: a multimodal imaging study. PLoS ONE **19**(3), e0299108 (2024). https://doi.org/10.1371/journal.pone.0299108
4. Pušica, M., Mijović, B., Leva, M.C., Gligorijević, I.: Machine learning performance in EEG-based mental workload classification across task types: a systematic review. Front. Neuroergonomics **6**, 1621309 (2025). https://doi.org/10.3389/fnrgo.2025.1621309
5. Das Chakladar, D., Roy, P.P.: Cognitive workload estimation using physiological measures: a review. Cogn. Neurodyn. **18**(4), 1445–1465 (2024). https://doi.org/10.1007/s11571-023-10051-3
6. Maldonado, S., et al.: Simultaneous feature selection and heterogeneity control for SVM classification: an application to mental workload assessment. Expert Syst. Appl. **143** (2020)
7. Gao, Z., et al.: Complex networks and deep learning for EEG signal analysis. Cogn. Neurodyn. **15**(3), 369–388 (2021)
8. Rahman, M.A., Hossain, M.F., Hossain, M., Ahmmed, R.: Employing PCA and t-statistical approach for feature extraction and classification from multichannel EEG signal. Egypt. Inform. J. **21**(1), 23–35 (2020)
9. Gong, S., Xing, K., Cichocki, A., Li, J.: Deep learning in EEG: advance of the last ten-year critical period. IEEE Trans. Cogn. Dev. Syst. **14**(2), 348–365 (2022)
10. Yedukondalu, J., Sharma, D., Sharma, L.D.: Subject-wise cognitive load detection using time-frequency EEG and Bi-LSTM. Arab. J. Sci. Eng. **49**, 4445–4457 (2024). https://doi.org/10.1007/s13369-023-08494-1
11. Jain, P., Yedukondalu, J., Chhabra, H., et al.: EEG-based detection of cognitive load using VMD and LightGBM classifier. Int. J. Mach. Learn. Cybern. **15**, 4193–4210 (2024). https://doi.org/10.1007/s13042-024-02142-2
12. Hussain, A., Keikhosrokiani, P., Asl, M.P.: Employee mental workload classification in industrial workplaces: a machine learning approach. In: Advances in Intelligent Computing Techniques and Applications. Springer (2024)
13. Ichige, K., Iwaki, M., Ishii, R.: Accurate estimation of minimum filter length for optimum FIR digital filters. IEEE Trans. Circ. Syst. II **47**(10), 1008–1016 (2000)

14. Hevner, A.R., March, S.T., Park, J., Ram, S.: Design science in information systems research. MIS Q. **28**(1), 75–105 (2004)
15. Peffers, K., Tuunanen, T., Rothenberger, M.A., Chatterjee, S.: A design science research methodology for information systems research. J. Manag. Inf. Syst. **24**(3), 45–77 (2007). https://doi.org/10.2753/MIS0742-1222240302
16. Wisniewski, M.G., Joyner, C.N., Zakrzewski, A.C., Makeig, S.: Finding tau rhythms in EEG: an independent component analysis approach. Hum. Brain Mapp. **45**(2) (2024)
17. Van, L.-D., Huang, P.-Y., Lu, T.-C.: Cost-effective and variable-channel FastICA hardware architecture and implementation for EEG signal processing. J. Signal Process. Syst. **82**(1), 91–113 (2016)
18. Mmeremikwu, V.O., Mbachu, C.B.: EEG signal improvement: comparison of different windows. World J. Innov. Res. **8**(4), 38–42 (2020)
19. Hart, S.G., Staveland, L.E.: Development of NASA-TLX (task load index): results of empirical and theoretical research. Adv. Psychol. **52**, 139–183 (1988)
20. Soldati, M., Laakso, I.: Effect of electrical conductivity uncertainty in assessment of electric fields induced in the brain at 50 Hz. IEEE Access **8**, 222297–222309 (2020)
21. Chaddad, A., Wu, Y., Kateb, R., Bouridane, A.: Electroencephalography signal processing: a comprehensive review and analysis of methods and techniques. Sensors **23**(14), 6434 (2023)
22. Coelli, S., et al.: Selecting methods for a modular EEG pre-processing pipeline: an objective comparison. Biomed. Signal Process. Control **90**, 105830 (2024)
23. Bigdely-Shamlo, N., Mullen, T., Kothe, C., Su, K., Robbins, K.A.: The PREP pipeline: standardized preprocessing for large-scale EEG analysis. Front. Neuroinform. **9**, 16 (2015)
24. Delorme, A., Makeig, S.: EEGLAB: an open source toolbox for analysis of single-trial EEG dynamics including independent component analysis. J. Neurosci. Methods **134**(1), 9–21 (2004)
25. Jung, T.-P., et al.: Removing electroencephalographic artifacts by blind source separation. Psychophysiology **37**(2), 163–178 (2000)
26. Hyvärinen, A., Oja, E.: Independent component analysis: algorithms and applications. Neural Netw. **13**(4–5), 411–430 (2000)
27. Welch, P.D.: The use of fast Fourier transform for the estimation of power spectra: a method based on time averaging over short, modified periodograms. IEEE Trans. Audio Electroacoust. **15**(2), 70–73 (1967)
28. Widmann, A., Schröger, E., Maess, B.: Digital filter design for electrophysiological data-a practical approach. J. Neurosci. Methods **250**, 34–46 (2015). https://doi.org/10.1016/j.jneumeth.2014.08.002

EH-FSL: Secure and Scalable Edge-Hosted Federated Split Learning in Data-Intensive Healthcare

Bilgehan Akdemir(✉) and Erkki Harjula

Centre for Wireless Communications (CWC), University of Oulu, 90570 Oulu, Finland
{Bilgehan.Akdemir,Erkki.Harjula}@oulu.fi

Abstract. Distributed Collaborative Machine Learning (DCML) has gained increasing attention as a means to reduce data exposure and communication overhead by enabling collaborative model training without centralizing data. Federated Learning (FL) and Split Learning (SL) represent two paradigms for decentralized model training, each offering complementary advantages. Their integration improves robustness against model inversion attacks while enabling the participation of resource-constrained devices across the Edge-Cloud Continuum (ECC), thereby enhancing system scalability. However, the application of DCML paradigms within a three-tier computing architecture for data- and compute-intensive medical workloads remains insufficiently explored. To address this gap, this concept paper investigates the integration of FL and SL within an Edge-Hosted Federated Split Learning (EH-FSL) framework to enable scalable, privacy-preserving model training for data-intensive medical imaging applications. We position EH-FSL as a unifying paradigm by analyzing existing FL, SL, and FSL approaches and examining their communication and computational trade-offs in healthcare settings. Furthermore, we highlight the feasibility of deploying an edge-hosted FSL architecture integrated with the distributed ECC as a conceptual paradigm for data-intensive digital healthcare scenarios.

Keywords: Digital Healthcare · Edge Computing · Distributed Learning · Federated Split Learning · Scalability

1 Introduction

We live in a rapidly evolving technology era where 400 million terabytes of data are generated every single day. Internet of Medical Things (IoMT) sensors and medical imaging devices are among the data generators that contribute to this volume. The data generated from the various sources is typically processed within the device itself, nearby local hardware, or remote servers. Centralized cloud computing resources been used for Deep Learning (DL)-based data analytics. However, challenges arise when transferring these tremendous volumes of data over networks, resulting in high latency, network congestion, and regulatory compliance restrictions on the sharing of patient data.

M. SäreStöniemi et al. (Eds.): NCDHWS 2026, CCIS 3010, pp. 418–427, 2026.
https://doi.org/10.1007/978-3-032-28819-6_26

Edge computing (EC) has enabled data to be processed closer to its source [11]. Among other EC approaches, Multi-access Edge Computing (MEC) is defined by the European Telecommunications Standards as extending cloud computing capabilities to the nearest mobile base stations. In healthcare and medical imaging, the growing adoption of Artificial Intelligence (AI) has significantly increased the demand for computing resources with Graphics Processing Units (GPUs), particularly for compute-intensive applications, e.g., advanced medical image analysis and reconstruction. Computational resources at the network edge provide efficient data processing, which can be achieved by addressing bandwidth (BW), latency, and privacy constraints inherent in digital healthcare.

Machine Learning (ML) and DL methods have demonstrated success in extracting meaningful patterns from imaging data. Modern DL models typically rely on Deep Neural Network (DNN) architectures, whose training processes are, as mentioned above, computationally expensive. As a result, the availability and placement of computational resources play a crucial role in enabling efficient model training and deployment. In the last decade, the emergence of EC and the increase in GPU-enabled local resources have boosted Distributed Collaborative Machine Learning (DCML) paradigms, which aim to leverage the use of decentralized data, improve resource utilization, and mitigate privacy and security concerns.

Two popular DCML approaches, Federated Learning (FL) and Split Learning (SL) have emerged as promising solutions to enable model training across decentralized data while keeping raw data local. The locally trained model parameters are shared at each FL communication round and aggregated by a central server to update the global model, a process that continues until the global model converges [5]. FL has already been applied in various domains, including digital healthcare and medical imaging [9]. The large volumes of data generated across geographically distributed locations motivate collaborative training of decentralized clients' models, which can lead to high-accuracy performance and generalizable representations.

DCML paradigms enhance network efficiency by reducing the communication burden on wireless networks via exchanging model parameters and intermediate data rather than raw data. SL is another DCML technique that addresses privacy concerns related to sensitive data by performing part of the training locally. This approach enables effective utilization of heterogeneous computing resources within a distributed edge–cloud architecture. However, training efficiency remains limited because each client interacts with the server sequentially that increases the overall training time [4]. The advantages of SL in utilizing low-power computing resources in edge-cloud continuum (ECC) with the parallel training capability of FL for improved scalability, as well as the improved privacy-preserving aspects with both approaches, can assist better resource utilization for data- and compute-intensive healthcare use cases.

Federated Split Learning (FSL) has been explored in different fields, such as resource-constrained IoMT [8] and Industrial Internet of Things (IIoT) [4]. However, its application in edge-hosted, resource-heterogeneous, intensive healthcare

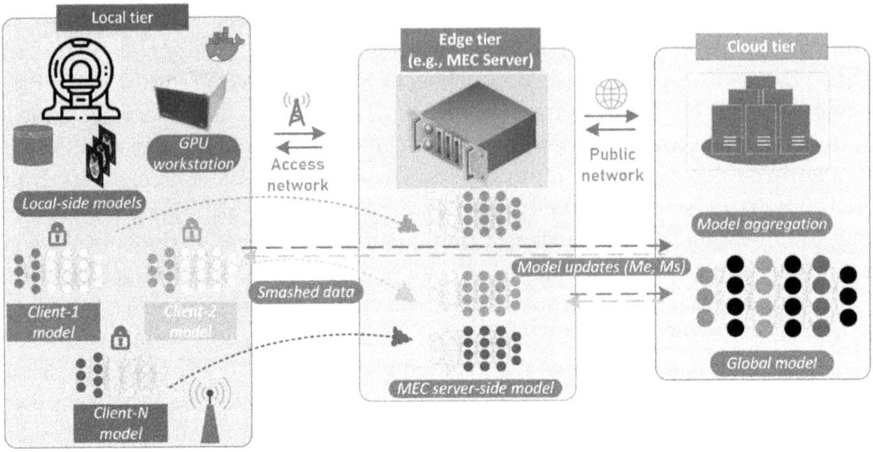

Fig. 1. EH-FSL Secure and Scalable Framework for Data-Intensive Healthcare.

environments remains largely underexplored. FSL reduces the long training time of SL by enabling the parallel training spirit of FL across numerous clients [4]. The study in [12] presents a comparative analysis of different DCML techniques and discusses how FSL outperforms other approaches in terms of network efficiency and privacy.

Traditionally, studies on FSL consider the server-side model interacting with many clients, which increases the storage and computational burden on the server [4]. In our proposed architectural concept, inspired by a 3-tier distributed ECC design as presented in Fig. 1, the nearest 5G/6G base station's MEC server acts as a paired server. This approach offloads computational workload to the MECs near the hospital, while the aggregator server in a remote cloud is used only for updating the global model. Therefore, in addition to balancing the workload, the nearest base station, in case it is provided by the hospital's private 5G network [2], also ensures a more secure environment.

The main contributions of this position paper are: (i) We present a conceptual DCML architecture that integrates FL and SL within an edge–cloud computing continuum, targeting low-power and resource-constrained environments. (ii) We propose leveraging MEC servers located at the nearest base stations (Private 5G) as computational resources for model training, while the remote cloud is used for model aggregation. (iii) We analyze and compare DCML paradigms presented in this work from a system-level perspective, highlighting the suitability of FSL for privacy-preserving and compute-efficient healthcare applications.

2 EH-FSL as a Secure and Scalable Learning Framework

While secure data processing is part of EH-FSL, using resources efficiently across the ECC is also essential for a large-scale DCML system. Compared to the FL,

Algorithm 1. EH-FSL: Proposed Edge-Hosted Framework

Initialization: Aggregator defines Global Model $\mathcal{M}$ and Split Point θ;
Partition $\mathcal{M}$ into Client-side M_e and MEC-side M_s sub-networks;
Broadcast M_e to Local Clients $\{C_1, \dots, C_K\}$ and M_s to MEC Nodes;
for each global synchronization round $t = 1, \dots, T$ **do**
  Tier 1: Local Edge Processing (Parallel)
  for all Clients $C_k \in \{1, \dots, K\}$ **do**
    Compute Smashed Data $Z_k = M_e(X_k; W_e^{(t)})$
    Offload $\{Z_k, Labels_k\}$ to Tier 2;
  end for
  Tier 2: MEC-Hosted Computation
  MEC Node receives $\{Z_k, Labels_k\}$ and manages concurrent requests:
  Perform Forward Pass: $\hat{Y}_k = M_s(Z_k; W_s^{(t)})$;
  Calculate Loss $\mathcal{L}(\hat{Y}_k, Labels_k)$ and local gradients ∇W_s;
  Backpropagate ∇Z_k to Client C_k for local update;
  Tier 3: Sync Global Model (Cloud/Aggregator)
  Collect updated sub-weights $\{W_e, W_s\}$ from Tiers 1 and 2;
  $W^{(t+1)} \leftarrow \text{FederatedAverage}(W^{(t)}, \Delta W)$;
  Broadcast updated parameters to all nodes;
end for

FSL leverages SL's reduced client-side computation within the framework to improve scalability in the resource-constrained edge-cloud. The EH-FSL natively mitigates privacy and security concerns by design. Additional privacy guarantees can be achieved through complementary techniques, such as differential privacy and homomorphic encryption techniques. The training phases of the EH-FSL concept are presented in Algorithm1. A detailed workflow of the algorithm is presented in Fig. 2.

2.1 Scalability Across Edge Nodes and Institutions

The scalability for DCML depends on heterogeneous edge nodes and involves several challenges. A uniform system, such as using imaging data from the same vendor and processing workstations from the same manufacturer, can facilitate scal-

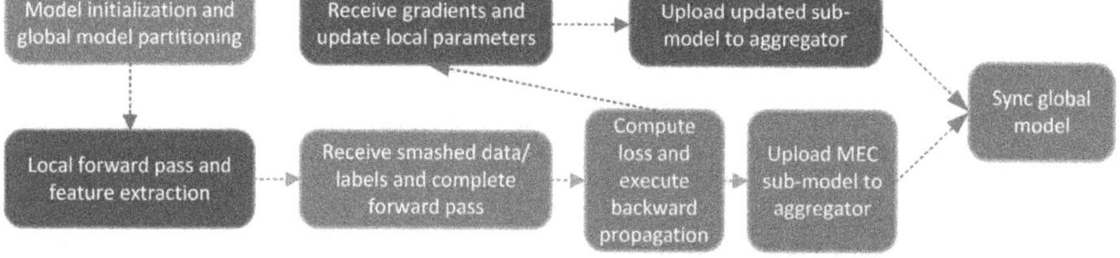

Fig. 2. EH-FSL training workflow. Gray color: Cloud, Orange: MEC-side, Blue: Client-side processes. (Color figure online)

Table 1. Qualitative and Technical Comparison of FL, SL, and FSL.

Metric	Description	FL	SL	FSL	Measurement Units
Computation Eff.	Client-side compute cost	Medium	Low	Medium	CPU and GPU utilization [%]
Training Eff.	Time to convergence	Medium	High	Medium	Communication rounds [#], training data size [samples]
Network BW Eff.	Bandwidth (BW) sensitivity	Medium	Low	Medium	Model update size [MB], network BW [Mbps]
Communication Freq.	Sync. rounds to convergence	Medium	High	Medium	Synchronization rounds [#]
Network Robustness	Tolerance to instability	Medium	Low	High	Accuracy degradation [%], packet loss rate [%]
Privacy and Security	Protection against raw data or model leakage	High	High	Very High	Network exposure risk [# of hostile nodes], leakage probability [%]
Local Resource Req.	Client hardware usage	High	Low	Low	RAM, GPU mem. usage [GB]
Scalability	Performance (# of clients)	Medium	Medium	High	Accuracy degradation [%]
Edge Cloud	Edge cloud compatibility	Medium	Low	High	Latency [ms], BW [Gbps]

ability to some extent. However, distributed healthcare systems encounter practical challenges, including non-IID data distribution, annotation consistency, and hardware heterogeneity across participating hospitals. The study in [4] experimented on the benchmarking dataset by increasing the number of participating clients in the DCML setup. The study shows that better scalability is achieved in the IID setting. The distributed EH-FSL approach leverages multiple computing nodes across the edge–cloud continuum, thereby naturally supporting horizontal scalability. By incorporating additional hospitals and sites, more data can be fed to the model, and computational resources can be scaled accordingly depending on the technical requirements. This flexibility enables efficient scaling of the system without relying on centralized solutions.

Vertical scalability can be achieved by increasing the computational capacity of each client at the local, edge, or cloud level. The DCML approaches, particularly for data-intensive imaging modalities, can benefit significantly from vertical scalability by enabling faster and more efficient training processes. However, integrating additional computational resources into an existing system is not always straightforward and often involves high costs. In this context, EH-FSL helps address this challenge by leveraging existing computing nodes for client-side model training, eliminating the need for costly hardware upgrades while still enabling efficient learning. Scaling up model training through DCML across multiple sites can introduce significant communication overhead. Therefore, to address this challenge, studies on model compression can be listed into three categories: model pruning, parameter quantization, and knowledge distillation, which show promising results for communication efficiency while preserving model performance for DCML techniques [4].

2.2 Network and Computational Overloads of DCML Approaches

We have presented some of the metrics with measurement units for DCML paradigms in Table 1.The qualitative ratings in this comparison are grounded in

Table 2. Popular Open-Source DCML Frameworks.

Framework	Main Focus	PyTorch	TensorFlow	FL	SL	FSL
Flower	Generic purpose FL	✓	✓	✓	∼	∼
PySyft	Privacy-preserving ML	✓	∼	✓	✓	∼
FATE	Industrial FL	∼	∼	✓	×	×
FedML	Distributed ML	✓	✓	✓	∼	∼
TensorFlow Federated	FL Research/Experiment	×	✓	✓	×	×
NVFlare	Research/Industrial	✓	✓	✓	✓	✓

✓: Full support, ∼: Partial support, ×: No support

the empirical trade-off analysis of privacy and communication efficiency established in [12]. The paper in [1] examines the technical requirements of data-intensive medical imaging, specifically the CBCT modality in a distributed 3-tier ECC environment. As it can be seen from the table, SL exhibits low client-side local resource requirements, as it leverages resource-rich MEC servers to perform of server-side model computation. In contrast, the computational efficiency of FL and FSL is rated as medium due to the partial or full execution of the model on client devices. Regarding network efficiency, FL and FSL demonstrate moderate efficiency, whereas SL requires a more robust network. This is because SL frequently exchanges activations and smashed data (intermediate gradients) during each forward and backward pass, rather than communicating model updates once per round as in FL. FSL leverages the spirit of FL on parallelizing the training process, which improves the network resource utilization.

There have been different distributed learning open-source frameworks for federated model training, which facilitate training processes of DCML approaches. These frameworks are widely used for general federated training, simulation, proof-of-concept (PoC), and real-world applications across various domains, including healthcare, finance, automotive, and IoT. A comprehensive survey on the open-source distributed learning frameworks is presented in [6], and Table 2 summarizes the popular frameworks used for decentralized model training. The purpose of this comparison is to demonstrate that the current DCML frameworks are technically to support the proposed EH-FSL paradigm.

3 Challenges and Research Directions

The popularity of FL can be attributed to the relative simplicity of the paradigm, the availability of mature frameworks supported by both academia and industry, and its ease of integration into existing DCML pipelines. In contrast, SL often introduces additional system and communication complexity. The FSL approach combines the benefits of FL and SL, which provides better outcomes. The heterogeneous resources in ECC for both networking and computing aspects present several key challenges.

3.1 Networking

Efficient networking is crucial in distributed model training [7]. Network bottlenecks affect synchronization overhead, especially in the case of a large number of participating clients in collaborative learning. To mitigate disruptions and enable uninterrupted and efficient training, robust communication technologies, such as emerging 6G networks, are essential. In FL, model updates are exchanged at each communication round; therefore, network latency and bandwidth limitations directly affect the server-side aggregation process, especially when model averaging is performed after receiving updates from all participating clients. The networking plays an even more critical role in SL, as activations and smashed data are exchanged every training iteration. This requires a stable and high-bandwidth connection, making SL more sensitive to network outages and increasing overall bandwidth consumption. In FSL, efficient networking remains a key requirement. However, by balancing local computation and communication, FSL reduces excessive data transfer while maintaining collaborative learning. With the continued evolution of wireless communication technologies, particularly 6G, emerging network capabilities are expected to better meet the stringent communication demands of large-scale DCML systems.

In the widely adopted FSL approach, the remote server handles the server-side models for multiple clients, which can lead to increased computational resource utilization as the number of clients grows. To address this limitation in large-scale systems, MEC servers located near base stations are employed to handle the server-side training workload and share the updated model parameters with a remote aggregator for global model updates. This approach also enhances privacy by reducing the exposure of data and AI models, as neither the clients nor the MEC servers possess a complete copy of the trained model.

3.2 Hardware and Software

Heterogeneity in distributed systems is one of the main challenges in collaborative learning environments [10]. Variations in hardware and software configurations can significantly affect model training performance. Even different versions of the same software tool may introduce notable inconsistencies. In DCML model training, computing devices across participating sites may differ substantially in terms of hardware capabilities, operating systems, and software dependencies, which complicates system integration and reproducibility. To mitigate these issues, adopting a unified software stack—such as a common Python framework (e.g., PyTorch), and carefully selecting suitable distributed learning frameworks (Table 2) can facilitate implementation. However, despite these efforts, achieving full uniformity across distributed environments remains challenging and needs more investigation. For efficient FSL implementation, having participating institutions share similar hardware and software infrastructures can facilitate the process. For example, collaboration among sites using the same computing resource vendors, identical CBCT scanners, or compatible medical IoT devices, or deployments within private hospital networks or governmental research hospitals.

3.3 Model Training

Model training time is an important parameter in DL-based systems. In conventional DL settings, support from GPU-enabled resources can significantly accelerate training time. However, in data- and computation-intensive scenarios, such as volumetric CBCT imaging can take a considerable amount of time to complete training. This causes a major challenge for efficient model development and deployment. The high computational requirements arise from the large amount of data, spatial resolution, and the volumetric nature of the CBCT scans, all of which increase memory usage and processing time. Thus, training of DNN models on such data requires robust computing infrastructure and stable system performance.

These challenges become even more prominent in DCML paradigms. In addition to local computation overhead, device heterogeneity, network latency, and communication delays further increase the overall training time, particularly when model updates must be exchanged frequently between clients and the remote server. Moreover, in SL, smashed data generated at the split/cut layer are transmitted repeatedly over the network, which can introduce communication bottlenecks and slow down the training process when many clients participating collaborative training. As a result, efficient resource management and communication-aware training strategies are essential for scalable and practical deployment of such systems. Due to clients computing only a part of the model, FSL is advantageous for low-power devices throughout ECC computing nodes, enabling them to participate in the training of heavy models.

3.4 Deployment at Edge–Cloud Continuum and Wireless Networks

The distributed edge cloud enables the deployment of DCML by providing scalable computing and networking resources [1]. The integration of advanced wireless networks, e.g., 5G and beyond, with GPU-supported MEC servers makes the deployment of decentralized model training more feasible and time/resource-efficient. Moreover, AI-powered wireless networks combined with rich hardware infrastructures enhance the robustness of DCML frameworks, enabling cost-effective and reliable medical data processing.

EH-FSL aims to leverage computational and networking resources in the ECC architecture more efficiently. The number of IoMT devices grows fast; thus, improper or inefficient use of these devices can lead to increased energy consumption and a large environmental footprint [3]. This, in turn, contributes to higher operational costs and negative environmental impact. Therefore, optimized resource utilization is a crucial aspect in implementing scalable and sustainable DCML systems.

4 Conclusion

In this paper, we proposed a conceptual edge-hosted framework of the use of federated split learning for a secure and scalable DCML approach in data- and compute-intensive healthcare applications. We presented the main comparison of FSL with FL and SL within a distributed edge–cloud architecture. We discussed the motivation behind the utilization of FSL alongside other DCML paradigms. The challenges and limitations, along with the impacts of these learning paradigms, were analyzed, with particular emphasis on key aspects such as scalability and secure data processing. Furthermore, we highlighted a comparison of DCML paradigms, including the different metrics, the role of open-source distributed learning frameworks, the integration of edge-cloud infrastructures, and the potential impact of distributed edge cloud and emerging mobile networks on digital healthcare. While this paper focuses on the architectural design, our future work will involve empirical validation to evaluate the efficiency of the EH-FSL approach in data-intensive healthcare environments.

Acknowledgments. This work was supported by Business Finland Tomohead project (Grant 8095/31/2022), the Research Council of Finland DigiHealth (Grant 326291), Profi6 (Grant 336449) and the 6G Flagship Programme (Grant 369116).

References

1. Akdemir, B., et al.: From technical prerequisites to improved care: distributed edge ai for tomographic imaging. IEEE Access **13**, 14317–14343 (2025). https://doi.org/10.1109/ACCESS.2025.3530297
2. Gimhana, S., Ahmad, I., Porambage, P., Harjula, E.: Kpis for evaluating the feasibility of private 5g networks in hospitals. In: 2024 IEEE Conference on Standards for Communications and Networking (CSCN), pp. 62–67 (2024). https://doi.org/10.1109/CSCN63874.2024.10849718
3. Heye, T., et al.: The energy consumption of radiology: energy- and cost-saving opportunities for ct and mri operation. Radiology **295**(3), 593–605 (2020). https://doi.org/10.1148/radiol.2020192084, pMID: 32208096
4. Jia, Y., et al.: Model pruning-enabled federated split learning for resource-constrained devices in artificial intelligence empowered edge computing environment. ACM Trans. Sen. Netw. (2024). https://doi.org/10.1145/3687478, just Accepted
5. McMahan, H.B., Moore, E., Ramage, D., Hampson, S., y Arcas, B.A.: Communication-efficient learning of deep networks from decentralized data (2023). https://arxiv.org/abs/1602.05629
6. Mehdi, M., Makkar, A., Conway, M.: A comprehensive review of open-source federated learning frameworks. Procedia Comput. Sci. **260**, 540–551 (2025). https://doi.org/10.1016/j.procs.2025.03.232, seventh International Conference on Recent Trends in Image Processing and Pattern Recognition (RTIP2R-2024)
7. Mills, J., Hu, J., Min, G.: Communication-efficient federated learning for wireless edge intelligence in iot. IEEE Internet Things J. **7**(7), 5986–5994 (2020). https://doi.org/10.1109/JIOT.2019.2956615
8. Ni, W., Ao, H., Tian, H., Eldar, Y.C., Niyato, D.: Fedsl: federated split learning for collaborative healthcare analytics on resource-constrained wearable iomt devices. IEEE Internet Things J. **11**(10), 18934–18935 (2024). https://doi.org/10.1109/JIOT.2024.3370985

9. Rieke, N., Hancox, J., Li, W., Milletari, F., Roth, H.R., Albarqouni, S., et al.: The future of digital health with federated learning. NPJ Digit. Med. **3**(119) (2020). https://doi.org/10.1038/s41746-020-00323-1
10. Schäfer, D., Edinger, J., VanSyckel, S., Paluska, J.M., Becker, C.: Tasklets: overcoming heterogeneity in distributed computing systems. In: 2016 IEEE 36th International Conference on Distributed Computing Systems Workshops (ICDCSW), pp. 156–161 (2016). https://doi.org/10.1109/ICDCSW.2016.22
11. Shi, W., Cao, J., Zhang, Q., Li, Y., Xu, L.: Edge computing: vision and challenges. IEEE Internet Things J. **3**(5), 637–646 (2016). https://doi.org/10.1109/JIOT.2016.2579198
12. Zhang, Z., Pinto, A., Turina, V., Esposito, F., Matta, I.: Privacy and efficiency of communications in federated split learning. IEEE Trans. Big Data **9**(5), 1380–1391 (2023). https://doi.org/10.1109/TBDATA.2023.3280405

Ethical Impact of AI Systems in Healthcare: A Survey of Recorded Incidents

Lauri Tuovinen(✉)

University of Oulu, Oulu, Finland
lauri.tuovinen@oulu.fi

Abstract. The real-world impact of artificial intelligence (AI) in healthcare involves major benefits but also substantial harms. To better understand the nature of these harms, a survey of recorded AI incidents in the health domain was carried out. The surveyed incidents were discovered by searching an online repository of AI incident reports for entries containing health-related keywords. 34 incidents were identified as relevant and analysed through inductive thematic coding to categorise them by the sector where the AI system was deployed, the purpose for which it was being used and the ethical requirement violated in the incident. The results of the analysis provide some indication of the nature and magnitude of the risks posed by AI systems in healthcare, but the tentative nature of the investigation necessitates further work using more comprehensive data and more rigorous methods. With the popularity of general-purpose AI tools increasing rapidly, future work should also address the risks of the public relying on them rather than human experts for health-related information.

Keywords: Artificial intelligence · AI ethics · AI incident · AI in healthcare

1 Introduction

Artificial intelligence (AI) in medicine has a history spanning half a century, starting with the earliest medical expert systems developed in the 1970s [1]. The then-dominant symbolic AI paradigm has since then been superseded by machine learning (ML); in medicine, ML systems introduce considerable opportunities to improve care but also substantial ethical and regulatory issues [2]. AI systems based on large language models, in which there has been a surge of interest in recent years, bring with them further challenges [3].

While there is abundant literature discussing the ethical concerns associated with the use of AI systems in healthcare, the same cannot be said of literature discussing actual verified harm inflicted by such systems in the real world. A part of the reason may be that suitable data has not been readily available, but the past few years have seen the emergence of several initiatives to collect and publish reports of AI incidents on the web. The results of these efforts vary

M. Särestöniemi et al. (Eds.): NCDHWS 2026, CCIS 3010, pp. 428–437, 2026.
https://doi.org/10.1007/978-3-032-28819-6_27

considerably in terms of quality and coverage, with the AI Incident Database (AIID) [4], the AI, Algorithmic and Automation Incidents and Controversies Repository (AIAAIC) [5] and the OECD AI Incidents and Hazards Monitor (AIM) [6] standing out as the most notable ones.

Researchers interested in the ethical impact of AI have now begun to exploit these new resources, and there are a handful of published papers using them to explore AI incidents in the health domain. These range in their level of granularity from the sectoral analysis of [7], where healthcare is one of the five sectors included, to the detailed examination of selected individual incidents in [8,9]. In between the extremes are [10], which provides an overview of health-related incidents found in the AIAAIC database, and [11], which uses data from the United States Department of Health and Human Services to examine data breach incidents specifically and discusses their implications to the use of AI in healthcare.

This paper adds a contribution to this underexplored research area by surveying recorded incidents in the health domain using the AIID as data source. The principal research question addressed by the survey is: *what characterises recorded incidents where the use of AI in healthcare has resulted in harm?* More specifically, the study aims to characterise the incidents in terms of the nature of the applications involved in the incidents as well as the nature of the harm inflicted. Research like this is needed in order to better understand the hazards of applying AI in a domain where the consequences of failure are potentially very severe, even fatal.

2 Materials and Methods

As a source of data on AI incidents, the AIAAIC is preferred by the most closely related previous work, particularly [10]. For this study, the AIID was selected because of its specific focus on AI incidents; the AIAAIC, as the name indicates, has a broader scope. The AIM was rejected because unlike the other two, it is not manually curated and suffers from issues such as duplicates and erroneously included incidents.

Besides using a different data source, this study differs methodologically from [10] to provide a complementary perspective on health-related AI incidents. The key differences are as follows:

- Only incidents involving the use of AI by organisations participating in the provision of health services are considered here. Other types of health-related AI incidents (e.g. ordinary individuals taking harmful medical advice from a general-purpose chatbot) are excluded.
- The studies have a partially different focus in terms of which aspects of the analysed incidents are considered; in particular, in this study the sector of deployment of the AI system is considered as one key characteristic of the incidents.
- Instead of using categorisations already present in the dataset, this study follows an approach where the categories are extracted inductively from the textual content of the database entries.

A search for relevant incidents was carried out in January 2026, at which time there were some 1300 incidents recorded in the AIID. For the search, a list of keywords was compiled, consisting of the following: health, medic* (for medicine, medical, medication), hospital, doctor, surg* (for surgeon, surgery, surgical), nurs* (for nurse, nursing), care, patient, diagnos* (for diagnose, diagnostic), treat* (for treat, treatment) and therap* (for therapy, therapist, therapeutic). By using a broad set of search terms relevant to the domain of interest, comprehensive coverage of relevant incidents was expected to be achieved.

The database was searched using each of the above terms in turn and the returned entries were classified based on their title and description as relevant, irrelevant or borderline. After the initial pass, the borderline cases were re-reviewed to determine whether they should be included; news articles about the incidents were consulted for additional details when necessary. The decision to include or exclude a given incident was made based on the application purpose and applier of the AI system involved, with no further discrimination done based on e.g. the type of the system or the nature of the harm inflicted.

The search and selection process resulted in a final dataset of 34 incidents reported between 1996 and 2025, listed in the Appendix. A single researcher (the author) read the AIID entries for the included incidents and inductively coded them to classify the incidents with respect to three aspects: the *sector* in which the incident occurred, the *purpose* for which the AI system was deployed and the ethical *requirement* violated. The results are presented in the next section.

3 Results

Table 1 presents a quantitative summary of the results of the analysis with respect to the sector where the AI system involved in the incident was deployed. As the table shows, the vast majority of the incidents fall into one of two categories: **patient care**, comprising hospitals and other such facilities, and **health administration**, comprising mainly government departments in charge of organising public healthcare. The other three categories have only 2–3 incidents each, with the unclear category used for incidents for which the sector could not be unambiguously determined from the information available in the database.

Table 1. Number of incidents by sector of deployment.

Sector	Incidents
Patient care	16
Health administration	11
Health insurance	3
Consumer products and services	2
Unclear	2

Table 2 presents a similar summary with respect to the purpose of the AI system. Six categories were identified here:

- **Resource allocation:** Systems designed to optimise the use of human, material or financial resources in healthcare; notable subcategories include allocation of medical practitioners' labour, distribution of vaccines and processing of insurance claims.
- **Medical practice:** Systems designed to help medical practitioners diagnose and/or treat patients more effectively.
- **Risk prediction:** Systems designed to assess the probability of various conditions or events occurring with patients.
- **Content authoring:** Systems designed to help produce various documents through prompting or speech-to-text conversion.
- **Advising:** Systems designed to interact with the user in natural language and provide advice on health-related topics.
- **Monitoring:** Systems designed to collect and analyse data over time to support decision-making or detect occurrences that require a response.

In the one uncategorised incident, the AI system was used to manage the IT infrastructure of a healthcare provider. Finally, Table 3 summarises the results of the analysis of the ethical requirements violated in the incidents. Four principal categories were identified:

- **Reliability:** The AI system fails to consistently produce outputs that are sufficiently accurate for the intended purpose of the system.
- **Fairness:** The AI system does not serve all subpopulations equally, performing more poorly for some races or ethnicities, for example.
- **Fundamental rights:** The AI system does not adequately protect individual rights such as privacy or autonomy.
- **Safety:** The AI system behaves in such a way that it poses a concrete threat to the health of patients or users.

There is some ambiguity in the classification, particularly among the reliability, fairness and safety categories. The fundamental rights category stands out

Table 2. Number of incidents by purpose of deployment.

Purpose	Incidents
Resource allocation	10
Medical practice	8
Risk prediction	7
Content authoring	4
Advising	2
Monitoring	2
Other	1

Table 3. Number of incidents by requirement violated.

Requirement	Incidents
Reliability	19
Fairness	8
Fundamental rights	4
Safety	3

as a more clearly distinct one, consisting of incidents involving data breaches, invasive monitoring and unethical research practices. Elements of more than one type of failure could be seen in several incident descriptions, but for the purposes of this overview study, it was deemed best to carry out a simple classification of the incidents based on what was perceived to be the principal failure type. As a result of this choice, transparency did not emerge in the analysis as a category, despite being a frequently raised concern in AI ethics.

4 Discussion

While the results give some indication of the relative frequency of different types of incidents, the generalisability of the results is necessarily limited by the fact that the coding was done by only one researcher. To reduce the inherent subjective element of this type of analysis, a more rigorous study with multiple coders should be carried out. For the current paper this was not feasible, but it can be justifiably argued that the results represent a valid perspective on the phenomenon studied and provide a starting point for further investigations.

The data is also likely to be biased in various ways, given that there are no guarantees that all relevant incidents will be included in the database. The AIID enables anyone to submit incident reports for review and possible inclusion in the database, but a URL pointing to a publicly available report (e.g. a news story) is required for each submission. This ensures that each candidate entry is backed up by evidence, but it also means that incidents of which no report has been published, such as those that have been covered up by the organisation(s) involved, are excluded by default. The AIAAIC follows a similar policy, only considering incidents that have already been covered by credible news outlets.

Even the definition of an AI incident is somewhat vague in practice; the AIID Editor's Guide defines it as "an alleged harm or near harm event to people, property, or the environment where an AI system is implicated", but many of the entries do not in fact pinpoint any specific event. For example, incident number 5 is actually a collection of thousands of cases where surgical robots have malfunctioned rather than an individual incident, and on the other hand, it is unclear whether AI actually played any role in controlling these robots. Under "About the Database", the AIID is compared to incident repositories in aviation and computer security, but the comparison is not entirely apt; the AIID could perhaps be better described as a collection of cases where AI systems have been associated with (near) harm in articles published by the mainstream media.

One notable indicator of possible bias in the data is the small number of incidents in the fundamental rights category. As seen in [11], data breach incidents in healthcare are certainly not uncommon, so it seems likely that there would be more such incidents involving healthcare AI specifically. Also interesting is the scarcity of incidents in the consumer products and services category, given the considerable popularity of consumer-oriented wellness AI products such as fitness and sleep trackers. In the health insurance category the number of incidents is likewise very small, but this may be at least partially explained by the sector being much more heavily regulated.

In this study the incidents were not classified by the severity of the harm inflicted, but a cursory examination of the incident descriptions corroborates the observation made in [10] that a substantial portion of the incidents are of high or critical severity. In three of the incidents, AI was explicitly linked with death: 5 (robotic surgery malfunctions, classification: patient care/medical practice/safety), 699 (gender bias in a suicide prevention algorithm, health administration/risk prediction/fairness) and 716 (algorithmic staffing failures in a care facility, patient care/resource allocation/safety). The diversity of categories shows that there are multiple different paths to potentially fatal harm, but no further analysis is feasible with such a small set of incidents.

For many incidents, assessing the level of harm is difficult because the AIID entry does not cite any concrete patient cases. Nevertheless, there is clearly significant potential for harm at the population level if, for instance, a bias in a medical AI system causes a serious condition to be underdiagnosed. It should be noted, though, that the issue of fairness is not ethically straightforward – it may be justifiable to deploy a system selectively for some groups rather than delay deployment until it performs equally well for the entire population, provided that the resulting inequity is addressed by other means [12].

Generative AI, though relatively recently popularised, already accounts for a significant subset of the incidents. In terms of the purpose categories in Table 2, all of the incidents in the content authoring and advising categories involve generative AI systems, and additionally there are some individual instances in other categories. In addition to these, there are the incidents involving "unofficial" use of generative AI e.g. for self-diagnosis; such cases were excluded from this study, but this should not be taken as a dismissal of the risks involved in this type of use. On the contrary, the increasing popularity of generative AI systems and the absence of expert supervision make it acutely important to monitor and mitigate the risks of individuals relying on them as sources of health-related information. While the systems may perform well against standard benchmarks, such performance does not automatically translate into good outcomes in real-world use [13], so there is a need for better understanding of how people actually interact with the systems and how this affects their safety as health consultants.

5 Conclusions

This paper presented a survey of incidents where the use of AI in healthcare has resulted in harm. Using the AI Incident Database as data source, 34 such incidents were discovered; these were characterised by examining the sector and purpose of deployment of the AI system and the principal ethical requirement violated in the incident. Almost 80% of the incidents occurred in the patient care and health administration sectors, with only a few incidents in other sectors such as health insurance. The most common purposes were resource allocation, medical practice and risk prediction, with these accounting for over 70% of the incidents. Reliability was the most frequently violated requirement, deemed to be the principal issue in more than half of the incidents.

Both the data used and the methodology applied are likely to have induced biases into the analysis results, and future work should address these to achieve more generalisable conclusions. While AI in healthcare promises great benefits to human wellbeing, it also introduces considerable risks, and effective mitigation of the risks requires that they are fully understood. Research on real-world AI incidents can yield valuable knowledge for this purpose, yet existing work in this area is scarce. Given the potential ethical and societal impact of AI systems in healthcare, more attention and effort should be directed here.

Appendix: AI Incidents Included in the Study

No.	Year	Title
5	2015	Collection of Robotic Surgery Malfunctions
42	1996	Inefficiencies in the United States Resident Matching Program
79	1999	Kidney Testing Method Allegedly Underestimated Risk of Black Patients
81	2020	Researchers find evidence of racial, gender, and socioeconomic bias in chest X-ray classifiers
91	2020	Frontline workers protest at Stanford after hospital distributed vaccine to administrators
104	2021	California's Algorithm Considered ZIP Codes in Vaccine Distribution, Allegedly Excluding Low-Income Neighborhoods and Communities of Color
110	2016	Arkansas's Opaque Algorithm to Allocate Health Care Excessively Cut Down Hours for Beneficiaries
123	2021	Epic Systems's Sepsis Prediction Algorithms Revealed to Have High Error Rates on Seriously Ill Patients
124	2019	Optum Algorithmic Health Risk Scores Reportedly Underestimated Black Patients' Needs
150	2018	Swedish Contraceptive App, Natural Cycles, Allegedly Failed to Correctly Map Menstrual Cycle
172	2020	NarxCare's Risk Score Model Allegedly Lacked Validation and Trained on Data with High Risk of Bias

(*continued*)

No.	Year	Title
173	2021	AI Tools Failed to Sufficiently Predict COVID Patients, Some Potentially Harmful
188	2018	Argentinian City Government Deployed Teenage-Pregnancy Predictive Algorithm Using Invasive Demographic Data
225	2017	IBM Watson for Oncology Criticized by Customers for Allegedly Unsafe and Inaccurate Cancer Treatment Recommendations
276	2022	Local South Korean Government's Use of CCTV Footage Analysis via Facial Recognition to Track COVID Cases Raised Concerns about Privacy, Retention, and Potential Misuse
449	2022	Startup Misled Research Participants about GPT-3 Use in Mental Healthcare Support
501	2019	Length of Stay False Diagnosis Cut Off Insurer's Payment for Treatment of Elderly Woman
535	2020	COVID-19 Detection and Prognostication Models Allegedly Flagged for Methodological Flaws and Underlying Biases
545	2023	Chatbot Tessa gives unauthorized diet advice to users seeking help for eating disorders
582	2023	Racial Bias in Lung Function Diagnostic Algorithm Leads to Underdiagnosis in Black Men
591	2023	Cigna Algorithm PXDX Allegedly Rejected Thousands of Patient Claims En Masse in Breach of California Law
603	2021	Algorithmic Allocation of Resources in Healthcare for Disabled and Elderly Care Services Allegedly Harming Patients
608	2023	UnitedHealth Accused of Deploying Allegedly Flawed AI to Deny Medical Coverage
685	2024	The WHO's S.A.R.A.H. Bot Reported to Provide Inconsistent and Inadequate Health Information
699	2024	VA Suicide Prevention Algorithm REACH VET Reportedly Prioritizes Men Over Women Veterans
716	2021	Algorithmic Staffing Failures Linked to Resident Deaths at Leading Assisted-Living Chain Brookdale
732	2024	Whisper Speech-to-Text AI Reportedly Found to Create Violent Hallucinations
827	2024	AI Transcription Tool Whisper Reportedly Inserting Fabricated Content in Medical Transcripts
1070	2025	Serviceaide AI Platform Implicated in Health Data Exposure Affecting 483,000 Catholic Health Patients
1084	2025	Federal 'Make America Healthy Again' Report Released with Multiple Reportedly Erroneous and Unverifiable Citations
1103	2025	Purported DOGE Contract Review Tool Cited in Reports of AI-Driven Misjudgments in VA Budget Cuts
1109	2021	Year-long AI Surveillance Pilot in Two South Australian Aged Care Facilities Reportedly Overwhelmed Staff with False Positives
1164	2024	Google Healthcare AI Model Med-Gemini Allegedly Produces Non-Existent 'Basilar Ganglia' Term in Published Output
1286	2025	Purportedly AI-Assisted Citation Errors Allegedly Found in Newfoundland and Labrador's 2025 Health Workforce Report by Deloitte

References

1. Kaul, V., Enslin, S., Gross, S.A.: History of artificial intelligence in medicine. Gastrointest. Endosc. **92**(4), 807–812 (2020). https://doi.org/10.1016/j.gie.2020.06.040
2. Mohammed, S., Malhotra, N.: Ethical and regulatory challenges in machine learning-based healthcare systems: a review of implementation barriers and future directions. BenchCouncil Trans. Benchmarks Stand. Eval. **5**(1), 100215 (2025). https://doi.org/10.1016/j.tbench.2025.100215
3. Ong, J.C.L., et al.: Ethical and regulatory challenges of large language models in medicine. Lancet Digit. Health **6**(6), e428–e432 (2024). https://doi.org/10.1016/S2589-7500(24)00061-X
4. The Responsible AI Collaborative: Artificial Intelligence Incident Database (nd). https://incidentdatabase.ai/. Accessed 29 Mar 2026
5. AIAAIC: AIAAIC Repository (nd). https://www.aiaaic.org/aiaaic-repository. Accessed 8 Jan 2026
6. OECD: OECD AI Incidents and hazards Monitor (nd). https://oecd.ai/en/incidents. Accessed 8 Jan 2026
7. Burema, D., et al.: A sector-based approach to AI ethics: Understanding ethical issues of AI-related incidents within their sectoral context. In: Proceedings of the 2023 AAAI/ACM Conference on AI, Ethics, and Society, pp. 705–714 (2023). https://doi.org/10.1145/3600211.3604680
8. Branley-Bell, D., Feiner, J., Prossnegg, S.: Ethical Implications of AI-Powered Chatbots: Considerations for the AI Act: A Case Study of Tessa. Jusletter IT, pp. 67–75 (2024). https://doi.org/10.38023/f8b4776d-12bd-4661-aadd-cf6e148ce73b
9. Denecke, K., Lopez-Campos, G., Rivera-Romero, O., Gabarron, E.: The unexpected harms of artificial intelligence in healthcare: reflections on four real-world cases. In: Healthcare of the Future 2025. Studies in Health Technology and Informatics, vol. 325, pp. 55–60 (2025). https://doi.org/10.3233/SHTI250219
10. Denecke, K., Lopez-Campos, G., May, R.: The unintended harm of artificial intelligence (AI): exploring critical incidents of AI in healthcare. In: MEDINFO 2025 — Healthcare Smart × Medicine Deep. Studies in Health Technology and Informatics, vol. 329, pp. 1013–1018 (2025). https://doi.org/10.3233/SHTI250992
11. Ugwu, A.O., Gao, X., Ugwu, J.O., Chang, V.: Ethical implications of AI in healthcare data: a case study using healthcare data breaches from the US Department of Health and Human Services breach portal between 2009–2021. In: 2022 International Conference on Industrial IoT, Big Data and Supply Chain (IIoTBDSC), pp. 343–349 (2022). https://doi.org/10.1109/IIoTBDSC57192.2022.00070
12. Vandersluis, R., Savulescu, J.: The selective deployment of AI in healthcare. Bioethics **38**(5), 391–400 (2024). https://doi.org/10.1111/bioe.13281
13. Bean, A.M., et al.: Reliability of LLMs as medical assistants for the general public: a randomized preregistered study. Nat. Med. **32**, 609—615 (2026). https://doi.org/10.1038/s41591-025-04074-y

Alternative Regulatory Strategies for AI Enabled Medical Devices in the EU

Alpo Värri[1(✉)] and Ilkka Juuso[2]

[1] Faculty of Medicine and Health Technology, Tampere University, Korkeakoulunkatu 3, 33720 Tampere, Finland
Alpo.Varri@tuni.fi
[2] SGS Fimko, Takomotie 8, 00380 Helsinki, Finland
ilkka.juuso@metavisual.fi

Abstract. The inclusion of artificial intelligence (AI) into the software of medical devices offers features that cannot be easily achieved by other means. To protect the health, safety and fundamental rights of the citizens in the European Union (EU), the European Parliament has approved the AI Act that regulates the use of AI within the EU. The AI Act introduces non-trivial requirements that apply to medical-device AI in parallel with the European Medical Device Regulation. Recently, the European Commission suggested revising the AI Act in a way that excludes medical devices from most of its discussion. This change appears to set the use of AI in different domains on separate paths, which in turn may leave manufacturers in uncertainty about how to address the requirements for products to be launched in the near future. This paper compares three different regulatory approaches to introducing AI-enabled medical devices to the market. The approaches differ in how thoroughly the manufacturer implements the requirements of the AI Act. As several international AI standards already exist, and many more are currently under late-stage development, it is advisable to consider what these standards can tell us the state of the art in the AI system design.

Keywords: Medical Devices · Artificial Intelligence · Regulation · AI Act

1 Introduction

The use of artificial intelligence (AI) in medical devices may provide functionality which is not easily provided via other means or at all. Training an AI model to a certain detection or classification task by using a large data set of labeled examples of past patient cases can result in a classifier that reaches a more accurate classification result than any deterministic rule set can achieve. The indeterministic behavior of AI models can, however, introduce risks which need to be managed appropriately. To protect the citizens of the European Union (EU) from unacceptable risks to health, safety and fundamental rights, the European Parliament has approved a law that imposes a lot of requirements particularly to the providers of high-risk AI systems, the AI Act in 2024 [1]. What is special in the AI Act is that it introduces requirements on how to protect the fundamental rights of citizens. The medical device manufacturers have not needed

M. Säreströniemi et al. (Eds.): NCDHWS 2026, CCIS 3010, pp. 438–444, 2026.
https://doi.org/10.1007/978-3-032-28819-6_28

to think about these aspects before and therefore every manufacturer should spend some time thinking and documenting about these.

The AI Act's definition of a high-risk AI system includes medical devices which are required to undergo a third-party conformity assessment which means medical devices in higher risk classes than one and in-vitro medical devices other than non-sterile Class A devices. The requirements for high-risk AI systems cover risk management, data and data governance, technical documentation, record-keeping, transparency and provision of information to deployers, human oversight, accuracy, robustness, cybersecurity, quality management system, documentation keeping, corrective actions, duty of information, cooperation with competent authorities, fundamental rights impact assessment, conformity assessment, CE marking, and registration of the product to an EU database. To make the requirements more concrete to follow, the EU Commission has issued a standardization request to the Joint technical committee 21 Artificial Intelligence of CEN and CENELEC to produce harmonized standards to the AI Act in ten areas of the above-mentioned requirements [2].

As the AI Act text is already available and the harmonized standards are expected to be published by the end of the year 2026, the manufacturers of the AI enabled medical devices know, in principle, what to do to get their products approved to the EU market. Another development, however, confuses the situation. In 2024, the European Parliament issued a request to the European Commission to alleviate the requirements of the EU medical device regulation in order to reduce the regulatory burden to medical device manufacturers [3]. The European Commission published its proposal to the European Parliament on 16.12.2025 [4]. This proposal included also a short change proposal to the AI Act, but this change was especially important to medical device manufacturers. It essentially proposes to lift the requirements introduced to high-risk AI systems from the medical device and in-vitro medical device manufacturers. The proposal would, however, give the possibility to the European Commission to issue implementation acts to re-introduce some part of high-risk AI system requirements to medical devices and in-vitro medical devices, too. It is necessary to mention that it is not yet certain that the European parliament and the Council will approve this 16.12.2025 proposal to change the AI Act in exactly this form. As the requirement alleviation request came from the EU Parliament itself, it would be logical that some form of alleviation would be approved by it, too.

2 Study Scenario

Given the above-mentioned regulatory uncertainty, the manufacturers of AI-enabled medical devices are left with the question, what will be the actual market entry and staying requirements for their products in the near coming years. What is certain is that the requirements of the Medical Device Regulation (MDR) [5] apply regardless of whether the device contains AI or not. The MDR requires that the design and manufacturing of the devices take into account the generally acknowledged state of the art. The question remains what the state of the art with respect to AI components of the devices is. This paper aims to address the regulatory approach in introducing an AI-enabled medical device into the EU market.

3 Results

3.1 Three Approaches to Conformity

Three alternative regulatory approaches are investigated here for medical device and in-vitro medical device manufacturers looking to include artificial intelligence features in their products.

3.1.1 Only the AI Regulation Applies

In this approach, the manufacturer assumes that only the AI Act applies to a medical device using artificial intelligence. For software that is not considered a medical device this would be a fair assumption, but for all other cases the manufacturer will soon discover that the assumption is false: all medical devices and in-vitro medical devices must meet the EU MDR and IVDR.

3.1.2 Both Regulations Apply in Full

In this approach, the manufacturer assumes that the requirements of the AI Act concerning high-risk AI systems will also apply as such to the medical devices of the manufacturer in full. The manufacturer then studies those articles in the AI Act carefully, acquires the set of harmonized standards to the AI Act and implements them.

The manufacturer must also address the fundamental rights of citizens in the context of its AI-enabled products. As this is a new topic for most existing and new medical device manufacturers this may mean engaging a consultancy for sufficient expertise.

If the manufacturer is new to medical devices, they will also similarly need to study the MDR or IVDR and meet the requirements therein. In effect they will need to develop their own synthesis of both regulations, fulfill the requirements of this synthesis, and stay current with new guidance for both regulations. The medical-device part of the equation is well known, and the AI part of the equation is currently evolving. If issues arise, they may come from collisions between the two domains, and it may not be immediately apparent which regulation takes precedence.

This approach leads to the least risk in passing conformity assessment activities of products, processes and documentation. The approach may, however, result in the highest resource expenditure or even the cancellation of product launch as some of the requirements are judged to be too costly or time-consuming to fulfill with a current product or the available training data for the AI model.

3.1.3 Something Borrowed and New

In this approach, the manufacturer assumes that fulfilling the requirements of the MDR will be sufficient for the regulatory approval of its products but that some new expectations may come out of the AI Act. The manufacturer assumes that the full set of high-risk AI system requirements will not be required from the AI-enabled medical devices, but that some additional requirements need to be taken into account. The manufacturer studies the requirements carefully, including the harmonized standards to the AI Act but does not fully implement them. To prepare for the conformity assessment, the manufacturer provides documentation where it lists all the requirements, how they have been addressed and records why certain requirements were not considered applicable to its AI-enabled medical device. The manufacturer does not seek external fundamental rights consultation but includes its own evaluation of the status of its products with respect to the fundamental rights. The manufacturer does, however, read the AI guidance from the Medical Device Coordination Group from June 2025 [6] and checks that its products and processes are compliant to it.

Similarly to the first approach, if the manufacturer is new to medical devices they need to learn and meet the requirements of the MDR or IVDR. The AI Act is an additional layer on top of the medical device expectations, but it is clear that the medical-device domain takes precedence over the AI domain, and thus any conflicts or uncertainties are resolved from that point of view.

The approach thus assumes that, for the most part, the manufacturing of AI-enabled medical devices will be business as usual – new expectations will be introduced, but these will always be applied to the existing medical-device framework and not an entirely new parallel system of expectations. The medical-device part of the equation is well known, and the AI part of the equation is currently evolving.

3.2 State of the Art Through Standards

In the above, we considered three different approaches to navigating the EU AI Act and the European Medical Device and In-Vitro Medical Device Regulations. In so doing, we came to the realization that while the framework of expectations for medical devices is at present quite well-established after several years of use, the expectations set for artificial intelligence are currently only taking shape. Thus, we need to merge both established and emerging thinking in some practical way.

A tool frequently used in medical devices, but not only there, to capture the evolving best practices around a specific topic is the concept of the state of the art. This concept refers to the commonly accepted best practice of accomplishing some task or running a specific activity, such as quality management, risk management, and clinical investigations. State of the art does not refer to the bleeding edge, or the very latest model for conducting some task, but instead it represents the consensus view of what is the right way to approach some task. This consensus view is quite naturally described in the international standards written by experts to represent the consensus view around a topic and the best way they see to structuring the activity under that topic. Typically, the standards used in this context are those which have been harmonized to a particular regulation, such as the EU MDR and IVDR, or as alluded to above, the EU AI Act. Note that for maximum applicability to AI-enabled medical devices, a standard should be harmonized to both EU MDR/IVDR and the AI Act. In the absence of harmonized standards, also other commonly accepted and used standards may qualify as a representation of the state of the art.

In identifying appropriate state of the art standards, a manufacturer should consider the evolving EU harmonization status of each document. The medical devices standards, for the most parts, come out of the ISO Technical Committee 210 which is also responsible for the global ISO 13485 standard on quality management and the ISO 14971 standard on risk management. The committee also produces guidance on how these industry standards are applicable to AI devices [7]. A great number of other AI-specific standards are developed by ISO and IEC Joint Technical Committee 1 Subcommittee 42 Artificial Intelligence [8] on topics including, for example, datasets, user interaction, transparency and governance. In addition to the above mentioned JTC 21, other standardization organizations to follow are HL7 [9] and IEEE [10, 11]. In fact, the number of AI standards is nowadays measured in hundreds, according to the AI Standards Hub [12].

In medical devices the core set of expectations is thus described by a handful of well-established medical device standards, while the emerging AI-specific standards are expected to provide further clarity on the best approaches within the topic AI. Thus, the state-of-the-art expectations for AI-enabled medical devices are also evolving. It should also be noted that each stakeholder—the manufacturer, the patients, the professional users, the notified body, the national competent authorities and the European Commission and Parliament will all have their own notions on what the state of the art is. In particular, the notified bodies are expected to assess a manufacturer's product in relation to that state of the art regardless of whether the manufacturer has labeled it state of the art or what standards they have claimed to observe. Thus, the question of what is the state of the art, and how a product or a manufacturer meets that definition, may be more pronounced than just which section of the AI Act medical devices fall under. State of the art, however, remains one of the most useful and practical concepts to track and apply for the sake safe and efficient devices and positive patient outcomes.

4 Discussion

The intentions of the EU AI Act are good, but fulfilling all its requirements is not trivial nor cheap to manufacturers whose products are classified as high-risk AI systems. It is not possible for lawmakers to foresee all the consequences of the requirements to all products that it affects. For this reason, it is important that there is sufficient flexibility in the requirements to allow simpler implementations when the thoroughly studied potential residual risks to health, safety and fundamental rights to the citizens are in reality minimal. It is hoped that this flexibility exists after the processing of the AI Act simplification proposal in the EU Parliament and the Council.

No manufacturer wants to see that their products hurt the patients due to the negligence of the manufacturer because it has all sorts of negative consequences to the reputation, legal status and finally profitability of the company. Manufacturers want to ensure the safety of the patients by fulfilling the requirements of the MDR or IVDR and that is often enough. Due to the novelty of the AI methodologies among the medical device design teams, some caveats may remain undetected by the manufacturers unless the state of the art is not studied sufficiently, for example from AI standards. This paper introduced some of these standards to begin with.

As the final form of the AI regulation for AI enabled medical devices is not yet available, it is important for the manufacturers to follow the legislation changes carefully. The reaction of the EU Parliament to the EU Commission AI Act change proposal is important. It is also important to follow the sentiments of the EU Commission about the need to issue implementation acts with the AI enabled medical devices and in-vitro medical devices in scope. The EU Commission's stand to sector specific "vertical" standards to the AI Act was negative in 2024, but the creation of an appropriately rigorous AI standard for medical and in-vitro medical devices may remove the need of an implementing act from the EU Commission. This standard could be developed, for example by CEN/TC251 Health informatics jointly with CENELEC/TC 62 Electrical equipment in medical practice. This standard could, instead of beginning from scratch, refer to (pieces of) other relevant AI standards.

It is worth noting that this paper has discussed medical devices that apply AI. The regulatory burden imposed by the AI Act is more dependent on the necessity of the notified body assessment than whether the device is regulated by the MDR or IVDR. There are other uses of AI in the health sector which are not medical devices. Many of these AI applications are not high-risk AI systems and then the regulatory requirements are much easier to comply with. Those AI systems that are kind of gatekeepers to health services may also fall into the high-risk class if the fundamental rights of the citizens are at stake.

5 Conclusions

The regulatory status of AI-enabled medical devices is currently somewhat uncertain and needs to be followed by the industry. In this situation the manufacturers can take various approaches to regulatory compliance. Whatever the result of AI regulation will be, the MDR requirement to apply the state of the art suggests the use of relevant standards in the design and governance of the AI enabled medical and in-vitro medical devices where they exist.

Disclosure of Interests. Author Värri is involved in standardization activities in CEN&CENELEC/JTC21 and CEN/TC251. Author Juuso is involved in standardization activities in CEN/TC251 and ISO/TC210 and works in a notified body although the thoughts expressed in this paper are not the official views of that notified body.

References

1. Regulation (EU) 2024/1689 of the European Parliament and of the Council of 13 June 2024 laying down harmonised rules on artificial intelligence and amending Regulations (EC) No 300/2008, (EU) No 167/2013, (EU) No 168/2013, (EU) 2018/858, (EU) 2018/1139 and (EU) 2019/2144 and Directives 2014/90/EU, (EU) 2016/797 and (EU) 2020/1828 (Artificial Intelligence Act). http://data.europa.eu/eli/reg/2024/1689/oj. Accessed 01 Feb 2026
2. European Commission C(2025)3871 - Standardisation request M/613, COMMISSION IMPLEMENTING DECISION of 23.6.2025 on a standardisation request to the European Committee for Standardisation and the European Committee for Electrotechnical Standardisation as regards high-risk AI-systems in support of Regulation (EU) 2024/1689 of the European Parliament and of the Council and repealing Implementing Decision C(2023)3215. https://ec.europa.eu/growth/tools-databases/enorm/mandate/613_en. Accessed 01 Feb 2026
3. European Parliament resolution of 23 October 2024 on the urgent need to revise the Medical Devices Regulation (2024/2849(RSP). http://data.europa.eu/eli/C/2025/485/oj. Accessed 01 Feb 2026

4. European Commission, Proposal for a regulation to simplify rules on medical and in vitro diagnostic devices, 16.12.2026. https://health.ec.europa.eu/publications/proposal-regulation-simplify-rules-medical-and-vitro-diagnostic-devices_en. Accessed 01 Feb 2026
5. Consolidated text: Regulation (EU) 2017/745 of the European Parliament and of the Council of 5 April 2017 on medical devices, amending Directive 2001/83/EC, Regulation (EC) No 178/2002 and Regulation (EC) No 1223/2009 and repealing Council Directives 90/385/EEC and 93/42/EEC. http://data.europa.eu/eli/reg/2017/745/2026-01-01/. Accessed 01 Feb 2026
6. MDCG 2025–6 Interplay between the Medical Devices Regulation (MDR) & In vitro Diagnostic Medical Devices Regulation (IVDR) and the Artificial Intelligence Act (AIA). June 2025. https://health.ec.europa.eu/medical-devices-sector/new-regulations/guidance-mdcg-endorsed-documents-and-other-guidance_en. Accessed 01 Feb 2026
7. ISO/TS 24971–2.2 Medical devices - Guidance on the application of ISO 14971, Part 2: Machine learning in artificial intelligence. https://www.iso.org/standard/87600.html. Accessed 01 Feb 2026
8. ISO/IEC JTC 1/SC 42 Artificial intelligence. https://www.iso.org/committee/6794475.html. Accessed 01 Feb 2026
9. HL7 AI. https://info.hl7.org/ai/. Accessed 01 Feb 2026
10. IEEE Autonomous and Intelligent Systems (AIS) Standards. https://standards.ieee.org/initiatives/autonomous-intelligence-systems/standards/. Accessed 01 Feb 2026
11. IEEE Artificial Intelligence Standards Committee. https://www.computer.org/volunteering/boards-and-committees/standards-activities/committees/artificial-intelligence-standards-committee/. Accessed 01 Feb 2026
12. AI Standards database. https://aistandardshub.org/ai-standards-search/. Accessed 01 Feb 2026

A HumanAI Digital Health Architecture for Scalable Visually Impaired People (VIP) Navigation

Babar Chaudary[1](✉), Petri Pulli[2], and Erkki Harjula[1]

[1] Faculty of Information Technology and Electrical Engineering, University of Oulu, Oulu, Finland
babar.chaudary@student.oulu.fi, erkki.harjula@oulu.fi
[2] Faculty of Technology, University of Oulu, Oulu, Finland
petri.pulli@student.oulu.fi

Abstract. Independent mobility is essential for autonomy and social participation among visually impaired people (VIP), yet most navigation aids remain device-centric and limited to isolated use. Rather than presenting new empirical results, this concept paper synthesizes longitudinal doctoral research to translate telepresence-based assistance into a scalable digital health service. We derive evidence-driven requirements and propose a HumanAI service architecture emphasizing continuity, structured handover, multi-caretaker coordination, and human-in-the-loop AI across an edge–cloud continuum. Navigation assistance is reframed as a longitudinal service that adapts to context, supports mentor–apprentice learning, and integrates community-based support. A user-centered evaluation framework is outlined to guide future real-world validation.

Keywords: digital health · edge–cloud continuum · handover · human-in-the-loop AI · mentor–apprentice learning · service architecture · telepresence · trust · visual impairment

1 Introduction

Visual impairment affects over two billion people globally and poses major challenges to independent living and social inclusion. Beyond clinical vision loss, difficulties in safe and confident navigation limit access to education, employment, healthcare, and public services, making independent mobility a key determinant of autonomy, dignity, and wellbeing [1–3].

Existing assistive navigation solutions—including smart canes, wearables, and mobile applications—primarily address obstacle detection or route guidance [4–8]. While effective in controlled settings, they often struggle in dynamic, socially complex environments where prioritization and interpretation are required [9]. Telepresence-based systems mitigate some limitations by enabling remote human assistance [10–12], yet typically rely on single-helper models and lack support for continuity, structured

M. Särestöniemi et al. (Eds.): NCDHWS 2026, CCIS 3010, pp. 445–454, 2026.
https://doi.org/10.1007/978-3-032-28819-6_29

handover, and learning over time. As a result, social factors such as trust, responsibility boundaries, and helper transitions remain underrepresented, limiting scalability and long-term adoption [13].

This paper translates longitudinal telepresence-based VIP navigation studies into evidence-driven requirements and a scalable HumanAI digital health architecture emphasizing continuity, structured handover, and multi-actor coordination.

This paper makes the following contributions: (i) reframing VIP navigation as a service-oriented digital health problem, (ii) proposing a HumanAI architecture enabling introducing a formalized zone–tier mapping framework, multi-actor coordination, and structured handover, (iii) introducing a formalized zone–tier mapping framework linking user context to system layers, and (iv) outlining a feasibility-oriented evaluation framework grounded in longitudinal observations.

The paper is structured as follows. Section 2 reviews related work and synthesizes longitudinal empirical findings from prior field studies. Section 3 presents the proposed HumanAI telepresence service architecture, including assistance orchestration and handover mechanisms. Section 4 outlines an evaluation plan aligned with functional, non-functional, and ethical requirements. Section 5 discusses implications for digital health transformation and concludes with directions for future research and deployment.

The empirical foundations of this work are drawn from prior longitudinal studies, and the proposed architecture represents a concept-driven design whose implementation and validation are part of future work.

2 Background: Existing Work and Empirical Foundations

2.1 Assistive Technologies for Visual Impairment

Assistive technologies and telepresence-based systems represent two complementary but distinct approaches to navigation support for VIP. Assistive mobility technologies span electronic travel aids, smart canes, wearable sensors, and mobile navigation applications. These systems focus on obstacle detection, route guidance, or object recognition and can improve situational awareness. However, reviews highlight persistent challenges related to robustness, usability, and real-world adoption, particularly in dynamic environments where semantics and safety-critical decisions matter [6–9].

Telepresence-based navigation systems enable a remote helper to provide real-time assistance through audio and video, leveraging human interpretation in ambiguous or socially complex situations [10–12]. While user experience can be positive, scalability remains limited due to helper availability, single-session designs, and insufficient support for multi-helper coordination and handover. Ethical, trust-related, and responsibility-boundary challenges further complicate large-scale deployment [13].

Table 1 compares existing approaches with the proposed HumanAI architecture, highlighting key differences across assistive technologies, telepresence systems, multimodal navigation, and digital health services.

Table 1. Comparison of assistive-device approaches, telepresence systems, and the proposed HumanAI service architecture, synthesized from prior reviews and digital-health service literature [4–9, 11]

Feature	Assistive Devices	Telepresence Systems	Proposed HumanAI Architecture
Assistance model	Device-centric	Single-helper	Multi-actor, service-oriented
Continuity over time	Limited	Session-based	Continuous, longitudinal
Multi-caretaker support	✗	✗	✓ (structured handover)
AI role	Detection/recognition	Minimal	Decision support (human-in-the-loop)
Context adaptation	Limited	Human-driven	Adaptive (AI + human)
Scalability	Device-bound	Helper-limited	Community + service scaling
Architecture	Standalone	Ad hoc	Local–Edge–Cloud continuum

2.2 Empirical Findings from Longitudinal Field Studies

This section primarily synthesizes longitudinal field studies conducted in prior longitudinal research on telepresence-based navigation assistance for visually impaired people [10, 14], complemented by relevant findings from the broader literature to situate and validate these observations.

Our longitudinal field studies indicate that acceptance of ICT-based navigation assistance among VIP is strongly shaped by individual needs, preferences, and context [10–14]. Adoption is higher when solutions align with everyday goals, adapt to users' capabilities, and demonstrate clear value in real settings, consistent with prior evaluations of electronic mobility aids emphasizing usability and perceived benefit [15]. The literature further highlights participatory and inclusive design approaches as critical for long-term relevance and uptake [16, 17].

Navigation assistance is inherently socio-technical and rarely an individual-only activity but is embedded within social routines and support networks. Studies on remote support show that sustained use depends not only on the primary user but also on the engagement and availability of support persons [9], aligning with the findings that caretakers' willingness to adapt routines materially influences feasibility and continuity of use [10, 14].

Table 2. Environment-aware zone model. Person in need of Assistance denotes the person receiving assistance i.e., VIP; Mentors are fully capable caretakers; Apprentices are trainee caretakers; Peer-Apprentices are VIPs learning assistance skills; Peer-Mentors are experienced caretakers acquiring new skills.

Role	Control Zone(Home/Office)	Familiar Zone	Discover Zone
Person in need of Assistance	Needs help in introduction to new space	Needs help if environment changes	Requires continuous assistance
Peer-Apprentice	Assists if available	Assists if available	Assists in familiar zone and learn
Peer-Mentor	No need	No need	Provides Assistance
Apprentice	Always assists	Always assists	Provides assistance and learn
Mentor	Assigns tasks to Peer-Apprentice	Assigns tasks to Peer-Apprentice	Mentors apprentice, Peer-Apprentice
Research Environment	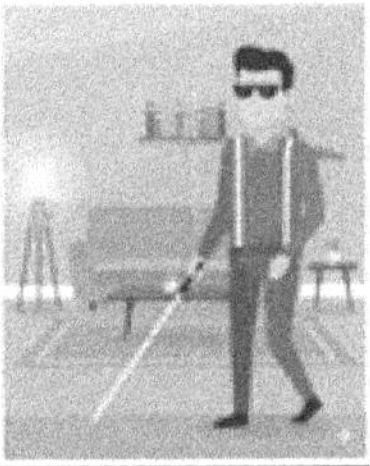	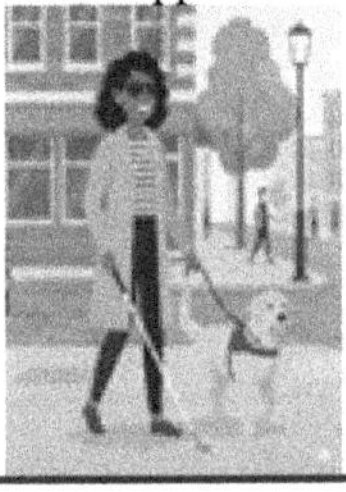	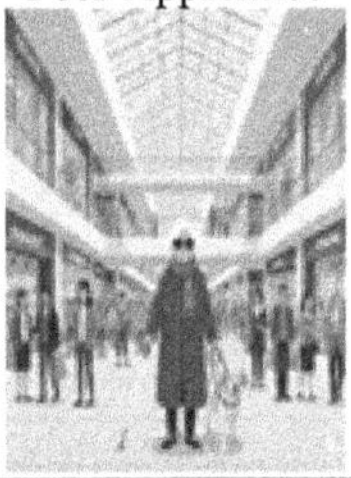

Assistance needs are highly context-dependent. Environmental and infrastructural factors significantly affect mobility, particularly in complex public spaces [18–20]. Longitudinal observations similarly showed that lighting, ambient noise, weather, and crowd density influence indoor and outdoor navigation differently. To structure this variability, the zone model in Table 2 links environmental familiarity to assistance intensity and escalation needs [10–14]. These observations are also consistent with guided participation and progressive skill development described in situated learning theory [24]. These role–zone relationships directly inform the service requirements in Sect. 2.4, particularly regarding adaptive assistance intensity, role allocation, and structured escalation across contexts. Prior reviews of multimodal navigation systems also emphasize context-sensitive modality selection and adaptive feedback for visually impaired users [21].

2.3 AI, Connectivity, and Edge–Cloud Technologies in Digital Health

The empirical findings in Sect. 2.2 imply infrastructure that supports real-time, adaptive, and trustworthy assistance. In digital health, AI is increasingly positioned as decision support rather than autonomous control to preserve human agency and accountability [22, 23, 25]. Wireless connectivity (4G/5G and emerging 6G) enables low-latency telepresence [26], while edge–cloud architectures support latency-sensitive processing near the user and longer-term coordination at the service level [27–31]. Distributed ledger technologies can further support auditable identity, consent, and session traceability for multi-actor assistance, complementing privacy and accountability requirements [32]. These technologies are rarely integrated into service-oriented designs grounded in longitudinal empirical use, motivating the architecture in Sect. 3.

2.4 Design Implications and Service Requirements

The findings indicate that effective navigation assistance for VIP should be designed as a service-oriented solution rather than a standalone device, supporting continuity over time. Such services must accommodate multi-actor involvement (family members, volunteers, professionals) and provide structured handover mechanisms to preserve contextual information during transitions. Assistance should adapt dynamically to environment and user state through multimodal interaction, while AI should function as a supporting and filtering component that preserves human oversight in safety-critical situations. Effective systems must also facilitate learning and increasing autonomy rather than permanent reliance on external support. Edge- and cloud-based healthcare services raise regulatory and deployment challenges related to privacy, accountability, and traceability [32], as well as large-scale deployment and integration [28–31].

Based on these implications, a scalable digital health service must support real-time bi-directional interaction, coordination among multiple helpers, and context-aware handover. Non-functional requirements include low latency, high reliability across environments, and robustness to network disruptions. Ethical and accessibility requirements include user consent, preservation of user agency, avoidance of cognitive overload, inclusive design, and clearly defined responsibility boundaries [13, 22, 23, 25, 31]. In contrast to prior device-centric and single-helper approaches, the proposed architecture explicitly integrates continuity, multi-actor coordination, and service-level orchestration, addressing key scalability and adoption limitations identified in existing systems.

3 Proposed Architecture: From Evidence to Digital Health Service Design

Based on the empirical requirements identified in Sect. 2—particularly the need for continuity, handover, and adaptive assistance—this section translates those findings into a concrete service architecture. The focus is on translating these constraints into architectural principles, system components, and orchestration mechanisms that support continuous assistance, multi-actor coordination, and adaptive HumanAI collaboration within a service-oriented digital health framework. This translation ensures traceability from empirical findings to architectural design decisions.

3.1 Conceptual HumanAI Assistance Model

The proposed assistance model follows a HumanAI cooperative paradigm in which the VIP remains the primary decision-maker. Human caretakers provide contextual interpretation and adaptive guidance in dynamic or unfamiliar environments, while AI functions as decision support within a human-in-the-loop paradigm supporting perception, information filtering, and prioritization without assuming autonomous control.

Assistance is continuous across environmental zones and over time. Guided by the validated zone-based model, assistance intensity and modality adapt to environmental familiarity and situational complexity. Repeated assisted navigation supports skill acquisition and confidence building, enabling a mentor–apprentice dynamic in which external support gradually decreases as user independence increases [24].

Scalability is achieved by integrating community and volunteer-based assistance alongside professional care, with clear roles and coordination to ensure accountability and availability. AI supports perception, prioritization, and routine context inference (e.g., scene summarization and anomaly detection), while decision authority remains with human caretakers. This distributes assistance capacity without replacing human judgment, enabling scalable and trustworthy HumanAI cooperation.

3.2 System Architecture

Service-Oriented Architectural Overview. As shown in Fig. 1, the architecture follows a three-tier design integrating intelligent local devices, edge computing, and cloud-based learning and analytics [11, 28]. Data processing originates at the Local tier and propagates toward Edge and Cloud for aggregation and learning, while assistance feedback flows downward from Cloud and Edge to Local devices for real-time user interaction. Table 3 formalizes the mapping between environment-aware user zones (Control, Familiar, Discover) and system tiers (Local, Edge, Cloud), clarifying how assistance logic and responsibility shift with contextual complexity. The design remains technology-agnostic at the component level to support heterogeneous deployments, with feasibility assessed through service-level KPIs (Sect. 4). From a system perspective, latency-sensitive processing is distributed to local and edge tiers (typically sub-100 ms), while cloud resources handle delay-tolerant learning and coordination. Bandwidth demands are managed through adaptive streaming and event-driven updates, enabling scalable operation under varying network conditions.

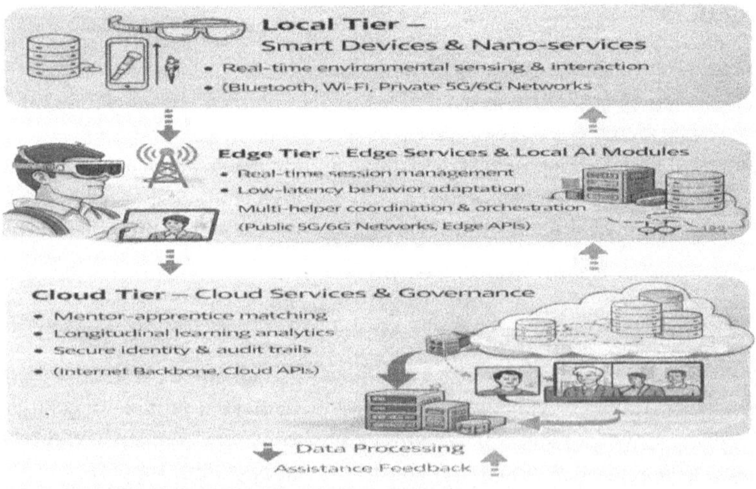

Fig. 1. HumanAI telepresence service architecture

Table 3. Dynamic mapping of user context zones to system tiers, illustrating the distribution of responsibilities across Local, Edge, and Cloud layers.

User Zone	Typical Context	Primary Tier	Key Functions
Control Zone	Predictable indoor spaces (home, workplace)	Local Tier	Real-time sensing, immediate feedback; edge coordination; cloud learning
Familiar Zone	Nearby outdoor or semi-structured environments	Edge Tier	Low-latency coordination; local sensing; cloud aggregation
Discover Zone	Unfamiliar, complex environments	Cloud Tier	Learning, analytics, identity; edge adaptation; local sensing

The zone–tier relationship is not a fixed one-to-one mapping but a dynamic distribution of responsibilities across all tiers. In each zone, Local, Edge, and Cloud tiers participate concurrently with varying functional emphasis depending on environmental complexity. The Local tier ensures real-time sensing and immediate interaction, the Edge tier supports low-latency coordination and adaptive processing, and the Cloud tier enables long-term learning, global coordination, and secure service management. This dynamic allocation allows the system to adapt to contextual demands while maintaining responsiveness, scalability, and continuity of assistance.

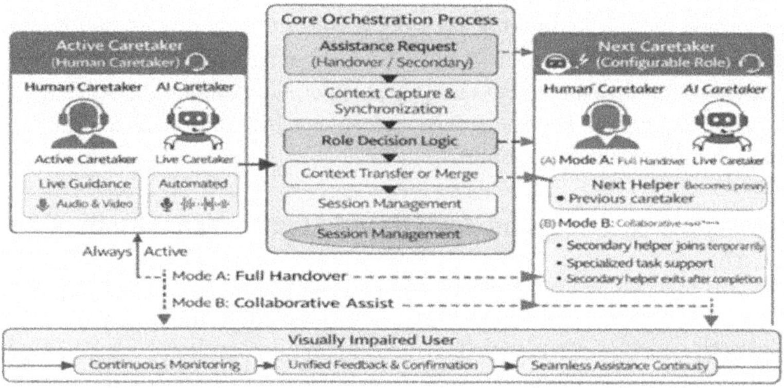

Fig. 2. Orchestration workflow for full and collaborative assistance handover.

Assistance Orchestration and Handover. Assistance orchestration is implemented as a unified, role-aware process supporting both full handover and collaborative assistance (Fig. 2). Contextual information—including environmental state, task progress, and interaction history—is synchronized at handover to preserve continuity. Users receive unified feedback regardless of caretaker transitions, reducing perceived disruption and supporting scalable HumanAI collaboration.

Data Flow, Security, and Accountability. Secure data exchange, identity management, and accountability mechanisms support trust and regulatory compliance [12]. Access control is role-based across VIPs and caretakers, with encrypted communication channels and auditable session logs. Distributed ledger mechanisms support identity verification, consent tracking, and traceability in multi-actor interactions.

4 Evaluation Plan

The evaluation plan defines a methodology for future validation of the proposed architecture, focusing on measurable service-level outcomes aligned with functional, non-functional, and ethical requirements. Functional performance is evaluated through indoor and outdoor field trials using realistic navigation tasks, with KPIs including task completion rate, time-to-completion, guidance errors, handover success rate, and continuity loss events during caretaker transitions. These KPIs capture whether assistance enables safe and efficient navigation, maintains continuity across transitions, and supports user trust and perceived usefulness.

Non-functional properties are assessed via end-to-end delay, interruption frequency/duration, recovery time under degraded connectivity, and helper availability under constrained conditions, as these directly affect perceived safety and confidence during navigation.

Ethical and accessibility requirements are evaluated through usability studies and qualitative interviews, complemented by standardized instruments where appropriate. KPIs include perceived control, trust in human and AI caretakers, cognitive workload, and perceived safety, as these dimensions capture how assistance is experienced rather than merely delivered. Longitudinal assessments track changes in autonomy, assistance frequency, and user confidence over time, providing evidence of learning effects and gradual reduction of dependency. As a concept paper, the evaluation emphasizes service feasibility, continuity, and user-perceived outcomes rather than clinical efficacy, which would require a separate, ethics-approved trial.

5 Discussion: Implications for Digital Health Transformation

This work reframes navigation assistance from a standalone assistive device into a distributed, service-oriented digital health system integrating human support, AI assistance, and networked infrastructure [4, 5, 23, 25]. While developed for VIP navigation, the underlying principles—human-in-the-loop decision making, continuity of support, and scalable service orchestration—are transferable to other assistive and care domains such as cognitive support, elderly care, and remote rehabilitation. By grounding architectural design in validated longitudinal empirical insights, the proposed framework provides a practical blueprint for deploying trustworthy, continuity-aware HumanAI services within future digital health ecosystems. The proposed approach has limitations, including reliance on network connectivity, the need for scalable caretaker coordination, and the absence of prototype validation at this stage. Practical deployment also requires addressing regulatory, ethical, and user adoption challenges in real-world digital health ecosystems. Future work will focus on large-scale real-world validation and deeper integration with public digital health infrastructures.

Acknowledgements. This paper was partially supported by the 6G Flagship programme (Grant No. 369116) funded by the Research Council of Finland. The work builds on doctoral research conducted at the University of Oulu within the OASIS research group. The authors gratefully acknowledge the contribution of visually impaired participants and caretakers.

References

1. World Health Organization: World Report on Vision. WHO, Geneva (2019)
2. European Commission: Digital Health and Care in the EU. European Commission (2020)
3. World Health Organization: Global Strategy on Digital Health 2020–2025. WHO, Geneva (2022)
4. Nguyen, H.N., Lasa, G., Iriarte, I., Atxa, A., Unamuno, G., Galfarsoro, G.: Human-centered design for advanced services: a multidimensional design methodology. Adv. Eng. Inform. **53**, 101720 (2022)
5. Kvedar, J.C., Fogel, A.L., Elenko, E., Zohar, D.: Digital medicine's march on chronic disease. Nat. Biotechnol. **34**(3), 239–246 (2016)
6. Bhowmick, A., Hazarika, S.M.: An insight into assistive technology for the visually impaired and blind people: state-of-the-art and future trends. IEEE Rev. Biomed. Eng. **10**, 195–207 (2017)
7. Reyes-Cruz, G., Fischer, J.E., Reeves, S.: Demonstrating interaction: the case of assistive technology. ACM Trans. Comput.-Hum. Interact. **29**(5), 1–37 (2022)
8. El-Taher, F.E.-Z., Taha, A., Courtney, J., McKeever, S.: A systematic review of urban navigation systems for visually impaired people. Sensors **21**(9), 3103 (2021)
9. Buchholz, M., Holmgren, K., Ferm, U.: Remote communication for people with disabilities: support persons' views on benefits, challenges, and suggestions for technology development. Technol. Disabil. **32**(2), 69–80 (2020)
10. Anonymous: Teleguidance-based remote navigation assistance for visually impaired and blind people: usability and user experience. Virtual Reality **27**(1), 141–158 (2023)
11. Almeida, L., Menezes, P., Dias, J.: Telepresence social robotics towards co-presence: a review. Appl. Sci. **12**(11), 5557 (2022)
12. Niemelä, M., Van Aerschot, L., Tammela, A., Aaltonen, I., Lammi, H.: Towards ethical guidelines for using telepresence robots in residential care. Int. J. Soc. Robot. **13**(3), 431–439 (2021)
13. Shneiderman, B.: Human-Centered AI. Oxford University Press, Oxford (2022)
14. Anonymous: Developing an ICT-based navigation assistance system for blind and visually impaired people. Doctoral Dissertation, University of Oulu (2022)
15. Roentgen, U.R., Gelderblom, G.J., Soede, M., de Witte, L.P.: User evaluation of two electronic mobility aids for persons who are visually impaired: a quasi-experimental study. Assist. Technol. **24**(4), 258–271 (2012)
16. Hersh, M.: The design and evaluation of assistive technology products and devices. Disabil. Rehabil.: Assisti. Technol. **8**(4) (2013)
17. Desmond, D., Layton, N., Bentley, J., et al.: Assistive technology and people: a position paper from the GREAT summit. Disabil. Rehabil. Assist. Technol. **13**(1), 1–6 (2018)
18. Montarzino, A., Robertson, B., Aspinall, P., et al.: The impact of environmental factors on the mobility of people with sight loss. Vis. Impair. Res. **9**(2), 67–85 (2007)
19. Barlow, J.M., Bentzen, B.L., Bond, T.: Blind pedestrians and complex signalized intersections: crossing behavior and alignment. Transp. Res. Rec. **1918**, 41–49 (2005)

20. Bentzen, B.L., Barlow, J.M., Franck, L.: Addressing orientation and mobility challenges at intersections for pedestrians who are blind. J. Vis. Impairment Blindness **98**(6), 347–362 (2004)
21. Kuriakose, B., Shrestha, A., Sandnes, F.E.: Multimodal navigation systems for users with visual impairments: a review. Multimodal Technol. Interact. **4**(3), 48 (2020)
22. Floridi, L., et al.: AI4People—an ethical framework for a good AI society. Mind. Mach. **28**, 689–707 (2018)
23. Amershi, S., et al.: Guidelines for human–AI interaction. In: Proceedings of the 2019 CHI Conference on Human Factors in Computing Systems. ACM (2019)
24. Lave, J., Wenger, E.: Situated Learning: Legitimate Peripheral Participation. Cambridge University Press, Cambridge (1991)
25. Okamura, K., Yamada, S.: Adaptive trust calibration for human–AI collaboration. PLoS ONE **15**(2), e0229132 (2020)
26. Saad, W., et al.: A vision of 6G wireless systems: applications, trends, technologies, and open research problems. IEEE Netw. **34**(3), 134–142 (2020)
27. Shi, W., et al.: Edge computing: vision and challenges. IEEE Internet Things J. **3**(5), 637–646 (2016)
28. Anonymous: Optimizing resource-aware service orchestration in edge–cloud continuum. In: 2025 IEEE Intelligent Mobile Computing (MobileCloud), pp. 44–50. IEEE (2025)
29. Kamruzzaman, M.M.: New opportunities, challenges, and applications of edge-AI for connected healthcare in smart cities. In: Proceedings of the IEEE Globecom Workshops (2021)
30. Rahmani, A.M., et al.: Exploiting smart e-health gateways at the edge of healthcare Internet of Things. Futur. Gener. Comput. Syst. **78**, 641–658 (2018)
31. Rancea, A., Anghel, I., Cioara, T.: Edge computing in healthcare: innovations, opportunities, and challenges. Future Internet **16**(9), 329 (2024)
32. European Union: General Data Protection Regulation (GDPR), Regulation (EU) 2016/679

Comparative Analysis: AI and Large Language Models in Healthcare - Tools for Professionals, Support for Citizens

Syed Ifham Qadri[1], Syed Rameem Zahra[1], Juha Röning[2], and Brejesh Lall[3](✉)

[1] Centre For Artificial Intelligence and Machine Learning, Sher-E-Kashmir University of Agricultural Sciences and Technology of Kashmir (SKUAST-K), Shalimar, Srinagar 190025, Jammu & Kashmir, India
[2] Biomimetics and Intelligent Systems Group, University of Oulu, 90014 Oulu, Finland
[3] Electrical Engineering Department, Indian Institute of Technology Delhi, New Delhi 110016, India
brejesh@ee.iitd.ac.in

Abstract. In healthcare sector, since the integration of large language models we are clear that it requires separate tools for professional clinic support and citizen assistance. So, in this paper we introduce a 5 phase deployment framework that alliance with these tools and with clinical risk levels. Professional diagnostic models like Med-PaLM 2 reach its 86.5% accuracy on USMLE like test, which surpasses human experts while intelligence solutions such as DAX copilot reduces documentation workload by 50% shows studies from 2023–2026. With 70% to 71% performance, age oriented, Probabilistic systems, like ADA health, focus on sensitivity to ensure safe escalation. Recent data shows we can cut hallucinations in generated content by over 40% with the help of RAG (Retrieval-Augmented Generation). With FDA's evolving predetermined change control plan (PCCP) and integrating these tech technologies give us a strategy for US healthcare to address the estimated $760 billion to $935 billion annual waste.

Keywords: Large Language Models (LLMs) · Healthcare AI · Professional Clinical Tools · Citizen Support Systems · 5-Phase Deployment Framework · Retrieval-Augmented Generation (RAG) · FDA Regulation

1 Introduction

Due to rising expenses, unstable workforce and unequal access to service, the modern healthcare system currently is facing polycrisis. Studies suggest that approximately 25% of total healthcare spending in United States which is between $760 billion and $935 billion is annually wasted [1]. This inefficiency is mainly caused by administrative complexity and failures of care delivery. Electronic Health Record (EHR) documentation consumes approximately two hours of a clinician's day for everyone over of direct patient care also physicians burnout rate has hovered near 50% leaving a sustained

M. Säreströniemi et al. (Eds.): NCDHWS 2026, CCIS 3010, pp. 455–466, 2026.
https://doi.org/10.1007/978-3-032-28819-6_30

strain on current human infrastructure of medicine [2]. Still AI has emerged as two distinct operational domains, each with unique performances risks and regulatory impact as response to these structural failures. Below, Table 1 shows a comparative analysis between the professional and citizen AI domains, highlighting their distinct user bases, operational goals, and regulatory pathways.

Table 1. Comparative Analysis of Professional vs. Citizen AI Domains.

Feature	Professional Clinical Tools	Citizen Support Systems
Primary User	Licensed Clinicians, Health Systems	Patients, Consumers
Operational Goal	Precision, Efficiency, Liability Management	Accessibility, Triage, Engagement
Key Metric	Diagnostic Accuracy (Specificity)	Triage Sensitivity (Risk Aversion)
Interaction Model	Human-in-the-loop (Augmentation)	Human-out-of-the-loop (Autonomous)
Regulatory Path	Class II (510k)/Class III (PMA)	Class I/Enforcement Discretion/Class II
Example Tools	Med-PaLM 2, DAX Copilot, GatorTron	Ada Health, Woebot, K Health

In this paper, using evidence from major clinical trials alongside regulatory filings, we propose a 5 phase deployment framework outlining how healthcare systems can progress from basic administrative automation to for more sensitive use of autonomous diagnostic agents. The choice of diagnostic accuracy as the primary metric for professional tools reflects the high-stakes clinical environment where false negatives carry serious liability. Triage sensitivity, on the other hand, is prioritised in citizen-facing systems because these tools operate without a physician present meaning the cost of missing a serious condition is higher than the cost of over referral. Patients too benefit from sensitivity focused design at this stage, as the goal is safe escalation rather than definitive diagnosis.

2 Professional Clinical Tools: The Era of the Augmented Physician

The professional domain mainly focuses on two objectives. One epistemic argumentation which is improving diagnostic reason and second operational efficiency which is reducing administrative burden so their validation relies on rigorous benchmarking against human standards.

2.1 Epistemic Engines: Med-PaLM 2 and Diagnostic Precision

Standard for medical AI competency has shifted from simple to complex clinical reasoning. Google Med-PaLM 2 is current best in this area. Google Med-PaLM 2 was made using a novel refinement promoting strategy which pass medical licensing exams unlike others and in controlled evaluations against MedQA dataset it achieve 86.5% accuracy and significantly surpasses human passing threshold which is approximately 60% [3]. It is first time an AI system has demonstrated performance comparable to expert test takers. As it did good in multiple choice accuracy but to check its clinical utility the generation of nuanced, safe and helpful long form answers are required. A panel of board certified physicians evaluated responses from Med-PaLM 2 against those generated by human physicians in an comparative study involving 1066 consumer medical questions and they preferred AI response over human physicians on 8 out of 9 evaluation axis, including scientific consensus, reasoning, quality, and low likelihood of harm [3].

2.2 Diagnostic Dialogue: The AMIE System

While Med-PaLM 2 perform good on static questions but clinical practice doesn't work that way, patient care is far more conversational and is often shaped by uncertainty. The articulate medical intelligence explorer (AMIE) was developed to handle the uncertainty and was involved in taking patients history. Its performance was assessed in a randomised, double blind crossover study using simulated patient actors, where AMIE was evaluated against board-certified primary care physicians (PCPs) [4]. The results showed that AI performance was statically better and specialist physicians rated AMIE higher the PCPs on 28 out of 32 clinical quality measures [4]. These measures covered areas like accuracy of the differential diagnosis, management decisions, communication, empathy. It also showed top 3 diagnostic accuracy, pointing to a lower tendency towards premature closure, a common cognitive bias in clinical decision making.

2.3 Operational Intelligence: DAX Copilot and the ROI of Time

Due to regulatory caution, the diagnostic AI remained largely in research phases but operational AI has already seen widespread commercial use. Nuance's DAX copilot (dragon ambient experience) is an example which uses ambient clinical intelligence, it listens to patient provider conversations turning them into structured clinical documentation with minimal clinical input. According to an industry report by Microsoft and Northwestern Medicine, data collected from real world use across thousands of clinicians show that DAX Copilot reduces documentation time by 50%, that means in a busy primary care practice approx. Seven minutes are saved per patient visit. Beyond the time savings 70% of users reported lower levels of burnout and fatigue [5]. Below, Table 2 summarizes the economic and operational impact of ambient clinical intelligence, illustrating the return on investment and time savings.

Table 2. Economic and Operational Impact of Ambient Clinical Intelligence

Metric	Outcome
Documentation Time	50% reduction (~7 min/visit)
Return on Investment	112% ROI (Year 1)
Patient Access	+5 appointments/provider/month
Revenue Capture	+3.4% Level of Service (LOS) coding
Clinician Burnout	70% reduction in fatigue feelings

However, the results are not same every time. However, an independent study published in NEJM Catalyst at Atrium Health found no short term productivity gains after rollout, this suggests that AI functions as a capacity creator, but realising ROI depends on whether organisations restructure workflows to utilise that newly available time [6].

2.4 Clinical NLP and Data Mining: GatorTron

Researchers at University of Florida developed GatorTron which is a large clinical language model trained on over 90 billion words of text to unlock insights from unstructured text in electronic health records (EHR's) which is in petabytes [7]. GatorTron gave superior performance in named entity recognition (NER) and relation extraction (RE) achieving an F1 score of 0.89964 for extracting clinical concepts and 0.96274, identifying drug adverse event relations [7]. These results clearly out form general domain models like BERT, proving that domain specific pretraining plays a critical role in achieving reliable performance in healthcare data mining.

3 Citizen Support Systems: Democratizing Triage and Therapy

The citizen domain follows a different logic prioritising scalability and safety in the absence of physician. As patients use these tools before consulting anyone, they must be highly sensitive to minimise the risk of missed serious illness.

3.1 Probabilistic Triage: Ada Health

ADA health takes a different approach from pure generative LLM, instead it relies on probabilistic reasoning that aims on safety and explainability. With a user base of over 14 million, the system draws on a large diverse pool of real world data. In a peer reviewed study published in rheumatology, Ada's triage performance was directly compared with that of a physician and it correctly identified inflammatory rheumatic disease with 71% sensitivity compare to 60% for primary care physicians [8]. Ada listed the correct diagnosis as its best suggestion in 54% of cases while physicians did it for 32% of cases. Similar results were seen in a separate emergency department study where Ada had the final discharge diagnosis within its top five suggestions in 70% of cases [9]. It was similar and closely matched to the average sensitivity of three independent board certified emergency physicians reviewing the same case. These results also suggested that modern symptom checkers are not experimental tools, and they appear mature enough to function as reliable tool for triage patients.

3.2 Digital Therapeutics: Woebot

Same as human therapist, Woebot creates a therapeutic relationship with user in just 3-5 days of use, it falls into the category of digital therapeutics or DTX software designed to treat diseases [10]. It has shown reduction in symptoms of depression and anxiety across range of populations in randomise controlled trials. Acknowledging woebot's potential to address a serious condition with limited treatment options, the US FDA granted woebot a designation of breakthrough device for its postpartum depression program [11].

3.3 Virtual Primary Care: K Health

K health has a massive dataset of anonymous medical records for comparisons. A large study published in mayo clinic proceedings: digital health, in which 102059 virtual patients were analysed and was found that AI generated differential diagnosis matched the clinicians final diagnosis in 84.2% of cases [12]. In early 60.9% of cases the clinician choose top ranked suggestion from AI and found no significant bias in performance across patient, age, gender, or ethnicity, suggesting Robust training data diversity. Below, Table 3 provides a side-by-side comparison of the key performance benchmarks for leading models in both the professional and citizen domains.

Table 3. Performance Benchmarks of Leading Medical AI Models [3, 4, 7, 8, 12].

Model	Domain	Primary Task	Key Performance Metric
Med-PaLM 2	Professional	Diagnostic QA	86.5% Accuracy (USMLE)
AMIE	Professional	Diagnostic Dialogue	Superior to Physicians on 28/32 axes
GatorTron	Professional	EHR Extraction	0.8996 F1 Score (NER)
Ada Health	Citizen	Symptom Triage	71% Sensitivity (Rheumatology)
K Health	Citizen	Primary Care	84.2% Provider Agreement

4 Technical Mitigation: The Hallucination Challenge and RAG

Hallucination is the confident generation of false and fabricated information, which is the biggest and main technical barrier in the adoption of generative AI in diagnostic decision support. Baseline studies suggest that without safeguard general purpose LLM's can hallucinate in more than 40% of complex clinical scenarios. However, to address this Retrieval-Augmented Generation (RAG) is a standard solution which rather than relying on what the model has learned during training, forces it to retrieve trusted knowledge base before generating an answer. Figure 1, illustrates the comparative efficacy of these architectures, highlighting the substantial error reduction achieved when moving from zero-shot models to RAG implementations.

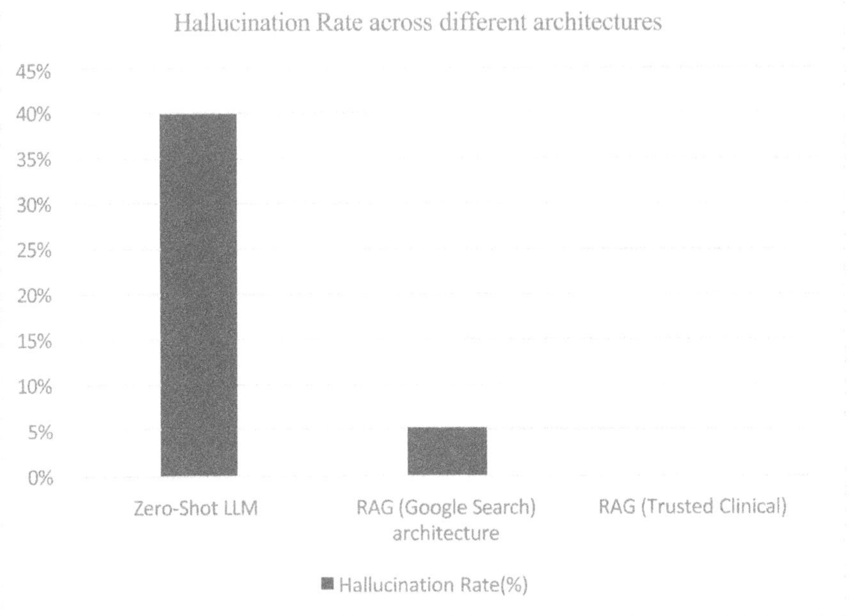

Fig. 1. Drastic reduction in medical hallucination rates when shifting from standard Large Language Models to Retrieval-Augmented Generation (RAG) grounded in trusted clinical databases [13, 14].

5 Algorithmic Bias and Health Equity

A valid deployment framework must consider how AI may enforce existing healthcare disparities. Study published in BMC, medical informatics and decision making (2025) looked at gender bias in summaries of long term care records produced by open source LLM's and found substantial variation across models. While Meta's Llama 3 showed no difference based on gender but Google Gemma produced summary and was using direct language for male patients while softening or omitting needs for female patients. This form of allocation harm where biased representations can influence decisions about care and resources must be mitigated through rigorous bias auditing [15, 16].

6 The 5-Phase Deployment Framework

Based on the performance metrics and risk profiles analysed above, we propose a phased deployment roadmap. Figure 2 illustrates this deployment roadmap, mapping the progression from low-risk administrative automation to high-stakes clinical autonomy.

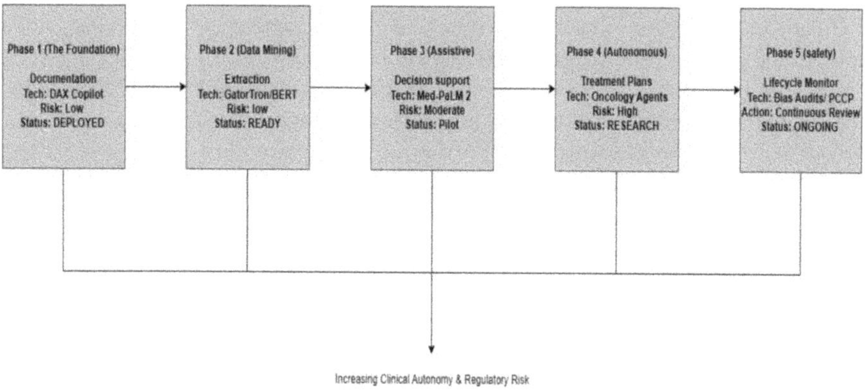

Fig. 2. The 5-Phase Deployment Framework for Clinical AI

- **Phase 1: Documentation & Administration (Immediate Deployment).** Technologies like DAX Copilot carry low clinical risk because they are purely administrative and always reviewed by a physician. With a validated 50% reduction in documentation time and potential for 112% ROI, this phase addresses the immediate burnout crisis [5].
- **Phase 2: Information Extraction & Synthesis (Year 1).** Tools like GatorTron can be deployed to mine existing EHR data for population health insights and to generate patient summaries. With F1 scores exceeding 0.89, these tools offer high reliability for retrospective analysis [7].
- **Phase 3: Assistive Diagnostic Decision Support (Years 2–3).** This phase involves the deployment of high performance models like Med-PaLM 2 as second opinions. Given the 86.5% accuracy benchmarks, these tools are capable of supporting clinicians but require human in the loop protocols and FDA Class II clearance [3].
- **Phase 4: Autonomous Triage & Treatment Planning (Years 3–5).** This phase involves systems like MEREDITH (Matching and Enabling Research and Evidence-based Drug Initiatives for Treatment in Haematology), an oncology clinical trial matching system developed to align patients with suitable treatment protocols using structured clinical data. Because hallucinations in treatment dosing can be fatal, this phase requires error rates below 0.1% and likely FDA Class III approval [17].
- **Phase 5: Continuous Monitoring & Lifecycle Management (Ongoing).** This phase aligns with the FDA's 2025 guidance on Predetermined Change Control Plans (PCCP), requiring manufacturers to monitor real world performance for concept drift and bias [18].

Across all five phases, the patient perspective must remain central. As AI involvement increases from Phase 1 to Phase 5, patients' trust, safety, and care experience become progressively more critical to monitor. In early phases, patients are largely unaffected by backend automation. However, from Phase 3 onward, where AI influences diagnostic suggestions, health systems should incorporate patient reported experience measures and informed consent protocols to ensure transparency about AI involvement in their care.

To contextualise this framework within existing literature, Table 4 provides a comparative analysis against three related frameworks: the AI Maturity Roadmap published in NEJM AI [18], the Healthcare AI Governance Readiness Assessment (HAIRA) published in npj Digital Medicine [19], and a systematic review of AI-CDSS implementation frameworks [20]. The key differentiator of our framework is its explicit bifurcation of professional and citizen AI domains, direct mapping of clinical risk to regulatory class per phase, and its grounding in LLM-specific performance benchmarks rather than general organisational maturity.

Table 4. Comparison of Proposed 5-Phase Framework with Existing Clinical AI Deployment Frameworks

Criterion	This Work	AI Maturity Roadmap (Microsoft/NEJM AI, 2024) [19]	HAIRA Model (npj Digital Medicine, 2026) [20]	AI-CDSS Implementation Review (PMC, 2024) [21]
Phases/Levels	5 Phases	5 Levels	5 Levels	4 Groups
Risk Stratification	Yes Low to High per phase	Partial	Partial	No
Regulatory Alignment	Yes FDA Class I/II/III + PCCP	No	Yes EU AI Act + FDA	Partial
LLM/GenAI Specific	Yes	Partial	No	No
Professional vs. Citizen Split	Yes explicit	No	No	No
Bias / Health Equity	Yes	Partial	Yes	Partial
Patient Perspective	Partial	No	Partial	No
Validation Type	Evidence-based review	Industry (50 + systems)	Systematic review	Narrative review

7 Analysis and Comparison to State of the Art

The data provided points to a gap between the performance of this framework and that of state of the arts and is usually defined in medical AI research. Majority of the existing literature tends to evaluate large language models as a single category which includes benchmark studies on GPT-4 on the USMLE primarily focusing on their ability to retrieve and reproduce medical knowledge. Our analysis indicates that "state of the art" is not fixed, but context dependent, splitting along two axes on one side clinical accuracy, and safety requirements of triage on other.

7.1 The Precision-Accessibility Trade-Off

Current state-of-the-art models like Med-PaLM 2 have reached 86.5% accuracy in professional licensing exams and that level of performance clearly exceeds the human expert threshold, our analysis points to a gap that is often neglected in academic benchmarks, strong diagnostic accuracy doesn't always mean safe patient triage. The difference becomes clear when these benchmarks are compared with citizen facing tools like Ada Health and its 71% sensitivity is lower than that of Med-PaLM's exam performance. This difference isn't failure of technology but a feature of design. Citizen-facing systems are built to prioritize recall so they catch every potential emergency even if that means being less precise about the final diagnosis. Unlike general purpose models like GPT-4 which may hallucinate a benign diagnosis for a serious condition, specialized probabilistic triage systems like Ada sacrifice specificity to maintain a safety net which aligns with the recent findings by Cen z et al regarding emergency department triage [3, 8, 9].

7.2 Hallucination Mitigation: RAG vs. Fine-Tuning

Until recently the default way to improve medical AI was to fine tune the model on more medical data like textbooks, guidelines, examples. Our meta analysis suggests that this strategy has largely run its course and even heavily fine tuned systems still hallucinate in roughly 5–10% of complex clinical cases. Across the studies we reviewed, including Chen .j et al (2025), the strongest gains come not from adding knowledge to the model but from changing how it reasons. Retrieval-Augmented Generation (RAG) marks a clear shift away from relying solely on what a model remembers. This change is structural instead of trusting internal weights alone, RAG forces models to validate their outputs against external trusted sources at inference time. Implementing RAG reduces hallucination rates from baseline levels near 40% to below 5% and this pattern is consistent with findings from the MEGA-RAG framework and points to a broader conclusion for Phase 3 diagnostic support architecture matters more than model size hence a smaller model paired with RAG can outperform a larger model operating without it [13].

7.3 Regulatory Realism vs. Theoretical Benchmarks

Much of the current literature focuses on human level performance as the end goal. Our 5 phase framework argues that this is the wrong target for deployment. Recent guidance from the FDA on Predetermined Change Control Plans (PCCP) points in the same direction suggesting that ma naging how a system evolves over time matters more than locking in a single static accuracy score [18]. While academic papers acknowledge a static score of 86.5% but real world state of the art depends on continuous monitoring for concept drift and demographic bias. Our findings on gender bias in models such as Gemma underscore this gap, headline accuracy numbers can easily hide allocational harm [15]. Therefore true SOTA is not defined by a USMLE benchmark but by systems that include ongoing bias auditing and lifecycle management as laid out in Phase 5 of the framework.

8 Regulatory Landscape

The FDA regulates medical AI under its software as a medical device, SaMD framework. Most diagnostic support tools including ADA health fall into class II requiring 510(k) clearance by demonstrating substantial equivalence to existing device and high risk diagnostic systems are likely to face class III premarket approval. Recent FDA guidelines on predetermined change control plans PCCPs gives flexibility allowing AI models to be updated over time without a new regulatory submission of every change as long as updates stay within an agree protocol which is essential for maintaining the relevance of AI models as medical knowledge evolves [18]. For deployments within the European Union, the regulatory landscape is governed by two complementary instruments. The EU Medical Device Regulation (MDR 2017/745) classifies AI based diagnostic software under the same risk tiered framework as physical medical devices, requiring clinical evaluation and post-market surveillance proportionate to risk class. Layered above this, the EU Artificial Intelligence Act (2024) introduces a horizontal risk framework specifically targeting AI systems, designating medical AI as high risk and mandating transparency, human oversight, and conformity assessments prior to deployment. For the Nordic healthcare context in particular, compliance with both MDR and the AI Act will be a prerequisite for any clinical AI deployment from Phase 3 onward [22][23].

9 Conclusion

The integration of AI into healthcare is not a singular event but a bifurcated process. Professional tools like Med-PaLM 2 and DAX Copilot are ready to address the nearly $1 trillion efficiency gap and offering expert level reasoning with substantial relief from administrative burden [3][5]. Meanwhile, citizen facing tools like Ada Health provide scalable triage with sensitivity comparable to physicians but only when they are kept within carefully defined safety limits. To bridge the gap between potential and practice, healthcare systems must adopt RAG architectures to mitigate hallucinations and adhere to a 5-Phase Framework that respects the distinct regulatory and safety requirements of each domain [13].

Disclosure of Interests. Authors declare no conflict of interest.

References

1. Shrank, W.H., Rogstad, T.L., Parekh, N.: Waste in the US Health care system: estimated costs and potential for savings. JAMA **322**(15), 1501–1509 (2019)
2. Sinsky, C., Colligan, L., Li, L., et al.: Allocation of physician time in ambulatory practice: a time and motion study in 4 specialties. Ann. Intern. Med. **165**(11), 753–760 (2016)
3. Singhal, K., et al.: Toward expert-level medical question answering with large language models. Nat. Med. **31**, 943–950 (2025)
4. Tu, T., et al.: Towards conversational diagnostic AI. arXiv preprint arXiv:2401.05654 (2024)
5. Microsoft & Northwestern Medicine. Northwestern Medicine Outcomes Study: DAX Copilot. Internal Epic Signal Data Report (2024)

6. Atrium Health. Impact of DAX on Provider Productivity and Satisfaction NEJM Catalyst (2024)
7. Yang, X., et al.: GatorTron: a large clinical language model to unlock patient information from unstructured electronic health records. arXiv preprint arXiv:2203.03540 (2022)
8. Knitza, J., et al.: Diagnostic accuracy of Ada and rheport: a randomized controlled crossover trial. Rheumatology **63**(4) (2024)
9. Cen, Z., et al.: Diagnostic accuracy of an ai symptom checker in the emergency department. JMIR Mhealth Uhealth **10**(9), e38364 (2022)
10. Fitzpatrick, K.K., Darcy, A., Vierhile, M.: Delivering cognitive behavior therapy to young adults with symptoms of depression and anxiety using a fully automated conversational agent (woebot): a randomized controlled trial. JMIR Ment. Health **4**(2), e19 (2017)
11. Woebot Health. Woebot Health Receives FDA Breakthrough Device Designation for Digital Therapeutic for Postpartum Depression. Business Wire (2021)
12. Zeltzer, D., et al.: Diagnostic accuracy of artificial intelligence in virtual primary care. Mayo Clin. Proc.: Digit. Health **1**(4), 480–489 (2023)
13. Xu, Y., et al.: MEGA-RAG: retrieval-augmented generation for medical question answering. arXiv preprint arXiv:2502.15040 (2025)
14. Chen, J., et al.: Benchmarking hallucinations in medical RAG systems. JMIR Cancer **11**, e70176 (2025)
15. Rickman, S., et al.: Evaluating gender bias in large language models for social care documentation. BMC Med. Inform. Decis. Mak. **25**, 45 (2025)
16. Zack, T., et al.: Assessing the potential of GPT-4 to perpetuate racial and gender biases in health care: a model evaluation study. The Lancet Digit. Health **6**(1), e12–e22 (2024)
17. Steele, B., et al.: Using natural language processing and machine learning to identify breast cancer local recurrence. BMC Bioinform. **22**(S1), 58 (2021)
18. FDA. Marketing submission recommendations for a predetermined change control plan for artificial intelligence-enabled device software functions. Guidance for Industry (2025)
19. The Health Management Academy, Microsoft & Nuance. The AI Maturity Roadmap: A Framework for Effective and Sustainable AI in Health Care. NEJM AI (2024)
20. Hussein, R., et al.: Advancing healthcare AI governance through a comprehensive maturity model based on systematic review. NPJ Digit. Med. **9** (2026)
21. Peek, N., Capurro, D., Rozova, V., van der Veer, S.N.: Bridging the gap: challenges and strategies for the implementation of artificial intelligence-based clinical decision support systems in clinical practice. Yearb. Med. Inform. **33**(1), 103–114 (2025)
22. European Parliament. Regulation (EU) 2017/745 on medical devices. Official Journal of the European Union (2017)
23. European Parliament. Regulation (EU) 2024/1689 laying down harmonised rules on artificial intelligence (Artificial Intelligence Act). Official Journal of the European Union (2024)

From Compatibility to Adoption: Unpacking the Psychological Mechanisms Mediating Human-AI Interaction in the UAE Healthcare Sector

Loubna Saad Saoud[1(✉)] and Omer Aftab Qureshi[2]

[1] The British University in Dubai, Dubai, United Arab Emirates
22001908@student.buid.ac.ae
[2] Adjunct Faculty Marketing and AI, Abu Dhabi University, Abu Dhabi, United Arab Emirates
Omer.i-adjunct@adu.ac.ae

Abstract. This study investigates the factors influencing the adoption of AI systems in the healthcare sector, with a focus on perceived human–AI compatibility (PHAIC) and the mediating roles of explainable AI (EXP), AI anxiety (AIA), and human–computer trust (HCT), as well as the moderating effect of speciesism (SP). Adopting a quantitative approach, the study draws on validated scales from prior literature through a survey of 287 healthcare professionals across hospitals in the United Arab Emirates (UAE). The findings reveal that while PHAIC positively influences explainability, trust, and anxiety, it does not directly affect AI adoption. Instead, emotional and relational factors particularly HCT and AIA serve as key mediators driving adoption. The results emphasize that clinicians' trust and emotional readiness are more critical than compatibility alone in fostering adoption behavior. Although explainability improves trust and reduces anxiety, its influence on adoption is indirect. Notably, speciesism did not demonstrate a significant moderating effect, suggesting that personal biases toward human versus AI systems play a limited role in healthcare adoption. These findings provide practical implications for developers and policymakers aiming to improve AI integration in clinical environments by emphasizing transparency, trust-building, and user-centered design.

Keywords: Artificial intelligence · Perceived human-AI compatibility · Human-computer trust · AI anxiety · AI explainability · Speciesism

1 Introduction

The integration of Artificial Intelligence (AI) into healthcare presents considerable potential for improving diagnostic accuracy, operational effectiveness, and overall patient care. The effective adoption of AI technologies relies not just on their technical ability but also on users' perceptions, emotional responses, and trust in these systems [1]. In the evolving data-centric healthcare environment, the perceived compatibility between people and AI systems is a crucial determinant influencing adoption decisions. Recent studies

M. Särestöniemi et al. (Eds.): NCDHWS 2026, CCIS 3010, pp. 467–489, 2026.
https://doi.org/10.1007/978-3-032-28819-6_31

emphasize the increasing significance of cognitive, emotional, and relational elements in determining AI acceptance [2, 3]. This paper presents a conceptual framework wherein Perceived Human–AI Compatibility acts as a primary antecedent to AI Adoption in healthcare sector in the UAE, mediated by three essential mechanisms: AI Anxiety, Explainable AI, and Human–Computer Trust (HCT). These mediators are represented in this study as the psychological, informational, and trust-related dynamics that either encourage or prevent user involvement with AI systems.

Drawing on the Technology Acceptance Model 3 (TAM3), the framework includes user-related factors such as anxiety and compatibility to clarify behavioral intents about AI. The model also utilizes Human–Computer Trust Theory [4] to highlight trust as a mediating variable, underscoring users' perceptions of the competence and integrity of AI systems. This work incorporates trust calibration theory to enhance that perspective, emphasizing the significance of system transparency and feedback in synchronizing user trust with actual system performance [5, 6]. This study particularly incorporates speciesism as a moderating variable. Speciesism, characterized as a bias favoring human intelligence over machine cognition, may affect users' perceptions, evaluations, and eventual adoption of AI technologies in medical settings. This ethical and socio-psychological element provides a new perspective for analyzing human-AI interaction [6, 7].

This study aims to examine the factors influencing the adoption of AI in healthcare, particularly focusing on the role of perceived human–AI compatibility, and the mediating effects of explainability, trust, and anxiety, as well as the moderating role of speciesism. To achieve this aim, the study suggested the following objectives:

1. To investigate the impact of perceived human–AI compatibility on AI adoption in healthcare.
2. To examine the mediating roles of explainable AI, human–computer trust, and AI anxiety in the relationship between compatibility and adoption.
3. To assess the moderating effect of speciesism on the relationship between the AI anxiety and explainability with AI adoption.
4. To provide theoretical contribution and practical implication in the context of AI adoption.

1.1 Significance of Study

Despite the growing integration of AI assistant diagnosis in treatment in clinical practice, healthcare practitioners remain cautious about embracing new technologies due to concerns over algorithmic capacity, explainability, data security, and legal accountability [8]. Previous research has mainly focused on behavioral characteristics such as trust and social impact, even within restricted clinical circumstances, so constraining wider applicability. It frequently disregards essential factors such as perceived risk and task-technology alignment, and it categorizes healthcare personnel as a homogeneous group, overlooking variations in role-specific perceptions. Moreover, the emotional and ethical dimensions of AI adoption are insufficiently addressed. Significant issues, including job displacement in highly automatable jobs, persist as primary sources of public anxiety [9]. In healthcare, ethical issues persist, particularly regarding AI assuming human responsibilities and managing personal health data [10]. Studies suggest that public trust in AI is closely influenced by factors like transparency, unbiased decision-making, regulatory clarity, and data protection [10, 11]. For instance, although certain research has explored state anxiety during AI interaction, they have not considered the effects of these emotions on long-term trust or adoption outcomes, nor has it investigated mediators like explainability or perceived competence [12]. Likewise, research concerning anxiety and dependency in adoption of AI has been conceptual and lack application in high-stakes domains like healthcare [13]. Investigations into explainable AI have often been tailored to specific professions, such as examining nurses and their innovation behavior, while neglecting its wider psychological impact across diverse clinical roles or on adoption intent [14]. These gaps highlight the need for a more holistic, ethically anchored, and psychologically informed framework for understanding AI adoption in healthcare.

2 Literature Review

2.1 AI in Healthcare Sector

Healthcare systems are constantly evolving to accommodate epidemiological, demographic, and social changes, with the objective of delivering cost-effective, efficient care in all regions [15]. These endeavors embrace the incorporation of innovative technologies such as AI for diagnostics, emergency response readiness, and preventive health programs. To facilitate this transformation, systems allocate resources to IT infrastructure, clinical trials, process optimization, and change management [16]. Healthcare is being transformed by artificial intelligence, specifically through machine learning (ML) and deep learning (DL), which allows for sophisticated diagnostics, improves medical imaging, and facilitates surgical procedures. [17] conducted a systematic review that underscored the potential of AI to enhance clinical decision-making and advance precision medicine by means of data insights and automation. Nevertheless, the enigmatic nature of AI models, which are frequently referred to as "black boxes" is a significant impediment to their widespread adoption. This is because they are not interpretable. This opacity is a contributing factor to the hesitation of healthcare providers and patients to accept AI-generated outcomes without perceiving the underlying rationale [18]. The UAE healthcare sector has made substantial progress in the integration of AI, particularly in the areas of predictive analytics, patient monitoring, and diagnostics [19].

2.2 Human-AI Compatibility

AI systems have been developed to operate according to specified goals, usually set by professionals, making the alignment of AI aims with human values a significant issue [20, 21]. Early AI work, grounded on cybernetics, embraced a comprehensive, interdisciplinary methodology but subsequently became constrained by military and corporate pressures. The difficulty of integrating human goals into AI systems, defined by Russell as the standard framework of AI, makes it essential for resolving human–AI compatibility [20]. Human-AI compatibility refers to the development of systems that are aligned with human values and objectives, ensuring they serve the interests of humanity without causing intentional or unintentional harm regardless of their level of intelligence [20]. [22] presents a new model for designing beneficial AI systems based on three basic concepts. First, AI systems should be fundamentally benevolent, aiming exclusively to satisfying human needs are inquiries. Second, they must exhibit humility by recognizing initial uncertainty around such preferences and deferring to human input as required. Third, AI must continuously acquire knowledge about human values by observing human behavior, using it as the principal source for understanding and responding to human requirements. These concepts are foundational to ensuring human–AI compatibility and ethical alignment in intelligent system design.

The progression of AI system design has shifted from a focus on technological performance to ethical and human-centered principles, leading to the emergence of Human-Compatible AI. This approach emphasizes the alignment of AI systems with human values, fostering individual and social welfare through equity, transparency, and governance [22]. The initial stages of AI development concentrated on Interpreted AI, which aimed to improve transparency and user comprehension of AI decisions [23]. Nonetheless, explainability alone was insufficient for addressing wider ethical issues such as bias and justice [24]. The notion of Socially Responsible AI emerged to address these limitations, seeking to reduce bias and enhance justice and trust in AI systems [25]. However, fairness is frequently established at a societal level, failing to consider individual variances in beliefs, needs, and cultural contexts crucial components for authentic human-centered design. These limitations have prompted the development of Human-AI Compatibility, which aims to align AI systems not only with ethical standards but also with individual human experiences [22].

2.3 Artificial Intelligence Anxiety (AIA)

AIA has developed as a unique psychological construct, expanding on established concepts such as computer anxiety and robot anxiety, which have been thoroughly examined in previous studies [26, 27]. Although previous studies have offered significant insights into technology-related anxieties, the specific features and effects of AIA are still insufficiently explored. AIA is characterized as a general emotional reaction characterized by anxiety or fear that prevents users from interacting with AI technologies [28]. It is considered as a multidimensional belief system rather than a situational or behavioral reaction, and current research treats it as an independent variable, independent from its antecedents or consequences. [29] defines AI as a system capable of thinking and acting both humanly and rationally, suggesting that anxiety toward AI may be more complicated than traditional computer fear. Computer anxiety itself is defined as the apprehension experienced when anticipating the use of computers [30].

2.4 AI Explainability

AI explainability (EXP) refers to the practice of making AI systems more understandable to humans by offering transparent explanations of their behavior [31]. Although the terms explainability sometimes used interchangeably in technical domains, possess significant differences. Explainability generally aims to make AI decisions transparent and understandable to end-users [32]. Perceived explainability is considered a crucial element in building initial trust in AI systems. Research in the social sciences highlights its mediating function between system affordances and user outcomes, especially in algorithmic contexts [33]. However, limited attention has been given to how users form perceptions of explainability before engaging with AI. In the healthcare sector, full transparency concerning AI system's operations may not always be accessible. [34] introduces the concept of contestability, asserting that explanations should not only clarify decisions but also enable users to challenge and potentially revise incorrect outputs.

2.5 Human Computer Trust Theory

Human–Computer Trust (HCT) refers to individuals' willingness to trust on AI systems for decision-making [35]. Trust is considered an attitudinal intention that affects technology acceptance by decreasing perceived risks and increasing perceived benefits [36]. In healthcare, studies show that perceived trust significantly predicts professionals' intention to adopt AI diagnostic tools [8, 36, 37]. As AI introduces new dynamics into medical settings, HCT has expanded beyond typical provider-patient relationships to include human–technology interaction [37]. Both user perceptions such as competence and risk influence the development of trust, forming a critical component in AI adoption [38].

2.6 Technology Acceptance Model 3 (TAM3)

The Technology Acceptance Model (TAM) was originally developed to predict individuals' adoption and use of information technologies. It suggests that behavioral intention is primarily influenced by two key beliefs: perceived usefulness that refers to the belief that using a technology improves job performance and perceived ease of use, which holds that using the technology involves minimal effort. TAM3 states that individuals' views of ease-of-use perceptions initially formed by their general computer beliefs, which are then adjusted through hands-on experience. Perceived usefulness can be shaped by social influence through compliance, identification, and internalization but perceived ease of use is more significantly influenced by individual characteristics and feelings, such as computer self-efficacy, computer playfulness, and computer anxiety. The impact of general notions like anxiety tends to decrease with time as people gain expertise. Rather, perceptions and usage behavior are shaped more by system-specific elements like objective usability and perceived enjoyment [39]. This study used TAM3 because it offers a strong theoretical foundation for understanding how individual experience, beliefs, and behavioral factors such as AI anxiety influence the adoption and application of intelligent technologies.

2.7 McKnight Trust Model

[4] offered a comprehensive model of trust building, identifying three key predictors of trust in technology adoption: disposition to trust, institution-based trust, and interpersonal trust. The Disposition to trust refers to an individual's general tendency to rely on others. Institution-based trust incorporates beliefs in supportive structures rather than

people and is composed of two key dimensions: structural assurance and situational normality [40]. Structural assurance indicates trust in institutional safeguards, such as legal frameworks or technological safety that maintain security and reliability in technology adoption [41]. In contrast, situational normality is the idea that the environment appears stable [42], routine, and predictable, supporting trust in that context [4]. Interpersonal trust focuses on trust beliefs acquire via interpersonal connection and includes four subdimensions: competence, benevolence, integrity, and predictability. Competence is the belief that the system has the essential capabilities to meet user needs, while benevolence reflects the perception that the system was developed with the user's best interests in mind. Integrity entails believing that the system behaves honestly and respects its commitments. Lastly, predictability refers to the belief that the system's behavior is predictable and consistent over time [43]. Recent studies have adopted this theory due to its relevance in the context of AI adoption [44, 45].

2.8 Trust Calibration Theory

Trust can be evaluated in terms of calibration, which refers to the alignment of an individual's trust in a system with the system's real trustworthiness or capabilities [46]. [47], using interpersonal trust literature, describes trustworthiness as an entity's capacity, benevolence, and honesty. Trust calibration has been extensively explored in the context of automation and AI to determine if users effectively change their trust based on system performance [48]. Researchers differentiate between dispositional trust, which is developed because of previous trust-related experiences, and history-based trust, which is formed through direct involvement with a particular system. As consumers gain more experience, their initial trust in automation frequently shifts from dispositional to history-based [49]. Users adjust their trust levels over time to better represent the automation's reliability and performance, demonstrating the dynamic nature of trust calibration [46].

3 Conceptual Framework and Hypothesis Development

This study focuses on how perceived human-AI compatibility influences adoption results, emphasizing key mediators such as AI anxiety, explainable AI, and human-computer trust. It also investigates the moderating effect of speciesism, a socio-ethical bias that can influence how consumers judge and accept AI. By the integration of these characteristics, the study provides a comprehensive framework (Fig. 1) for better understanding the psychological and contextual factors influencing AI adoption in healthcare.

Perceived human–AI compatibility, defined as the extent to which users feel that AI systems align with their needs and values, plays a critical role in influencing AI adoption in healthcare. A review of AI-infused systems highlights that compatibility improves trust, enhances usability, and significantly improves user AI adoption [50]. This is particularly crucial in healthcare settings where trust in AI-driven decisions is essential. This is supported by research on human–AI teaming in medical settings, which demonstrates that healthcare professionals are more likely to work with AI when systems are designed with high compatibility, which results in better diagnostic outcomes [51]. According to similar findings from domains like algorithmic matchmaking indicate that when users perceive computed compatibility, they are more likely to perceive the AI system as effective and worthwhile [2]. Furthermore, compatibility influences users' perceptions of system behavior in addition to having a direct impact on adoption. Explainability, a crucial feature that improves transparency and facilitates accurate decision-making, is more likely to be requested and valued by users who feel more aligned with AI systems [52]. Therefore, compatibility promotes both a demand for understandable system outputs and trust in the system's decisions, especially in high-stakes industries like healthcare. Consequently:

H1: Perceived human–AI compatibility has a positive and significant influence on AI adoption in healthcare.

H2: Perceived human–AI compatibility has a positive and significant influence on perceptions of explainable AI.

Perceived human–AI compatibility can significantly influence both AI anxiety and Human–Computer Trust, when AI systems align with user expectations and needs, they tend decrease psychological discomfort such as fear of job replacement, privacy attack, and loss of control, which are the core of AI anxiety [53, 54]. Supporting this, research in healthcare shows that when nurses perceive AI as a possible substitute, heightened AI anxiety mediates the cooperation intentions [55]. This leads to the following hypothesis:

H3: Perceived human–AI compatibility has an influence on AI anxiety.

Conversely, compatibility enhances trust by providing familiarity and predictability that are the key antecedents of HCT. Research show that disclosing AI involvement can reduce perceived authenticity and trust, particularly when AI feels fake or misaligned; compatibility provides a buffer by creating a sense of alignment [56]. In educational settings, students' trust in AI teaching assistants rises when AI demonstrates attributes such as competence, benevolence, and integrity traits reinforced by perceived compatibility [57]. Hence:

H4: Perceived human–AI compatibility has a significant and positive influence on human–computer trust.

Explainability, trust, and anxiety are critical factors in the adoption of AI, particularly in healthcare environments where decisions have significant consequences. Explainable AI not only clarifies decision-making but also significantly increases users' willingness to adoption. In a structural equation modelling study involving 368 Chinese nurses, medical EXP was shown to enhance innovation behavior by boosting AI self-efficacy and decreasing AI anxiety, underscoring the empowering effects of explainability [58]. Similar, research that examined the explainability effect on physicians' intention to use AI discovered that physicians who received transparent, contextually detailed explanations of AI-generated recommendations reported significantly stronger adoption intentions than those who received no explanation [59]. In total, these results highlight the significance of explainability in building the trust and willingness of healthcare professionals to adopt AI-driven systems. Thus, we hypothesize:

H5: Explainable AI has a significant and positive influence on AI adoption in healthcare.

Human–computer trust (HCT) consistently emerges as a strong predictor of AI adoption in healthcare. A study in the dental healthcare sector has analyzed 343 dental professionals, it revealed that Human-computer trust in AI notably influenced by social influence and expectancy, and it significantly mediated the relationship between beliefs about AI's usefulness and intention to adopt it [8]. Similarly, another study found that HCT in AI had a strong positive correlation with nurses' behavioral intention toward AI adoption. These findings confirm that when healthcare workers perceive an AI system as reliable and trustworthy, they are far more inclined to adopt it [60]. Consequently, we propose:

H6: Human–computer trust has a significant and positive influence on AI adoption in healthcare.

AI anxiety encompassing has been shown to significantly impact continuous adoption of AI, particularly among healthcare professionals. In a cross-sectional study involving 550 primary care nurses, their findings highlighting that anxiety erodes sustained adoption unless trust is actively built [61]. Complementing this, a study among 264 nursing students revealed a strong negative correlation between AI anxiety and positive attitudes toward AI, emphasizing the detrimental effect of anxiety on adoption intention [62]. These findings reinforce the expectation that higher levels of AI anxiety are associated with lower intention to adopt AI in healthcare contexts. Consequently:

H7: AI anxiety has a negative influence on AI adoption in healthcare.

3.1 The Mediating Role of HTC, EXP, and AIA

Trust is a fundamental bridge that consistently links compatibility with adoption intentions. The willingness of users to adopt an AI system is directly influenced by their perception that it is consistent with their values and expectations, which in turn increases their trust in the system [55]. In a study that emphasizes the mediating role of HCT in the relationship between social influence which was based on perceived compatibility and AI adoption intention, found that increased HTC levels lead to increasing intentions to incorporate AI into clinical practice [8]. Thus, we hypothesize that:

H8: Human–computer trust mediates the relationship between perceived human–AI compatibility and AI adoption in healthcare.

Perceived human-AI compatibility enhances users' expectations for explainability, which in turn enhance trust and adoption. Shin (2020) revealed that when personalized AI systems are perceived as fair and explainable, users consider them significantly more trustworthy and useful. Similarly, [64] discovered that when AI evaluations result in disappointment especially negative feedback about users experience for lack of transparency anxiety, a psychological barrier that decreases perceived fairness and user acceptance. These findings suggest that explainability not only strengthens perceived compatibility but also reduces transparency-related anxiety, making it a critical psychological link through which compatibility enhances AI adoption in clinical settings. Thus, we hypothesize that:

H9a: Explainable AI mediates the relationship between perceived human–AI compatibility and AI adoption in healthcare.

Empirical evidence highlights AI anxiety as a crucial psychological mechanism that can undermine adoption unless properly addressed. Recent study found that organizational trust and AI trust fully mediated the negative impact of AI anxiety on continuous AI use, suggesting that managing anxiety is essential for sustaining adoption behaviors [61]. Similarly, research involving nursing students revealed that while perceptions of AI reduce anxiety, increased anxiety strongly and negatively correlates with both attitudes toward AI and intention to use [63]. Mediation analysis confirmed that anxiety plays as a significant mediator between perceived human capability and adoption intention [65]. These findings illustrate that users' AI anxiety decreases when they perceive AI systems as compatible, thus creating a psychological pathway that encourages the adoption of AI in healthcare. Thus, we hypothesize that:

H10a: AI anxiety mediates the relationship between perceived human–AI compatibility and AI adoption in healthcare.

3.2 The Moderator Role Speciesism

Speciesism refers to the psychological and ethical concept that denotes bias or discrimination in Favor of humans over non-human entities [66]. In a field study of 249 patients conducted during the COVID-19 pandemic, researchers discovered that the acceptance of medical AI was significantly increased by explainable and assistive AI systems [67]. However, this effect was significantly weaker among participants with high speciesism, who strongly believed in human superiority [67]. In fact, the positive impact of system transparency (a central component of EXP) on users' willingness to adopt AI was reduced by high speciesism, particularly when AI systems acted in an independent decision-making role. These results suggest that even strong explainability may not be sufficient to completely dismantle deep-rooted biases against non-human intelligence. This gives validity to the hypothesis:

H9b: Speciesism moderates the relationship between EXP and AI adoption in healthcare.

Anxiety that individuals experience regarding AI innovations, such as ethical implications or concerns about autonomy, is likely to have a more significant deterrent influence on their adoption intentions when they hold strong speciesism beliefs, preferring human intelligence over AI. Research indicates that the involvement of medical personnel in the development of AI systems substantially enhances acceptance by fostering ownership and reducing biases [68]. Nevertheless, individuals who exhibit a high degree of speciesism may continue to be resistant, even when they are actively involved, as their bias may exacerbate anxieties and undermine participatory efforts. Thus, even participatory strategies may not be sufficient for relieving AI anxiety to facilitate adoption when speciesism is high. On the other hand, when speciesism is low, anxiety is less likely to impede adoption, and participatory design entirely enhances acceptance [67]. This gives validity to the hypothesis:

H10b: Speciesism moderates the relationship between AI anxiety and AI adoption in healthcare.

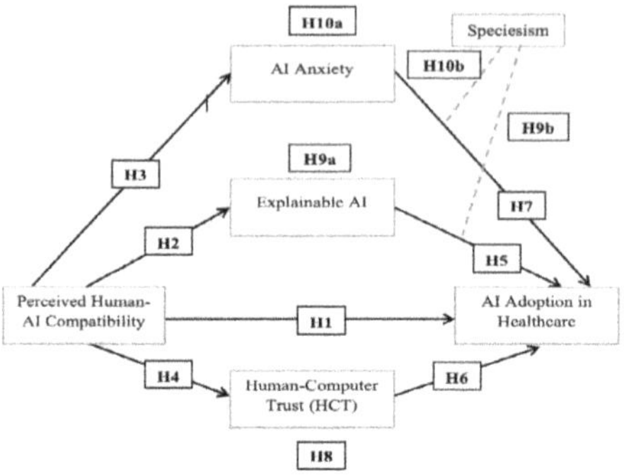

Fig. 1. Conceptual framework developed by the authors

4 Method

The existing literature was used to ensure the reliability and validity of the measurement items. The items assessing perceived human AI compatibility were adapted from [69], for AI adoption and human-computer trust from [8], AI anxiety from [39], and explainable AI from [70]. As for speciesism to be used as a moderator, the items were adapted from [71]. A total of 21 items were utilized for this research, assessed using a five-point Likert scale, with response options ranging from 1 (strongly disagree) to 5 (strongly agree).

All questions were contextualized within the healthcare service sector to align with the specific environment in which respondents' AI adoption behaviors were examined. It was important to maintain context-specific AI adoption, as it not only demonstrates high explanatory power in research models [72], but also enhances comprehensibility [73]. Hence, this research approach aligns with the previous research conducted by [73–77], ensuring context-specific AI adoption within the healthcare sector.

This study utilized data from the UAE to validate the proposed research model, leveraging country's advanced technological infrastructure and its progressive approach towards digital transformation in healthcare [78]. The UAE [79] accentuates the sector's continued investment in technology, with strategic commitments extending through 2031. Recent developments in artificial intelligence further emphasize the transformative role of data in reshaping and revolutionizing the healthcare sector [80]. In addition, rising healthcare expenses driven by technological progress and price inflation highlight the sector's evolving dynamics [81].

Using snowball sampling across UAE hospitals, eligible respondents with prior knowledge or experience of using AI enabled healthcare systems were invited to complete an online questionnaire. Of approximately 870 individuals approached, 291 responded, but 4 responses were excluded due to incomplete information or uniform answers across all items, to minimize potential bias. This resulted in a final sample of 287 healthcare professionals with a response rate of 33%. All the respondents were asked to reflect on the AI system they used most frequently in the past month. The study's purpose was clearly explained to encourage honest participation.

A total of 287 healthcare professionals participated, predominantly female (57%), aged between 28 and 47 (50%), and primarily based in Dubai and Abu Dhabi (61%). Most held roles as doctors, medical assistants, or nurses, with over half having 6–17 years of experience. The majority (52%) worked in in large institutions with over 500 employees. Demographic details are presented in Table 1.

Table 1. Demographic details of the respondents

Respondents		N = 287	
Category	Sub-category	Frequency	Percentage
Gender	Male	123	43%
	Female	164	57%
Age	18 to 27	51	18%
	28 to 37	73	25%
	38 to 47	71	25%
	48 to 57	60	21%
	58 and above	32	11%
Position	Doctors/Physicians	89	31%
	Medical Assistants	74	26%
	Nurses	60	21%
	Nurse Practitioners	62	22%
	Others	2	1%
Years of experience	0 to 5	75	26%
	6 to 11	84	29%
	12 to 17	76	26%
	18 and above	52	18%
Location	Abu Dhabi	56	20%
	Dubai	118	41%
	Sharjah	44	15%
	Ajman	20	7%
	Ras al Khaimah	23	8%
	Fujairah	15	5%
	Umm al Quwain	11	4%
Company size	1 to 249	20	7%
	250 to 499	119	41%
	500 and above	148	52%

5 Results

This research applied Partial Least Squares Structural Equation Modelling (PLS-SEM) as the primary analytical technique due to its effectiveness in explaining theoretical relationships and overseeing complex research models [82]. PLS-SEM is particularly well-suited for studies involving multiple latent variables and indicators, allowing for the concurrent assessment of both measurement and structural models [82, 83]. Its flexibility regarding sample size and scale assumptions further supports its use in applied research context [82–84]. The analysis was conducted using SmartPLS 4.0, with all variables treated as reflective.

5.1 Measurement Model

To assess the quality and consistency of the measurement model, both convergent and discriminant validity were examined [82, 85]. Convergent validity was evaluated through item reliability, composite reliability, and average variance extracted (AVE). Internal consistency was supported by Cronbach's alpha and Dijkstra-Henseler's rho (ρC), with all values exceeding the recommended threshold of 0.70 [86, 87]. Similarly, all AVE values were above 0.50 [88], whereas the individual item loadings were greater than 0.70 indicating that each item closely reflected its intended construct [82, 84]. These results confirm that the model measures its intended concepts accurately and consistently, as illustrated in Table 2.

Table 2. Reliability and convergent validity

Construct	Cronbach's alpha	Composite reliability	Average variance extracted (AVE)
AI Adoption	0.922	0.926	0.927
AI Anxiety	0.755	0.890	0.802
Explainable AI	0.894	0.926	0.758
Human-Computer Trust	0.934	0.950	0.791
Perceived Human-AI Compatibility	0.933	0.948	0.751
Speciesism	0.892	0.949	0.903

Discriminant validity on the other hand assesses whether measures of different constructs are sufficiently discrete from one another [89]. In this research, each item loaded highest on its intended construct, as illustrated in Table 3, hence supporting construct distinctiveness.

Table 3. Discriminant validity: Cross-loadings and outer-loadings

	ADI	AIA	EXP	HCT	PHAIC	SP
ADI1	**0.966**	0.649	0.601	0.650	0.562	0.548
ADI2	**0.960**	0.607	0.561	0.611	0.534	0.474
AIA1	0.622	**0.913**	0.685	0.757	0.674	0.430
AIA2	0.543	**0.878**	0.719	0.653	0.565	0.393

(continued)

Table 3. (*continued*)

	ADI	AIA	EXP	HCT	PHAIC	SP
EXP1	0.488	0.698	**0.883**	0.699	0.742	0.431
EXP2	0.492	0.625	**0.846**	0.640	0.695	0.388
EXP3	0.547	0.687	**0.875**	0.630	0.657	0.396
EXP4	0.575	0.711	**0.879**	0.670	0.699	0.388
HCT1	0.523	0.643	0.619	**0.869**	0.651	0.491
HCT2	0.552	0.679	0.635	**0.892**	0.675	0.463
HCT3	0.608	0.718	0.644	**0.886**	0.644	0.487
HCT4	0.600	0.734	0.729	**0.909**	0.751	0.492
HCT5	0.624	0.733	0.731	**0.890**	0.774	0.511
PHAIC1	0.522	0.610	0.752	0.655	**0.894**	0.368
PHAIC2	0.494	0.623	0.714	0.700	**0.868**	0.420
PHAIC3	0.531	0.638	0.687	0.724	**0.838**	0.447
PHAIC4	0.466	0.573	0.613	0.660	**0.822**	0.368
PHAIC5	0.482	0.615	0.712	0.699	**0.886**	0.342
PHAIC6	0.458	0.551	0.683	0.663	**0.888**	0.405
SP1	0.515	0.464	0.464	0.557	0.457	**0.952**
SP2	0.496	0.409	0.409	0.488	0.402	**0.948**

Note: Bold numbers represent the loadings on their respective construct. ADI = AI Adoption; AIA = AI Anxiety; EXP = Explainable AI; HCT = Human-Computer Trust; PHAIC = Perceived Human-AI Compatibility; SP = Speciesism

Additionally, the Fornell and Larcker criterion (Table 4) was applied as a complementary test, whereby the square root of each construct's AVE exceeded its correlations with other constructs, as recommended by Henseler et al. (2016), indicating that the model demonstrates adequate discriminant validity [88].

Table 4. Discriminant validity: Fornell and Larcker criterion

	ADI	AIA	EXP	HCT	PHAIC	SP
ADI	**0.963**					
AIA	0.653	**0.896**				
EXP	0.604	0.782	**0.871**			
HCT	0.656	0.791	0.758	**0.889**		
PHAIC	0.569	0.696	0.802	0.790	**0.867**	
SP	0.532	0.460	0.460	0.550	0.453	**0.950**

5.2 Structural Model

After verifying the measurement model, the evaluation of structural model was assessed to check its accuracy and overall model fit. The coefficient of determination (R^2) is a key metric for assessing the structural model, reflecting the predictive power of exogenous variables on endogenous outcome [82, 84]. According to Henseler et al. (2016), values below 0.25 are considered weak, between 0.25 and 0.50 moderate, and above 0.50 strong. In this study, the R^2 value for AI adoption in healthcare is 0.524, indicating a substantial explanatory power of the exogenous variables on the endogenous variable, i.e., AI adoption, thus meeting the threshold for a strong model fit. Furthermore, the collinearity statistics were assessed using the variance inflation factor (VIF), as recommended by [84], and all variables remained well below the threshold value of 5, indicating no multicollinearity concerns based on standard evaluation criteria.

Table 5. Structural model evaluation

Hypothesis	Path	Type	(β)	t-Stat	p-Value	Remarks
H1	PHAIC → ADI	Direct	0.008	0.093	0.926	Not supported
H2	PHAIC → EXP	Direct	0.802	26.429	0.000	Supported
H3	PHAIC → AIA	Direct	0.696	17.585	0.000	Supported
H4	PHAIC → HCT	Direct	0.790	23.108	0.000	Supported
H5	EXP → ADI	Direct	0.094	0.855	0.392	Not supported
H6	HCT → ADI	Direct	0.233	2.169	0.030	Supported
H7	AIA → ADI	Direct	0.291	2.680	0.007	Supported
H8	PHAIC → HCT → ADI	Mediating	0.184	2.116	0.034	Supported
H9a	PHAIC → EXP → ADI	Mediating	0.075	0.850	0.395	Not supported
H9b	SP*EXP → ADI	Moderating	-0.001	0.021	0.983	Not supported
H10a	PHAIC → AIA → ADI	Mediating	0.202	2.618	0.009	Supported
H10b	SP*AIA → ADI	Moderating	0.048	0.707	0.479	Not supported

Note: Alpha = 0.05; Confidence interval = 95%; t-stat = 1.96

The structural model results (Table 5) indicate that Perceived Human-AI Compatibility (PHAIC) significantly influences Explainable AI (EXP), AI Anxiety (AIA), and

Human-Computer Trust (HCT), supporting H2, H3, and H4. However, PHAIC does not have a significant direct effect on AI Adoption (ADI), and thus H1 is not supported. Among the mediators, only HCT and AIA show significant direct effects on ADI (H6 and H7), while EXP does not (H5 not supported). Mediation analysis further reveals that HCT and AIA significantly mediate the relationship between PHAIC and ADI (H8 and H10a supported), whereas EXP does not (H9a not supported). Additionally, neither speciesism as a moderator of EXP (H9b) nor AIA (H10b) significantly influences ADI, indicating no significant moderation effects. Below Fig. 2 is the visual representation of the overall structural model.

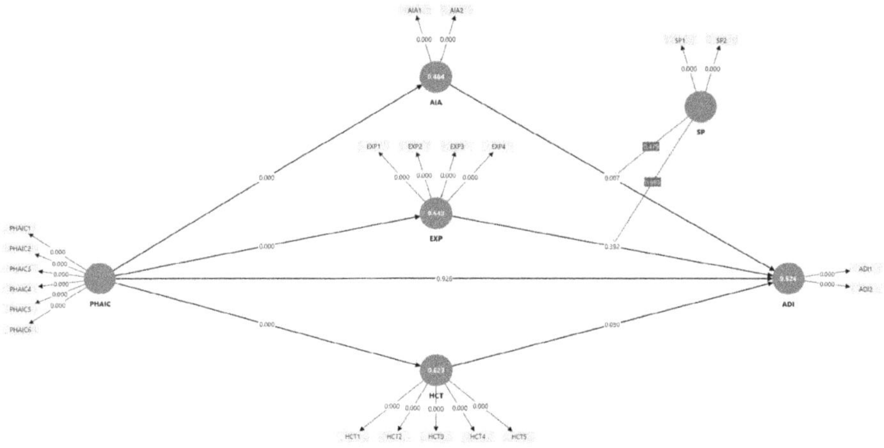

Fig. 2. Structural Model

6 Discussion and Implications

6.1 Discussion of the Findings

Our results confirm that Perceived Human-AI Compatibility (PHAIC) significantly enhances users' experiences with Explainability (EXP), AI Anxiety (AIA), and builds Human-Computer Trust (HCT), aligning with previous qualitative work showing clinicians requiring AI explanations to feel comfortable and trusting in real-world use [90, 91]. However, the absence of a direct PHIAC to AI adoption underlines that compatibility alone is not sufficient; instead, successful AI adoption (AIA) hinges on emotional and relational mechanisms, such as reducing anxiety and establishing trust, echoing clinical findings that cognitive trust and emotional readiness are crucial for the acceptance of AI systems for healthcare professionals [50].

Only HCT and AIA showed direct, significant effects on AI adoption, highlighting trust and emotional comfort as central to healthcare professionals' willingness to adopt AI [58]. This aligns with the research published by [92], which shows that trust in AI systems depends primarily on their transparency, reliability, and relevance rather than any inherent professional bias. Similarly, our data support growing evidence that EXP enhances healthcare professionals trust and reduces anxiety but requires trust to directly translate into adoption [91].

The mediation analysis confirms that HCT and AIA fully mediate the effect of PHAIC on AIA, but EXP does not, suggesting that explanations only facilitate adoption when they build trust and alleviate anxiety [60]. Additionally, speciesism (SP) was not a significant moderator, indicating that personal bias toward human versus AI systems has minimal impact in healthcare adoption contexts. This further echoes findings from [91] that users' trust and concerns over ethical/legal aspects play a larger role than innate biases.

6.2 Contributions and Implications

This study extends the Technology Acceptance Model 3 (TAM3) by examining AI adoption in healthcare and demonstrating that adoption is shaped not only by cognitive evaluations but also by emotional and relational mechanisms. While TAM3 traditionally emphasizes perceived usefulness and ease of use, the findings show that Perceived Human–AI Compatibility does not directly predict AI adoption. Instead, its influence is indirect, operating through AI anxiety and human–computer trust. This highlights the importance of users' emotional readiness and perceived harmony with AI systems, particularly in complex and safety-critical healthcare environments. Drawing on the Hybrid Trust framework and Trust Calibration Theory, the study underscores the central role of well-calibrated trust in fostering effective human–AI collaboration. Human–computer trust significantly mediates the relationship between compatibility perceptions and adoption intention, indicating that trust must accurately reflect AI system capabilities. When trust is appropriately calibrated—neither excessive nor insufficient—healthcare professionals are more likely to engage with AI technologies. These findings reinforce the need for explainable and transparent AI systems that enable users to form realistic and informed trust judgments. The results further validate Human–Computer Trust Theory by demonstrating that trust is not a secondary outcome of system performance but a foundational determinant of AI adoption. Trust emerges from both system characteristics, such as explainability, and human factors, including emotional comfort and perceived fit, confirming its multidimensional cognitive, emotional, and social nature.

From a practical perspective, AI adoption in healthcare is driven primarily by emotional and relational factors, notably AI anxiety, trust in AI, and explainability, rather than ideological biases such as speciesism. Accordingly, healthcare organizations should prioritize human-centered AI design, incorporating intuitive interfaces, transparent feedback, and alignment with clinical workflows. Training, simulation, and structured onboarding can further reduce anxiety and strengthen trust. At the policy level, regulatory frameworks should mandate explainability, transparency, and trustworthiness standards, supporting the responsible and collaborative integration of AI into clinical practice.

6.3 Limitations and Future Research

Although this study provides valuable insights into AI adoption in healthcare, several limitations should be acknowledged. First, the use of a quantitative, cross-sectional design restricts the ability to establish causal relationships or examine how perceptions of trust, anxiety, and AI adoption evolve over time. Future research would benefit from longitudinal or mixed method approaches to capture dynamic changes in user attitudes as exposure to AI increases. Second, the reliance on snowball sampling, while effective for accessing healthcare professionals, may have introduced sampling bias and limited respondent diversity. Future studies should consider random or stratified sampling techniques to enhance representativeness across professional roles and levels of AI experience. Additionally, as the study was conducted within the UAE, further research in different cultural and institutional contexts is needed to assess the generalizability of the findings.

Building on these limitations, future research should explore additional psychological and contextual factors influencing AI adoption. Constructs such as AI self-efficacy may play a critical role in shaping users' confidence and behavioral intentions. Incorporating perceived usefulness and ease of use could also extend the explanatory power of TAM3. Moreover, ethical alignment reflecting the extent to which AI systems are perceived to uphold medical values may act as a moderating factor in adoption decisions. Finally, examining organizational and practical challenges, including readiness, training constraints, workflow integration, and resistance to change, from the perspectives of multiple stakeholders, would help bridge the gap between theoretical models and real-world AI implementation in healthcare.

7 Conclusion

In conclusion, this research offers a comprehensive framework for understanding AI adoption in the UAE healthcare sector by integrating TAM 3, hybrid trust, calibration insights, and Human-Computer Trust Theory. By highlighting the mediating roles of AI anxiety, explainable AI, and human-computer trust, examining speciesism as a non-significant moderator, it moves beyond traditional models to capture the emotional and relational dimensions of adoption. The findings highlight the importance of trust, clarity, and user compatibility in facilitating AI acceptance, providing both theoretical insights and practical guidance for designing AI systems that align with the needs and expectations of healthcare professionals in complex, data-driven environments.

Acknowledgments. The authors acknowledge using generative AI and Grammarly to enhance the language, and they ensured that all revised text is reviewed.

References

1. Roppelt, J.S., Schuster, A., Greimel, N.S., Kanbach, D.K., Sen, K.: Towards effective adoption of artificial intelligence in talent acquisition: a mixed method study. Int. J. Inf. Manage. **82**, 1–18 (2025). https://doi.org/10.1016/j.ijinfomgt.2025.102870
2. Paul, A., Ahmed, S.: Computed compatibility: examining user perceptions of AI and matchmaking algorithms. Behav. Inf. Technol. **43**, 1002–1015 (2024). https://doi.org/10.1080/0144929X.2023.2196579
3. Aldholay, A., Abdullah, Z., Isaac, O., Mutahar, A.M.: Perspective of Yemeni students on use of online learning: extending the information systems success model with transformational leadership and compatibility. Inf. Technol. People **33**, 106–128 (2020). https://doi.org/10.1108/ITP-02-2018-0095

4. McKnight, D.H., Choudhury, V., Kacmar, C.: Developing and validating trust measures for e-commerce: an integrative typology. Inf. Syst. Res. **13**, 334–359 (2002). https://doi.org/10.1287/isre.13.3.334.81
5. Saoud, L.S., Romman, A.A.: AI-powered chatbots in the telecommunications industry in the UAE: studying the factors impacting consumer adoption. In: 2024 15th International Conference on Information and Communication Technology Convergence (ICTC), pp. 1549–1553. IEEE (2024). https://doi.org/10.1109/ICTC62082.2024.10827670
6. Qureshi, O.A., Saad Saoud, L.: From perception to action: empowering ai-human-centric project management through the mediating role of consumer trust. Presented at the (2025). https://doi.org/10.56889/yfrk1589
7. Qureshi, O.A., Wilkins, S., Iqbal, H.: Chatbots: can they satisfy customers in the banking sector? Presented at the (2024). https://doi.org/10.1007/978-3-031-56121-4_34
8. Cheng, M., Li, X., Xu, J.: Promoting healthcare workers' adoption intention of artificial-intelligence-assisted diagnosis and treatment: the chain mediation of social influence and human-computer trust. Int. J. Environ. Res. Public Health **19**, 13311 (2022). https://doi.org/10.3390/ijerph192013311
9. Grassini, S.: Development and validation of the AI attitude scale (AIAS-4): a brief measure of general attitude toward artificial intelligence. Front. Psychol. **14** (2023). https://doi.org/10.3389/fpsyg.2023.1191628
10. Morley, J., et al.: The ethics of AI in health care: a mapping review (2020). https://doi.org/10.1016/j.socscimed.2020.113172
11. Middleton, S.E., Letouzé, E., Hossaini, A., Chapman, A.: Trust, regulation, and human-in-the-loop AI. Commun. ACM **65**, 64–68 (2022). https://doi.org/10.1145/3511597
12. Yang, H., Sundar, S.S.: AI anxiety: explication and exploration of effect on state anxiety when interacting with AI doctors. Comput. Hum. Behav.: Artif. Hum. **3**, 100128 (2025). https://doi.org/10.1016/j.chbah.2025.100128
13. Frenkenberg, A., Hochman, G.: It's scary to use it, it's scary to refuse it: the psychological dimensions of ai adoption—anxiety, motives, and dependency. Systems. **13** (2025). https://doi.org/10.3390/systems13020082
14. Li, X., Zong, Q., Cheng, M.: The impact of medical explainable artificial intelligence on nurses' innovation behaviour: a structural equation modelling approach. J. Nurs. Manag. **2024** (2024). https://doi.org/10.1155/2024/8885760
15. Figueroa, C.A., Harrison, R., Chauhan, A., Meyer, L.: Priorities and challenges for health leadership and workforce management globally: a rapid review (2019). https://bmchealthservres.biomedcentral.com/articles/10.1186/s12913-019-4080-7, https://doi.org/10.1186/s12913-019-4080-7
16. Bednarz, A.L., Borkowska-Bierć, M., Matejun, M.: Managerial responses to the onset of the covid-19 pandemic in healthcare organizations project management. Int. J. Environ. Res. Public Health **18**, 12082 (2021). https://doi.org/10.3390/ijerph182212082
17. Li, F., Ruijs, N., Lu, Y.: Ethics & AI: a systematic review on ethical concerns and related strategies for designing with AI in healthcare (2023). https://www.mdpi.com/2673-2688/4/1/3, https://doi.org/10.3390/ai4010003
18. Aliu, J., et al.: Towards a new paradigm of project management: a bibliometric review (2023). https://www.mdpi.com/2071-1050/15/13/9967, https://doi.org/10.3390/su15139967
19. Al Badi, F.K., Alhosani, K.A., Jabeen, F., Stachowicz-Stanusch, A., Shehzad, N., AMANN, W.: Challenges of AI adoption in the UAE healthcare. Vision. **26**, 193–207 (2022). https://doi.org/10.1177/0972262920988398
20. Russell, S.: Human-compatible artificial intelligence (2021)
21. Brundage, M.: Taking superintelligence seriously. Superintelligence: paths, dangers, strategies by Nick Bostrom (Oxford University Press, 2014). Futures. **72**, 32–35 (2014). https://doi.org/10.1016/j.futures.2015.07.009

22. Kido, T., Takadama, K.: The challenges for GenAI in social and individual well-being (2024)
23. Kido, T., Takadama, K.: The challenges for interpretable AI for well-being -understanding cognitive bias and social embeddedness-. In: CEUR Workshop Proceedings (2019)
24. Kido, T., Takadama, K.: The challenges for fairness and well-being - how fair is fair? Achieving well-being AI - how F. In: CEUR Workshop Proceedings (2022)
25. Kido, T., Takadama, K.: The challenges for socially responsible AI for well-being. In: CEUR Workshop Proceedings, pp. 211–212 (2023)
26. Haring, K.S., Mougenot, C., Ono, F., Watanabe, K.: Cultural differences in perception and attitude towards robots. Int. J. Affect. Eng. **13**, 149–157 (2014). https://doi.org/10.5057/ijae.13.149
27. Wang, Y.Y., Wang, Y.S.: Development and validation of an artificial intelligence anxiety scale: an initial application in predicting motivated learning behavior. Interact. Learn. Environ. **30**, 619–634 (2022). https://doi.org/10.1080/10494820.2019.1674887
28. Kaya, F., Aydin, F., Schepman, A., Rodway, P., Yetişensoy, O., Demir Kaya, M.: The roles of personality traits, ai anxiety, and demographic factors in attitudes toward artificial intelligence. Int. J. Hum. Comput. Interact. **40**, 497–514 (2024). https://doi.org/10.1080/10447318.2022.2151730
29. Russell, S., Norivg, P.: Artificial Intelligence: A Modern Approach (Global Edition). Artificial Intelligence: A Modern Approach (2021)
30. Maurer, M.M., Simonson, M.R.: Development and validation of a measure of computer anxiety (1984)
31. Floridi, L., et al.: AI4People—an ethical framework for a good ai society: opportunities, risks, principles, and recommendations. Minds Mach. (Dordr) **28**, 689–707 (2018). https://doi.org/10.1007/s11023-018-9482-5
32. Minh, D., Wang, H.X., Li, Y.F., Nguyen, T.N.: Explainable artificial intelligence: a comprehensive review. Artif. Intell. Rev. **55**, 3503–3568 (2022). https://doi.org/10.1007/s10462-021-10088-y
33. Xie, X., Du, Y., Bai, Q.: Why do people resist algorithms? From the perspective of short video usage motivations. Front. Psychol. **13**, 941640 (2022). https://doi.org/10.3389/fpsyg.2022.941640
34. Lipton, Z.C.: The mythos of model interpretability. Commun. ACM **61**, 36–41 (2018). https://doi.org/10.1145/3233231
35. Madsen, M., Gregor, S.: Measuring human-computer trust. In: Proceedings of Eleventh Australasian Conference on Information Systems, pp. 6–8 (2000)
36. Liu, P., Yang, R., Xu, Z.: Public acceptance of fully automated driving: effects of social trust and risk/benefit perceptions. Risk Anal. **39**, 326–341 (2019). https://doi.org/10.1111/risa.13143
37. Gerli, P., Clement, J., Esposito, G., Mora, L., Crutzen, N.: The hidden power of emotions: how psychological factors influence skill development in smart technology adoption. Technol. Forecast. Soc. Change. **180**, 121721 (2022). https://doi.org/10.1016/j.techfore.2022.121721
38. Alagarsamy, S., Mehrolia, S.: Exploring chatbot trust: antecedents and behavioural outcomes. Heliyon. **9** (2023). https://doi.org/10.1016/j.heliyon.2023.e16074
39. Venkatesh, V., Bala, H.: Technology acceptance model 3 and a research agenda on interventions. Decis. Sci. **39**, 273–315 (2008). https://doi.org/10.1111/j.1540-5915.2008.00192.x
40. Oluyinka, S., Shamsuddin, A., Wahab, E.: Regions of trust to technological know-how structured for banking customers (2015)
41. Yousafzai, S.Y., Pallister, J.G., Foxall, G.R.: Strategies for building and communicating trust in electronic banking: A field experiment (2005). https://onlinelibrary.wiley.com/doi/10.1002/mar.20054, https://doi.org/10.1002/mar.20054

42. Saoud, L.S., Suleimani, M.A., Eid, J.: The impact of organizational learning on business continuity through the moderating effect of organizational culture: a study of UAE's public sector organizations. In: BUiD Doctoral Research Conference, pp. 393–407. Springer, Cham (2024). https://doi.org/10.1007/978-3-031-84371-6_32
43. Mcknight, D.H., Carter, M., Thatcher, J.B., Clay, P.F.: Trust in a specific technology: an investigation of its components and measures. ACM Trans. Manag. Inf. Syst. **2** (2011). https://doi.org/10.1145/1985347.1985353
44. Cigdem, E., Toker, C.A., Coşkun, A.: Association for information systems association for information systems AIS electronic library (AISeL) AIS electronic library (AISeL) understanding finfluencer engagement: a conceptual framework understanding Finfluencer engagement: a conceptual framework of attitude development and continued usage in video of attitude development and continued usage in video consumption consumption (2023)
45. Alkhalifah, A.: Exploring trust formation and antecedents in social commerce. Front. Psychol. **12** (2022). https://doi.org/10.3389/fpsyg.2021.789863
46. Lee, J.D., Katrina, A: Trust_in_Automation_Designing. **46**, 50–80 (2004). https://doi.org/10.1518/hfes.46.1.50_30392
47. Mayer, R.C., Davis, J.H., Schoorman, F.D.: An integrative model of organizational trust. Acad. Manage. Rev. **20** (1995). https://doi.org/10.5465/amr.1995.9508080335
48. Okamura, K., Yamada, S.: Adaptive trust calibration for human-AI collaboration. PLoS One. **15** (2020). https://doi.org/10.1371/journal.pone.0229132
49. Naiseh, M., Al-Thani, D., Jiang, N., Ali, R.: How the different explanation classes impact trust calibration: the case of clinical decision support systems. Int. J. Hum. Comput. Stud. **169**, 102941 (2023). https://doi.org/10.1016/j.ijhcs.2022.102941
50. Ismatullaev, U.V.U., Kim, S.H.: Review of the factors affecting acceptance of AI-infused systems. Hum. Factors **66**, 126–144 (2024). https://doi.org/10.1177/00187208211064707
51. Reverberi, C., et al.: Experimental evidence of effective human–AI collaboration in medical decision-making. Sci. Rep. **12**, 14952 (2022). https://doi.org/10.1038/s41598-022-18751-2
52. Shin, D.: The effects of explainability and causability on perception, trust, and acceptance: Implications for explainable AI. Int. J. Hum. Comput. Stud. **146**, 102551 (2021). https://doi.org/10.1016/j.ijhcs.2020.102551
53. Li, J., Huang, J.S.: Dimensions of artificial intelligence anxiety based on the integrated fear acquisition theory. Technol. Soc. **63**, 1–10 (2020). https://doi.org/10.1016/j.techsoc.2020.101410
54. Kim, J., et al.: AI anxiety: a comprehensive analysis of psychological factors and interventions. SSRN Electron. J. 3993–4009 (2023). https://doi.org/10.2139/ssrn.4573394
55. Fan, J., Zhang, L., Li, N., Man, S.: How the perceived substitution of AI technology hinders nurses' innovation behavior: the mediating role of AI anxiety and human-AI cooperation intention and the moderating role of organizational AI readiness. BMC Nurs. **24**, 832 (2025). https://doi.org/10.1186/s12912-025-03265-9
56. Kučinskas, G.: Negative effects of revealing ai involvement in products: mediation by authenticity and risk, moderation by trust in AI and familiarity with AI (2024)
57. Peng, Z., Wan, Y.: Human vs. AI: exploring students' preferences between human and AI TA and the effect of social anxiety and problem complexity. Educ. Inf. Technol. (Dordr). **29**, 1217–1246 (2024). https://doi.org/10.1007/s10639-023-12374-4
58. Li, X., Zong, Q., Cheng, M.: The impact of medical explainable artificial intelligence on nurses' innovation behaviour: a structural equation modelling approach. J. Nurs. Manag. **2024**, 104884 (2024). https://doi.org/10.1155/2024/8885760
59. Liu, C.F., Chen, Z.C., Kuo, S.C., Lin, T.C.: Does AI explainability affect physicians' intention to use AI? Int. J. Med. Inform. **168** (2022). https://doi.org/10.1016/j.ijmedinf.2022.104884

60. Chen, C.H., Lee, W.I.: Exploring nurses' behavioural intention to adopt AI technology: the perspectives of social influence, perceived job stress and human-machine trust. J. Adv. Nurs. **81**, 3739–3752 (2025). https://doi.org/10.1111/jan.16495
61. Zhou, Q., et al.: The mediation of trust on artificial intelligence anxiety and continuous adoption of artificial intelligence technology among primacy nurses: a cross-sectional study. BMC Nurs. **24**, 724 (2025). https://doi.org/10.1186/s12912-025-03406-0
62. Ayed, A., et al.: Insights into the relationship between anxiety and attitudes toward artificial intelligence among nursing students. BMC Nurs. **24**, 812 (2025). https://doi.org/10.1186/s12912-025-03490-2
63. Shin, D.: User perceptions of algorithmic decisions in the personalized AI system: perceptual evaluation of fairness, accountability, transparency, and explainability. J. Broadcast. Electron. Media **64**, 541–565 (2020). https://doi.org/10.1080/08838151.2020.1843357
64. Lopez, A., Garza, R.: Consumer bias against evaluations received by artificial intelligence: the mediation effect of lack of transparency anxiety. J. Res. Interact. Mark. **17**, 2040–7122 (2023). https://doi.org/10.1108/JRIM-07-2021-0192
65. Cho, K.A., Seo, Y.H.: Dual mediating effects of anxiety to use and acceptance attitude of artificial intelligence technology on the relationship between nursing students' perception of and intention to use them: a descriptive study. BMC Nurs. **23** (2024). https://doi.org/10.1186/s12912-024-01887-z
66. Horta, O.: What is speciesism? J. Agric. Environ. Ethics **23**, 243–266 (2010). https://doi.org/10.1007/s10806-009-9205-2
67. Huo, W., et al.: Speciesism and preference of human–artificial intelligence interaction: a study on medical artificial intelligence. Int. J. Hum. Comput. Interact. **40** (2024). https://doi.org/10.1080/10447318.2023.2176985
68. Huo, W., Yuan, X., Li, X., Luo, W., Xie, J., Shi, B.: Increasing acceptance of medical AI: the role of medical staff participation in AI development. Int. J. Med. Inform. **175**, 105073 (2023). https://doi.org/10.1016/j.ijmedinf.2023.105073
69. Martin, C.L.: The customer compatibility scale: measuring service customers' perceptions of fellow customers. J. Consum. Stud. Home Econ. **19**, 299–311 (1995). https://doi.org/10.1111/j.1470-6431.1995.tb00552.x
70. Hu, P., Zeng, Y., Wang, D., Teng, H.: Too much light blinds: the transparency-resistance paradox in algorithmic management. Comput. Human Behav. **161**, 1–15 (2024). https://doi.org/10.1016/j.chb.2024.108403
71. Huo, W., Yuan, X., Li, X., Luo, W., Xie, J., Shi, B.: Increasing acceptance of medical AI: the role of medical staff participation in AI development. Int. J. Med. Inform. **175**, 1–10 (2023). https://doi.org/10.1016/j.ijmedinf.2023.105073
72. Venkatesh, V., Morris, M.G., Davis, G.B., Davis, F.D.: User acceptance of information technology: toward a unified view. MIS Q. **27**, 425–478 (2003). https://doi.org/10.2307/30036540
73. Hung, S.Y., Tsai, J.C.A., Chuang, C.C.: Investigating primary health care nurses' intention to use information technology: an empirical study in Taiwan. Decis. Support. Syst. **57**, 331–342 (2014). https://doi.org/10.1016/j.dss.2013.09.016
74. Ahmed, M.H., et al.: Intention to use electronic medical record and its predictors among health care providers at referral hospitals, north-West Ethiopia, 2019: Using unified theory of acceptance and use technology 2(UTAUT2) model. BMC Med. Inform. Decis. Mak. **20**, 1–11 (2020). https://doi.org/10.1186/s12911-020-01222-x
75. Alkhwaldi, A.F.: Understanding the acceptance of business intelligence from healthcare professionals' perspective: an empirical study of healthcare organizations. Int. J. Organ. Anal. **32**, 2135–2163 (2024)

76. Karahoca, A., Karahoca, D., Aksöz, M.: Examining intention to adopt to internet of things in healthcare technology products. Kybernetes **47**, 742–770 (2018). https://doi.org/10.1108/K-02-2017-0045
77. Zhan, X., Abdi, N., Seymour, W., Such, J.: Healthcare voice AI assistants: factors influencing trust and intention to use. Proc. ACM Hum. Comput. Interact. **8**, 1–37 (2024). https://doi.org/10.1145/3637339
78. Khatib, M.E., Zitar, R.A., Al-Nakeeb, A.: The effect of AI on project and risk management in health care industry projects in the United Arab Emirates (UAE). Int. J. Appl. Eng. Res. (Netherlands) **6**, 1–11 (2021)
79. MoE, U.A.E.: Investing in healthcare in the UAE (2019). https://doi.org/10.31826/9781463240134-toc
80. Report, B.C.: U.A.E. healthcare sector (2024)
81. Koornneef, E., Robben, P., Blair, I.: Progress and outcomes of health systems reform in the United Arab Emirates: a systematic review. BMC Health Serv. Res. **17**, 1–13 (2017). https://doi.org/10.1186/s12913-017-2597-1
82. Hair, J.F., Risher, J.J., Sarstedt, M., Ringle, C.M.: When to use and how to report the results of PLS-SEM. Eur. Bus. Rev. **31**, 1–25 (2019). https://doi.org/10.1108/EBR-11-2018-0203
83. Chin, W.W.: The Partial Least Squares Approach to Structural Equation Modeling: Modern Methods for Business Research. Lawrence Erlbaum Associates, New Jersey (1998)
84. Hair, J.F., Sarstedt, M., Ringle, C.M., Mena, J.A.: An assessment of the use of partial least squares structural equation modeling in marketing research. J. Acad. Mark. Sci. **40**, 414–433 (2012). https://doi.org/10.1007/s11747-011-0261-6
85. Gefen, D., Straub, D.W., Boudreau, M.-C., Gefen, D., Straub, D.W., Boudreau, M.: Structural equation modeling and regression: guidelines for research practice. Commun. Assoc. Inf. Syst. **4**(1), 7 (2000)
86. Henseler, J., Hubona, G., Ray, P.A.: Using PLS path modeling in new technology research: updated guidelines. Ind. Manag. Data Syst. **116**, 2–20 (2016). https://doi.org/10.1108/IMDS-09-2015-0382
87. Teo, T.S.H., Lim, V.K.G., Lai, R.Y.C.: Intrinsic and extrinsic motivation in Internet usage. Omega (Westport). **27**, 25–37 (1999). https://doi.org/10.1016/S0305-0483(98)00028-0
88. Fornell, C., Larcker, D.F.: Evaluating structural equation models with unobservable variables and measurement error. J. Mark. Res. **18**, 39 (1981). https://doi.org/10.2307/3151312
89. Campbell, D.T., Fiske, D.W.: Convergent and discriminant validation by the multitrait-multimethod matrix. Psychol. Bull. **56**, 81–105 (1959). https://doi.org/10.1037/h0046016
90. Bienefeld, N., et al.: Solving the explainable AI conundrum by bridging clinicians' needs and developers' goals. NPJ Digit. Med. **6**, 1–7 (2023). https://doi.org/10.1038/s41746-023-00837-4
91. Rosenbacke, R., Melhus, Å., McKee, M., Stuckler, D.: How explainable artificial intelligence can increase or decrease clinicians' trust in ai applications in health care: systematic review. JMIR **3**, 1–30 (2023). https://doi.org/10.2196/preprints.53207
92. Oyekunle, D., Matthew, U.O., Preston, D., Boohene, D.: Trust beyond technology algorithms: a theoretical exploration of consumer trust and behavior in technological consumption and AI projects. J. Comput. Commun. **12**, 72–102 (2024). https://doi.org/10.4236/jcc.2024.126006

Physiotherapy Professionals' Perspectives on AI-Based Tools for Future Practice: A Thematic Analysis

Tuulikki Sjögren[1(✉)], Hilkka Korpi[1,2,3], Sanna Laine[1], and Ville Heilala[4]

[1] Faculty of Sport and Health Sciences, University of Jyväskylä, Jyväskylä, Finland
{tuulikki.sjogren,sanna-mari.k.laine}@jyu.fi,
hilkka.korpi@helsinki.fi

[2] School of Wellbeing and Culture, Oulu University of Applied Sciences, Oulu, Finland

[3] Faculty of Medicine, University of Helsinki, PL 63, 00014 Helsinki, Finland

[4] Faculty of Humanities and Social Sciences, University of Jyväskylä, Jyväskylä, Finland
ville.s.heilala@jyu.fi

Abstract. Artificial intelligence (AI) transforms the traditional roles, competencies, and operational practices of physiotherapists. The aim of this study is to examine how Finnish Physiotherapy professionals intend to use AI-based tools in their future work, based on a survey developed for physiotherapy professionals. A mixed-methods survey was conducted among Finnish Physiotherapy professionals, including students, between October and December 2025. A future-oriented open-ended question using a metaphor was formulated as follows: "If you could have any superpowers with the help of artificial intelligence that would support you in your work as a Physiotherapy professional, what would they be?" answered 141 experts (n = 141; 77 % women; mean age 47.7 years). The dataset comprises 1,407 words of transcribed text. The data were analyzed using inductive thematic analysis.

A total of 214 meaning units were identified. The analysis yielded five overarching themes with 12 subthemes. AI as a tool for physiotherapists included strengthening clinical expertise, evidence-based decision-making, and holistic understanding of the human body. AI in supporting clients included enhancing rehabilitation client agency and motivation, personalized and meaningful rehabilitation, and accessible physiotherapy services. AI in supporting administrative work included freeing time for core tasks and improving documentation quality and efficiency. AI in research and development included enhancing the use of research evidence and effectiveness-based practice. AI-positive work culture included continuous professional learning and the perception of work as meaningful. In addition, the findings indicate uncertainty and concerns among participants regarding AI-based support. The results underscore that the adoption of AI as a work tool is not solely a matter of technological implementation but also requires new competencies and skills at the individual, organizational, and societal level.

Keywords: Artificial intelligence · Physiotherapy professionals · Future needs · Survey · Thematic analysis · Change in professional practice culture

M. Säreströniemi et al. (Eds.): NCDHWS 2026, CCIS 3010, pp. 490–507, 2026.
https://doi.org/10.1007/978-3-032-28819-6_32

1 Introduction

There is a clear need for change in the work of physiotherapists, as societal re-sources are expected to remain unchanged or decrease, while the demand for rehabilitation is increasing substantially at both national and international levels [1]. The increasing use of artificial intelligence (AI) may represent one potential solution to this challenge. However, at this stage, based on international systematic reviews, research on AI and physiotherapy has mainly focused on the production of physiotherapy content for rehabilitation clients [e.g. 3, 4] and only a limited number of studies have examined physiotherapists' experiences of using AI in their work [5–7].

International research has not specifically addressed how AI as a work tool influences the development of professional expertise, emerging competence requirements, or work culture, including aspects such as work productivity, perceived well-being at work, or the organization of work [see 5–7]. Nonetheless, some previous studies suggest that AI has the potential to transform physiotherapists' work by enabling professionals to allocate more time to direct rehabilitation clients interaction, guidance and counselling, functional assessment, as well as the delivery of therapeutic interventions [8–10].

In Finland, research related to AI in physiotherapy and rehabilitation remains largely absent [see, e.g., 11–15], despite emerging indications that AI may be beginning to influence physiotherapists' work, including aspects of professional expertise, operational culture, leadership, and work organization. To our knowledge, future-oriented expectations regarding the use of artificial intelligence in physiotherapy have not yet been examined in Finland [see 12, 13].

The aim of this study was to examine how Finnish physiotherapy experts would like to use AI-based tools in their future work. The present study addresses this gap and contributes to the existing literature by providing novel insights into how such expectations are articulated. A key methodological innovation of this study is the use of an open-ended, future-oriented question, which enables respondents to move beyond current practices and articulate prospective visions of AI use.

2 Material and Methods

Artificial Intelligence and Future Opportunities in Physiotherapy study: University of Jyväskylä and Finnish Association of Physiotherapists are collaboratively conducting a study entitled *"The Use of Artificial Intelligence and Future Opportunities in Physiotherapy: From Evidence-Based Knowledge to National Recommendations."*

The aim of this comprehensive study is to examine how artificial intelligence can be utilized as a tool in physiotherapists' work, as well as in the development of AI-related expertise and work culture, while considering leadership and work organization across different career stages in physiotherapy. The study will generate societal-, sectoral- and workplace-level recommendations and policy actions regarding the use of artificial intelligence as a professional tool in physiotherapy. Data collection is conducted through three sub-studies: 1) a survey of physiotherapy professionals, 2) an interview study with Physiotherapy professionals and students, and 3) a Delphi expert panel study involving physiotherapy professionals, experts in social and healthcare and rehabilitation, specialists in technology and artificial intelligence, and individuals in decision-making positions. The study is funded by the Finnish Work Environment Fund (2025–2026). This article presents preliminary findings derived from an open-ended question employing a future-oriented, metaphor-based approach.

A Survey for Physiotherapy Professionals: A survey was conducted between October and December 2025. The survey was distributed via the Finnish Association of Physiotherapists, the research group's website, and the researchers' personal networks and social media, and responses were collected anonymously. The questionnaire included 11 AI-related questions, of which nine were common to all participants, including one open-ended question that was identical for all respondents. Two additional questions were tailored to respondents' study or work roles (e.g., students, clinical work, supervisory roles, management, education and training, and research, development, and innovation activities). The nine common AI-related questions, along with their response scales and follow-up items, are described in detail in Supplementary Table 1.

Participants: A total of 141 experts responded (77 % women; mean age 47.7 years, SD 13.8). The respondents represented a diverse range of physiotherapy-related backgrounds. These included bachelor-level physiotherapy students (n = 17; 12.0 %), master's-level physiotherapy students (n = 16; 11.4 %), physiotherapists engaged in client work (n = 60; 60 %), individuals in supervisory or departmental management positions (n = 16; 11.3 %), professionals working in education or training roles (n = 7; 5.0 %), and those involved in research, development, and/or innovation activities (n = 14; 9.9 %). In addition, 11 respondents (7.8 %) reported working in other fields. These other occupations included, for example, positions in non-governmental organizations, entrepreneurship within the rehabilitation sector, and retirement. The respondents had an average of 20,3 (SD 13.4) years of work experience related to physiotherapy, with a range of 0,33–56,0 years. In terms of specialization, musculoskeletal physiotherapy (n = 73; 52.8 %), neurological physiotherapy (n = 47; 33.3 %), and gerontological physiotherapy (n = 34; 24 %) were the most represented. The survey respondents did not represent the most experienced Physiotherapy professionals in AI, as fifty-eight percent of respondents indicated that they require training related to the use of AI.

A Future-Oriented Open-Ended Question Using a Metaphor: In the present study, the data consisted of written responses to a future-oriented, metaphor-based open-ended question: *"If you could have any superpowers with the help of AI that would support you in your work as a Physiotherapy professional, what would they be?"* Written responses were provided by 101 participants (72 %). The dataset comprises 1,407 words of transcribed text. The question was deliberately designed to orient respondents toward future perspectives and the expanding scope of AI utilization in physiotherapy. The use of future-oriented, metaphor-based questioning can enable respondents to move beyond the immediate constraints of everyday practice, including resource- and system-level limitations. Such an approach also provides analytical insight into how the profession is conceptualized and the kinds of roles and expectations attributed to it. Moreover, metaphors function as a means of accessing more nuanced and layered understandings of the multidimensional nature of physiotherapy and its evolving relationship with AI (see e.g.,

16–18]. Prior research in the field of education has similarly employed metaphor-based approaches; for example, Chounta et al. 2022 [19] conceptualized artificial intelligence through the metaphor of a "future-oriented superpower."

Thematic Analysis of Qualitative Data: The data were analyzed using an inductive thematic analysis approach [20]. Thematic analysis was conducted using investigator triangulation and proceeded in a stepwise manner. The analysis began with a thorough familiarization with the dataset, followed by initial coding of meaningful units (TS). Codes were then organized and grouped into broader categories, which facilitated the development of preliminary themes and subthemes (TS). These themes were subsequently refined, reviewed, and named to ensure they accurately captured the content of the data (TS, HK). Finally, the results were systematically described and reported, providing a comprehensive representation of the participants' perspectives (TS, HK, SL, VH). The most significant competence gaps were related to understanding guidelines and regulations issued at the European Union level and addressing data security–related problem situations. Self-assessed AI competence was strongest in areas concerning professional responsibility, transparency of use, consent, and data protection.

For the present study, the data consisted of written responses to a future-oriented, metaphor-based open-ended question: "If you could have any superpowers with the help of AI that would support you in your work as a Physiotherapy professional, what would they be?" Written responses were provided by 101 participants (72 %). The dataset comprises 1,407 words of transcribed text.

The analysis began with a thorough familiarization with the dataset, followed by initial coding of meaningful units. Codes were then organized and grouped into broader categories, which facilitated the development of preliminary themes and subthemes. These themes were subsequently refined, reviewed, and named to ensure they accurately captured the content of the data. Finally, the results were systematically described and reported, providing a comprehensive representation of the participants' perspectives.

3 Results

A total of 214 meaning units were identified in the dataset, which were analyzed according to the principles of thematic analysis. The analysis yielded five overarching dimensions: AI as a tool for physiotherapists, AI support for rehabilitation clients, AI in supporting administrative work, AI in supporting research and development activities, An AI-positive work culture. These main themes emerged from 12 subthemes. Appendix Table 2. Provides a detailed overview of the results of the thematic analysis, including the main and subthemes, along with examples of meaning units.

The results are organized into main themes and subthemes that describe Physiotherapy professionals' expectations and perceptions regarding the role of AI in their work. Sections 3.1–3.6 present these themes in detail, illustrating how AI is anticipated to support clinical practice, rehabilitation clients, administrative work, research and development, and the development of an AI-positive expert culture. Each section further elaborates the corresponding subthemes to provide a comprehensive understanding of the identified areas. Finally, Sect. 3.6 describes participants' uncertainty and concerns regarding AI support.

3.1 AI as a Tool for Physiotherapists

Finnish Physiotherapy professionals and students express an intention to use AI-based tools in their future work as a means of enhancing clinical expertise, support evidence-based physiotherapy, supports holistic rehabilitation clients understanding.

AI is expected to support physiotherapy holistically by improving clinical insight, diagnostic accuracy, decision-making, and individualized therapy planning and monitoring, while also enhancing evaluation, rehabilitation clients safety, and the prediction of rehabilitation outcomes. Furthermore, AI is anticipated to support evidence-based physiotherapy by improving access to reliable research, synthesizing key evidence, and providing up-to-date recommendations to guide clinical decision-making. In addition, AI is expected to support physiotherapy through advanced data utilization, holistic rehabilitation clients understanding, and improved assessment processes, while also enhancing communication, multidisciplinary collaboration, and rehabilitation client-centered rehabilitation in diverse and complex context.

Below are verbatim quotations from the dataset that illustrate the participants' reflections on the identified theme.

> *"Clinical assessment and support for reasoning. The development of speech-based programs, particularly to assist documentation and, to a limited extent, preliminary conclusions."*
>
> *"It would be great if artificial intelligence could analyze a patient's movement using video or sensors and provide suggestions for appropriate exercises. It could also anticipate potential problems and offer the physiotherapist evidence-based recommendations."*
>
> *"Artificial intelligence would work best if it brought the latest research knowledge to the physiotherapist in a compiled and efficient way. I do not wish for artificial intelligence to start replacing personal interaction and individualized rehabilitation, or to create rehabilitation programs and such for clients solely using AI."*
>
> *"I would like to master the human body as a whole, to be able to correctly integrate its functions, and to reflect together with artificial intelligence on what the best treatment is for each physiotherapeutic problem. Improving the quality of human life = improving the well-being of our society."*

3.2 AI Support for Rehabilitation Clients

From the rehabilitation clients perspective, AI is anticipated to strengthening agency, motivation, and the individualization and meaningfulness of rehabilitation as well as the accessibility of physiotherapy. AI is expected to enhance physiotherapy by improving rehabilitation clients motivation, adherence, and understanding, while supporting effective, impactful care and long-term outcomes such as healthy ageing. AI is also expected to enhance physiotherapy by supporting personalized meaningful rehabilitation, improving understanding of health and pain, facilitating guidance and navigation, and strengthening rehabilitation clients motivation and engagement. In addition, AI is expected to enhance access to physiotherapy by enabling timely need identification, improving rehabilitation clients pathways, and supporting the availability and visibility of services.

Below are verbatim quotations from the dataset that illustrate the participants' reflections on the identified theme.

"The ability to see inside the human body would facilitate practice, as would the ability to guess in what way phrasing things would motivate the client to take responsibility for their part in the rehabilitation process."

"I would be able to create for the patient a clear, visual, and personalized biopsychosocial understanding of their own pain history. This would help them find better personal functional capacity."

"I would want to be present for the 'patients' when the need is greatest, that is, most often outside of working hours."

3.3 AI in Supporting Administrative Work

In administrative tasks, AI is expected to free up time for core physiotherapy work while enhancing the quality and efficiency of documentation. Physiotherapy professionals expect AI to support their work by automating routine administrative tasks, particularly documentation, reporting, scheduling, and communication processes. AI is anticipated to streamline and structure clinical documentation, reduce manual workload, and facilitate efficient information management. These efficiencies are expected to enable greater focus on rehabilitation client-centered rehabilitation and rehabilitation. In addition, AI is expected to enhance documentation by supporting efficient writing, speech-to-text processing, and structured, high-quality reporting.

Below are verbatim quotations from the dataset that illustrate the participants' reflections on the identified theme.

"I would like an artificial intelligence superpower that would help with patient documentation and reduce manual writing. It could suggest ready-made text templates and automatically check grammar. In addition, artificial intelligence could assist in the planning and monitoring of exercise programs, thereby freeing up more of the physiotherapist's time for patient care."

"With the help of artificial intelligence, I would like a superpower that would automate routine tasks such as documentation, reporting, and appointment scheduling. This way, I could spend more time on patient interaction and rehabilitation."

"Artificial intelligence could act as a personal work partner that monitors the patient's progress, suggests appropriate exercises, provides reminders, and assists with documentation. It would be like an invisible colleague who makes everyday work smoother and more efficient ☺."

3.4 AI in Supporting Research and Development Activities

In the future, AI is anticipated to play a supportive role in research and development, particularly by enhancing the use of research evidence and promoting effectiveness-based practice. Physiotherapy professionals expect AI to support research utilization by enabling efficient access to and critical appraisal of evidence. AI is anticipated to facilitate the identification of knowledge gaps, streamline literature search and synthesis, and support the rapid evaluation and integration of new research findings. In addition, AI is expected to enable the rapid processing and analysis of large datasets, facilitating real-time generation and reporting of effective data. Overall, AI is anticipated to strengthen evidence-based and outcome-oriented practice by supporting the evaluation of rehabilitation effectiveness, ultimately contributing to improved quality and reliability of physiotherapy services.

Below are verbatim quotations from the dataset that illustrate the participants' reflections on the identified theme.

> *"Extracting patient background information from texts without manual work. Data collection and analysis of operational activities without manual work directly from the source system."*

> *"I would be able to extract information from different systems about the impact of physiotherapy/rehabilitation on the client's/patient's life, for example on work ability, service needs, etc. The information needs concern both short-term effects and long-term effects."*

> *"Speed in checking the reliability of source materials and in summarizing the core message of extensive reviews, as well as in highlighting potential gaps."*

3.5 An AI-Positive Work Culture

In the future, an AI-positive expert culture is expected to emerge, encompassing continuous professional development and the perception of work as meaningful through AI-supported practice. Physiotherapy professionals expect AI to support continuous professional development by facilitating access to up-to-date research evidence, clinical guidelines, and evidence-based interventions. AI is anticipated to enhance learning and expertise by assisting in information synthesis, clarifying complex concepts, and providing timely answers to clinical questions. In addition, Physiotherapy professionals expect AI to support meaningful and human-centered work by acting as a collaborative partner in daily practice. AI is anticipated to enhance work efficiency and smoothness, reduce physical and cognitive workload, and foster professional well-being. Furthermore, AI is expected to promote innovation, support challenging work situations, and encourage the adoption of new practices within physiotherapy and rehabilitation services.

Below are verbatim quotations from the dataset that illustrate the participants' reflections on the identified theme.

> *"I would wish for an artificial intelligence superpower that would help me continuously develop in my work. It could provide new research, clinical guidelines, and evidence-based exercises for different patient groups easily and quickly"*

> *"So-called "strengthening of multidisciplinary competence" in unexpected situations: how to guide the client forward (e.g., various applications and forms: which authority can assist, etc.)."*

"From a management perspective, I would need superpowers to motivate staff to use artificial intelligence in rehabilitation and functional capacity support services..."

3.6 Participants' Uncertainty and Concerns Regarding AI Support

In addition to the themes described above, some responses indicated that participants did not yet understand, or could not specify, how AI could support their work. Furthermore, certain responses reflected a negative attitude toward AI. These perspectives highlighted concerns related to fundamental principles of AI, as well as factors influencing its reliability and the exercise of professional expertise.

Below are verbatim quotations from the dataset illustrating participants' reflections on this theme.

"I don't know what artificial intelligence could enable, so I cannot answer the question.."

"On principle, I consider the use of artificial intelligence wrong, and I want to stay away from it as long as possible."

"A physiotherapist who needs artificial intelligence for expertise is then not an expert themselves, but rather transfers their expertise to AI. I would replace the therapist myself, who would have to ask AI for instructions on treating my condition."

4 Discussion

The aim of this study is to examine how Finnish Physiotherapy professionals would like to use AI-based tools in their future work. The results underscore that the adoption of AI as a work tool is not solely a matter of technological implementation but also requires new competencies and skills at the individual, organizational, and societal level. Specifically, AI has the potential as a tool for physiotherapists to enhance clinical reasoning, support evidence-based decision-making, and facilitate a holistic understanding of the human body, aligning with physiotherapists' professional expertise. Beyond clinical practice, AI is also expected to play an important role in supporting rehabilitation clients, administrative work, research and development, and fostering an AI-positive work culture.

The thematic analysis presented in Table 1 highlights the multifaceted roles that AI may assume in physiotherapy. These roles have implications not only for professional practice and organizational structures, but also for education, research and development activities as well as across the broader professional and organizational culture. The findings further revealed a hierarchical, multilayered structure of aspirations, with future-oriented hopes addressing individual-level concerns as well as organizational and societal dimensions. Consistent with previous research, most studies have focused primarily on either clients/rehabilitation clients [3, 4] or physiotherapists [5–7]. However, such a narrow focus overlooks the broader context of physiotherapy and its complex, multidimensional ecosystem, which encompasses professional practice, organizational structures, education, and research and innovation activities.

The results also highlight the diverse future competence needs of physiotherapy professionals, which relate not only to five main thematic areas but also to the management of the broader ecosystem. The study's thematic findings may inform the development of physiotherapy programs at undergraduate, graduate, and doctoral levels, as well as continuing education initiatives The study results, which highlight future-oriented visions and needs, also further contribute to and guide the development of AI guidelines relevant to physiotherapy and rehabilitation, providing valuable evidence to inform the creation of such guidelines at the national level, which represents a central objective of this broader project.

Although the dataset was relatively small, it was rich in content. This richness was reflected, for example, in the wide range of potential future use cases identified for physiotherapy across diverse professional contexts, including clinical practice, administrative work, research and development, and the development of an AI-positive professional culture. In addition, the data revealed a distinct theme highlighting concerns and resistance regarding the increasing use of artificial intelligence. The results further indicate that the design of a future-oriented open-ended question using a metaphor elicited rich and detailed responses; however, alongside positive future perspectives, it also revealed participants' uncertainty and concerns regarding AI support.

The data also exhibited clear signs of saturation, particularly in themes related to clinical practices and administrative work. A substantial proportion of the meaningful units identified in the dataset were categorized under these domains. In future the findings will be further validated as part of a larger national study on telerehabilitation [12, 13], in which follow-up cohort measurements are currently underway.

Although digitalization and remote physiotherapy have largely been understood as real-time guidance delivered via digital platforms [12, 13], our findings suggest that AI has the potential to extend beyond these practices and transform work organization, leadership, and professional culture across different career stages. Taken together, the results indicate that, in order to meet future expectations and emerging needs within physiotherapy, a more comprehensive and strategic implementation of AI is required. Such implementation should be supported by targeted skill development, structured guidance, and collaborative practices to fully realize the potential of artificial intelligence in physiotherapy.

When considering changes to the organizational culture related to AI, it is essential to recognize the diversity of experiences and perspectives. While the current data predominantly reflected positive future visions, any discussion of hopes and opportunities should also account for skepticism, critical attitudes, and even resistance, as these elements are integral to understanding and guiding cultural transformation.

Critical Reflections and Methodological Considerations

While the novelty of this study constitutes an important contribution, the findings should be interpreted with appropriate caution. Existing research on AI in physiotherapy has largely focused on the development of AI-generated content for rehabilitation clients [e.g., 3–4] or on physiotherapists' experiences of AI use in clinical practice [5–7]. By including physiotherapy students, physiotherapists, physiotherapy managers and administrative staff, educators, and experts engaged in research, development, and innovation, the present study broadens the scope of inquiry. The heterogeneity of the participants can be considered a strength of this study, as it enabled the generation of diverse and meaningful insights at the individual, community, and societal levels. This diversity provided a comprehensive understanding of the broad field of physiotherapy, as well as its future development, including the emerging AI ecosystem within physiotherapy. At the same time, such heterogeneity may contribute to variability in perspectives, reflecting differences in professional roles, levels of AI familiarity, and contextual constraints.

The use of metaphors in research questions require careful consideration, as unconventional question framing may confuse respondents or even distort the findings. In this study, the term 'superpower' was deliberately employed in the formulation of the question, as the aim was to elicit responses that would be detached from the current context of physiotherapy and established practices. A potential risk associated with this formulation was that respondents might assume their answers should be exclusively positively oriented. As metaphors are not neutral, they may, for example, unduly direct respondents' thinking [e.g., 16]. However, despite the positive framing of the question, respondents in this study also expressed more critical perspectives on the future use of artificial intelligence in physiotherapy (see Sect. 3.6, Participants' uncertainty and concerns regarding AI support). This finding is important, as it reflects the intended aim of the research question design, which sought to access more nuanced and layered understandings of the multidimensional nature of physiotherapy and its evolving relationship with AI, as highlighted in previous research [see, e.g., 16–19].

The relatively small qualitative dataset (1,407 words) may limit the depth and richness of the thematic analysis, as well as the transferability of the findings. Although the results highlight future-oriented aspirations and expectations regarding AI in physiotherapy, these should not be interpreted as representative of the profession as a whole. Rather, the findings reflect a set of themes and subthemes that capture emerging meanings and perspectives situated within specific professional and organizational contexts. To enhance the trustworthiness of these interpretations, future research should incorporate data triangulation by integrating findings from other components of the broader survey. Additionally, more in-depth qualitative approaches are needed to further explore how professional roles, career stages, and organizational contexts shape these themes, as well as to examine tensions between enthusiasm, skepticism, and resistance toward AI-driven transformation in physiotherapy practice.

Acknowledgments. The study is based on the research project funded by the Finnish Work Environment Fund, "The Use of Artificial Intelligence and Future Opportunities in Physiotherapy – From Evidence-Based Knowledge to National Recommendations and Action Proposals" (2025–2026).

Disclosure of Interests. The authors have no competing interests to declare that are relevant to the content of this article.

Appendix

Table 1. The key artificial intelligence–related questions included in the survey questionnaire

Artificial intelligence related questions [scale] / Follow-up questions
1. In your opinion, to what extent is artificial intelligence currently applicable in physiotherapy practice? Scale: 0–7 [0 = cannot say / do not know, 1 = strongly disagree, 7 = strongly agree] in the following contexts: 1] Client work, 2] Supervisory or managerial work, 3] Sector-level leadership, 4] Teaching and training, 5] Research, development, and innovation [RDI] activities, 6] Expert roles [e.g., work in professional organizations or other specialist roles], 7] Bachelor's-level studies, 8] Independent professional development, 9] Short courses or continuing professional education, 10] Master's-level postgraduate studies, 11] Doctoral-level studies, 12] Leisure activities related to the profession, 13] Other physiotherapy-related work – please specify what and how?
2. Are you aware of any artificial intelligence–related guidelines currently in use within your wellbeing services county/region? [Scale: Yes / No / Do not know] 1] General guidelines or recommendations on the use of artificial intelligence are currently in place within the wellbeing services county, 2] These guidelines or recommendations are intended for social and healthcare professionals, 3] Rehabilitation is addressed in the wellbeing services county's guidelines or recommendations, 4] Physiotherapy is addressed in the wellbeing services county's guidelines or recommendations, 5] Are you aware of any other guidelines or recommendations related to the use of artificial intelligence at, for example, the organizational or unit level within your wellbeing services county?
3. In your opinion, what is the need for guidelines related to the use of artificial intelligence in social and healthcare, including rehabilitation and physiotherapy? Scale: 0–7 [0 = cannot say / do not know, 1 = strongly disagree, 7 = strongly agree] in the following contexts: 1] There is a need for common, AI-related general guidelines or recommendations for social and healthcare professionals across wellbeing services counties, 2] There is a need for common guidelines or recommendations that take into account the perspective of rehabilitation across wellbeing services counties, 3] There is a need for common guidelines or recommendations that take into account the perspective of physiotherapy across wellbeing services counties, 4] Physiotherapy-related guidelines or recommendations should take into account the different specialties within physiotherapy [e.g., geriatric physiotherapy, paediatric physiotherapy, neurological physiotherapy, psychophysical physiotherapy, cardiovascular and respiratory physiotherapy, musculoskeletal physiotherapy, occupational health physiotherapy], 5] Physiotherapy-related guidelines or recommendations should consider the various contexts in which physiotherapy is delivered [e.g., primary healthcare, specialized healthcare, occupational health services, private sector, third sector].

(*continued*)

Table 1. (*continued*)

Physiotherapy-related guidelines or recommendations should take into account different stages of career development [e.g., students, physiotherapists, administrative staff, teaching personnel, and those working in research, development, and innovation roles] / **Follow-up question:** What additional aspects should be considered in physiotherapy-related guidelines?

4. Have you participated in any training related to the use of artificial intelligence during the past two years? [Scale: Yes / No / Do not know] / **Follow-up question a:** If you answered "No" or "I don't know," please specify the reasons for not participating in such training. **Follow-up question b:** If you answered "Yes," please specify the provider and duration of the training: 1] I have participated in AI-related education or training as part of physiotherapy degree or postgraduate studies, 2] I have participated in AI-related training or events organized by my wellbeing services county, 3] I have participated in AI-related training or events organized by my organization, 4] I have participated in other AI-related training or events.

5. Do you perceive a need for education or training on artificial intelligence in the context of physiotherapy? Please select the option that best reflects your current view [Scale: Yes / No / Do not know] / **Follow-up question:** If you answered "Yes," please describe in more detail what kind of AI-related training you consider necessary.

6. Please assess your competence related to the use of artificial intelligence in physiotherapy: Scale: 0–7 [0 = cannot say / do not know, 1 = strongly disagree, 7 = strongly agree] in the following contexts: 1] I understand professional responsibility related to the use of artificial intelligence, 2] I understand the requirements for transparency and openness in the use of artificial intelligence, 3] I understand that the use of artificial intelligence requires the consent of the client/patient, 4] I understand the data protection requirements related to AI applications or tools that process personal data, 5] I understand the regulations governing medical devices that utilize artificial intelligence [Medical Device Regulation, MDR], 6] I understand the different roles of AI-based applications or tools in my work, 7] I understand the basic principles of algorithms used in artificial intelligence, 8] I understand sustainability considerations related to AI-based technologies, 9] I am able to critically evaluate research related to artificial intelligence, 10] I am familiar with terminology related to artificial intelligence, 11] I am able to manage risks related to information security in artificial intelligence, 12] I understand the principles of intellectual property rights and copyright related to artificial intelligence, 13] I understand the guidelines in accordance with the European Union [EU] Artificial Intelligence Act, 14] I am able to verify the accuracy of information generated by artificial intelligence, 15] I am able to act appropriately if information security issues are identified in AI-based systems [applications or tools] / **Follow-up question:** Please describe any thoughts or reflections the above statements elicited.

(*continued*)

Table 1. *(continued)*

7. Perceived added value of artificial intelligence in my work: I believe that artificial intelligence could enhance… [Scale: 0–7 [0 = cannot say / do not know, 1 = strongly disagree, 7 = strongly agree] 1] …referrals to physiotherapy within care pathways, 2] …provision of physiotherapy services , 3] …availability of physiotherapy services, 4] …accessibility of physiotherapy services, 5] …equity among rehabilitation clients/patients, 6] …participation of rehabilitation clients/patients, 7] …client-/patient-centeredness in rehabilitation, 8] …work productivity, 9]…effectiveness of work, 10]…meaningfulness of work, 11] …physiotherapists' perceived well-being at work, 12]…physiotherapists' perceived work ability, 13]…work-related safety /**Follow-up question:** Please describe any thoughts or reflections the above statements elicited.
8. Please assess how your perception of the potential of artificial intelligence in physiotherapy has changed compared to your views six months ago compared to your perceptions six months ago [Scale: 1–7] 1] My perceptions have become significantly more negative, 2] My perceptions have become clearly more negative, 3] My perceptions have become slightly more negative, 4] My perceptions have remained unchanged, 5] My perceptions have become slightly more positive, 6] My perceptions have become clearly more positive, 7] My perceptions have become significantly more positive
9. If you could have any "superpowers" enabled by artificial intelligence to support your work as a physiotherapy expert, what would they be?

Table 2. Roles of artificial intelligence in physiotherapy, thematic analysis

Main themes	Sub-themes	Meaningful units
1) AI as a tool for physiotherapists	1) Enhancing clinical expertise	Enables visualization inside the human body, X-ray-like vision, Radiographic vision, Provides understanding of movement in subcutaneous structures, Provides understanding of biomechanics, Supports a deeper understanding of biomechanics, Provides information on anatomy, Analyzes patient movement using video or sensors, Assists in identifying anatomical structures and landmarks, Supports acupuncture and fascial manipulation, Enables precise analysis of symptoms
		Provides rapid support in demanding tasks (e.g., identification of symptoms and related risks in rare conditions), Assists in out-of-the-box thinking when addressing problems and challenges
		Produces rapid and accurate physiotherapy diagnoses, Generates preliminary diagnostic options, Supports diagnosis, Identifies symptoms and related risks in rare conditions, Serves as a diagnostic tool for physiotherapists, Forms diagnoses based on clinical findings, Enables client digitalization, Supports the formulation of physiotherapy diagnoses, Accelerates the diagnostic process
		Clinical reasoning, Supports treatment principles based on anamnesis and clinical findings, Clarifies clinical reasoning, Assists in making rapid conclusions, Supports rapid decision-making, Assists in the selection of rehabilitation interventions, Supports clinical assessment and reasoning, Supports preliminary conclusions, Supports physiotherapy-related conclusion
		Supports physiotherapy planning, Assists in the selection of therapy methods, Supports the development of individualized exercises for clients, Accelerates the creation of instructions for clients
		Supports the ideation of exercise programs, Assists in exercise program planning, Provides suggestions for appropriate exercises, Assists in selecting exercises and repetitions, Supports the creation of exercises, Supports the development of exercise programs, Assists in creating more graphical exercise instructions, Produces targeted exercises
		Assists in monitoring exercise programs, Tracks patient progress, Classifies symptoms, Identifies correct therapeutic directions, Determines exercises and their dosage, Supports evaluation, Assists in assessing physiotherapy effectiveness, Oversees the implementation of physiotherapy
		Prevention, Anticipates potential problems, Ensures patient safety, Provides support in unexpected situations
		Assists with uncooperative patients, Helps turn resistant patients into receptive ones, Assists in structuring interviews
		Assists in predicting rehabilitation success, Supports forecasting rehabilitation outcomes, Predicts therapy effectiveness, Anticipates future developments
	2) Support evidence-based physiotherapy	Access to research evidence, Verification of source material reliability, Summarization of key messages from extensive reviews, Utilization of research evidence, Selection of effective interventions, Provides physiotherapists with evidence-based recommendations, Provides the latest recommendations on various topics, Summarizes recommendations needed in practice, Generates easily evidence-based rehabilitation recommendations for specific conditions, Shared AI-generated recommendations for physiotherapy
	3) Supports holistic client/rehabilitees understanding	Generates necessary information for physiotherapy use, Extracts patient background information, Collects operational data, Analyzes operational data from source systems, Retrieves data, Analyzes data, Organizes operations, Supports holistic consideration, Supports understanding
		Comprehensive consideration of functional capacity, Considers the patient's biomechanics, physiological load, rehabilitation process, and various medical conditions

(continued)

Table 2. *(continued)*

		Assists in seeing the bigger picture, Supports holistic management of the human body, Aids in identifying psychophysical exercises and activities, Suggests appropriate exercises, Supports assessment of work ability impact, Supports evaluation of service needs
		Supports a humane and meaningful life, Enhances quality of human life
		Strengthens multidisciplinary expertise, Guides clients forward; Observes clients' changing situations
		Acts as an interpreter and communication aid in multicultural settings, Translates patient instructions into different languages, Ensures that patients understand the content of instructions, Functions as a "sensory interpreter" in physiotherapy when working with neurological and disabled patients, Able to accurately interpret patients' bodily signals and expressions
2) AI support for rehabilitation clients	4) AI support for rehabilitation clients	Clarity of language used, Engagement in exercise, Supports healthy ageing, Assists in motivating clients, Supports client/patient life through impactful physiotherapy, Identifies root causes of clients' complaints, Motivates patients to participate in rehabilitation, Ability to support clients in fulfilling their part of the rehabilitation process
	5) Strengthening individualization and meaningfulness of rehabilitation	Clarifies the impact of medical history on the current condition, Supports patients in achieving better functional capacity, Assists in determining the appropriate physiotherapeutic treatment for each individual, Creates a biopsychosocial understanding of pain history for the patient, Provides a clear and personalized understanding of pain history, Acts as an interpreter of the patient's understanding, Provides information on disease manifestations, Provides information on interactions between diseases and medications
		Enables an interactive exercise program, Supports the development of enjoyable physical activities, Personalized therapy, Provides individual support, Highlights short-term and long-term effects
		Guides the client forward, Assists in selecting applications and forms, Directs to the appropriate supporting authority
		Supports the realization of human rights in physiotherapy, Supports the development of collaboration between physiotherapist and client, Provides tailored rehabilitation instructions, Supports the development of the patient's intrinsic motivation, Enhances client motivation for engaging in physiotherapy, Ability to anticipate how to motivate the client
	6) Accessible physiotherapy	Guides referral to physiotherapists, Rapid identification of the need for rehabilitation interventions, Enables physiotherapy for all Finnish residents, Enables free physiotherapy, Facilitates easy delivery of physiotherapy, Access to physiotherapy outside office hours, Supports marketing of physiotherapy, Could assist in marketing, Could assist in directing suitable patients considering my expertise
3) AI in supporting administrative work	7) Freeing up time for core physiotherapy work	Automates routine tasks, Automates documentation, Automates reporting, Automates scheduling, Sends reminders, Automatic dictation for documentation, Automatic text structuring, Automatic task tracking, Automatic monitoring of workspaces, Automatic summary of the patient's key health history, Automation of routine work tasks (orders, work shift planning), Planned and scheduled work

(continued)

Table 2. (*continued*)

		Supports documentation, Documentation assistance, Provides help with visit documentation, Facilitates documentation, Accelerates documentation, Speeds up documentation, Eases documentation, Performs documentation, Documentation, Speeds up documentation, Speeds up documentation, Speeds up documentation, Assists in documentation, Streamlines documentation, Documentation streamlining, Accelerates documentation, Streamlines and structures documentation, Streamlines and structures other written texts
		Considering ICF classification, Assists in creating summaries, Speeds up statement/report writing, Supports patient documentation, Reduces manual documentation, Provides ready-made text templates, Exports documentation to patient information systems, Would accelerate work, Speeds up work
		Responds to inquiries and calls from other professionals regarding services, Screens calls that do not concern the individual, Directs calls appropriately, Guides collaborators to intranet resources, Frees up time for patient work, Provides more time for patient interaction and rehabilitation, Supports physiotherapy documentation, Brings additional time to patient work, Saves time for essential tasks, Provides more time for working with clients, Adds time for physiotherapy implementation
	8) Enhancing documentation quality and efficiency	Assists in creating tables, Assists in documentation, Provides support for report entry, Automatically checks grammar, Transcribes speech, Facilitates writing, Identifies condition from speech, Records results from speech into predefined templates, Saves reports, Enables smooth writing (memos, reports, plans, process diagrams)
4) AI in supporting research and development activities	9) Enhancing the use of research evidence	Highlights gaps in reviews, Assists in development, Enables reliable and rapid source evaluation, Reliable AI, Facilitates reading of research, Supports mastering of extensive research knowledge, Enhances the search for new information, Accelerates evaluation of new studies, Online tool for synthesizing research evidence, Online tool for gathering sources
	10) Promoting effectiveness-based practice	Rapid processing of massive datasets, Drawing conclusions from massive datasets, Accelerates information retrieval Real-time compilation of effectiveness data, Real-time reporting of effectiveness data
		Promoting the effectiveness of physiotherapy, Mining data from systems on physiotherapy/rehabilitation effectiveness, Supports outcome-based work, Enables rapid rehabilitation, Aspiration for AI to support the quality of physiotherapy, Aspiration for AI to support the reliability of physiotherapy
5) AI-positive work culture	11) Continuous professional development	AI-related training, Supports continuous professional development in my work, Aspiration for AI to support physiotherapists' expertise
		Facilitates structuring of thoughts, Clarifies thinking, Provides answers to physiotherapists' questions, Synthesizes information
		Provides clinical guidelines, Offers new research, Provides evidence-based exercises for different patient groups easily and rapidly, Delivers new knowledge from the field, Provides the latest research evidence from the field, Brings the most recent research evidence to physiotherapists in a concise and efficient manner
	12) Meaningful work through AI-supported practice	Supports humane and meaningful work, Provides a sense of contributing to societal well-being, Acts as a personal work partner, Functions as an invisible colleague, Makes everyday work smoother and more efficient, Promotes calmness, judgment, and patience in the worker, Supports innovation in physiotherapy practice, Performs the physically most demanding physiotherapy tasks, Assists in managing challenging staffing situations, Inspires physiotherapy staff, Encourages the use of AI in rehabilitation, Encourages the use of AI in services supporting functional capacity

References

1. Cieza, A., Causey, K., Kamenov, K., Hanson, S. W., Chatterji, S., Vos, T.: Global estimates of the need for rehabilitation based on the global burden of disease study 2019: a systematic analysis. Lancet **396**(10267), 2006–2017 (2021). https://doi.org/10.1016/S0140-6736(20)32340-0
2. Heino, P., Mäkinen, J., Seppänen-Järvelä, R.: Vaativan lääkinnällisen kuntoutuksen lain muutoksen vaikutus kuntoutuksen kohdentumiseen: rekisteritutkimus vuosien 2014, 2016 ja 2017 kuntoutuspäätöksistä. Helsinki: Kela, Sosiaali- ja terveysturvan raportteja **23** (2020)
3. Ravali, R.S., et al.: A systematic review of artificial intelligence for pediatric physiotherapy practice: past, present, and future. Neurosci. Inform. **2**(4), 100045 (2022). https://doi.org/10.1016/j.neuri.2022.100045
4. Sumner, J., Lim, H.W., Chong, L.S., Bundele, A., Mukhopadhyay, A., Kayambu, G.: Artificial intelligence in physical rehabilitation: a systematic review. Artif. Intell. Med. **146**, 102693 (2023). https://doi.org/10.1016/j.artmed.2023.102693
5. Hegazy, F., Aboelnasr, E., Abuzaid, M., Elshami, W., Tekin, H.: The impact of artificial intelligence (AI) in physiotherapy practice: a study of physiotherapists' willingness and readiness [Congress abstract] (2023). https://world.physio/congress-proceeding/impact-artificial-intelligence-ai-physiotherapy-practice-study-0#:~:text=Conclusions%3A%20Implementation%20of%20AI%20into,results%20for%20patients%20and%20providers
6. Shawli, L., Alsobhi, M., Chevidikunnan, M.F., Rosewilliam, S., Basuodan, R., Khan, F.: Physical therapists' perceptions and attitudes towards artificial intelligence in healthcare and rehabilitation: a qualitative study. Musculoskelet. Sci. Pract. **73**, 103152 (2024). https://doi.org/10.1016/j.msksp.2024.103152
7. Merolli, B., Ahmed, O., McCreesh, K., Remedios, L., Butler-Henderson, K.: Are physiotherapists expected to be competent in digital health practice? Meta-synthesis of international physiotherapy practice competency standards. Physiotherapy Theory Pract., 1–12 (2024). Ahead-of-print
8. Bills, A., Basheer, R.: Embracing the digital revolution: exploring the acceptance and potential of artificial intelligence in physiotherapy. Int. J. Res. Med. Sci. **13**(1), 571–575 (2024). https://doi.org/10.18203/2320-6012.ijrms20244172
9. Naqvi, W.M., Shaikh, S.Z., Mishra, G.V.: Large language models in physical therapy: time to adapt and adept. Front. Public Health **12**, 1364660 (2024). https://doi.org/10.3389/fpubh.2024.1364660
10. Scheper, M.C., van Velzen, M., van Meeteren, N.L.U.: Towards responsible use of artificial intelligence in daily practice: what do physiotherapists need to know, consider and do? J. Physiother. **70**, 81–84 (2024). https://doi.org/10.1016/j.jphys.2023.07.012
11. DigiFinland. Esiselvitystyön loppuraportti, maaliskuu 2024 (2024)
12. Hellstén, T., Arokoski, J., Sjögren, T., Jäppinen, A.M., Kettunen, J.: The current state of remote physiotherapy in Finland: cross-sectional web-based questionnaire study. JMIR Rehabil Assist Technol **9**(2), e35569 (2022). https://doi.org/10.2196/35569
13. Hellstén, T., Arokoski, J., Sjögren, T., Jäppinen, A., Kettunen, J.: Remote physiotherapy in Finland—suitability, usability and factors affecting. Eur. J. Physiotherapy (2023).https://doi.org/10.1080/21679169.2023.2233560
14. Kaasalainen, K., Ruohonen, T., Neittaanmäki, P.: Interventiot ja tekoäly terveydenhuollossa. Loppuraportti Vol. 3: Value From Public Health Data With Cognitive Computing (VFH) ja Watson Health Cloud Finland (WHC) -hankkeiden (2016–2019) loppuraportti, vol.1–4. Jyväskylän yliopiston IT-tiedekunta, Jyväskylä (2019)
15. SOTE-tekoälyn ekosysteemi (2024). https://digifinland.fi/sote-tekoalyn-ekosysteemi/

16. Carpenter, J.: Metaphors in qualitative research: shedding light or casting shadows? Res. Nurs. Health **31**, 274–282 (2008). https://doi.org/10.1002/nur.20253
17. Khadpe, P., Krishna, R., Li, F-F., Hancock, J.Y., Bernstein, M.S.: Conceptual metaphors impact perceptions of Human-AI collaboration. Proc. ACM Hum.-Comput. Interact. **4**(CSCW2), 163 (2020). 26 pages. https://doi.org/10.1145/3415234
18. Steele, R., Baird, J., Davies, B.: Using metaphors to make research findings meaningful. Can. J. Nurs. Res. **54**(2), 99–100 (2022). https://doi.org/10.1177/08445621221085555
19. Chounta, I.A., Bardone, E., Raudsep, A., Pedaste, M.: Exploring teachers' perceptions of artificial intelligence as a tool to support their practice in Estonian K-12 education. Int. J. Artif. Intell. Educ. **32**, 725–755 (2022). https://doi.org/10.1007/s40593-021-00243-5
20. Braun, V., Clarke, V.: Using thematic analysis in psychology. Qual. Res. Psychol. **3**(2), 77–101 (2006). https://doi.org/10.1191/1478088706qp063oa

Generating BPMN Healthcare Process Models Using LLMs

Adam Grík[1], Silvia Putekova[2], Anna Petrulova[3], Marek Rabincak[4], Karol Nemoga[5], and Fedor Lehocki[1(✉)]

[1] Faculty of Informatics and Information Technologies, Slovak University of Technology in Bratislava, Bratislava, Slovakia
{xgrik,fedor.lehocki}@stuba.sk
[2] Faculty of Health Care and Social Work, Trnava University, Trnava, Slovakia
[3] National Institute of Cardiovascular Diseases, Bratislava, Slovakia
[4] Psychiatric Hospital Michalovce, Michalovce, Slovakia
[5] Mathematical Institute SAS, Bratislava, Slovakia

Abstract. Business Process Model and Notation (BPMN) is widely used in healthcare to formalize clinical workflows, clinical pathways, and organizational procedures. In practice, however, these processes are primarily documented in extensive, unstructured textual artifacts such as clinical guidelines and standardized healthcare procedures. Transforming such documents into BPMN models typically requires substantial manual effort in the early modeling phases, which can reduce time efficiency. Recent advances in LLM-based chatbots offer promising capabilities for analyzing and synthesizing complex textual documents. Nevertheless, existing BPMN generation approaches typically depend on intermediate representations and deterministic parsers, introducing additional architectural complexity and reducing practical usability. This paper proposes a multi-step LLM-based workflow for directly generating BPMN process models encoded in XML from unstructured healthcare procedure documents using a conversational chatbot. The workflow combines multiple prompting techniques and strategies to improve generation robustness and technical correctness. The approach is evaluated on five official healthcare procedure documents issued by the Ministry of Health of the Slovak Republic from the domains of psychology and psychiatry. The generated BPMN models are assessed using a dual evaluation strategy that combines qualitative expert evaluation with objective XML-based metrics. Experimental results demonstrate that the proposed workflow consistently produces formally correct, complete, and clear BPMN models, outperforming a zero-shot prompting baseline according to the evaluated quality criteria. The findings indicate that the proposed approach is well suited for supporting early-stage process modeling from complex healthcare documents.

Keywords: BPMN · healthcare · large language models · chatbots · process modeling

M. Särestöniemi et al. (Eds.): NCDHWS 2026, CCIS 3010, pp. 508–524, 2026.
https://doi.org/10.1007/978-3-032-28819-6_33

1 Introduction

1.1 Motivation and Problem

Business Process Model and Notation (BPMN) is accepted as a notation in healthcare for representing clinical workflows, clinical pathways, and organizational procedures in a structured and interpretable form. In practice, however, healthcare processes are primarily described in extensive textual documents such as standardized procedures and clinical guidelines. Manually analyzing these documents and transforming them into formal process models can be time-consuming and typically requires close collaboration with domain experts.

Recent advances in large language model (LLM)–based chatbots, such as ChatGPT, demonstrate strong capabilities in analyzing and synthesizing complex textual documents. Prior research highlights the potential of conversational AI systems to support healthcare services by assisting in the interpretation and processing of medical documentation [1]. These capabilities make LLM-based chatbots a promising tool for supporting the early stages of process modeling from textual healthcare documents as well as support educational efficiency by targeting healthcare professional's knowledge gaps related to application of clinical pathways in practice [2].

Empirical studies indicate that LLMs can perform document analysis tasks substantially faster than human analysts while achieving comparable qualitative coverage [3]. In this context, LLM-based chatbots are not intended to replace domain experts, but rather to accelerate initial phases of process modeling, such as document analysis and the generation of preliminary BPMN drafts, which can subsequently be refined and validated by experts.

Despite this potential, the direct application of LLM-based chatbots to structured process modeling raises several open challenges.

One major challenge is that existing approaches for applying LLMs to process modeling predominantly rely on intermediate representations, such as parser-based abstractions, tabular or schema-driven representations, or domain-specific process modeling languages. These additional transformation layers increase the overall complexity of the solution and introduce dependencies on auxiliary tools and environments, which can limit the practical accessibility of such approaches in applied settings. Approaches that attempt direct generation of BPMN process models encoded in XML from natural language documents remain limited. Consequently, there is a lack of systematic methodologies for directly generating BPMN process models from unstructured healthcare procedure documents.

Another important challenge arises from inherent limitations that complicate their use for structured process modeling tasks. Their outputs are non-deterministic and sensitive to prompt formulation, with measurable variability observed even under deterministic decoding settings [4]. This variability poses challenges for generating consistent, complete, and technically valid BPMN models, particularly in the context of complex healthcare processes, and therefore necessitates explicit mechanisms for controlling and stabilizing the generation process.

Together, these challenges highlight the need for structured approaches that enable BPMN model generation directly from textual healthcare documents using LLM-based systems, while incorporating controlled prompting strategies to guide the generation process.

1.2 Related Work

Recent research has explored the use of LLMs to support process-oriented reasoning in the healthcare domain, particularly for extracting, interpreting, and navigating clinical workflows from textual sources.

In [5] authors investigate the automated extraction of clinical pathway information from guideline documents using LLMs, proposing a conceptual intermediate model that bridges unstructured text and formal process representations. Their findings demonstrate the suitability of LLMs for supporting early-stage pathway extraction from clinical text.

Similarly, [6] demonstrates the use of LLMs for generating diagnostic pathways through sequential decision-making prompts, effectively modeling clinical reasoning processes for differential diagnosis. Their results show that the use of structured prompting strategies substantially improves the quality and coherence of the generated diagnostic pathways.

The inverse problem is addressed in [7] by focusing on the interpretation and querying of existing clinical process models using LLMs, demonstrating that LLMs can reliably understand and navigate complex clinical pathway graphs.

Complementary findings are reported in [8], demonstrating that LLMs can effectively comprehend and reason over BPMN models. Similarly, [9] explores the use of LLMs for generating process descriptions from BPMN models, further supporting the notion that LLMs possess inherent understanding of BPMN structure and process semantics.

Beyond healthcare, multiple approaches have investigated the generation of BPMN models using LLMs in general process modeling contexts.

Most LLM-based BPMN generation approaches do not produce BPMN process models encoded in XML directly, but instead rely on intermediate representations (e.g., structured text, JSON, tabular formats) that are later transformed into BPMN using deterministic parsers, introducing additional architectural complexity [10–15].

Direct generation of BPMN process models encoded in XML using LLMs without intermediate representations has been explored only to a limited extent. In [16], a zero-shot prompting approach for direct BPMN XML generation is proposed; however, it does not address the challenges posed by complex, unstructured documents nor the need for generation stability and consistency.

Finally, the evaluation of BPMN models generated by LLMs remains an underexplored area. A systematic approach to this problem is introduced in [17] through the 3C framework, which evaluates such models beyond syntactic validity. This framework represents one of the first efforts to assess the quality of LLM-generated BPMN models in a more comprehensive manner.

In summary, existing research demonstrates that LLMs are capable of understanding, extracting, and reasoning about process-related information, and can support process modeling tasks in both healthcare and general domains. However, current approaches to BPMN model generation largely employ multi-stage pipelines based on intermediate representations, while direct generation of BPMN process models encoded in XML from unstructured documents remains insufficiently explored, particularly in real-world healthcare settings. These gaps motivate the workflow-based approach and evaluation strategy proposed in this work.

1.3 Contributions

This work presents a multi-step LLM-based workflow for directly generating executable BPMN XML from complex, unstructured healthcare documents, combining structured information extraction, schema-guided prompting, and repair strategies. The applicability of the workflow is demonstrated on official healthcare procedure documents from the domain of psychology and psychiatry. A dual evaluation approach is introduced, combining qualitative 3C-based assessment with objective XML-based metrics to assess both visual and formal properties of LLM-generated BPMN models. Finally, the proposed workflow is empirically compared with a zero-shot prompting baseline.

2 Materials and Methods/Study Scenario

2.1 LLM-Based BPMN Generation Workflow

The proposed workflow represents a sequence of multiple steps used to generate BPMN process models in XML format from structured textual documents. Instead of relying on a single prompt, the workflow decomposes the generation task into several steps, each corresponding to a specific prompting strategy applied during the generation process.

The workflow consists of a sequence of clearly defined steps, as illustrated in Fig. 1.

Role-based Prompting serves as the initial step of the workflow. In this step, the chatbot is explicitly instructed to assume the role of an expert in BPMN process modeling. By defining the model's role upfront, this step establishes a consistent modeling perspective and constrains the model's responses to the domain of process modeling. The primary purpose of this step is to promote the use of domain-specific terminology and structural reasoning aligned with BPMN principles.

RAG[1] **Initialization** is performed to load and provide the relevant healthcare documents used as input for the BPMN generation process. In this step, the structured textual documents describing the target process are made available to the large language model as contextual information. This ensures that

[1] RAG stands for *Retrieval-Augmented Generation.*

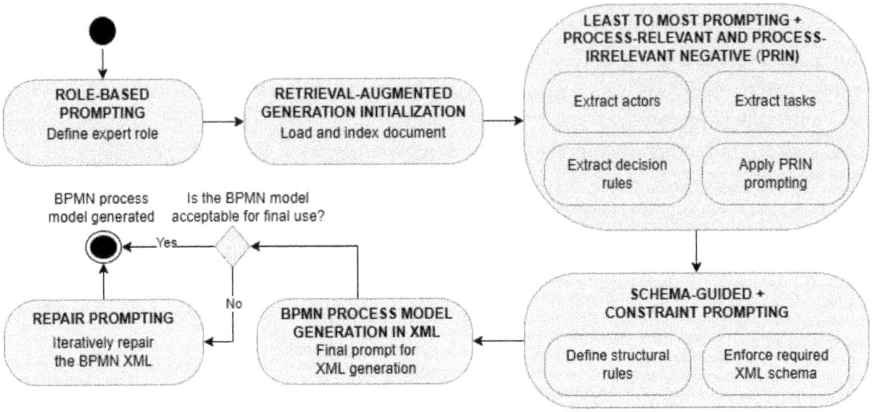

Fig. 1. Multi-step workflow

subsequent steps are grounded in the source documents from which the process model is generated.

Least-to-Most Prompting with PRIN[2] applies an incremental prompting strategy to decompose the process modeling task into a sequence of smaller and more manageable sub-tasks. Instead of generating the complete process model at once, the workflow progressively extracts individual process elements step-by-step. Specifically, the model is prompted to extract process actors, tasks, and decision points in separate steps. During each extraction step, a PRIN-inspired prompting strategy is applied by explicitly requesting both elements that belong to the target process and elements that are present in the source documents but should be excluded from the final process model [18]. This strategy helps clarify decision boundaries and reduce ambiguity in the generated outputs.

Schema-Guided and Constraint-Based Prompting introduces explicit structural guidance to ensure that the generated BPMN representation conforms to the expected XML format. In this step, an example of a valid BPMN XML structure is provided to the model, which helps align the model's output with the expected schema and establishes the required syntactic layout and mandatory elements. In addition, explicit constraints are applied to enforce the inclusion of required diagram and layout information, ensuring that the final process model is not only syntactically valid but also structurally complete. Together, schema guidance and constraint-based prompting ensure alignment of the generated BPMN XML with the expected structural and syntactic requirements.

BPMN XML Generation generates the final BPMN process model in XML format using all information, constraints, and intermediate results obtained from the preceding workflow steps.

[2] PRIN stands for *Process-Relevant and Process-Irrelevant Negative prompting.*

Repair Prompting is applied after a manual review and execution check of the generated BPMN process model, when syntactic, structural, or layout-related issues are identified. The workflow does not prescribe explicit repair rules, a fixed number of repair iterations, or strict acceptance thresholds for determining when a model is considered sufficiently complete or correct. Instead, the application of repair prompting is guided by expert judgment based on the observed issues.

Furthermore, the decision to apply repair prompting is context-dependent and considers practical aspects such as time efficiency and the complexity of the required modifications. In cases where identified issues are minor, for example limited to layout adjustments or simple structural refinements, manual correction of the BPMN model may be more efficient than invoking additional LLM-based repair iterations.

2.2 Evaluation Methodology

The 3C-Based Evaluation Framework was originally proposed in [17]. In this work, the framework is adapted and applied to assess the visual quality of BPMN process models generated by the proposed LLM-based workflow. The evaluation is performed manually by a human expert and is based solely on visual inspection of the rendered BPMN diagrams, without considering the underlying XML structure.

The framework evaluates LLM-generated process models across three dimensions: Correctness, Completeness and Clarity. *Correctness* reflects the semantic and logical validity of the generated BPMN process model, including the correctness of control flow and decision logic. *Completeness* assesses the extent to which the generated model captures all relevant process elements and control-flow paths described in the source document. *Clarity* evaluates the readability and interpretability of the BPMN model from a human perspective, focusing on the transparency of the process structure and flow.

Within each dimension, the framework defines multiple evaluation criteria with assigned importance levels (High, Moderate, Low) and corresponding weights. Each criterion is assessed using a binary true/false evaluation, indicating whether the generated model satisfies the criterion or not. Each generated BPMN process model is evaluated independently for each of the three dimensions. The final score for each dimension is computed as a weighted average of the individual criteria, resulting in a value in the range $\langle 0,1 \rangle$.

For the purposes of this evaluation, only a subset of the original 3C criteria was applied, as some criteria are not applicable in the context of the proposed workflow. Examples include criteria that assume explicitly defined control-flow elements in the prompt or criteria that require comparison against a reference (gold-standard) process model, neither of which are available in our setting.

Together, these dimensions enable a qualitative assessment of BPMN models that captures semantic correctness and human interpretability, which cannot be fully evaluated using purely syntactic or structural metrics.

While the 3C-based framework provides a structured approach to model quality assessment, it also exhibits certain limitations. In particular, the evaluation relies on expert judgment, which introduces an inherent degree of subjectivity.

Objective XML-Based Metrics are introduced to complement the qualitative 3C-based evaluation by providing a quantitative and reproducible assessment of generated BPMN process models. In contrast to visually driven evaluations in the original 3C framework, the proposed metrics operate directly on the BPMN XML representation and are independent of visual layout and human interpretation. This allows the assessment to focus on structural correctness, formal completeness, and minimal technical prerequisites for model clarity.

To maintain conceptual consistency with the qualitative evaluation, the objective metrics are organized according to the same three dimensions—Correctness, Completeness, and Clarity—and evaluated using a set of ratio-based measures derived from the BPMN XML representation, as summarized in Table 1.

All metrics are computed as ratio-based measures, yielding values in the range $\langle 0,1 \rangle$. For each evaluation dimension, the final dimension score is computed as the arithmetic mean of all metrics belonging to that dimension, with equal importance assigned to each metric.

Table 1. Objective XML-based metrics

Dimension	Metric	Formula
Correctness	Element connectivity	$\frac{\text{connected elements}}{\text{total elements}}$
	Balanced gateways	$\frac{\text{balanced gateways}}{\text{total gateways}}$
	Valid sequence flows[a]	$\frac{\text{valid sequence flows}}{\text{total sequence flows}}$
Completeness	Task coverage	$\frac{\text{tasks in XML}}{\text{tasks extracted}}$
	Decision coverage	$\frac{\text{decisions in XML}}{\text{decisions extracted}}$
Clarity	Labeled elements (name+id)	$\frac{\text{labeled elements}}{\text{total elements}}$
	Labeled outgoing flows	$\frac{\text{labeled outgoing flows}}{\text{total outgoing flows}}$
	BPMN-DI[b] coverage	$\frac{\text{elements with BPMN-DI}}{\text{total elements}}$

[a] A *sequenceFlow* is a BPMN element defining the execution order between connected flow nodes [19].
[b] BPMN Diagram Interchange [19]

For correctness-oriented metrics, connected elements denote BPMN tasks, gateways, and events that are referenced as either source or target in at least one sequenceFlow element. Balanced exclusive gateways refer to *exclusive (XOR) gateways* that are structurally well-formed with at least one incoming and at least two outgoing sequence flows, or as merge points with at least two incoming and one outgoing sequence flow. Valid sequence flows are defined as sequenceFlow elements whose source and target references correspond to existing BPMN elements.

Completeness-oriented metrics measure coverage with respect to elements identified during the extraction steps, without penalizing additional elements present in the generated model. In this study, completeness is assessed using task coverage and decision coverage, where decisions correspond to exclusive (XOR) gateways in the BPMN process model.

Clarity-oriented metrics focus on minimal technical prerequisites for readability, including the presence of element labels and corresponding BPMN-DI representations.

While the objective XML-based metrics provide a reproducible and expert-independent assessment of structural and formal properties, they do not capture semantic correctness or higher-level interpretability of BPMN models. For this reason, they are used as a complementary evaluation alongside the qualitative 3C-based framework.

2.3 Study Scenario

The proposed workflow was evaluated using a set of official healthcare procedure documents issued by the Ministry of Health of the Slovak Republic [20–24]. The selected documents originate from the domain of psychology and psychiatric care and include standardized procedures and comprehensive psychological management guidelines, describing process steps such as diagnosis, intervention, treatment, and prevention. The source documents are used in Tables 2 and 3 and are referenced throughout the study using anonymized identifiers DOC1–DOC5[3] [20–24]. The complete original versions of all evaluated documents are publicly available in a dedicated GitHub repository[4].

Each document was processed independently using the proposed LLM-based BPMN generation workflow. The same workflow configuration and prompting strategies were applied across all provided documents to ensure consistent experimental conditions. All experiments were conducted using ChatGPT (version 5.2) as the underlying LLM. The generated BPMN XML models were imported into Camunda Modeler for rendering and inspection, ensuring that all evaluated models were executable and visually interpretable in a standard BPMN environment.

For comparison, the same document set was also processed using a single-step zero-shot prompting baseline inspired by the approach reported in [16].

All generated BPMN process models were evaluated using both the qualitative 3C-based framework and the objective XML-based metrics described in the previous section.

[3] DOC1 – Comprehensive Psychological Management of an Adult Patient with Chronic Pain; DOC2 – Comprehensive Psychological Management of a Patient with a Somatic Disease; DOC3 – Agoraphobia; DOC4 – Post-Traumatic Stress Disorder; DOC5 – Comprehensive Psychological Management of an Adult Patient with Depressive Disorder and Recurrent Depressive Disorder.

[4] https://github.com/xgrik/llm-bpmn-generation-artifacts.

2.4 Prompt Building

This section outlines representative examples and skeleton formulations of the prompting strategies that constitute the proposed workflow. The original and exact prompt formulations, as used in the experiments, are publicly available in a dedicated GitHub repository.[5]

Role-Based Prompting strategy is used to initialize the interaction context by explicitly defining the modeling perspective and scope of the LLM before any process extraction or generation is performed. A representative example of the role-based prompt is shown in Listing 1.1.

Listing 1.1. Representative role-based prompt

```
You are an expert in BPMN 2.0 process modeling with experience in
    healthcare workflows and system-oriented process automation.

Your task is to support the transformation of structured healthcare
    documents into formal BPMN process models that capture both human
    and system-supported activities.

Constraints:
- strictly follow BPMN modeling principles,
- use precise process-oriented and healthcare terminology,
- ground all modeled elements in the provided source documents,
- do not introduce assumptions or unsupported process steps,
- focus on structured process modeling rather than narrative
    descriptions.
```

RAG Initialization prompting strategy presents the source healthcare document to the LLM and instructs it to assess whether the document is suitable for BPMN-based process modeling. A representative example of the RAG initialization prompt is provided in Listing 1.2.

Listing 1.2. Representative RAG initialization prompt

```
The following document describes a healthcare-related procedure titled:
"[DOCUMENT_TITLE]".

Your task is to carefully read and analyze the document and decide
    whether it contains sufficient procedural information to be
    represented as a BPMN process model.

In your assessment, focus on whether the document:
- describes a sequence of activities or actions,
- includes decision points, roles, or responsibilities,
- implies control-flow relations between steps.
```

[5] https://github.com/xgrik/llm-bpmn-generation-artifacts.

```
Do not generate any BPMN elements at this stage. Only analyze the
    document and state whether it is suitable for BPMN-based process
    modeling, with a brief justification.
```

Least-to-Most Prompting with PRIN strategy operationalizes the incremental extraction of process elements by applying the same PRIN-based prompt structure across multiple extraction steps (actors, tasks, and decision points), while varying only the targeted element type. A representative example of the PRIN-based extraction prompt is shown in Listing 1.3.

Listing 1.3. Representative PRIN-based extraction prompt

```
Based on the provided healthcare process document, identify all
    [PROCESS_ELEMENT_TYPE] that should be included in the BPMN process
    model.

Include only elements that:
- actively influence the execution or control flow of the process,
- represent concrete responsibilities, actions, or decisions,
- are explicitly supported by the source document.

For each identified element:
- provide a brief description,
- reference the part of the document it is derived from.

Additionally, identify elements mentioned in the document that should
    NOT be included as [PROCESS_ELEMENT_TYPE] in the BPMN model.

These may include:
- contextual or informational mentions,
- high-level goals or recommendations,
- assessments or statements that do not affect process execution.

For each excluded element, briefly justify why it is not relevant for
    BPMN modeling.
```

Schema-Guided and Constraint-Based Prompting strategy constrains the XML generation step by providing an explicit BPMN schema template and a set of structural constraints that the model must satisfy when producing the final BPMN process representation. A representative example of the schema-guided and constraint-based prompt is shown in Listing 1.4.

Listing 1.4. Representative schema-guided and constraint-based prompt

```
Use the provided BPMN 2.0 XML schema example as a mandatory structural
    reference
for generating the BPMN process model.
```

```
The schema example includes:
- [INSERT XML SCHEMA HEADER AND NAMESPACES, e.g., Camunda-compatible
    BPMN definitions],
- [INSERT MINIMAL EXECUTABLE PROCESS STRUCTURE],
- [INSERT BASIC BPMN-DI ELEMENTS REQUIRED FOR DIAGRAM RENDERING].

The generated BPMN XML must comply with the structure and namespaces
    defined in the provided schema example.

The model must additionally satisfy a set of explicit structural and
    modeling constraints, such as:
- [INSERT REQUIRED STRUCTURAL, CONSISTENCY OR DIAGRAMMATIC
    CONSTRAINTS, e.g., executable process definition, valid sequence
    flow references, BPMN-DI coverage]

Do not introduce any process elements that were not identified in
    previous extraction steps. Use the schema and constraints to guide
    the generation, ensuring that the resulting BPMN XML is
    structurally complete and executable. But do not generate any BPMN
    elements at this stage.
```

BPMN XML Generation step synthesizes all previously extracted process elements and constraints into a single, executable BPMN process model, instructing the LLM to generate only the final XML representation without additional explanations. A representative example of the BPMN XML generation prompt is shown in Listing 1.5.

Listing 1.5. Representative BPMN XML generation prompt

```
Generate the final BPMN 2.0 process model in XML format using
    exclusively the process elements and control-flow logic identified
    in previous workflow steps.

Synthesize all extracted actors, tasks, decision points, and
    constraints into a single, coherent, and executable BPMN process
    model.

Requirements:
- use only previously identified process elements,
- do not introduce any new actors, tasks, events, or gateways,
- reflect both human-performed and system-supported activities,
- ensure the output is executable and suitable for deployment.

Return only the final BPMN XML without explanations or additional text.
```

Repair Prompting strategy serves as a corrective fallback mechanism that can be invoked when validation tools or manual inspection reveal issues in the generated BPMN XML, such as schema violations or diagram rendering problems. A representative example of a repair prompting formulation is provided in Listing 1.6.

Listing 1.6. Representative repair prompt

```
The following BPMN XML contains errors identified during validation or
    manual inspection.

[INSERT VALIDATION ERRORS, EXECUTION ERRORS, OR LAYOUT ISSUES HERE]

Your task is to repair the existing BPMN XML while preserving the
    original process structure and semantics.

Requirements:
- fix only the reported issues,
- do not introduce new process elements,
- do not remove valid existing elements,
- preserve all previously identified actors, tasks, and decision
    points,
- ensure the repaired model remains executable and structurally
    consistent.

Return only the corrected BPMN XML without explanations or additional
    text.
```

3 Results and Discussion

The primary focus is on evaluating the effectiveness and robustness of the proposed multi-step LLM-based BPMN generation workflow using both the qualitative 3C-based framework and the objective XML-based metrics. A baseline zero-shot prompting approach is included as a reference point to contextualize the observed improvements and highlight the contribution of the proposed workflow. Both approaches were evaluated on the same set of five healthcare procedure documents.

For evaluation purposes, only BPMN models generated prior to the application of repair prompting were considered, in order to assess the baseline performance of the generation workflow without iterative post-hoc corrections.

An example of a final BPMN process model generated from DOC1, including the complete process representation and a brief descriptive explanation, is provided in a dedicated GitHub repository[6].

3.1 3C-Based Results

The 3C-based evaluation provides a qualitative, expert-driven assessment of the visual clarity, perceived correctness, and completeness of BPMN process models generated by an LLM, as summarized in Table 2.

[6] https://github.com/xgrik/llm-bpmn-generation-artifacts.

Table 2. 3C-based results

	Weight	WORKFLOW					ZERO-SHOT				
Clarity		DOC 1	DOC 2	DOC 3	DOC 4	DOC 5	DOC 1	DOC 2	DOC 3	DOC 4	DOC 5
No unlabeled elements	3	☑	☑	☑	☑	☑	X	☐	☐	☑	☐
No diagram layout issues (eg. spacing, zigzag)	2	☑	☐	☐	☐	☑	X	☑	☑	☐	☐
No overlapping flows	2	☐	☐	☐	☐	☐	X	☐	☐	☐	☐
All outgoing arcs of (X)OR splits have labels	1	☑	☑	☑	☑	☑	X	☐	☐	☑	☐
		0.75	**0.5**	**0.5**	**0.5**	**0.75**	**X**	**0.25**	**0.25**	**0.5**	**0.38**
Correctenss											
No syntactical and behavioral correcteness violations (eg. deadlocks)	3	☑	☑	☑	☑	☑	X	☐	☐	☑	☐
No structural correctness violations (eg. disconnected elements or paths)	3	☑	☑	☑	☑	☑	X	☐	☐	☑	☐
No reduntant flows/elements (no hallucinations introduced)	2	☑	☑	☑	☑	☐	X	☐	☐	☑	☐
		1.0	**1.0**	**1.0**	**1.0**	**0.75**	**X**	**0.0**	**0.0**	**1.0**	**0.0**
Completness											
No missing start/end events	3	☑	☑	☑	☑	☑	X	☐	☑	☑	☑
No missing decision outcomes (eg. Both 'Yes' and 'No' paths are modeled)	2	☑	☑	☑	☑	☑	X	☐	☐	☑	☑
		1.0	**1.0**	**1.0**	**1.0**	**1.0**	**X**	**0.0**	**0.6**	**1.0**	**1.0**

Across all evaluated documents, the workflow achieves consistently high scores in the Correctness and Completeness dimensions, indicating that the generated BPMN models are structurally sound, free of disconnected elements and deadlocks, and capture all essential process components, including decision outcomes and start/end events.

The Clarity dimension exposes the primary limitation of the generated models. While all models consistently contain labeled elements and properly labeled outgoing decision flows, recurrent issues related to diagram layout and overlapping sequence flows are observed. This indicates that the main challenge for the LLM does not lie in conceptual or structural process modeling, but rather in the visual arrangement and routing of BPMN elements. These issues are purely visual in nature and do not affect the logical correctness or completeness of the underlying process models.

The zero-shot prompting baseline exhibits substantially lower and less stable performance across the evaluated dimensions. In particular, deficiencies in diagram layout generation and incomplete or missing BPMN-DI information frequently hinder meaningful qualitative assessment. In one evaluated case (DOC 1), the generated BPMN XML did not satisfy the minimal requirements for visual interpretability, as the model lacked BPMN-DI information required to render the process diagram. As a result, the process model could not be visually inspected, which directly affected both Clarity and Correctness evaluations.

This qualitative evaluation, which follows the 3C framework, was conducted using a subset of its original criteria, excluding those that require a reference process model, explicit control-flow specifications in the prompt, or lane-based modeling.

3.2 XML-Based Results

Table 3 presents the results of the objective XML-based evaluation, which provides a quantitative assessment of the formal structure, completeness, and minimal technical prerequisites of the generated BPMN models, independent of visual inspection.

Table 3. XML-based results

	WORKFLOW					ZERO-SHOT				
Clarity	DOC 1	DOC 2	DOC 3	DOC 4	DOC 5	DOC 1	DOC 2	DOC 3	DOC 4	DOC 5
Labeled elements	1.0	1.0	1.0	1.0	1.0	1.0	1.0	1.0	1.0	1.0
Labeled outgoing flows	1.0	1.0	1.0	1.0	1.0	1.0	1.0	0.0	1.0	0.0
BPMN-DI Coverage	1.0	1.0	1.0	1.0	1.0	0.0	0.17	0.56	1.0	0.85
	1.0	**1.0**	**1.0**	**1.0**	**1.0**	**0.66**	**0.72**	**0.52**	**1.0**	**0.62**
Correctenss										
Element connectivity	1.0	1.0	1.0	1.0	1.0	1.0	1.0	1.0	1.0	1.0
Balanced getaways	1.0	1.0	1.0	1.0	1.0	1.0	1.0	1.0	1.0	1.0
Valid sequence flow	1.0	1.0	1.0	1.0	1.0	1.0	1.0	1.0	1.0	1.0
	1.0	**1.0**	**1.0**	**1.0**	**1.0**	**1.0**	**1.0**	**1.0**	**1.0**	**1.0**
Completness										
Task coverage	0.94	0.92	1.0	1.0	1.0	-	-	-	-	-
Decision coverage	0.83	0.71	0.75	0.91	1.0	-	-	-	-	-
	0.89	**0.82**	**0.88**	**0.96**	**1.0**	-	-	-	-	-

Across all evaluated documents, the proposed workflow achieves consistently maximal scores in both the Correctness and Clarity dimensions. These results indicate the formal soundness and technical completeness of the workflow-generated BPMN XML.

In terms of Completeness, the workflow exhibits minor variability. This indicates that while the workflow successfully transfers the majority of previously extracted process elements into the final BPMN model, some information loss may occur during the multi-step generation process. Nevertheless, completeness scores remain consistently high across all documents.

In contrast, the zero-shot prompting approach shows pronounced deficiencies in the Clarity dimension. In particular, incomplete or missing BPMN-DI information and inconsistently labeled outgoing decision flows are observed across multiple documents. These findings align with the qualitative 3C-based evaluation and demonstrate that the limitations of zero-shot prompting are not purely perceptual but are reflected in the underlying XML structure.

Correctness metrics reach perfect scores for the zero-shot models, indicating syntactically valid BPMN XML. However, the absence of reliable BPMN-DI information significantly limits the practical usability and visual interpretability of the generated models.

Completeness metrics were not evaluated for the zero-shot approach, as no explicit extraction of process elements was performed.

3.3 Discussion

Although both approaches can generate syntactically valid BPMN XML, notable differences emerge in their stability, completeness, and suitability for practical BPMN modeling.

The workflow demonstrates a high degree of robustness across all evaluated documents, yielding consistently structured, fully visualizable BPMN models with complete BPMN-DI information. In contrast, the zero-shot approach exhibits pronounced variability: some generated models achieve acceptable structural quality, while others suffer from incomplete diagram information or missing visual representations altogether. This variability significantly limits the reliability of zero-shot prompting for systematic BPMN model generation.

A key distinction lies in the consistent generation of BPMN-DI data. The proposed workflow reliably produces models that can be directly visualized and manipulated in standard BPMN modeling tools, which is essential for practical adoption by domain experts and process modelers. Although zero-shot prompting can generate formally valid XML, the absence or incompleteness of BPMN-DI information frequently renders the resulting models difficult or impossible to interpret visually, reducing their applicability in real-world modeling scenarios. Our presented approach is subject to several limitations that should be considered when interpreting the results. Use of specific large language model for process model generation - while it can provide useful insights at the given point in time the results can change as the technology continues to evolve. The selection was motivated by community adoption and its' extensive coverage in recent studies. Another limitation is focus on the processes in single clinical domain that can create bias toward specific process types. Furthermore, the study is based on a single LLM (ChatGPT), which may limit the generalizability of the results across different model architectures [25]; future work will therefore explore comparative evaluations involving multiple LLMs. Additionally, LLM-based generation is inherently sensitive to prompt formulation, where even minor changes in wording can lead to variations in output [4]; to mitigate this, the exact prompts used in the experiments are provided to ensure transparency and reproducibility.

Overall, the results indicate that the primary strength of the proposed workflow lies not only in formal correctness, but in its ability to consistently generate complete, executable, and tool-compatible BPMN models. At the same time, the observed layout-related issues suggest that visual optimization remains a challenging aspect of LLM-based process modeling and represents a direction for further improvement.

4 Conclusion

This work investigated the use of LLM-based chatbots to support process modeling from complex healthcare documents and introduced a multi-step workflow for directly generating BPMN process models encoded in XML. The results demonstrate that the proposed workflow produces structurally correct, complete, and consistently visualizable BPMN models, outperforming a zero-shot prompting baseline in terms of stability, clarity, and practical usability.

Despite these improvements, limitations remain. In particular, the visual layout quality of generated diagrams is not always optimal, and semantic correctness with respect to clinical intent is not formally verified and still requires expert review. Future work will therefore focus on validating generated process models against the original clinical procedures in collaboration with domain experts, enabling a systematic assessment of clinical fidelity and differences between workflow-based and zero-shot generation. Additional directions include improving layout-aware generation strategies, incorporating expert feedback into the workflow, and extending evaluation with reference models to support deeper semantic validation of generated BPMN models.

Acknowledgements. This work was funded by the European Union through the NextGenerationEU initiative under the Recovery and Resilience Plan for Slovakia, project No. 09I05-03-V02-00084, *Digital solutions in support of mental health in patients with CHF (DigiMent)*. The research was also supported by EU's DEP Sustainable Healthcare with Digital Health Data Competence and by the NATO Science for Peace and Security Program under project SPS G8765 - "PerRsonalised Micro Environmental change Alert - PRIME Alert".

References

1. Javaid, M., Haleem, A., Singh, R.P.: ChatGPT for healthcare services: an emerging stage for an innovative perspective. BenchCouncil Trans. Benchmarks Stand. Eval. (2023)
2. Udvardi, O., Sikula, M., Batalik, P., Lang, J.: Personalized learning support. In: 2025 IEEE Digital Education and MOOCS Conference (DEMOcon), pp. 1–6 (2025)
3. Prescott, M.R., et al.: Comparing the efficacy and efficiency of human and generative AI: qualitative thematic analyses. JMIR AI (2024)
4. Atil, B., Chittams, A., Fu, L., Ture, F., Xu, L., Baldwin, B.: LLM stability: a detailed analysis with some surprises (2024)
5. Grathwol, D., van der Aa, H., López, H.A.: Automating pathway extraction from clinical guidelines: a conceptual model, datasets and initial experiments. In: International Conference on Cooperative Information Systems. Springer (2024)
6. Castagnari, E., Muyama, L., Coulet, A.: Prompting large language models for supporting the differential diagnosis of anemia. In: 2024 2nd International Conference on Foundation and Large Language Models (FLLM). IEEE (2024)
7. Yu, Y., et al.: Using large language models to retrieve critical data from clinical processes and business rules. Bioengineering (2024)
8. Kourani, H., et al.: Leveraging large language models for enhanced process model comprehension. Decis. Support Syst. (2025)
9. Gomes, F.C.: Generating process descriptions from BPMN models: towards an approach with large language models (2024). https://lume.ufrgs.br/handle/10183/287897
10. Kourani, H., Berti, A., Schuster, D., van der Aalst, W.M.: Process modeling with large language models. In: International Conference on Business Process Modeling, Development and Support. Springer (2024)
11. Kourani, H., Berti, A., Schuster, D., van der Aalst, W.M.: Evaluating large language models on business process modeling: framework, benchmark, and self-improvement analysis. Softw. Syst. Model. (2025)
12. Köpke, J., Safan, A.: Efficient LLM-based conversational process modeling. In: International Conference on Business Process Management. Springer (2024)

13. Grohs, M., Abb, L., Elsayed, N., Rehse, J.-R.: Large language models can accomplish business process management tasks. In: International Conference on Business Process Management. Springer (2023)
14. Nour Eldin, A., Assy, N., Anesini, O., Dalmas, B., Gaaloul, W.: Nala2bpmn: automating BPMN model generation with large language models. In: International Conference on Cooperative Information Systems. Springer (2024)
15. Daclin, N., Mallek-Daclin, S., Zacharewicz, G.: Generative AI for business model generation (GAI4BM): from textual description to business process model. In: The 10th International Food Operations and Processing Simulation Workshop (2024)
16. Toxtli, C., Li, W.: Automating automation: using LLMs to generate BPMN workflows for robotic process automation. In: World Congress in Computer Science, Computer Engineering & Applied Computing. Springer (2024)
17. Drakopoulos, P., Malousoudis, P., Nousias, N., Tsakalidis, G., Vergidis, K.: Do LLMs speak BPMN? An evaluation of their process modeling capabilities based on quality measures. Computation **14**(1), 10 (2026)
18. Ahn, J.J., Yin, W.: Prompt-Reverse Inconsistency: LLM Self-Inconsistency Beyond Generative Randomness and Prompt Paraphrasing. arXiv preprint arXiv:2504.01282 (2025)
19. Object Management Group (OMG). Business Process Model and Notation (BPMN) Version 2.0.2 (2014)
20. Ministry of Health of the Slovak Republic. Agorafóbia (2021)
21. Ministry of Health of the Slovak Republic. Komplexný psychologický manažment dospelého pacienta s chronickou bolesťou (2021)
22. Ministry of Health of the Slovak Republic. Komplexný psychologický manažment dospelého pacienta s depresívnou poruchou a recidivujúcou depresívnou poruchou (2021)
23. Ministry of Health of the Slovak Republic. Komplexný psychologický manažment pacienta so somatickým ochorením (2021)
24. Ministry of Health of the Slovak Republic. Posttraumatická stresová porucha (2021)
25. Liang, P., et al.: Holistic evaluation of language models. arXiv preprint arXiv:2211.09110 (2022)

Delegating Tasks to AI: Current State in Dental Healthcare

Ville Tuominen[1,2](✉), Jaakko Vuolasto[3], and Kari M. Koskinen[4]

[1] Entteri Professional Software Oy, Tampere, Finland
Ville.Tuominen@entteri.fi
[2] University of Antwerp, Antwerpen, Belgium
[3] University of Jyväskylä, Jyväskylä, Finland
[4] Aalto University, Espoo, Finland

Abstract. Various software solutions that use artificial intelligence (AI) have been introduced in the healthcare sector. These solutions aim to improve aspects such as the quality and efficiency of providing health care across the different stages of the process. At the same time, research has identified several obstacles that must be addressed for these solutions to achieve the desired outcomes. This research focuses on dental healthcare and examines the current situation in the area regarding the use of AI-based solutions. It adopts the view of task delegation and looks into which tasks of dental healthcare workers AI-based solutions are seen as most promising and beneficial, and what kinds of potential challenges these solutions face. The research draws on qualitative data from group and individual interviews with sector professionals and identifies two primary areas for the use of AI-based solutions: documentation and information retrieval, and diagnostics. While both areas show potential for the use of AI-based solutions, there are also concerns in them that not only need to be addressed but also have implications for how these solutions are to be deployed.

Keywords: AI delegation · task delegability · healthcare AI adoption · trust · risk · dental care

1 Introduction

The rapid development of machine learning, natural language processing, and computer vision models over the past decade has created unprecedented opportunities to reallocate routine, information-intensive, and even some demanding cognitive tasks from humans to artificial intelligence (AI) systems. Large health technology systems already use AI to flag sepsis, prioritise radiology worklists, and predict emergency department surges, yet at scale, only a fraction of potentially "delegable" work is actually being handed over to these solutions [1]. In dentistry, reviews already identify applications in radiographic interpretation, diagnosis support, treatment planning, prediction, and administrative uses, suggesting substantial technical potential for AI-enabled delegation [2–4]. Current research is consistently showing that the majority of AI pilots fail to translate into routine clinical workflows because delegation barriers outweigh perceived

M. Säreströniemi et al. (Eds.): NCDHWS 2026, CCIS 3010, pp. 525–537, 2026.
https://doi.org/10.1007/978-3-032-28819-6_34

benefits [5, 6]. High-profile failures, such as Google's Med-Gemini "basilar ganglia" hallucination in August 2025, fuel skepticism by highlighting accuracy and accountability risks [7].

Broader trends in digital technology development and servitization provide a crucial backdrop for understanding why healthcare organizations struggle with AI task delegation. Digitalization has transformed how value is created and delivered, re-shaping expectations, relationships, and interactions across industries [8, 9]. While digitalisation opens opportunities for innovation, efficiency, and ecosystem-based value creation, it is also fraught with paradoxical tensions. Organizations must balance flexibility with stability, pursue profitability while absorbing high upfront costs, and reconcile diverging perceptions between executives and frontline professionals regarding digital initiatives [10, 11]. These paradoxes mirror the dilemmas in AI delegation: the promise of efficiency versus fears of risk, the challenge of automation versus threats to professional identity, and the opportunities of collaboration versus the realities of regulatory and infrastructural constraints.

At the same time, the development of AI technologies has advanced in great leaps over the past decade, raising interest in its more extensive use in a range of industries and sectors. The healthcare sector, and within that, dental healthcare, represents a particularly intriguing empirical setting for studying task delegation for AI-based solutions: it is data-rich, highly regulated, safety-critical, and culturally professionalized.

Importantly, delegating tasks to AI is rarely a single actor's choice in dental healthcare. It is a multi-level decision shaped by both the individual clinician who must trust and rely on the system in patient work, and the organization (e.g., a dental chain or public provider) that procures technologies, governs data access, defines documentation policies, and carries reputational and legal exposure. In this sense, AI delegation is simultaneously a matter of professional judgement and organizational control over processes, accountability, and infrastructure.

Against this background, our study investigates the status of delegating healthcare tasks to AI in dental care. Additionally, we are interested in the current and future barriers and opportunities for delegation. Drawing on qualitative empirical data from interviewees working in different roles in dental healthcare sector and with AI-based solutions for the sector, we aim to answer the following question:

- RQ1. What tasks are currently delegated to AI?
- RQ2. What are the current barriers and opportunities for delegation?

This paper contributes by conceptualizing AI delegation in dental healthcare as a bounded, task-specific, and multi-level phenomenon. Rather than assuming that adoption follows directly from technical capability, we examine how clinician judgement, workflow realities, and organizational governance jointly shape which tasks are currently perceived as delegable and which remain firmly under human control.

2 Theoretical Background

Delegation is classically defined as the transfer of decision authority from a principal to an agent [12]. In a human-AI context, the agent is a software system whose level of autonomy can vary from mere reflexive to fully autonomous decision-making [13]. This level of autonomy is tied to the role of the human in relation to the software system, particularly with respect to the extent of oversight and control the human retains. These dynamics depend on factors such as the artefact's presumed capabilities and the types of tasks it is expected to carry out [13].

According to Baird and Maruping [13], whether a task can be delegated to a technological artefact depends on its action requirements, complexity, and decomposability—the types of actions involved, the level of uncertainty and interdependence, and the extent to which the task can be broken into smaller parts. Lubars & Tan describe four antecedents that shape perceived delegability: motivation, difficulty, risk, and trust, and jointly determine whether humans are willing to transfer control [12].

Recent managerial discourse extends the idea beyond individuals to organisational processes, arguing that "AI delegation" is fast becoming a critical leadership competence [14]. In healthcare, however, high task complexity, life-and-death stakes and tightly coupled workflows make the delegation especially sensitive to risk and trust dimensions [1, 15].

Prior research has looked into the barriers of task delegation in the healthcare sector. By reviewing existing research on the topic, Ahmed et al. [5] reveals six persistent barrier clusters for delegating healthcare tasks for AI, which are summarized in Table 1.

Issues regarding trust towards the AI-based solution and the risks that those pose emerge as pivotal levers. As a result, without credible assurances on safety, explainability, and accountability, it is argued that clinicians will not delegate tasks to these solutions, regardless of potential efficiency gains or other benefits they might entail.

In this sense, these issues act as clear barriers to adoption, even though the question is also related to how much risk can be tolerated, depending on the task in question. In addition, these risks can possibly also be mitigated in some manner, such as using AI-based solutions more as supporting one's tasks, but without giving it clear decision-making roles or allowing those to function without active human supervision. This, however, affects the amount of gain these solutions can deliver.

2.1 Task Characteristics and Healthcare-Specific Barriers

In this regard, explainability is repeatedly cited as the single most influential determinant of clinician trust [16]. Lack of model transparency contradicts evidence-based medicine norms and hinders error tracing when adverse events occur. Conversely, even partial explanations, such as saliency maps, counterfactuals, or confidence scores, can increase acceptance by 5–8 percentage points in controlled experiments [16].

Yet explainability alone is insufficient. High-profile faults, such as Med-Gemini's fabricated "basilar ganglia", remind practitioners that AI may be brittle in novel clinical contexts [7]. Robust post-deployment monitoring, transparent update logs, and clinician override mechanisms are therefore essential complements to algorithmic explanation if task delegation is to be considered safe. Recent evidence on generative AI in clinical contexts reinforces this point. Even when such systems appear helpful for summarization or drafting, clinicians remain concerned about hallucinated details, silently propagated errors, and unclear responsibility for reviewing outputs [19, 20]. Higher technical capability, therefore, does not remove the need to ask which tasks are appropriate to delegate and under what safeguards.

Table 1. Thematic barriers (modified from [5])

Barrier cluster	Illustrative mechanisms	Key evidence	Delegability dimension
Technical reliability & accuracy	Model mis-calibration, data drift, hallucinations	[7]; [5]	Risk
Explainability & transparency	"Black-box" logic undermines auditability	[16]	Trust
Regulatory & liability ambiguity	Unclear malpractice allocation, device classification hurdles	[1]; [17]	Risk
Data governance & privacy	Secondary use of sensitive patient data GDPR/AI-Act compliance	[1]; [17]	Trust
Professional identity & workflow fit	Fear of deskilling, loss of clinical autonomy; workflow misalignment	[18]	Motivation
Infrastructure & resourcing	Integration with legacy EHRs, cost of maintenance, training gaps	[6]	Difficulty

In addition to risk and trust factors, delegation may also be impacted by the altered professional boundaries. Qualitative work with allied-health clinicians shows concerns that AI may "erode craft skill" or produce role displacement if introduced without co-design and up-skilling [18]. Resistance is amplified where practitioners perceive a threat to their moral accountability for patient outcomes. Training, participatory design, and clear liability frameworks can mitigate these identity tensions.

In addition to identifying areas for use of AI-based solutions in dental healthcare, we also aim to understand the extent to which barriers, as well as other factors, currently play a role in hindering the adoption of the solutions.

3 Materials and Methods

We conducted a qualitative study of AI task delegation in dental care using two complementary datasets. Dataset 1 by Kukkola and Saxen [21] available at Fairdata.fi, comprises a workshop-style group interview (May 2024) with six dental professionals (three dentists and three dental hygienists). Dataset 2 comprises seven semi-structured individual interviews (October-December 2025) with professionals involved in dental work and dental health-IT implementation (e.g., clinical roles and product/implementation lead). Three of the interviewees had experience in public and private sector organizations, and four were mainly from the private sector. All interviewees had experience in both the managerial and clinical workflows of dental clinics.

All sessions were audio-recorded and transcribed (Microsoft Teams). The workshop transcript (dataset 1) is content-focused rather than verbatim.

All participants received information about the study purpose, voluntary participation, confidentiality, and their right to withdraw without consequence. Identifiers were removed from transcripts, quotations were translated and lightly edited for readability, and data will be stored in Fairdata.fi online archive.

Material analysis was based on the principles of deductive theory-informed thematic analysis [22].

We analyzed the seven individual interviews using iterative qualitative coding informed by our theoretical background on task delegability and socio-technical adoption barriers. The workshop material was first used to validate and calibrate this theoretical lens and to refine an initial coding frame. We then coded the interview transcripts, applying and refining codes that captured the two focal delegation areas (documentation/information retrieval; diagnosis) and cross-cutting constraints (trust/verification burden, workflow integration, professional autonomy, organizational risk).

To report the coding concisely, we present a cross-actor synthesis table (Table 2) summarizing how each theme was framed by clinicians versus chain stakeholders, and an evidence map (Table 3) indicating where themes were salient across datasets and interview IDs. The evidence map links individual interviews and, for workshop data, to whether the topic was mentioned or discussed in detail.

We addressed trustworthiness through triangulation across two datasets, comparison of clinician and organizational perspectives, and an explicit audit trail from theoretical constructs to codes to synthesis tables. Coding decisions were discussed among the three authors, and any discrepant interpretations were resolved in meetings prior to final synthesis.

To preserve double-blind review, we present quotations as translated excerpts and identify sources only by workshop dataset (WS) and interview ID (INT1–INT7).

4 Results

4.1 Overview of Current Delegation Patterns

Across the workshop and seven individual interviews, delegation discussions clustered around two main task areas. Participants consistently identified (1) documentation and information retrieval as the first functions they would delegate to AI, and (2) imaging interpretation as acceptable primarily as a second opinion rather than an autonomous decision-maker. Table 2 summarizes how these themes were framed by clinicians versus chain/vendor actors, and Table 3 maps their salience across the two datasets.

The remaining themes in our analysis (trust and verification burden, governance and regulation, workflow integration, and professional autonomy) help explain why some areas were framed as easier to delegate and others as harder.

Answering RQ1, the current delegation is concentrated in assistive roles: documentation support (e.g., transcription/drafting and summarization) and information retrieval, alongside imaging tools that highlight suspected findings. Delegation beyond these areas remains limited and is typically framed as pre-visit support (e.g., symptom-based triage) or operational optimization (e.g., scheduling/resource planning), rather than autonomous clinical decision-making.

Table 2. Interview coding synthesis across actor groups (dentists/hygienists vs chain/vendor).

Theme (coded)	Dentists/hygienists: how it was framed	Chain/vendor: how it was framed	Implication for delegation (Area 1 vs Area 2)
Documentation & information retrieval as 'first delegable' targets (Area 1)	High-value time saver; reduces "detective work" and end-of-day charting; acceptable if clinician can quickly review/correct outputs	Strong fit with standardization and productivity goals; interest in scalable documentation support, but dependent on integration and governance of what enters records	Easier to delegate because outputs are reversible/auditable if provenance + low-friction review are in place
Imaging AI as 'second opinion', not autonomous (Area 2)	Acceptable as a second reader that marks suspected findings; clinician remains responsible for final judgement; concern about over-trust and rare harmful errors	Adoptable primarily as decision support; emphasis on validation, monitoring, regulatory classification, and liability when scaling across sites/devices	Harder to delegate beyond second opinion due to accountability, higher perceived risk, and need for chain-level governance at scale
Trust / verification burden	Core limiter: if AI adds checking work or produces uncertain outputs, clinicians disengage; worries about hallucinations and calibration over time	Need for audit trails, performance monitoring, update management, and clear responsibility allocation	Determines whether Area 1 scales (verification must be cheap); constrains Area 2 autonomy (over-trust risk requires safeguards)
Workflow integration	Adoption depends on seamless fit into chairside routines; extra steps or switching systems undermines use	Integration with record systems/imaging infrastructure, access control, logging, and procurement constraints are prerequisites	Precondition for both areas; without integration, delegation remains experimental rather than routine

(continued)

Table 2. (*continued*)

Theme (coded)	Dentists/hygienists: how it was framed	Chain/vendor: how it was framed	Implication for delegation (Area 1 vs Area 2)
Professional autonomy	Strong autonomy and "my way of working" shapes uptake; judgement-heavy tasks trigger identity and control concerns	Difficult to mandate adoption; variability across clinics and clinicians complicates rollout and standard operating models	Reinforces why Area 2 stays bounded (judgement/identity); Area 1 is less identity-threatening and more standardizable
Organizational risk	Risk framed as responsibility for patient harm and reputational loss if AI is wrong or misused	Compliance (e.g., device classification), liability, information governance, and reputational exposure across the chain	Raises the bar for Area 2; in Area 1, risk is lower but can still gate scaling if record-entry rules are unclear

Table 3. Evidence map showing salience of themes across data

Theme (coded)	Dentists/hygienists (IDs)	Chain/vendor (IDs)	Workshop (WS)
Documentation & information retrieval as 'first delegable' targets (Area 1)	INT1, INT2	INT4, INT6, INT7	discussed
Imaging AI as 'second opinion', not autonomous (Area 2)	INT1, INT2	INT4, INT6, INT7	discussed
Trust / verification burden	INT1, INT2	INT4, INT6	discussed
Workflow integration	INT1, INT2	INT4, INT5, INT6	mentioned
Professional autonomy	INT1, INT2,INT3	INT4, INT5	mentioned
Organizational risk	INT1	INT5, INT6, INT7	discussed

4.2 Documentation and Information Retrieval as 'First Delegable' Targets (Area 1)

Participants described documentation and information retrieval as high-value, low-hanging fruit for AI delegation. They emphasized the time spent reviewing prior notes and assembling a coherent view of the patient's history, as well as the burden of producing detailed clinical documentation under time pressure. Automation was viewed as acceptable when it reduced documentation workload (e.g., speech-to-text, drafting structured notes, summarizing prior visits), while leaving clinicians responsible for review and sign-off. Even in this 'first delegable' area, trust was conditional: participants expressed concern about fabricated or misplaced details and emphasized that AI output must be clearly attributable and easy to verify (e.g., traceable to source notes) before it can be entered into the patient record.

Organizationally, documentation delegation also aligned with chain-level goals such as standardizing records, improving throughput, and reducing variation in note quality. However, participants stressed implementation prerequisites: integration into existing systems, clear rules for data access (including patient record infrastructure), and governance processes that define how AI output can be used in official documentation. This governance also functions as a boundary-setting mechanism: chains can enable delegation only within approved workflows and accountability arrangements, while individual clinicians retain discretion over what is ultimately signed and recorded.

These factors help explain why delegation appeared easier in area 1 than in area 2. Documentation and retrieval benefits are immediate and measurable, and errors can be detected and corrected locally. By contrast, delegation in diagnostic domains introduces higher stakes, harder-to-audit reasoning, and greater legal and reputational exposure, particularly for dental chains that aim to standardize quality across sites. The contrast also reflects professional autonomy: clinicians can adopt documentation aids opportunistically, whereas diagnostic delegation is more likely to be resisted as it touches core expertise and liability. Answering RQ2, documentation and retrieval are perceived as easier to delegate because benefits are immediate and measurable, outputs are auditable and locally correctable, and clinical risk is comparatively low, provided that provenance and workflow integration reduce verification work.

4.3 Imaging AI is Acceptable as a 'Second Opinion', not as an Autonomous Decision-Maker (Area 2)

First, clinicians were generally willing to use imaging AI as a second reader: a tool that marks potential caries or other findings and prompts closer attention. Acceptance depended on a human-in-the-loop workflow in which the clinician can inspect the evidence, override suggestions, and remain the accountable decision-maker.

Second, imaging carries a higher perceived clinical risk and accountability. Interviewees emphasized that rare but consequential errors could quickly undermine trust and create ambiguity about who is responsible when AI output is wrong. These concerns were amplified by expectations around validation, continuous performance monitoring, and compliance processes that can slow deployment in organizational settings. Participants also linked resistance to professional identity and patient trust: clinicians feared over-reliance, deskilling, and difficult conversations if an AI-driven judgement conflicts with clinical assessment.

In short, imaging support was viewed as valuable when it augments professional perception (e.g., highlighting suspected findings) while keeping decision authority, documentation, and patient communication with the clinician. Moving beyond a second-opinion role triggers barriers that participants described as qualitatively different from those associated with administrative delegation. For dental chains, this increases perceived organizational risk because an autonomous tool would need to be defensible across sites, devices, and patient groups, not only in individual cases. Answering RQ2, imaging is harder to delegate beyond a 'second opinion' because stakes and accountability are higher, over-trust risks are salient, and organizational governance (e.g., device classification, monitoring, and liability) must scale across sites and patient groups (Table 4).

Table 4. Task areas, current delegation status, and socio-technical conditions shaping delegability

	Task area 1 Documentation& information retrieval	Task area 2 Imaging interpretation
Current status (RQ1)	Emerging/partial use; strong near-term demand	In use/piloting as decision support in some settings
Typical delegation form	Drafting/transcription; summarization; clinician review and sign-off	Second reader highlighting findings; clinician decides
Opportunities enabling delegation	Clear time savings; reversible outputs; auditability if linked to source notes; supports standardization	Perceptual augmentation (markings); potential throughput gains; aligns with human-in-the-loop accountability
Dominant barriers (why harder)	Hallucinations/accuracy concerns; verification burden; integration into record systems; governance of what can enter the patient record	Over-trust/deskilling concerns; liability/safety case; device classification and regulatory requirements; monitoring at scale
Level most salient	Clinician and organization	Organization (risk) and clinician (accountability)
Example evidence	INT1–INT2; WS	WS; INT7

5 Discussion

Our findings support the view that AI delegation in healthcare is best understood as a bounded, task-specific phenomenon rather than a general attitude toward AI. This aligns with Baird and Maruping's [13] argument that delegability depends on task characteristics and with digital servitization research showing that digital technologies create value only when they fit organizational processes and governance arrangements [23, 24]. In dental care, the relevant boundary is not simply technical capability but the combination of reviewability, accountability, and workflow fit.

The first boundary concerns documentation and information retrieval. Recent work on clinical natural language processing and AI scribes suggests that documentation support can reduce administrative burden, but only when outputs remain easy to verify and correct [25]. Our findings are consistent with the literature: participants saw documentation as more delegable, not because it is risk-free, but because errors are comparatively local, reversible, and auditable when provenance is visible and human sign-off remains mandatory.

The second boundary concerns imaging AI. Reviews of AI in dental radiology show clear technical promise, yet both professionals and patients tend to prefer human oversight and adjunctive use rather than autonomous interpretation [26, 27]. Our results fit this pattern. Imaging support was accepted as a second opinion, but participants resisted more extensive delegation because the task is more closely tied to professional accountability, patient communication, and the consequences of rare but serious errors.

A further contribution of this study is the explicit multi-level framing of delegation. For individual dentists and hygienists, the boundary is shaped by workflow fit, autonomy, and the practical cost of verification. For dental chains and public providers, the boundary is shaped by scaling concerns, including integration with record systems, monitoring requirements, device classification, data governance, and liability exposure across sites. This echoes broader implementation research showing that clinical acceptance and organizational readiness must align before AI can become routine [17, 28].

These findings also sharpen the practical meaning of explainability. In our data, participants were less interested in abstract model transparency than in operational traceability: what source material the system used, how a recommendation can be checked, and who remains responsible for the outcome. This interpretation is consistent with recent healthcare AI literature that treats trust as a product of usable oversight mechanisms rather than as blind confidence in model outputs [16, 28].

For practice, the implication is not to indiscriminately maximize autonomy, but to design for bounded delegation. AI tools are more likely to be adopted when they support reversible, auditable tasks, fit existing record and imaging workflows, make human oversight explicit, and are paired with governance arrangements that clarify responsibility, validation, and acceptable use. This also means that implementation should involve clinicians early and address organizational concerns about compliance, liability, and cross-site consistency from the outset [1, 17].

Taken together, these findings add to an emerging but still limited literature on AI use in dentistry by focusing specifically on delegation boundaries. The contribution of this study is to show how the same technology may be perceived differently depending on whether it affects documentation work, diagnostic interpretation, or organizational control over risk.

This study has limitations. The sample is small and purposive. The study focuses on providing insight into complex phenomena and investigates the topic from multiple perspectives. Further studies could focus on providing deeper insight into individual organizational roles. Future work could examine how delegation boundaries vary across specialties, organizational forms, and more mature AI deployments. Longitudinal studies are needed to explain how AI delegation changes over time once the technology matures and acceptance grows.

6 Conclusions

This study examined why and how dental professionals and organizations resist or limit the delegation of tasks to AI. We found that the current delegation is concentrated in two areas: documentation and information retrieval, and imaging tools used as a second opinion rather than an autonomous decision-maker. Documentation/retrieval is perceived as the most delegable because it offers immediate efficiency gains, and outputs can be reviewed, corrected, and audited, especially when systems provide provenance and seamless integration. Imaging support is valued, but delegation remains constrained by higher perceived clinical stakes, risks of over-trust, and the need for chain-level governance around validation, monitoring, and liability. Overall, our results suggest that progress in AI-enabled dental care will depend as much on socio-technical conditions: verification work, workflow integration, professional autonomy, and organizational risk management as on algorithmic performance alone.

Disclosure of Interests. The authors have no competing interests. The first author is employed by Entteri Oy, a manufacturer of digital services for healthcare.

References

1. Hassan, M., Kushniruk, A., Borycki, E.: Barriers to and facilitators of artificial intelligence adoption in health care: scoping review. JMIR Hum. Factors **11**, e48633 (2024)
2. Shan, T., Tay, F.R., Gu, L.: Application of artificial intelligence in dentistry. J. Dent. Res. **100**(3), 232–244 (2021). https://doi.org/10.1177/0022034520969115
3. Khanagar, S.B., et al.: Developments, application, and performance of artificial intelligence in dentistry: a systematic review. J. Dent. Sci. **16**(1), 508–522 (2021). https://doi.org/10.1016/j.jds.2020.06.019
4. Mörch, C.M., et al.: Artificial intelligence and ethics in dentistry: a scoping review. J. Dent. Res. **100**(13), 1452–1460 (2021). https://doi.org/10.1177/00220345211013808
5. Ahmed, M.I., Spooner, B., Isherwood, J., Lane, M., Orrock, E., Dennison, A.: A systematic review of the barriers to the implementation of artificial intelligence in healthcare. Cureus **15**(10), e46454 (2023)
6. Scipion, C.E.A., Manchester, M.A., Federman, A., et al.: Barriers to and facilitators of clinician acceptance and use of artificial intelligence in healthcare settings: a scoping review. BMJ Open **15**(4), e092624 (2025)
7. Field, H.: Google's healthcare AI made up a body part—what happens when doctors don't notice? The Verge (2025)
8. Verhoef, P.C., et al.: Digital transformation: a multidisciplinary reflection and research agenda. J. Bus. Res. **122**, 889–901 (2021). https://doi.org/10.1016/j.jbusres.2019.09.022
9. Lähteenmäki, I., Nätti, S., Saraniemi, S.: Digitalization-enabled evolution of customer value creation: an executive view in financial services. J. Bus. Res. **146**, 504–517 (2022). https://doi.org/10.1016/j.jbusres.2022.03.037
10. Gebauer, H., Fleisch, E., Lamprecht, C., Wortmann, F.: Growth paths for overcoming the digitalization paradox. Bus. Horiz. **63**(3), 313–323 (2020). https://doi.org/10.1016/j.bushor.2020.01.005
11. Qin, R.: Overcoming the digital transformation paradoxes: a digital affordance perspective. Manag. Decis. **61**(6), 1985–2007 (2023). https://doi.org/10.1108/MD-05-2022-0576
12. Lubars, B., Tan, C.: Ask not what AI can do, but what AI should do: towards a framework of task delegability. arXiv preprint: arXiv:1902.03245 (2019)
13. Baird, A., Maruping, L.M.: The next generation of research on IS use: a theoretical framework of delegation to and from agentic IS artifacts. MIS Q. **45**(1), 315–341 (2021)
14. Marr, B.: AI delegation: the one skill you will need to succeed in the future. Forbes (2023)

15. Fechner, P., Lämmermann, L., Lockl, J., Röglinger, M., Urbach, N.: Toward triadic delegation: how agentic IS artifacts affect the patient-doctor relationship in healthcare. J. Assoc. Inf. Syst. **26**(6), 1703–1736 (2025)
16. Amann, J., Blasimme, A., Vayena, E., Frey, D., Madai, V.I.: Explainability for artificial intelligence in healthcare: a multidisciplinary perspective. BMC Med. Inform. Decis. Mak. **20**, 310 (2020)
17. Chen, Y., Stavropoulou, C., Narasinkan, R., Baker, A., Scarbrough, H.: Professionals' responses to the introduction of AI innovations in radiology and their implications for future adoption: a qualitative study. BMC Health Serv. Res. **21**, 813 (2021). https://doi.org/10.1186/s12913-021-06861-y
18. Hoffman, J., Wenke, R., Angus, R.L., Shinners, L., Richards, B., Hattingh, L.: Overcoming barriers and enabling artificial intelligence adoption in allied health clinical practice: a qualitative study. Digital Health **11**, 20552076241311144 (2025)
19. Templin, T., Perez, M.W., Sylvia, S., Leek, J., Sinnott-Armstrong, N.: Addressing 6 challenges in generative AI for digital health: a scoping review. PLOS Digital Health **3**(5), e0000503 (2024). https://doi.org/10.1371/journal.pdig.0000503
20. Palm, E., Manikantan, A., Mahal, H., Belwadi, S.S., Pepin, M.E.: Assessing the quality of AI-generated clinical notes: validated evaluation of a large language model ambient scribe. Front. Artif. Intell. **8**, 1691499 (2025). https://doi.org/10.3389/frai.2025.1691499
21. Kukkola, K., Saxén, H.: Tekoälyn hyödyntäminen hammashoidossa [dataset]. Oulun yliopisto (2024). https://doi.org/10.23729/31d074f4-f93e-4e96-bb94-101d4132277f
22. Gale, N.K., Heath, G., Cameron, E., Rashid, S., Redwood, S.: Using the framework method for the analysis of qualitative data in multi-disciplinary health research. BMC Med. Res. Methodol. **13**, 117 (2013). https://doi.org/10.1186/1471-2288-13-117
23. Gebauer, H., Paiola, M., Saccani, N., Rapaccini, M.: Digital servitization: crossing the perspectives of digitization and servitization. Ind. Mark. Manage. **93**, 382–388 (2021). https://doi.org/10.1016/j.indmarman.2021.01.005
24. Struyf, B., Galvani, S., Matthyssens, P., Bocconcelli, R.: Toward a multilevel perspective on digital servitization. Int. J. Oper. Prod. Manag. **41**(5), 668–693 (2021). https://doi.org/10.1108/IJOPM-08-2020-0538
25. Hassan, H., Zipursky, A.R., Rabbani, N., et al.: Clinical implementation of artificial intelligence scribes in health care: a systematic review. Appl. Clin. Inform. **16**(4), 1121–1135 (2025). https://doi.org/10.1055/a-2597-2017
26. Mohammad-Rahimi, H., et al.: Deep learning for caries detection: a systematic review. J. Dent. **122**, 104115 (2022). https://doi.org/10.1016/j.jdent.2022.104115
27. Mertens, S., Krois, J., Garcia Cantu, A., Arsiwala, L.T., Schwendicke, F.: Artificial intelligence for caries detection: randomized trial. J. Dent. **115**, 103849 (2021). https://doi.org/10.1016/j.jdent.2021.103849
28. Hogg, H.D.J., et al.: Stakeholder perspectives of clinical artificial intelligence implementation: systematic review of qualitative evidence. J. Med. Internet Res. **25**, e39742 (2023). https://doi.org/10.2196/39742

Feasibility of Deep Learning-Based Classification of Lumbar T_2-Weighted MRIs in Subjects With and Without Low Back Pain Symptoms

Mustafa Al-Rubaye[1(✉)], Satu I. Inkinen[1,2], Jaro Karppinen[1,4,5], Miika T. Nieminen[1,3,4], and Juuso H. J. Ketola[1,2]

[1] Research Unit of Health Sciences and Technology, University of Oulu, Oulu, Finland
Mustafa.Al-Rubaye@oulu.fi
[2] HUS Diagnostic Center, Radiology, University of Helsinki and Helsinki University Hospital, Helsinki, Finland
[3] Department of Diagnostic Radiology, Oulu University Hospital, Oulu, Finland
[4] Medical Research Center Oulu, Oulu University Hospital and University of Oulu, Oulu, Finland
[5] Wellbeing Services County of South Karelia, Lappeenranta, Finland

Abstract. Background: Low back pain (LBP) is a prevalent condition. Magnetic resonance imaging (MRI) enables visualization of lumbar spinal structures, but the relationship between MRI findings and symptoms is complex, as degenerative changes are also frequently observed in asymptomatic individuals.

Purpose: This study investigates the feasibility of deep learning for automated classification of lumbar spine MRIs into symptomatic and asymptomatic cases. The aim was to assess whether symptom-related information can be learned from T_2-weighted MRI data.

Study Design: A deep learning-based classification approach using a pre-trained ResNet50 convolutional neural network (CNN) was developed to distinguish between symptomatic and asymptomatic cases.

Methods: Sagittal T_2-weighted MRIs from the Northern Finland Birth Cohort 1966 dataset were used to train, validate, and test the ResNet50-based model for LBP classification. The impact of varying the number of sagittal slices per subject was also evaluated.

Results: The best classification performance was achieved using a modified pre-trained ResNet50 network. The model attained a Balanced Accuracy of 0.713 ± 0.014, an Average Precision of 0.494 ± 0.013, and an Area Under the Receiver Operating Characteristic Curve (AUC-ROC) of 0.724 ± 0.004. Binary classification was more effective in predicting asymptomatic cases, while incorporating Pfirrmann grading improved symptomatic case predictions.

Conclusions: Deep learning-based analysis of lumbar spine MRI showed modest ability to distinguish symptomatic and asymptomatic cases in this cohort. The results support the feasibility of this exploratory approach while highlighting important clinical limitations.

M. Säreströniemi et al. (Eds.): NCDHWS 2026, CCIS 3010, pp. 538–556, 2026.
https://doi.org/10.1007/978-3-032-28819-6_35

Keywords: Deep Learning · Image Classification · Magnetic Resonance Imaging · Lumbar Spine · Low Back Pain

1 Introduction

Low back pain (LBP) is a significant public health problem [12], and up to 84% of people will experience LBP during their lives [5]. Based on the National Institute of Neurological Disorders and Stroke (NINDS), LBP is the leading cause of work disability [26].

LBP is a multifactorial symptom, and the relationship between structural findings in the spine and patient-reported pain is complex [3,9]. Degenerative findings such as intervertebral disc (IVD) degeneration, annular tears, and endplate lesions may be associated with LBP at the population level, but are also frequently observed in asymptomatic individuals [11,24,25,39–41]. Clinically, LBP is often categorized into specific and non-specific pain, where non-specific LBP represents the majority of cases and lacks a clearly identifiable pathoanatomical cause [3,9,19].

Diagnostic imaging methods can be used to identify pathoanatomical changes in selected LBP patients. MRI provides detailed visualization of the lumbar spine and surrounding soft tissues without ionizing radiation [8,30,35,42]. However, routine MRI is generally not recommended for non-specific LBP, as imaging findings may not explain symptoms or alter management [30,35]. The advantage of using MRI over other imaging techniques is that it can visualize spinal structures such as the vertebrae and the intervertebral discs as well as the surrounding tissues with an excellent soft tissue contrast, while conventional radiography and computed tomography (CT) offer limited contrast between different soft tissues [3]. Therefore, MRI is the preferred method for diagnostics of, e.g. degenerative changes, nerve root entrapment, and lumbar disc herniation [15].

In MRI scans of the spine, images with T_1- and T_2-weighted contrast are typically acquired. In spine imaging, T_1-weighted contrast is useful for identifying fatty tissue and obtaining morphological information as fluid causes a low signal on T_1-weighted sequence, making it appear dark in these images [6]. T_2-weighted contrast is used to detect edema and inflammation and reveal white matter lesions as the fluid has a high signal intensity in T_2-weighted sequences. [6]. Vertebral endplates and intervertebral discs can be clearly visualized in T_2-weighted MRI [1], and fat infiltration, which is associated with LBP, is also visible in T_2-weighted MRI [18]. From T_2-weighted images, intervertebral disc degeneration, which is associated with LBP, can be assessed with the five-grade Pfirrmann scoring method, as signal loss and nonuniformity of the disc correlates with the progressive degenerative changes [31,36,37]. Pfirrmann scoring is performed on T_2-weighted midsagittal fast spin-echo images [31].

In recent years, the use of machine learning (ML), and its sub-field deep learning (DL) [20], in medical data analysis has increased substantially [2,13,33]. ML has been successfully applied for the detection, diagnosis, and prognosis of spinal diseases and LBP [28]. LBP detection from MRI is a very challenging task since the pain is often non-specific, but recently, a population-based study on the Northern Finland Birth Cohort 1966 (NFBC1966) [38] data employing radiomics texture analysis suggested that texture statistics extracted from T_2-weighted MRI may contain information associated with LBP status [16].

Neural network applications have been developed for LBP and spinal degeneration assessment from non-imaging data. [2] developed an LBP classification system using neural networks on kinematic data, which can classify LBP from dynamic back motion with 85% accuracy. Another study showed that neural network techniques could effectively categorize patients with acute and chronic LBP based on electronic symptom diary and activity meter data [21]. Other approaches to study LBP include using human balance and body sway performance during standing trials to detect chronic LBP using DL [13].

For an imaging data-based DL assessment of spine degeneration, the SpineNet DL model was developed to assess MR images [14]. SpineNet can be used to predict Pfirrmann grading, disc narrowing, upper or lower endplate defects, upper or lower bone marrow (Modic) changes, spondylolisthesis, and central canal stenosis. The method is able to automatically produce radiological gradings of spinal lumbar MRIs and also predict pathology location, with results exhibiting near human performance level [14]. An external validation was done to the SpineNet model by predicting disc degeneration using Pfirrmann classification and Modic changes from the NFBC1966 data [22].

In this study, we investigated how DL using convolutional neural networks (CNNs) can be applied to identify MRI-derived patterns associated with symptomatic and asymptomatic cases from lumbar spine T_2-weighted MRI data. We evaluated binary classification accuracy when: 1) different numbers of input MRI sagittal images from the spine region were fed into the network, 2) data augmentation was applied, and 3) Pfirrmann grading was added to the model classification layer. In the first evaluation, three different dataset inputs were compared: i) the mid-sagittal slice from each MRI study, ii) the mid-sagittal slice images ± 4 mm (3 slices), and iii) mid-sagittal slice images ± 4 mm and ± 8 mm (5 slices). Finally, data augmentation and Pfirrmann grading were added to the best-performing model from the first evaluation (See Fig. 1).

2 Materials and Methods

2.1 Dataset

In this study, we used the Northern Finland Birth Cohort 1966 dataset (NFBC1966) [38] (1966). During 2012–2014, cohort members at the age of 46–48 living within 100 km from the city of Oulu in Northern Finland ($N = 1\ 988$) were invited to undergo lumbar MRI examinations of the spine, where ($N = 1$ 540) attended the examinations. The NFBC1966 data collection was described by [27] until the age of 46 years in a cohort profile article. Examinations were carried out using the Signa HDxt 1.5 T MRI system (GE Healthcare, Chicago, IL, USA). The subjects also replied to a health questionnaire that included questions related to LBP. The first question was: "Have you had any aches or pains

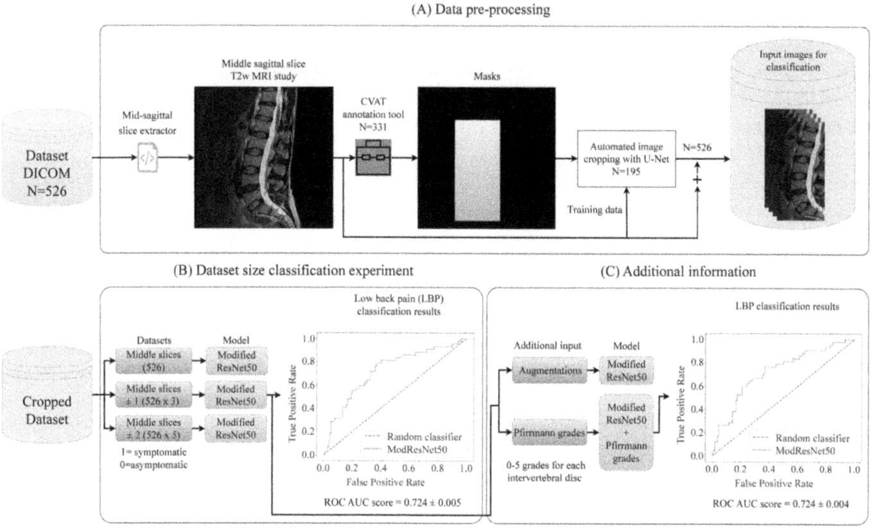

Fig. 1. The workflow of the classification process designed in the present study.

in your low back?", where there were only two responses (1) no, and (2) yes. In order to pinpoint the correct anatomical area, drawings were used. If the answer was yes, the next question would be: "How often have you had aches or pains during the last 12 months?", where the options were (1) 1–7 days, (2) 8–30 days, (3) more than 30 days, and (4) daily. The intensity of the pain was assessed by asking if the individuals reported pain during the past 12 months using a Likert scale from 0 (no pain) to 10 (extremely severe or bothersome pain).

Based on questionnaire answers, the subjects were divided into two groups for binary classification as follows: Individuals with clinically relevant pain (frequency $\geq$30 days and intensity $\geq$6/10), and no clinically relevant pain (frequency $\leq$ 7 days, intensity $\leq$3/10, and no previous pain episodes in the follow-up period). Altogether 526 MRI studies ($N = 113$ (21%) symptomatic and $N = 413$ (79%) asymptomatic cases) met these criteria. In addition, Pfirrmann grading of lumbar IVDs was performed for selected subjects based on MRI studies by two physicians who were experienced with spine MRI (Table 1).

In order to have a clear visualization of the lumbar spine and its surrounding anatomy, sagittal T_2-weighted images were chosen for image classification [6]. They were acquired using a fast spin-echo sequence (TE = 112.7 ms, TR = 3 500 ms, ETL = 27, slice thickness = 4 mm, matrix size = 512 × 512, and FOV = 280 mm × 280 mm).

Table 1. Pfirrmann changes statistics of asymptomatic and symptomatic cases from the dataset used in this study. The values are for each Pfirrmann grade at each intervertebral disc (IVD), where the percentage is calculated individually for each IVD. The overall number of cases and the percentage of each Pfirrmann grade are shown in the last column.

Case	Changes	L1-L2	L2-L3	L3-L4	L4-L5	L5-S1	Overall
Asymptomatic	Pfirrmann 0	2 (<1%)	2 (<1%)	2 (<1%)	2 (< 1%)	2 (<1%)	10 (<1%)
$N = 413$	Pfirrmann 1	0 (0%)	0 (0%)	1 (<1%)	1 (<1%)	0 (0%)	2 (<1%)
(79%)	Pfirrmann 2	361 (87%)	333 (81%)	265 (64%)	154 (37%)	128 (31%)	1241 (60%)
	Pfirrmann 3	41 (10%)	66 (16%)	105 (25%)	126 (31%)	100 (24%)	438 (21%)
	Pfirrmann 4	8 (2%)	11 (3%)	37 (9%)	112 (27%)	142 (34 %)	310 (15%)
	Pfirrmann 5	1 (< 1%)	1 (< 1%)	3 (1%)	18 (4%)	41 (10%)	64 (3%)
Symptomatic	Pfirrmann 0	0 (0%)	0 (0%)	0 (0%)	0 (0%)	0 (0%)	0 (0%)
($N = 113$	Pfirrmann 1	0 (0%)	0 (0%)	0 (0%)	0 (0%)	0 (0%)	0 (0%)
(21%)	Pfirrmann 2	93 (82%)	79 (70%)	67 (59%)	26 (23%)	23 (20%)	288 (51%)
	Pfirrmann 3	17 (15%)	25 (22%)	26 (23%)	35 (31%)	26 (23%)	129 (23%)
	Pfirrmann 4	3 (3%)	9 (8%)	18 (16%)	41 (36%)	42 (37%)	113 (20%)
	Pfirrmann 5	0 (0%)	0 (0%)	2 (2%)	11 (10%)	22 (19%)	35 (6%)

2.2 Data Preprocessing

A custom Python script was developed to automatically select the sagittal slice image from the center of the spinal canal. These images were denoted as mid-sagittal images. The selection of images was done by choosing the most similar images to a couple of template middle-slice images that were chosen manually by the author. The similarity was estimated by computing the maximum correlation between the images from the convolution of the template images and each slice in the MRI study using the fast Fourier transform algorithm [4]. After annotation/extraction, the middle images were manually verified to ensure that the images were from the center of the spinal canal. A total of 510 out of 526 were correctly extracted/annotated, and the rest had to be corrected manually.

2.3 Lumbar Cropping

An automated deep learning pipeline for image cropping was developed to obtain a bounding box/mask of the lumbar spine area (Fig. 1 Masks). The mask was used in image cropping of the input images which were fed as input to the classification network.

First, a subset of data (312 middle slices) was manually annotated using the CVAT-annotation tool [34]. These annotated masks were made by drawing a rectangle covering the lumbar spine in each middle image in each MRI study. As the lumbar spine size varies from one person to another, the initial mask sizes were different for each image. In order to have masks of the same size, the center location of the initial mask was used to extract fixed-sized masks of

100 × 200. These masks were used for localization of the lumbar region. For the classification task, a larger crop of 400 × 200 pixels was extracted around the estimated lumbar center to retain more anatomical context.

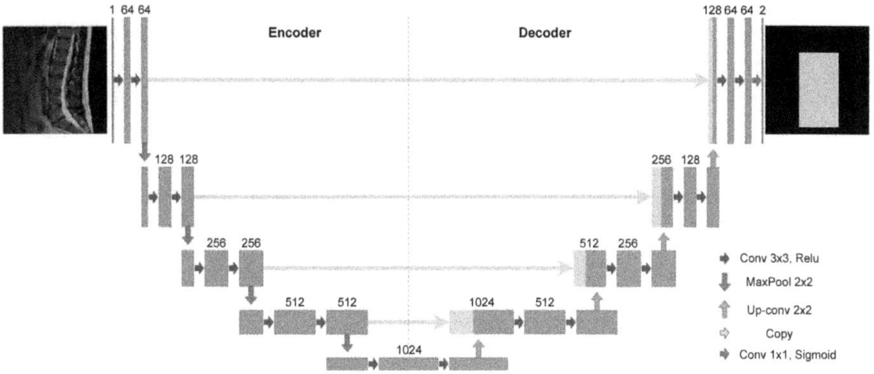

Fig. 2. Illustration of the applied U-Net architecture. The input size was (16×512×512×1), and the network produced an output mask. The term Conv stands for convolution, and ReLU for rectified linear unit activation function.

The mask segmentation pipeline was developed in PyTorch v.1.7.0 [29]. ImageNet pre-trained U-Net convolutional neural network model was trained with annotated masks ($N = 312$) [32]. The ImageNet pre-trained model was trained for 100 epochs and was optimized by minimizing the single-label binary cross-entropy loss function (Fig. 2). 5-fold cross-validation was implemented on the training dataset for hyperparameter tuning (four for training and one for validation). The dice coefficient was used to evaluate the performance of the model [7]. The average Dice score of all the 5-folds was calculated to assess the pipeline's performance on the validation dataset. After defining the optimal hyperparameters (number of epochs 100, learning rate 0.0001, weight decay 0.001, batch size 16, number of workers 20, and milestones where the learning rate is reduced by a factor of ten at 20 and 40 epochs) the training and validation data were combined and used to train the final network model which was used for mask segmentation for the rest of the images.

2.4 Classification

Pytorch machine learning framework v.1.7.0 [29] was used in Python v.3.8 to build DL-based classification pipelines. For the classification task, we chose an ImageNet pre-trained ResNet50 convolutional neural network model [10] with modifications to the last fully-connected classification layers. ResNet50 is a CNN model that is formed from stacks of residual blocks on top of each other. The model is 50 layers deep, consisting of 48 convolutions, 1 max pool, and 1 average pool layer. This model was selected as a robust and widely adopted baseline architecture in medical imaging. The rationale for this choice and possible future improvements are further discussed in Sect. 4.

Two different model architectures were experimented with. In the first model architecture, the last fully-connected layer was replaced with a binary (pain/no pain) classification. In the second model architecture, the last fully-connected layer was replaced with two branches i.e. fully-connected layer for the binary (pain/no pain) classification and a separate fully-connected layer for Pfirrmann grading/classification. This branch configuration was inspired by the previous work by Jamaludin et al. [14], which suggested that the utilization of multiple branches in spine degeneration classification provides additional information for the model. The branches ($N = 6$) consist of 5-Pfirrmann branches ($N = 5$, one for each IVD) and one binary (pain/no pain) branch allowing parameter sharing (Fig. 3).

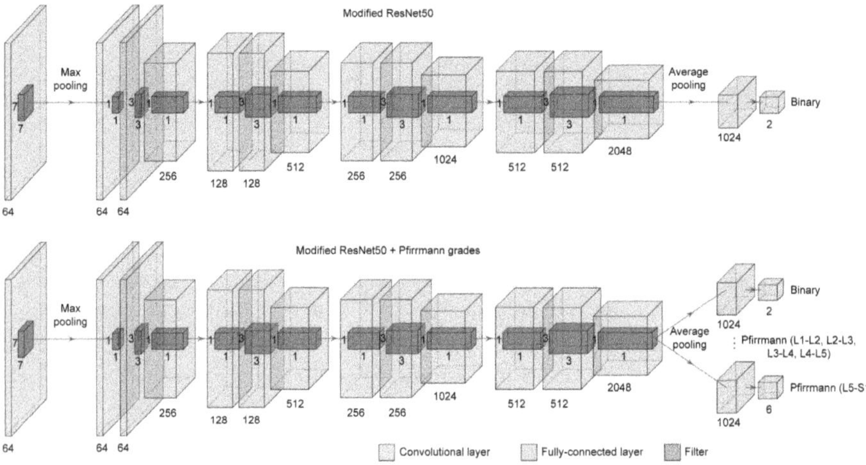

Fig. 3. Diagram representation of the modified ResNet50 and modified ResNet50 + Pfirrmann grading branch architectures. The model input were two-dimensional 400×200 images. Convolution kernels were 7×7, 3×3, and 1×1. ReLU activation function was used between layers.

Model Inputs. The cropped 400×200 pixel sagittal T_2-weighted images were used as the input data for the model, such that the MRI slice (a grayscale image) was copied to 3 channels as the pre-trained model required a three-channel image as input. As the dataset size was small ($N = 526$ studies), different dataset size configurations were experimented with to assess the effect of using more than one 2D sagittal image of an MRI stack. Three approaches were investigated: *i)* only the middle sagittal image slice was fed as input ($N = 526$), *ii)* mid-sagittal slice image and two adjacent slice images (middle slice $\pm$ 1 slice images) were added to the dataset ($N = 526 \times 3 = 1578$), *iii)* mid-sagittal slice images and four adjacent slice images (middle slice ± 2 slice images) were added to the dataset ($N = 526 \times 5 = 2630$). In the ii) and iii) approaches, each MRI study was considered symptomatic if the DL model would predict pain in one of the slices. Images were standardized before feeding them to the network, and light data augmentations were employed during training. The augmentations were padding to 410 × 210 pixels, random horizontal flipping, cropping to 400 × 200 pixels, and rotating ± 10 degrees. The model architecture using the Pfirrmann branch ($N = 5$) (one for each IVD) was applied to mid-sagittal slice images ± 1 slice image input only. This slice-based strategy was motivated by dataset size limitations and by the fact that Pfirrmann grading is typically assessed on midsagittal images. However, restricting the analysis to central slices may miss laterally located abnormalities, such as foraminal or paracentral disc herniations, and therefore represents a simplification of the full lumbar MRI examination.

Dataset Splitting and Model Training. Data were split into training-validation (90%) and test (10%) datasets. Stratified group K-Fold ($K = 10$) was used to split training-validation data during training. This type of split was used to preserve the percentage of symptomatic and asymptomatic cases at each fold, and also images from the same MRI study would be at the same fold. The model for each input approach was individually trained for 100 epochs. The initial learning rate of 0.0001 was reduced by a factor of ten after 30 epochs. The pre-trained ImageNet weights were frozen before the fully-connected layer and run for 40 epochs before completely unfreezing in training. For binary branches (binary classification), binary cross-entropy loss was used and cross-entropy loss was used in the Pfirrmann branches (multi-class classification). Adam optimization (learning rate of 0.0001–0.001 and weight decay of 0.001) algorithm was used to optimize the models by updating network weights [17]. Early stopping was implemented where the model stops after 10 epochs if the loss does not decrease.

The hyperparameters were chosen based on the validation results and the maximum difference of predicted probabilities between symptomatic and asymptomatic populations. As our dataset was imbalanced the optimal threshold for binary classification was chosen based on the validation data and the threshold of 0.22 was used in the testing phase of the 1-slice dataset, 0.24 for the 3-slice, 0.18 for the 5-slice, 0.21 for 3-slice + Pfirrmann, and 0.26 for the 3-slice + augmentations. The threshold was computed from the optimal threshold for the ROC curve. The training process was repeated five times using different seeds to ensure generalization. The model with the best five Matthews Correlation Coefficient (MCC) results before the minimum loss epoch was saved each time (one from each seed). The average classification threshold of the five trained models was calculated to assess the performance of the test dataset.

2.5 Model Performance Assessment

Model performance was evaluated on the test set, which contained 39 asymptomatic and 14 symptomatic subjects. The Receiver operating characteristic

Table 2. The metrics that are used in the present study. Where metrics are defined in terms of TP = True Positives (predicted as positive as was correct) FP = False Positives (predicted as positive but was incorrect), FN = False Negatives (failed to predict an object that was there), and TN = True Negatives (predicted as negative as was correct).

Name	Equation	Range of values
Average Precision score	$AP = \sum_{n}(Recall_n - Recall_{n-1})Precision_n$	$[0, 1]$
ROC AUC score	$ROC - AUC = \int_0^1 TPR(FPR)\, dFPR$	$[0, 1]$
Precision score	$Precision = \frac{TP}{TP+FP}$	$[0, 1]$
Negative predictive value	$NPV = \frac{TN}{TN+FN}$	$[0, 1]$
Recall score	$Recall = \frac{TP}{TP+FN}$	$[0, 1]$
Specificity score	$TNR = \frac{TN}{TN+FP}$	$[0, 1]$
Balanced accuracy score	$BACC = \frac{1}{2}(\frac{TP}{TP+FN} + \frac{TN}{TN+FP})$	$[0, 1]$
Matthews correlation coefficient	$MCC = \frac{TN \cdot TP - FP \cdot FN}{\sqrt{(TN+FN)(FP+TP)(TN+FP)(FN+TP)}}$	$[-1, 1]$
False positive rate	$FPR = \frac{FP}{FP+TN}$	$[0, 1]$
True positive rate	$TPR = \frac{TP}{TP+FN}$	$[0, 1]$

(ROC) curve, Precision-Recall curve, and confusion matrix were computed. Furthermore, several metrics were determined to assess model performance (Table 2).

3 Results

3.1 Segmentation of Lumbar Region

By using 331 sagittal middle slice images to train the model, the Dice Coefficient averaged over 5-folds was 0.97 ± 0.01 (mean $\pm$ standard error of the mean). After that, we used the pipeline to segment the rest ($N = 195$) of the images.

3.2 Classification

The baseline model using only one slice for classification yielded the lowest classification scores apart from the specificity score (TNR) (Table 3, Fig. 5 a, b, and c). When adjacent slices were included in the dataset in the 3-slice approach, Area Under Curve of the Receiver Operating Characteristic (ROC AUC) increased to 0.724, Average Precision score (AP) increased to 0.469 and balanced accuracy score (BACC) increased to 0.709, with similar increases in other classification scores apart from a slight decrease in TNR (Table 3, Fig. 4).

Adding Pfirrmann classification to the model further increased AP to 0.494 and BACC to 0.713, while ROC AUC remained at 0.724, Negative predictive value (NPV) and Recall increased, and precision score, TNR, and Matthews correlation coefficient (MCC) decreased compared to the 3-slice approach (Table 3, Fig. 4). Including augmentations increased AP to 0.526 and ROC AUC to 0.778

Table 3. The results (mean ± standard error of the mean) of different approaches using different metrics. AP stands for the average precision score, ROC AUC for the Area Under Curve of the Receiver Operating Characteristic score, precision score, NPV for the negative predictive value score, Recall score, TNR for the specificity score, BACC for the balanced accuracy score, and MCC for the Matthews correlation coefficient.

Metrics	1-slice	3-slice	5-slice	3-slice + Pfirrmann	3-slice + Augmentations
AP	0.403 ± 0.007	0.469 ± 0.017	0.369 ± 0.004	0.494 ± 0.013	0.526 ± 0.019
ROC AUC	0.667 ± 0.008	0.724 ± 0.005	0.619 ± 0.004	0.724 ± 0.004	0.778 ± 0.006
Precision	0.500 ± 0.101	0.571 ± 0.019	0.393 ± 0.017	0.440 ± 0.035	0.467 ± 0.036
NPV	0.755 ± 0.019	0.846 ± 0.003	0.880 ± 0.006	0.893 ± 0.012	0.816 ± 0.017
Recall	0.143 ± 0.111	0.571 ± 0.027	0.786 ± 0.027	0.786 ± 0.081	0.500 ± 0.073
TNR	0.949 ± 0.050	0.846 ± 0.014	0.564 ± 0.039	0.641 ± 0.063	0.795 ± 0.061
BACC	0.546 ± 0.032	0.709 ± 0.006	0.675 ± 0.011	0.713 ± 0.014	0.647 ± 0.023
MCC	0.153 ± 0.073	0.418 ± 0.006	0.309 ± 0.020	0.377 ± 0.016	0.289 ± 0.041

(Fig. 5 g, h, and i) while other classification scores decreased compared to the 3-slice approach (Table 3). Finally, the 5-slice approach decreased all classification scores apart from increased recall and NPV compared to the 3-slice approach (Table 3, Fig. 5 d, e, and f).

Comparing the 3-slice approach with and without Pfirrmann scoring, the standard 3-slice approach resulted in less true positives but also less false positives in the test set, while with Pfirrmann scoring in the model, the amount of true positives increased at the cost of increased false positives as well (Fig. 4). To gain insight into the model's decision-making process, we visualized Class Activation Maps (CAMs) for selected symptomatic subjects, as shown in Fig. 6. These examples illustrate both interpretable and ambiguous activation patterns, highlighting the strengths and limitations of CAM-based interpretability in LBP classification.

4 Discussion

The features of T_2-weighted MR images were analyzed in this study using a deep learning-based classification method. Our method investigated subjects from a subset of the NFBC1966 [38] data ($N = 526$) using a modified ResNet50 architecture. While ResNet50 is a general-purpose classification model, it is a robust and extensively validated network commonly used as a baseline in medical imaging due to its transfer learning capabilities and strong generalization on small datasets. The primary contribution of this study is an exploratory evaluation of whether symptom-related information can be learned from lumbar MRI data, and whether incorporating Pfirrmann grading improves classification performance.

Our results show that DL-based LBP classification is able to identify symptomatic cases from the NFBC1966 data considerably better than a random classifier. The best performance was achieved using the 3-slice approach and the 3-

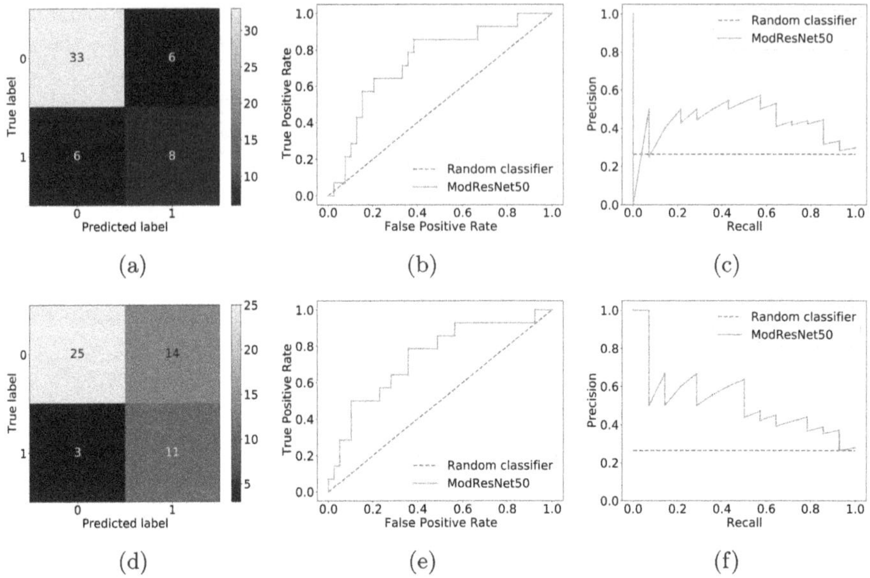

Fig. 4. (a) Confusion matrix of the 3-slice approach, (b) ROC curve of the 3-slice approach, (c) Precision-Recall curve of the 3-slice approach, (d) confusion matrix of the 3-slice + Pfirrmann approach, (e) ROC curve of the 3-slice + Pfirrmann approach, and (f) Precision-Recall curve of the 3-slice + Pfirrmann approach.

slice model augmented with Pfirrmann grading. Based on Table 1, symptomatic cases did not contain any discs graded as Pfirrmann 0 or 1, while a small number of such grades were observed in asymptomatic subjects. However, the frequency was insufficient to use these grades as a definitive indicator for classification.

Adding Pfirrmann grading appeared to improve sensitivity by correctly identifying more symptomatic cases, but it also increased the number of false positives. This is logical since disc degeneration, quantified by Pfirrmann grading, is also prevalent among asymptomatic individuals. Consequently, specificity and precision decreased when Pfirrmann branches were added, although recall improved.

The 1-slice baseline model, which used only the mid-sagittal slice from each MRI study, yielded the lowest classification performance. This is likely due to the limited anatomical context in a single slice. Expanding the input to a 3-slice configuration significantly improved performance. Interestingly, adding even more slices (5-slice) did not yield further benefits and instead reduced accuracy, likely due to the inclusion of image regions with less diagnostic relevance.

The 3-slice approach was more effective at identifying asymptomatic subjects, while the Pfirrmann-enhanced model performed better at detecting symptomatic individuals. Both models exhibited a substantial number of misclassifications. In clinical diagnostics, a false positive is generally more acceptable than a false negative to ensure cases do not go unnoticed. However, in LBP diagnostics, where degenerative changes are also common in healthy individuals, this trade-off becomes more complex. These findings should be interpreted primarily as evidence of limited but non-random association between MRI-derived image features and symptom status in this cohort, rather than as evidence of immediate clinical applicability.

Our approach differs fundamentally from SpineNet, a state-of-the-art deep learning model designed for radiological grading of lumbar disc degeneration features such as Pfirrmann classification and Modic changes. SpineNet uses a multitask architecture trained on T_2-weighted MRIs to provide detailed structural assessments at each disc level. Its performance has been externally validated on the same NFBC1966 dataset used in our study, showing strong agreement with expert raters for Pfirrmann grading (Cohen's kappa = 0.68) and Modic changes (Cohen's kappa = 0.74) [22,23]. In contrast, our model focuses on subject-level symptomatic classification, predicting the presence or absence of low back pain symptoms, rather than detailed structural grading. As such, our approach is more lightweight and modular, and was intended as an exploratory feasibility study of subject-level symptom classification rather than as a clinically deployable screening tool.

A direct performance comparison between SpineNet and our method is not meaningful due to the differing tasks and prediction targets. Moreover, SpineNet operates on disc-level annotations, while our model performs classification at the subject level. Nonetheless, SpineNet's utility in radiological grading could be complementary to our model in a multi-stage diagnostic framework, where structural assessment is used to support or interpret symptom classification.

Our model used only the mid-sagittal slice and its immediate neighbors rather than the full MRI volume. While this choice was motivated by dataset size limitations and common clinical grading practices, it reduces anatomical coverage and may miss laterally located abnormalities. This limitation likely impacts both model performance and clinical interpretability. Future work should consider full-volume or 3D approaches.

Compared to previous texture-analysis-based ML approaches applied to the same NFBC1966 data [16], the classification results in this work showed lower scores, except for slightly higher precision in the 3-slice model. However, in the present work, we used a larger region of interest, including the entire lumbar spine with some surrounding tissues, instead of segmenting the vertebrae and IVDs specifically. Moreover, the present work was intended to streamline the multi-phase approach of the previous work by replacing the data processing pipeline (segmentation, texture analysis, principal component analysis, logistic regression classification) with a single convolutional neural network that could automatically process lumbar MRI data.

We also experimented with additional branches for Modic changes and pain scale inputs (data not shown). Modic changes correlate with the Pfirrmann and modified Pfirrmann grades of disc degeneration in lumbar degenerative disease [43]. Five Modic branches similar to Pfirrmann were tested, but they did not show any improvement. This may be because only T_2-weighted images were used, whereas T_1-weighted images are usually needed to detect Modic changes. In addition, multi-class classification using the pain scale as an input was implemented both individually and with binary outputs to support binary classification, but it did not improve the results, likely due to a low number of high-pain cases in the dataset.

The synthetic minority oversampling technique (SMOTE) was also tested, where augmented copies of the original images were added to increase the number of symptomatic cases. Many augmentation techniques, including random noise, random rotations in the range $(-10, 0)$ degrees, padding between 5–10 pixels followed by cropping, contrast-limited adaptive histogram equalization (CLAHE), and slight blurring, were tested both individually and in combination. However, none showed a notable improvement in classification performance.

We introduced Class Activation Mapping (CAM) to improve model interpretability. CAMs were used to generate heatmaps highlighting areas within the image that contributed most strongly to the classification output. Several examples where the activation maps aligned well with known anatomical features, such as narrowed disc spaces or signal changes at intervertebral disc levels, were selected and included in the supplementary material. CAMs highlighted image regions contributing to model predictions, and in some cases overlapped with plausible anatomical structures. However, activations were often diffuse or difficult to interpret clinically, reflecting the complex relationship between MRI findings and symptoms. These results should therefore be interpreted cautiously.

Future work could explore more spine-specific or task-specific architectures to improve performance. This includes adopting 3D convolutional neural networks to leverage volumetric context from MRI stacks or implementing spine-specialized frameworks such as SpineNet, which has shown strong performance in spinal grading tasks. Additionally, a hybrid approach combining localization, segmentation, and classification could offer a more holistic solution for automatic LBP assessment.

This study has several limitations. The dataset was relatively small and imbalanced, and the test set size was limited. Only T_2-weighted images were used, which may reduce sensitivity to certain pathologies. Furthermore, only mid-sagittal slices were analyzed, which do not fully represent the 3D anatomy of the lumbar spine and may miss clinically relevant lateral abnormalities. Importantly, LBP is a multifactorial condition influenced by biological, psychological, and social factors [9], and cannot be reliably determined from MRI alone. MRI is also not routinely recommended for non-specific LBP, and the present work should therefore be interpreted as an exploratory methodological study rather than a clinical diagnostic solution.

To conclude, feature analysis of lumbar spine MRI data using DL suggests that lumbar MRI may contain limited information associated with symptom status at the cohort level, but does not establish clinical utility for diagnosing LBP from imaging alone.

In the future, we aim to include anatomical references for the most relevant image features using improved interpretability tools. We also plan to incorporate T_1-weighted and fat-saturated sequences, explore the classification of Modic changes, and eventually implement a fully 3D classification framework to utilize volumetric MRI data more effectively.

5 Conclusion

This study evaluated the feasibility of deep learning-based classification of lumbar spine T_2-weighted MRI in subjects with and without low back pain symptoms. The best performance was achieved using 3-slice approaches with and without Pfirrmann grading. While these models showed modest ability to distinguish between groups, the results highlight the complexity of linking MRI findings to symptoms. The present work should therefore be interpreted as an exploratory methodological study. Future work should incorporate broader anatomical coverage, additional MRI sequences, and clinically more direct outcome targets.

Supplementary Information

This article includes supplementary files containing additional figures supporting the main results. The supplementary material provides extended visualizations of performance metrics, including confusion matrices, ROC curves, and Precision–Recall curves for different experimental settings.

Acknowledgments. We thank Antti Isosalo for the technical support during the study. We also thank Dr. Juhani Määttä for assistance in processing the clinical MRI data. The project was funded by the Technology Industries of Finland Centennial Foundation and Jane & Aatos Erkko Foundation.

Ethics Statement. The study was conducted in accordance with applicable ethical standards and regulations governing the use of patient data.

Conflict of Interest. The authors declare that they have no conflicts of interest.

Data Availability. The Northern Finland Birth Cohort (NFBC) 1966 dataset is not publicly available due to personal data content under the EU General Data Protection Regulation (679/2016) and the Finnish Data Protection Act. The data can be requested for research collaboration projects with the University of Oulu from the NFBC scientific committee.

A Supplementary Material

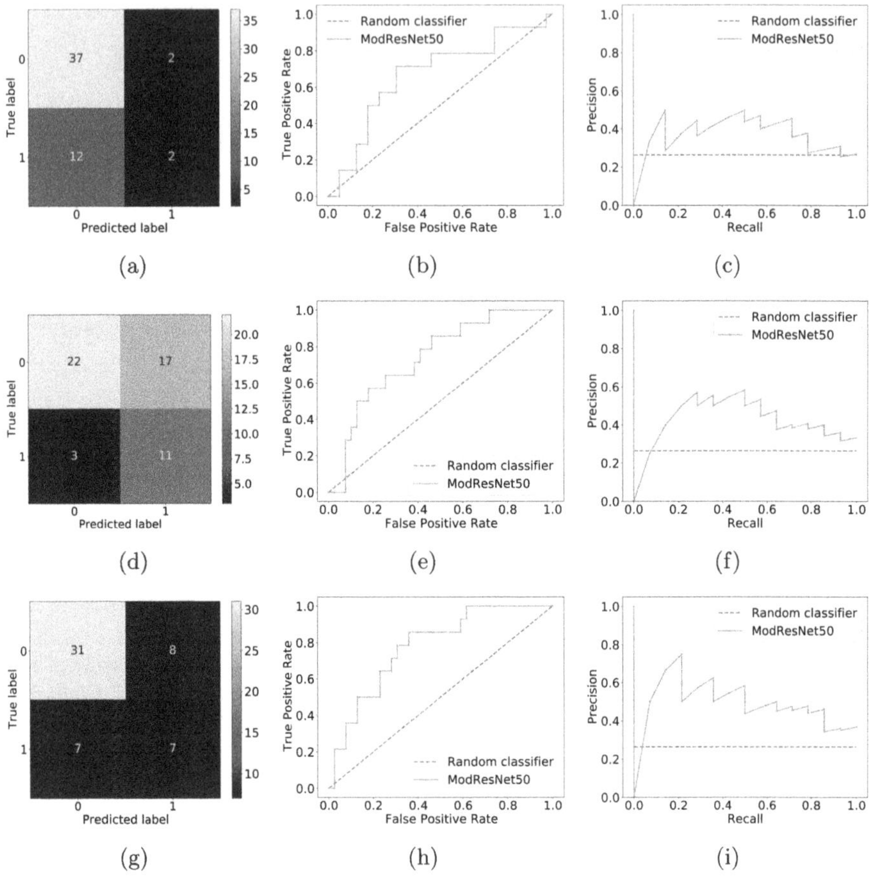

Fig. 5. (a) Confusion matrix of the 1-slice approach, (b) ROC curve of the 1-slice approach, (c) Precision–Recall curve of the 1-slice approach, (d) confusion matrix of the 5-slice approach, (e) ROC curve of the 5-slice approach, (f) Precision–Recall curve of the 5-slice approach, (g) confusion matrix of the 3-slice + augmentations approach, (h) ROC curve of the 3-slice + augmentations approach, and (i) Precision–Recall curve of the 3-slice + augmentations approach.

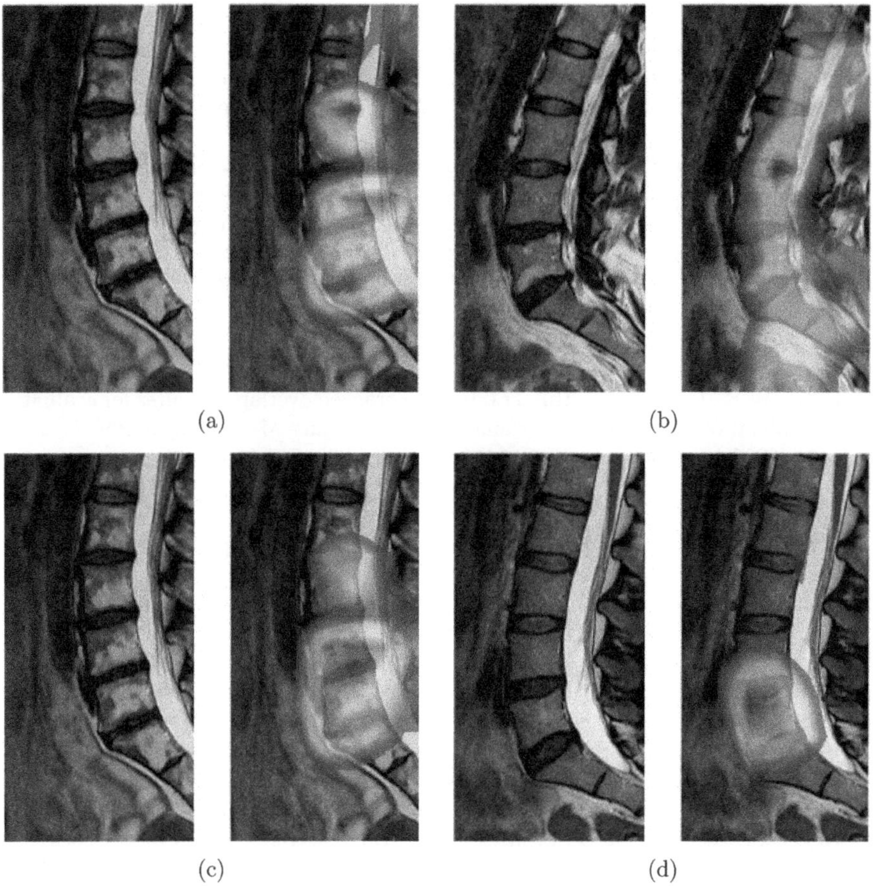

Fig. 6. Example Class Activation Maps (CAMs) from selected symptomatic subjects. (a) Correctly classified case with partially interpretable activations near intervertebral discs. (b) Correctly classified case where the rightmost slice shows plausible focus on a degenerated level. (c) Correctly classified case with activation highlighting disc-level features generally consistent with clinical expectations. (d) Incorrectly classified symptomatic case predicted as no pain, with concentrated activation on a single disc level with limited clinical plausibility according to expert review. These examples illustrate both the potential and limitations of CAM-based interpretability in deep learning for low back pain classification.

References

1. Beattie, P.: Current understanding of lumbar intervertebral disc degeneration: a review with emphasis upon etiology, pathophysiology, and lumbar magnetic resonance imaging findings. J. Orthop. Sports Phys. Therapy **38**(6), 329–340 (2008). https://doi.org/10.2519/jospt.2008.2768
2. Bishop, J., Szpalski, M., Ananthraman, S., McIntyre, D., Pope, M.: Classification of low back pain from dynamic motion characteristics using an artificial neu-

ral network. Spine **22**(24), 2991–2998 (1997). https://doi.org/10.1097/00007632-199712150-00024
3. Braun, J., Baraliakos, X., Regel, A., Kiltz, U.: Assessment of spinal pain. Best Pract. Res. Clin. Rheumatol. **28**(6), 875–887 (2014). https://doi.org/10.1016/j.berh.2015.04.031
4. Burrus, S.C., Parks, T.W.: DFT/FFT and Convolution Algorithms: Theory and Implementation, 1st edn. John Wiley & Sons Inc., USA (1991)
5. Cassidy, J.D., Carroll, L., Côté, P.: The saskatchewan health and back pain survey. the prevalence of low back pain and related disability in saskatchewan adults. Spine **23**, 1860–1866 (1998). https://doi.org/10.1097/00007632-199809010-00012
6. Cousins, J.P., Haughton, V.M.: Magnetic resonance imaging of the spine. JAAOS - J. Am. Acad. Orthop. Surg. **17**, 22–30 (2009). https://doi.org/10.5435/00124635-200901000-00004
7. Crum, W.R., Camara, O., Hill, D.L.G.: Generalized overlap measures for evaluation and validation in medical image analysis. IEEE Trans. Med. Imaging **25**(11), 1451–1461 (2006). https://doi.org/10.1109/TMI.2006.880587
8. Grover, V.P., Tognarelli, J.M., Crossey, M.M., Cox, I.J., Taylor-Robinson, S.D., McPhail, M.J.: Magnetic resonance imaging: principles and techniques: Lessons for clinicians. J. Clin. Exp. Hepatol. **5**(3), 246–255 (2015). https://doi.org/10.1016/j.jceh.2015.08.001
9. Hartvigsen, J., et al.: Lancet low back pain series working group: what low back pain is and why we need to pay attention. Lancet (London, England) **391**(10137), 2356—2367 (2018). https://doi.org/10.1016/s0140-6736(18)30480-x
10. He, K., Zhang, X., Ren, S., Sun, J.: Deep residual learning for image recognition (2015)
11. Herlin, C., et al.: Modic changes-their associations with low back pain and activity limitation: a systematic literature review and meta-analysis. PLoS ONE **13**(8), 1–27 (2018). https://doi.org/10.1371/journal.pone.0200677
12. Hoy, D., Brooks, P., Blyth, F., Buchbinder, R.: The epidemiology of low back pain. Best Pract. Res. Clin. Rheumatol. **24**(6), 769–781 (2010). https://doi.org/10.1016/j.berh.2010.10.002
13. Hu, B., Kim, C., Ning, X., Xu, X.: Using a deep learning network to recognize low back pain in static standing. Ergonomics **61**, 1–22 (2018). https://doi.org/10.1080/00140139.2018.1481230
14. Jamaludin, A., Kadir, T., Zisserman, A.: Spinenet: automated classification and evidence visualization in spinal mris. Med. Image Anal. **41**, 63–73 (2017). https://doi.org/10.1016/j.media.2017.07.002
15. Jarvik, J., Hollingworth, W., Heagerty, P., Haynor, D., Deyo, R.: The longitudinal assessment of imaging and disability of the back (laidback) study. Spine **26**, 1158–66 (2001). https://doi.org/10.1097/00007632-200105150-00014
16. Ketola, J.H.J., Inkinen, S.I., Karppinen, J., Niinimäki, J., Tervonen, O., Nieminen, M.T.: T2-weighted magnetic resonance imaging texture as predictor of low back pain: A texture analysis-based classification pipeline to symptomatic and asymptomatic cases. J. Orthop. Res. **39**(11), 2428–2438 (2021). https://doi.org/10.1002/jor.24973, https://onlinelibrary.wiley.com/doi/abs/10.1002/jor.24973
17. Kingma, D.P., Ba, J.: Adam: a method for stochastic optimization (2017). https://doi.org/10.48550/arXiv.1412.6980
18. Kjaer, P., Bendix, T., Sorensen, J., Korsholm, L., Leboeuf-Yde, C.: Are mri-defined fat infiltrations in the multifidus muscles associated with low back pain? BMC Medicine **5**, 2 (2007). https://doi.org/10.1186/1741-7015-5-2

19. Koes, B., Tulder, M., Thomas, S.: Diagnosis and treatment of low back pain. BMJ (Clinical research ed.) **332**, 1430–4 (2006). https://doi.org/10.1136/bmj.332.7555.1430
20. LeCun, Y., Bengio, Y., Hinton, G.: Deep learning. Nature **521**, 436–44 (2015). https://doi.org/10.1038/nature14539
21. Liszka-Hackzell, J., Martin, D.: Categorization and analysis of pain and activity in patients with low back pain using a neural network technique. J. Med. Syst. **26**, 337–47 (2002). https://doi.org/10.1023/A:1015820804859
22. McSweeney, T.P., et al.: External validation of spinenet, an open-source deep learning model for grading lumbar disc degeneration MRI features, using the Northern Finland Birth Cohort 1966. Spine **48**, 484–491 (2023). https://doi.org/10.1097/BRS.0000000000004572
23. McSweeney, T., et al.: External validation of spinenet, a deep learning model for automated grading of lumbar disc degeneration mri features, using the northern Finland birth cohort. Osteoarthritis Cartilage **30**(Supplement 1), S86 (2022). https://doi.org/10.1016/j.joca.2022.02.106
24. Munir, S., Freidin, M.B., Rade, M., Määttä, J., Livshits, G., Williams, F.M.K.: Endplate defect is heritable, associated with low back pain and triggers intervertebral disc degeneration: a longitudinal study from twinsuk. Spine **43**(21), 1496—1501 (2018). https://doi.org/10.1097/brs.0000000000002721
25. Määttä, J., Wadge, S., MacGregor, A., Karppinen, J., Williams, F.: Issls prize winner: vertebral endplate (modic) change is an independent risk factor for episodes of severe and disabling low back pain. Spine **40**, 1187–1193 (2015). https://doi.org/10.1097/BRS.0000000000000937
26. National Institutes of Health: Low back pain fact sheet (2020). https://www.ninds.nih.gov/Disorders/Patient-Caregiver-Education/Fact-Sheets/Low-Back-Pain-Fact-Sheet
27. Nordström, T., et al.: Cohort Profile: 46 years of follow-up of the Northern Finland Birth Cohort 1966 (NFBC1966). Int. J. Epidemiol. **50**(6), 1786–1787j (2021). https://doi.org/10.1093/ije/dyab109
28. Parisa, A., Taravat, Y., C., B.E., Nayeb, A.H., Shirzad, A., Sohrab, S., Ali, M.: A review on the use of artificial intelligence in spinal diseases. Asian Spine J. **14**(4), 543–571 (2020). https://doi.org/10.31616/asj.2020.0147, http://www.asianspinejournal.org/journal/view.php?number=1194
29. Paszke, A., et al.: Pytorch: an imperative style, high-performance deep learning library. In: Wallach, H., Larochelle, H., Beygelzimer, A., d'Alché-Buc, F., Fox, E., Garnett, R. (eds.) Advances in Neural Information Processing Systems, vol. 32, pp. 8024–8035. Curran Associates, Inc. (2019). http://papers.neurips.cc/paper/9015-pytorch-an-imperative-style-high-performance-deep-learning-library.pdf
30. Patel, N.D., et al.: ACR appropriateness criteria low back pain. J. the Am. Coll. Radiol. **13**(9), 1069–1078 (2016). https://doi.org/10.1016/j.jacr.2016.06.008, https://www.sciencedirect.com/science/article/pii/S1546144016304409
31. Pfirrmann, C., Metzdorf, A., Zanetti, M., Hodler, J., Boos, N.: Magnetic resonance classification of lumbar intervertebral disc degeneration. Spine **26**, 1873–8 (2001). https://doi.org/10.1097/00007632-200109010-00011
32. Ronneberger, O., Fischer, P., Brox, T.: U-net: convolutional networks for biomedical image segmentation. In: Navab, N., Hornegger, J., Wells, W., Frangi, A. (eds.) Medical Image Computing and Computer-Assisted Intervention – MICCAI 2015. MICCAI 2015. LNCS 9351, vol. 9351, pp. 234–241. Springer, Cham (2015). https://doi.org/10.1007/978-3-319-24574-4_28

33. Schmidhuber, J.: Deep learning in neural networks: An overview. Neural Netw. **61**, 85–117 (2015). https://doi.org/10.1016/j.neunet.2014.09.003
34. Sekachev, B., Manovich, N., Zhavoronkov, A.: Computer vision annotation tool (2019). https://doi.org/10.5281/zenodo.3497106
35. Sheehan, N.: Magnetic resonance imaging for low back pain: indications and limitations. Postgrad. Med. J. **86**, 374–8 (2010). https://doi.org/10.1136/ard.2009.110973
36. Takatalo, J., Karppinen, J., Niinimaki, J., Taimela, S., Mutanen, P., Sequeiros, R., Nayha, S., Jarvelin, M.R., Kyllonen, E., Tervonen, O.: Association of modic changes, schmorl's nodes, spondylolytic defects, high-intensity zone lesions, disc herniations, and radial tears with low back symptom severity among young finnish adults. Spine **37**(14), 1231–1239 (2012). https://doi.org/10.1097/BRS.0b013e3182443855
37. Takatalo, J., Karppinen, J., Niinimaki, J., Taimela, S., Nayha, S., Mutanen, P., Sequeiros, R., Kyllonen, E., Tervonen, O.: Does lumbar disc degeneration on mri associate with low back symptom severity in young finnish adults? Spine **36**(25), 2180–2189 (2011). https://doi.org/10.1097/BRS.0b013e3182077122
38. University of Oulu: Northern finland birth cohort 1966. http://urn.fi/urn:nbn:fi:att:bc1e5408-980e-4a62-b899-43bec3755243, university of Oulu
39. Videman, T., Battie, M., Gibbons, L., Maravilla, K., Manninen, H., Kaprio, J.: Associations between back pain history and lumbar mri findings. Spine **28**(6), 582–588 (2003). https://doi.org/10.1097/01.BRS.0000049905.44466.73
40. Videman, T., Nurminen, M.: The occurrence of anular tears and their relation to lifetime back pain history: a cadaveric study using barium sulfate discography. Spine **29**, 2668–76 (2004). https://doi.org/10.1097/01.brs.0000146461.27105.2b
41. Wang, Y., Videman, T., Battié, M.C.: Issls prize winner: lumbar vertebral endplate lesions: associations with disc degeneration and back pain history. Spine **37**(17), 1490–1496 (2012). https://doi.org/10.1097/brs.0b013e3182608ac4
42. Westbrook, C., Talbot, J.: MRI in Practice, 5th edn. Wiley Publishing, Hoboken (2018)
43. Yu, L.P., Qian, W.W., Yin, G.Y., Ren, Y.X., Hu, Z.Y.: MRI assessment of lumbar intervertebral disc degeneration with lumbar degenerative disease using the pfirrmann grading systems. PLOS ONE **7**(12), 1–7 (2012). https://doi.org/10.1371/journal.pone.0048074

Real-Time Thermal Monitoring and Respiratory Analytics on Edge AI for Remote Healthcare

Christian Schuss(✉), Kari Remes, Atte Koskela, and Tapio Fabritius

Optoelectronics and Measurement Techniques (OPEM) Research Group, University of Oulu, 90014 Oulu, Finland
christian.schuss@oulu.fi

Abstract. Contactless respiratory monitoring is increasingly relevant for remote healthcare, infection-control workflows, and continuous assessment in non-clinical environments. Thermal imaging provides an unobtrusive modality for respiratory sensing, yet most existing systems rely on high-frame-rate or radiometric cameras that limit scalability. This work presents a real-time, edge-deployable thermal monitoring system that performs respiratory-rate estimation, temperature extraction, and multi-person tracking using a low-cost FLIR C5 camera despite its low temporal resolution. The pipeline integrates YOLO-based person detection, persistent ID tracking, and a robust temperature-scale extraction method using OCR with temporal smoothing and outlier rejection. Respiratory signals are derived from nostril-level thermal fluctuations using motion-gated sampling, adaptive resampling, FIR band-pass filtering, and Welch spectral analysis, with a spectral-coherence check to suppress unstable estimates. The full system runs on an NVIDIA Jetson Orin NX with real-time visualisation and per-person logging. Preliminary results show that reliable respiratory-rate estimation is achievable under low-frame-rate constraints, demonstrating the feasibility of low-cost thermal sensors for scalable, privacy-preserving remote health monitoring.

Keywords: Thermal imaging · Respiratory rate monitoring · Edge AI

1 Introduction

Respiratory rate (RR) is a clinically informative vital sign associated with early physiological deterioration, respiratory infections, and postoperative complications. Numerous studies have shown that abnormal RR is one of the earliest indicators of patient decline and is included in most early-warning scoring systems [1,2]. Continuous temperature monitoring has also demonstrated clinical value, with recent prospective trials showing that temperature trends can reveal postoperative infections earlier than routine assessments [3]. These findings highlight the growing importance of unobtrusive, continuous monitoring technologies in both clinical and non-clinical environments. Such capabilities are increasingly

M. Särestöniemi et al. (Eds.): NCDHWS 2026, CCIS 3010, pp. 557–572, 2026.
https://doi.org/10.1007/978-3-032-28819-6_36

essential for remote-healthcare workflows, where scalable, low-burden sensing solutions can support early detection and continuous follow up outside traditional clinical settings.

Contactless sensing has emerged as a promising approach for enabling such continuous monitoring. Techniques based on RGB remote photoplethysmography (rPPG) [4], depth sensing, and radar [5] have shown potential for extracting vital signs without physical contact, though these modalities often remain sensitive to illumination, occlusions, or ambient noise. Thermal imaging offers an attractive alternative because it directly captures temperature fluctuations around the nostrils during inhalation and exhalation, operates independently of lighting conditions, and preserves privacy by omitting identifiable facial texture. Recent reviews and technical studies highlight significant advances in thermal respiration monitoring, including multi-resolution and phase-sensitive signal processing for robust RR extraction [6], and comprehensive analyses of thermal cameras for continuous vital-sign assessment [7]. The feasibility of fully embedded, real-time thermal-based RR monitoring has also been demonstrated on compact edge hardware [8]. Together, these developments indicate growing momentum towards practical, privacy-preserving thermal monitoring systems.

Despite these advances, most thermal respiratory-monitoring approaches rely on high-performance radiometric sensors operating at frame rates around 30 Hz, as exemplified by early clinical systems [9], or on lower-cost radiometric devices constrained to approximately 9 Hz by export-control limitations. Such sensors remain costly and inconvenient for large-scale or home-based deployment. Low-cost consumer devices such as the FLIR C-series offer only low temporal resolution and non-radiometric, palette-encoded outputs, introducing challenges including irregular frame timing, unstable temperature scales, limited spatial detail, and greater susceptibility to motion artefacts. These limitations contrast with the more stable sensing conditions available to prior high-end modalities such as rPPG [4], radar-based respiration [5], and radiometric thermography [9,10]. Robust respiratory-rate estimation under these constraints remains an open engineering challenge, with relatively few studies addressing the combination of low-FPS thermal input, non-radiometric colour mapping, and real-time embedded deployment.

This work addresses these limitations by presenting a real-time, edge-based thermal respiratory analytics system designed specifically for low-FPS, non-radiometric thermal cameras. The system integrates lightweight YOLO-based multi-person detection informed by recent deep-learning approaches to thermal monitoring [11], and builds upon clinical insights from prior thermal RR analysis [12,13]. Persistent ID tracking is combined with a robust temperature-scale extraction mechanism that leverages optical character recognition (OCR), temporal smoothing, and outlier rejection to stabilise the colour-mapped temperature output of low-cost devices. Respiratory signals are derived from nostril-level thermal fluctuations using motion-gated sampling, adaptive resampling, finite-impulse-response (FIR) band-pass filtering, and Welch power spectral density (PSD) estimation [14], with a spectral-coherence check to suppress motion-corrupted windows. The complete system runs on an NVIDIA Jetson Orin NX (16 GB) and supports real-time visualisation, per-person signal processing, and continuous logging for embedded digital-health applications.

By demonstrating that reliable respiratory-rate estimation is achievable even under the severe constraints of low-frame-rate, non-radiometric thermal imaging, this work contributes to the development of scalable, privacy-preserving, and cost-effective sensing solutions for digital health. In contrast to prior nostril-centric or high-FPS radiometric approaches [6–8], the proposed system operates on commodity hardware, supports multi-person tracking, and retains fully on-device computation suitable for edge deployment. These capabilities provide a foundation for future multimodal extensions and for integrating higher-fidelity thermal hardware as such sensors become increasingly accessible, advancing continuous, unobtrusive health monitoring in home and clinical environments.

2 Related Work

2.1 Thermal Imaging for Respiratory Monitoring

Thermal imaging has emerged as an effective modality for non-contact RR estimation, capturing periodic temperature fluctuations around the nostrils without requiring physical instrumentation. Early clinical studies demonstrated that radiometric thermal cameras can produce reliable respiratory waveforms even in challenging environments such as neonatal care [13]. More recent developments have improved robustness under motion and environmental variability. For example, Shu et al. employed a YOLOv3-based detector to track the nostril region in low-resolution thermal sequences, achieving RR errors below 2% across diverse breathing patterns [11]. Complementary advances include multi-resolution and phase-sensitive thermal signal-processing frameworks for stable RR extraction under motion [6], as well as broader analyses highlighting thermal cameras as practical tools for continuous, hygienic vital-sign monitoring in both clinical and home environments [7]. The feasibility of fully embedded thermal-based RR monitoring has also been demonstrated on compact edge hardware through nostril-focused detection and adaptive time-domain analysis [8]. Despite this progress, nearly all existing systems assume single-person monitoring with a stable, isolated region of interest (ROI), limiting applicability in real-world settings where multiple individuals may appear simultaneously. These constraints, combined with reliance on high-frame-rate or radiometric cameras, motivate the need for methods that operate reliably on low-cost, low-FPS thermal sensors.

2.2 Deep Learning for ROI Detection in Thermal Imagery

Deep learning has become a central component in stabilising ROI extraction for thermal respiratory monitoring, particularly in scenarios involving motion, occlusion, or low-resolution sensors. Shu et al. demonstrated that YOLOv3-based nostril tracking substantially improves robustness compared with classical template-matching approaches, enabling accurate RR estimation even in low-quality thermal sequences [11]. While such methods highlight the value of deep detectors for single-person thermal monitoring, they typically assume radiometric cameras and relatively high frame rates. Existing approaches also focus on isolated ROI tracking rather than broader scene understanding. In contrast, the present work extends this line of research by employing a lightweight YOLO-based multi-person detector optimised for embedded execution. This enables simultaneous ROI extraction across multiple individuals and supports real-time operation on low-FPS, non-radiometric thermal hardware, addressing practical constraints that remain underexplored in prior literature.

2.3 Signal Processing for Thermal Respiratory Waveforms

Extracting stable respiratory waveforms from thermal imagery requires signal-processing methods that suppress noise, handle motion, and enhance the periodic structure of breathing. Prior work typically applies temporal filtering to stabilise nostril-temperature trajectories before estimating the respiratory rate. Shu et al. used a Butterworth low-pass filter on YOLO-tracked nostril signals to achieve accurate RR estimation in low-resolution thermal sequences [11], while clinical studies with radiometric cameras similarly rely on filtering and spectral analysis to obtain reliable rhythms [13]. Broader investigations have emphasised preprocessing to mitigate environmental and physiological variability [12]. Frequency-domain estimation is commonly performed using Welch's method, which improves robustness through windowed averaging of the power spectral density [14]. However, these approaches generally assume adequate frame rates and stable radiometric output, offering limited guidance for extracting respiratory signals from low-FPS, non-radiometric thermal sensors. To address this gap, the present work employs motion-gated sampling, adaptive resampling, FIR band-pass filtering, and spectral-coherence validation to ensure stable RR extraction under embedded-hardware constraints.

2.4 Embedded and Edge-Based Thermal Analytics

Thermal respiratory monitoring has demonstrated strong potential in clinical and research settings, yet most existing systems rely on offline processing pipelines or high-end radiometric cameras that limit their practicality for real-world deployment. Studies reporting accurate thermal RR estimation typically assume stable imaging conditions, controlled environments, and sufficient frame rates to support conventional filtering and spectral analysis [11,13]. Broader investigations into thermal vital-sign monitoring have similarly emphasised algorithmic robustness but seldom address the computational constraints of embedded platforms [12]. As a result, the literature provides limited guidance on achieving reliable multi-person respiratory analytics using low-FPS, non-radiometric sensors operating directly at the edge. Addressing this gap requires efficient ROI detection, motion-robust signal processing, and system-level optimisation to ensure real-time performance under constrained hardware resources. The present work contributes to this underexplored area by delivering a fully integrated, real-time thermal analytics pipeline on the NVIDIA Jetson Orin NX, enabling practical deployment in embedded and remote-health monitoring scenarios.

3 Methods

This work introduces a real-time, edge-optimised pipeline designed for low-FPS, non-radiometric thermal cameras. The system integrates lightweight YOLO-based multi-person detection, persistent identity (ID) tracking, and robust extraction of the temperature scale to support reliable nostril-level signal acquisition under embedded constraints. Motion-gated sampling, adaptive resampling, and FIR band-pass filtering enhance the periodic structure of the thermal waveform, while Welch spectral analysis provides stable respiratory-rate estimates. The full pipeline runs on an NVIDIA Jetson Orin NX, enabling multi-person monitoring and real-time visualisation suitable for practical digital-health deployment.

3.1 System Overview

The proposed system is designed as a modular, real-time edge-AI architecture that transforms low-FPS, non-radiometric thermal video into stable RR estimates for multiple individuals. As illustrated in Fig. 1, the architecture comprises four tightly integrated components: (i) lightweight YOLO-based multi-person detection executed directly on the embedded GPU; (ii) persistent ID tracking for maintaining temporal continuity across sparse detections; (iii) on-device temperature-scale extraction and nostril-level signal acquisition using OCR with temporal smoothing and outlier rejection; and (iv) motion-aware signal processing and spectral analysis for per-person RR estimation. To minimise latency, detection is performed every few frames, OCR is throttled using monotonic timing, and motion-gated sampling suppresses unstable windows. All computation is performed entirely on the NVIDIA Jetson Orin NX without cloud connectivity, providing inherent privacy preservation and eliminating communication overhead. This integrated edge-AI architecture enables continuous monitoring, multi-window visualisation, and per-person logging using only a low-cost FLIR C5 thermal sensor, supporting practical deployment in embedded and remote-health monitoring scenarios.

3.2 Detection and Tracking

Person detection is performed using a lightweight YOLOv8n model executed directly through a PyTorch runtime on the NVIDIA Jetson Orin NX. To reduce computational load under the low-FPS thermal input of the FLIR C5, YOLO inference is invoked every $N = 3$ frames, while intermediate frames rely solely on the tracking module. This strategy enables substantial savings in GPU usage

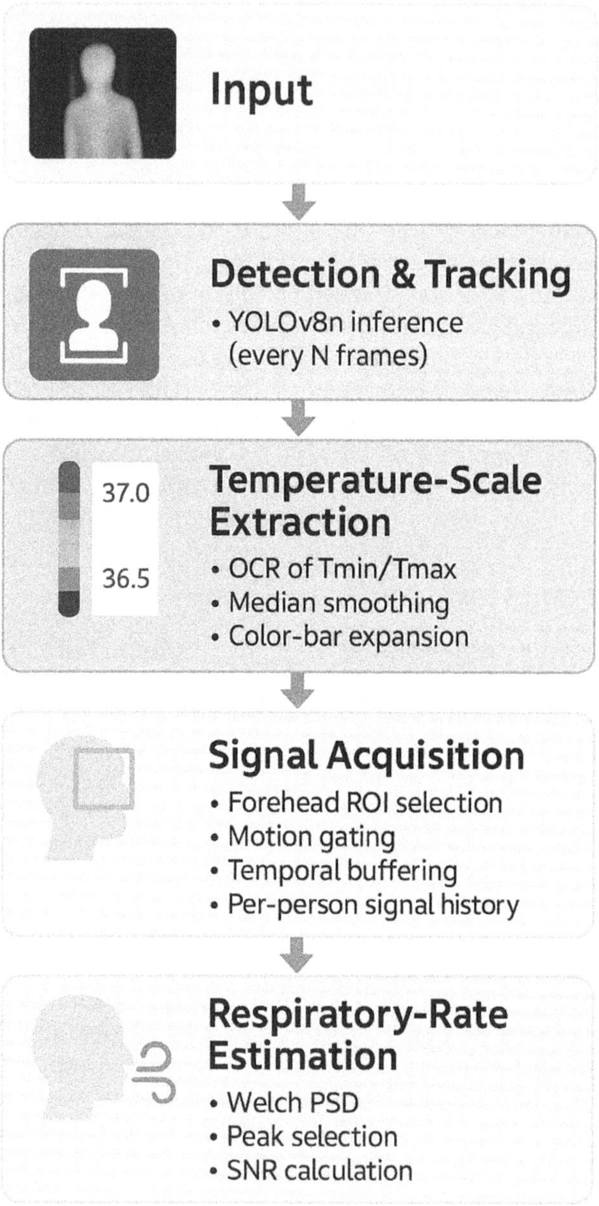

Fig. 1. Edge-AI system architecture for real-time thermal respiratory analytics.

without compromising temporal continuity, as detections are refreshed at a sufficient rate for the slow thermal scene dynamics.

Tracking is implemented using a greedy intersection-over-union (IoU)-based data-association algorithm. For each new frame, pairwise IoU scores are computed between existing tracks and the latest detections, sorted in descending order, and matched greedily whenever the IoU exceeds a threshold of 0.30. Unmatched detections spawn new tracks, while unmatched tracks are aged and removed after 30 missed frames. No motion model or appearance embedding is used; instead, spatial proximity and bounding-box overlap ensure stable identity maintenance even under partial occlusion or intermittent detector updates.

The YOLOv8n model is used without thermal-domain retraining. Although trained on RGB images, YOLO models are known to generalise well to human silhouettes in thermal imagery due to the strong temperature-based contrast. We performed qualitative validation on a collection of representative thermal frames under varying illumination, temperature, and multi-person conditions, confirming that the model reliably produced person bounding boxes suitable for downstream respiratory analysis.

Each tracked individual is associated with a dedicated state structure containing temporal buffers for temperature values, motion estimates, and respiratory-signal history. This modular design ensures that detection latency does not propagate through the pipeline and that per-person trajectories remain stable throughout real-time operation.

3.3 Temperature-Scale Extraction and Signal Acquisition

Temperature-scale extraction is performed by combining OCR-based readings of the FLIR C5 colour-bar endpoints with a robust colour-matching procedure. Optical character recognition is implemented using the Tesseract engine (via the `pytesseract` interface), configured with a digit-only whitelist and Otsu thresholding to ensure reliable parsing of low-contrast thermal labels. To limit computational load, OCR queries are throttled using monotonic timing, and the extracted $T_{\min}$ and $T_{\max}$ values are median-filtered to suppress transient outliers.

For each tracked person, a forehead-level region of interest is isolated using geometric offsets relative to the detected bounding box. Pixel intensities within this region are matched against the expanded colour-bar profile in CIE LAB space, producing a robust estimate of the local temperature without requiring radiometric calibration. The warmest percentile of pixels is used to stabilise the estimate under low spatial contrast and sensor noise. These per-frame temperature values form the raw temporal signal used for respiratory analysis, and motion-gated sampling is applied to discard frames exhibiting excessive displacement or instability.

3.4 Signal Processing and Respiratory-Rate Estimation

The temperature-derived waveform for each tracked individual is processed using a sequence of filtering and spectral-analysis steps optimised for low-FPS thermal data. An exponential moving average stabilises the raw signal prior to resampling. The sampling rate is estimated from timestamp differences and clamped to a feasible range before uniform resampling. A linear-phase FIR band-pass filter isolates the respiratory band (0.10–0.70 Hz), and the resulting signal is normalised to suppress amplitude drift. RR estimation is performed using Welch's method with overlapping segments, providing a low-variance power spectral density. The dominant peak within the respiratory band is selected as the RR estimate, subject to a coherence check that requires agreement between the spectral peaks of the first and second halves of the window. This combination of motion gating, adaptive resampling, and coherence-validated spectral analysis yields stable respiratory-rate estimates under the constraints of non-radiometric, low-frame-rate thermal imaging.

3.5 Real-Time Implementation

The complete pipeline is implemented on an NVIDIA Jetson Orin NX using a PyTorch-based runtime. YOLO inference runs directly on the GPU, while all other components, including OCR, tracking, temperature-scale extraction, and respiratory-signal processing, execute on the CPU. A multi-stage architecture coordinates frame acquisition, inference, OCR cadence control, and signal processing, allowing each module to operate asynchronously with minimal blocking. Shared memory buffers propagate detections, temperature estimates, and respiratory-signal samples between modules. The system supports simultaneous monitoring of multiple individuals and provides real-time visualisation through separate windows for the thermal feed, the hottest-temperature history, the filtered respiratory waveform, and per-person statistics. This PyTorch-driven design enables reliable real-time performance on embedded hardware and forms the basis for the empirical evaluation presented in the next chapter.

3.6 System Latency and Real-Time Behaviour

Although the current implementation is not fully optimised, the proof-of-concept pipeline achieves consistent real-time performance. Based on logged timestamps during operation, the end-to-end processing loop runs at approximately 40–70 ms per iteration under steady conditions, corresponding to an internal update rate of 14–25 Hz. This measurement includes frame acquisition, OCR, detection (when invoked), temperature extraction, and respiratory-signal processing. Since the thermal camera delivers frames at approximately 1 Hz, the edge pipeline introduces negligible additional latency. The system processes all incoming frames without backlog or buffering, confirming that on-device inference and signal processing are sufficiently fast for responsive edge operation.

4 Results

4.1 Experimental Setup

To evaluate the feasibility and robustness of the proposed thermal respiratory-monitoring system, we conducted a series of experiments across four representative real-world scenarios, including several deliberately non-ideal conditions. In all cases, the FLIR C5 thermal camera was positioned approximately 1 m from the participant(s) at eye level and connected to an NVIDIA Jetson Orin NX, where the full processing pipeline executed on-device. The raw thermal frame from the FLIR C5 is first processed for person detection, ROI localisation, and temperature-scale extraction. Under these nominal conditions, the system reliably detects the person, assigns a persistent identity, and automatically extracts both the temperature scale and the nostril-level region of interest required for respiratory analysis. The acquisition geometry was chosen so that the face and upper torso were fully visible while remaining within the effective field of view of the thermal sensor.

4.2 Use Case 1: Normal Indoor Environment

A baseline scenario was recorded in a normally illuminated room ($E_v = 500\,\text{lx}$), with the participant standing 1 m from the camera at eye level. This scenario provides the first demonstration of the complete on-device processing pipeline running on the NVIDIA Jetson Orin NX. Under these nominal conditions, the system reliably detects the person, assigns a persistent identity, and automatically extracts both the temperature scale and the nostril-level region of interest required for respiratory analysis. Figure 2 illustrates the thermal-only person detection and ROI localisation, including the extracted temperature scale used for subsequent signal normalisation. The corresponding per-person physiological statistics, temperature, respiratory rate, and signal-to-noise ratio (SNR), are shown in Fig. 3(a). Figure 3(b) presents the hottest-point tracking used to stabilise the temperature reference, while the extracted breathing waveform and spectral respiratory-rate estimate are depicted in Fig. 3(c). Together, these outputs demonstrate that the system produces a clean respiratory signal and stable RR estimate under standard indoor conditions, forming the reference point for the subsequent non-ideal scenarios.

4.3 Use Case 2: Complete Darkness

To assess system performance without any visible-light cues, the same measurement setup was repeated in a fully darkened room ($E_v = 0\,\text{lx}$). Under these conditions, the FLIR MSX visible-light overlay becomes unavailable, leaving only the raw thermal signal for processing. Despite the absence of illumination, the system maintained reliable person detection and identity tracking due to the thermal-only processing pipeline. Figure 4 shows the thermal frame in complete darkness, including successful detection and temperature-scale extraction

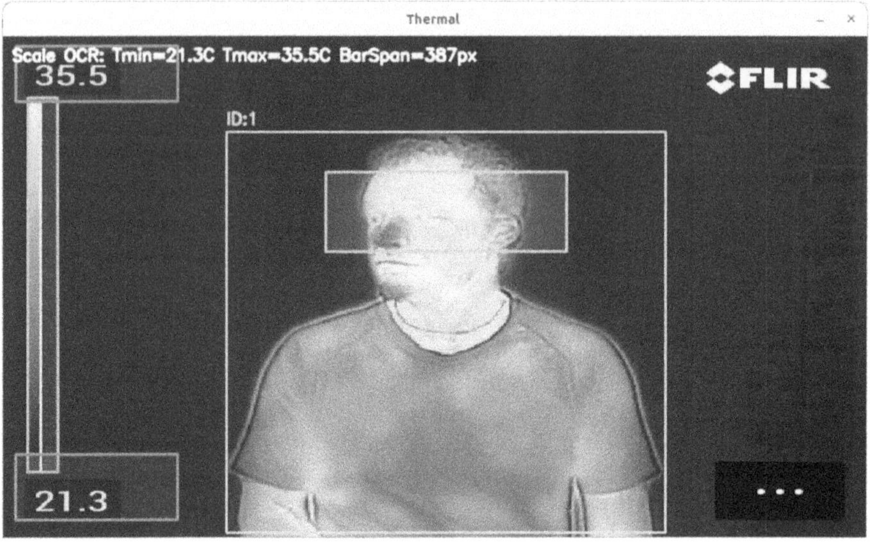

Fig. 2. Use Case 1: Thermal image with detection, ID, and temperature scale.

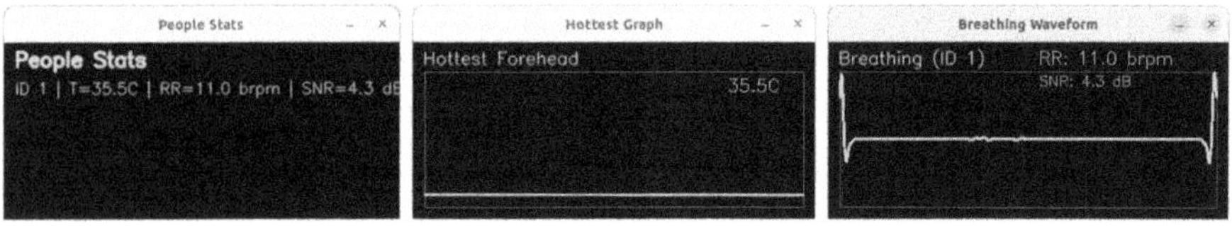

Fig. 3. On-device analysis outputs for Use Case 1: (a) per-person physiological statistics (temperature, RR, SNR); (b) hottest-point tracking used for temperature-scale stabilisation; (c) extracted breathing waveform with spectral RR estimate.

even as the participant moves away from the centre of the field of view. The corresponding on-device analysis outputs are grouped in Fig. 5, demonstrating that per-person physiological statistics, hottest-point tracking, and respiratory waveform extraction remain stable in the absence of visible-light information. This scenario confirms that the proposed pipeline operates robustly under zero-illumination conditions, relying solely on thermal contrast for ROI localisation and respiratory-rate estimation.

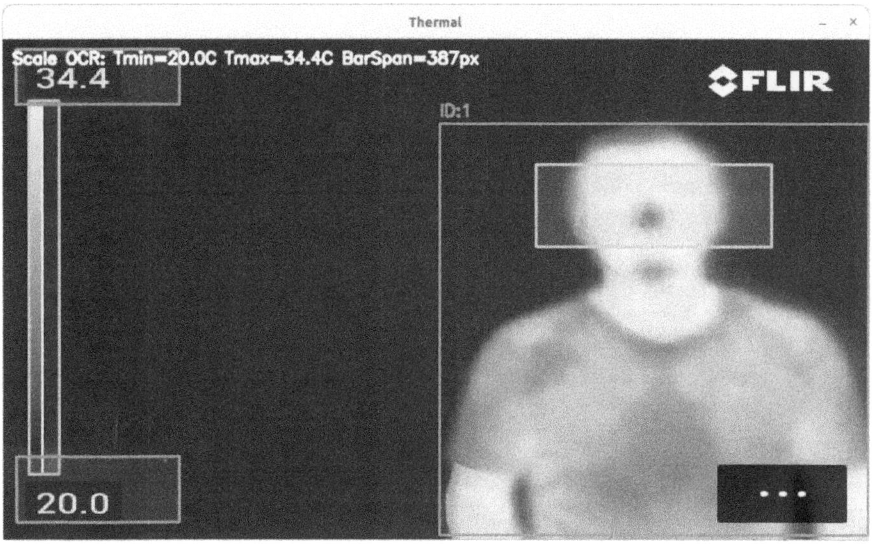

Fig. 4. Use Case 2: Thermal image with detection, ID, and temperature scale.

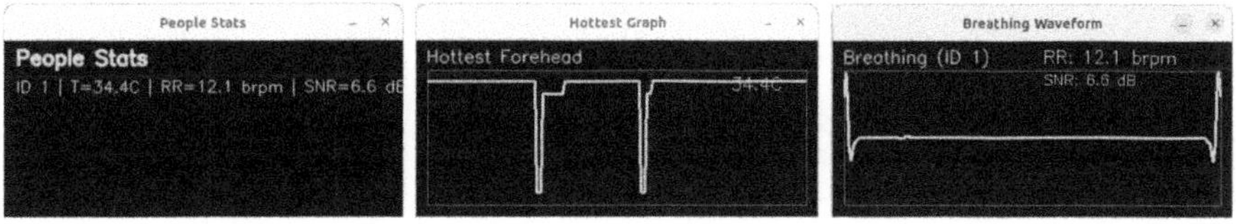

Fig. 5. On-device analysis outputs for Use Case 2.

4.4 Use Case 3: Cold-to-Warm Transition

To evaluate the robustness of the system under rapidly changing thermal conditions, a participant first remained outdoors in cold winter weather (-15° C) and then entered the measurement space. Upon entry, the thermal dynamic range widened substantially due to cooled clothing and skin surfaces, resulting in a markedly broader temperature scale and reduced contrast in the facial region. In addition, the participant wore a winter cap that partially occluded the forehead and upper facial area. Figure 6 shows the thermal frame immediately after the participant entered the room, illustrating the broadened temperature scale and the reduced thermal contrast caused by the cold exposure. Despite these non-ideal conditions, the system maintained stable person detection and identity tracking. The corresponding on-device analysis outputs are grouped in Fig. 7, demonstrating that hottest-point tracking, temperature-scale extraction, and respiratory waveform estimation remain functional even when the thermal distribution is dominated by cold surfaces. Reliable respiratory-rate estimates were obtained throughout the transition period, confirming the robustness of the proposed pipeline under strong temperature perturbations and partial occlusion.

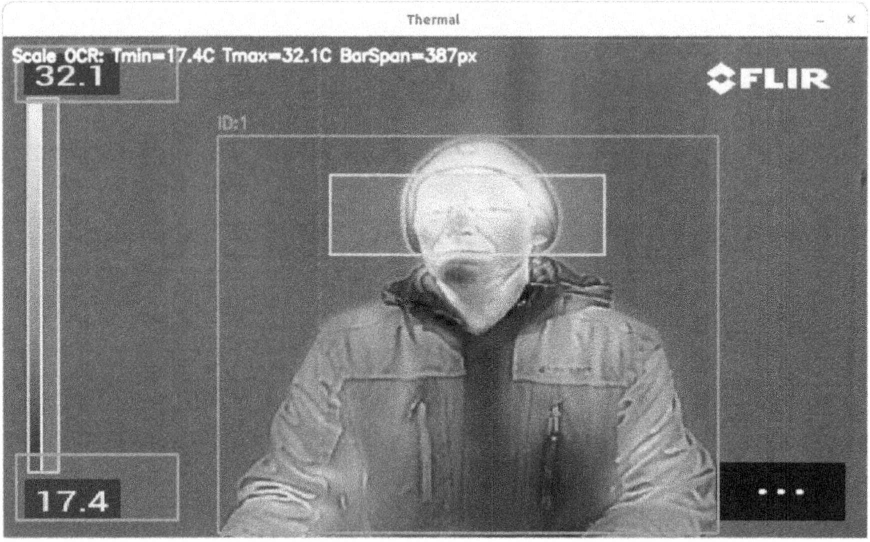

Fig. 6. Use Case 3: Thermal image with detection, ID, and temperature scale.

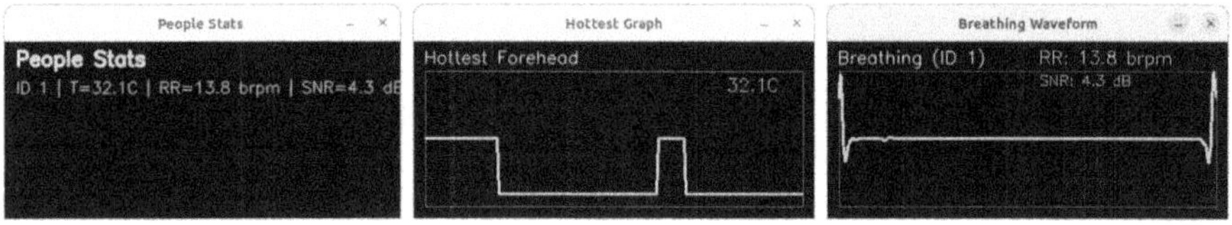

Fig. 7. On-device analysis outputs for Use Case 3.

4.5 Use Case 4: Multi-person Scenario with Speech-Induced Motion

To assess performance in a more realistic social setting, two participants were present simultaneously in the measurement space. The individuals exhibited different thermal characteristics, including distinct maximum temperatures and varying clothing insulation. One participant engaged in brief conversation, introducing additional facial motion and local temperature fluctuations around the mouth region. Figure 8 shows the thermal frame with both participants detected and assigned persistent identities. Despite the presence of multiple people, differing temperature maxima, and speech-related motion, the system maintained stable tracking and correctly associated each respiratory signal with the corresponding identity. The grouped analysis outputs in Fig. 9 demonstrate that per-person physiological statistics, hottest-point tracking, and respiratory waveform extraction remain reliable even in multi-person conditions. This scenario confirms that the pipeline supports simultaneous monitoring of multiple individuals without cross-contamination of respiratory signals or loss of identity consistency.

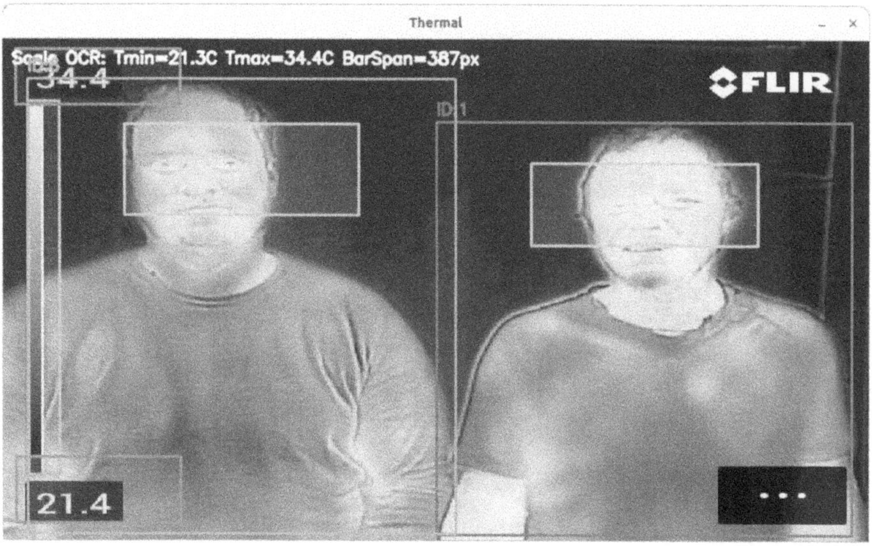

Fig. 8. Use Case 4: Thermal image with detection, ID, and temperature scale.

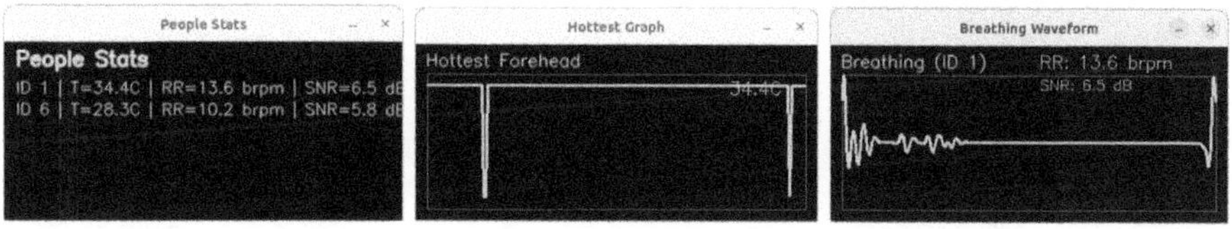

Fig. 9. On-device analysis outputs for Use Case 4.

4.6 Reference Measurement with a Respiration Belt

To obtain an independent reference for respiratory activity, a Vernier Respiration Monitor Belt was connected to a Vernier Gas Pressure Sensor (GPS-BTA). The output voltage of the pressure sensor was digitised using the 16-bit ADC of a National Instruments (NI) myDAQ and recorded in a custom LabVIEW programme. The recording duration was 60 s, during which the thermal signal was acquired simultaneously. Figure 10 shows the resulting voltage trace, capturing the periodic pressure fluctuations associated with thoracic expansion and contraction. Peak counting over the reference signal (threshold voltage at 2.240 V) yielded ten respiratory cycles, corresponding to a breathing rate of about 10 brpm. The thermal-based respiratory-rate estimates (see Figs. 11 and 12) fluctuated between 10.08 brpm (SNR: 4.14 dB) and 10.62 brpm (SNR: 4.07 dB) across the same interval. This close agreement between the reference belt measurement and the thermal pipeline demonstrates the reliability of the proposed method under controlled conditions.

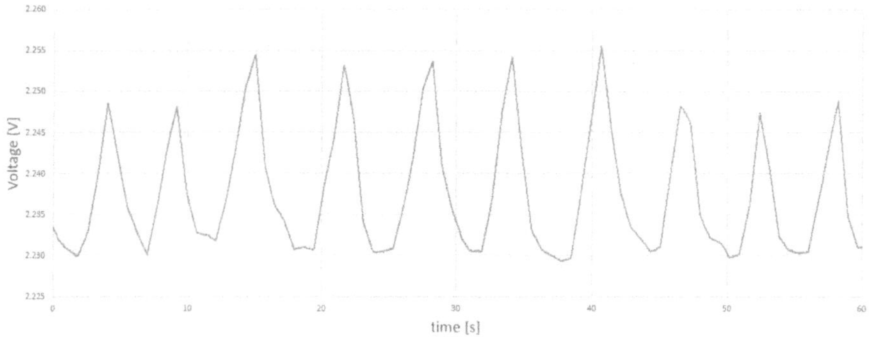

Fig. 10. Averaged voltage signal recorded over 60 s using an NI myDAQ.

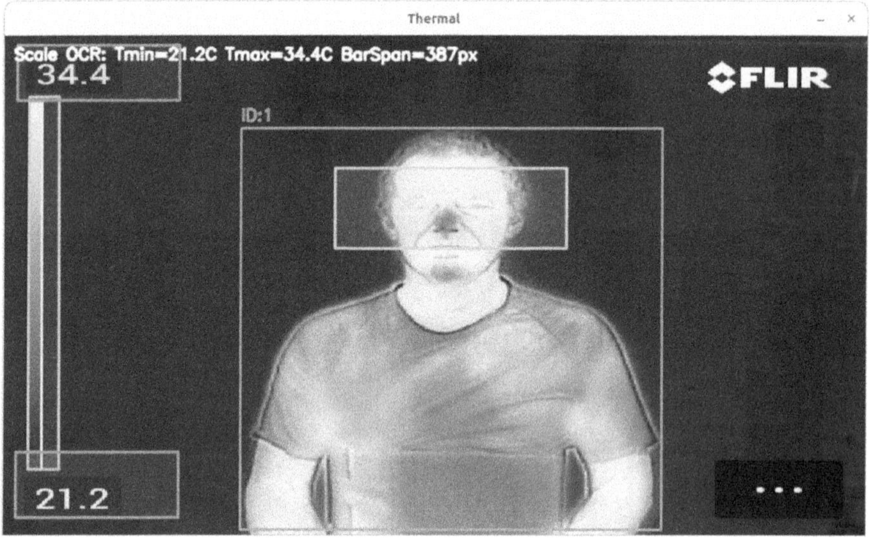

Fig. 11. Verification: Thermal image with detection, ID, and temperature scale.

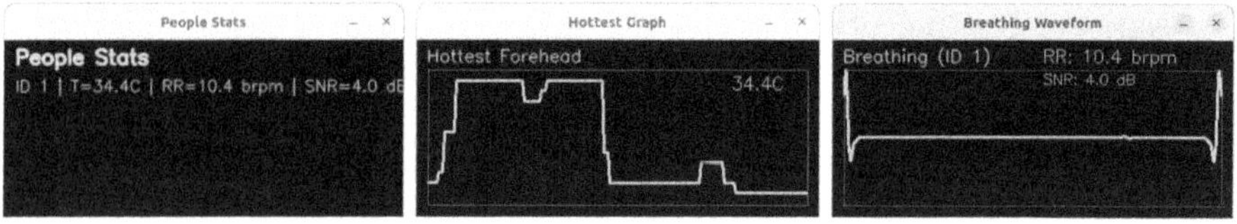

Fig. 12. On-device analysis outputs for verfication.

5 Discussion and Conclusion

The four use cases collectively demonstrate that the proposed thermal respiratory-monitoring system operates reliably under a wide range of real-world conditions. The pipeline maintained stable person detection, identity tracking, and respiratory-rate estimation across variations in illumination, temperature dynamics, occlusion, and multi-person interaction. These scenarios represent common challenges in practical deployments, particularly in clinical triage, occupational safety, and public-health monitoring.

In complete darkness, the thermal-only processing pipeline remained fully functional, confirming that the system does not rely on visible-light information. During the cold-to-warm transition, the broadened temperature scale and reduced facial contrast did not compromise respiratory-rate estimation, highlighting the robustness of the temperature-scale extraction and hottest-point tracking modules. The multi-person scenario further demonstrated that the system can maintain identity consistency and avoid cross-contamination of respiratory signals, even when individuals exhibit different thermal characteristics or engage in speech-induced motion.

The results indicate that low-resolution thermal sensors, when combined with lightweight on-device processing, can provide reliable respiratory monitoring without requiring controlled environmental conditions. The entire pipeline runs in real time on an embedded NVIDIA Jetson Orin NX platform, underscoring the feasibility of deploying the system in portable or battery-powered settings.

Future work will focus on extending the system to handle larger crowds, improving robustness under rapid head motion, and integrating additional physiological cues such as heart-rate estimation from thermal micro-variations, which typically requires higher frame rates. Another promising direction is the incorporation of a stereo-camera setup to obtain depth information, enabling more accurate head-pose compensation and improving signal stability during natural movement. Nevertheless, the present findings demonstrate that thermal imaging, combined with efficient on-device processing, offers a practical and scalable approach for unobtrusive respiratory monitoring in diverse environments.

Acknowledgments. This work has been supported by the SUSA project, funded by the European Union's Digital Europe Programme (DEP) under grant agreement No 101190010.

Disclosure of Interests. The authors declare no competing interests.

AI Use and Tools. Artificial intelligence tools were used for language editing during the preparation of this manuscript. All content was reviewed and approved by the authors.

References

1. Cretikos, M.A., Bellomo, R., Hillman, K., Chen, J., Finfer, S., Flabouris, A.: Respiratory rate: the neglected vital sign. Med. J. Aust. **188**(11), 657–659 (2008)
2. Jagadev, P., Giri, L.I.: Non-contact monitoring of human respiration using infrared thermography and machine learning. Infrared Phys. Technol. **104**, 103117 (2020)

3. Schäfer, L., et al.: Early detection of postoperative infections using continuous temperature monitoring: a prospective clinical trial. J. Clin. Monit. Comput. 1–13 (2025)
4. Sinhal, R., Singh, K., Raghuwanshi, M.M.: An overview of remote photoplethysmography methods for vital sign monitoring. In: Gupta, M., Konar, D., Bhattacharyya, S., Biswas, S. (eds.) Computer Vision and Machine Intelligence in Medical Image Analysis. AISC, vol. 992, pp. 21–31. Springer, Singapore (2019). https://doi.org/10.1007/978-981-13-8798-2_3
5. Wang, Y., et al.: Fine-grained contactless human respiratory measurement using millimeter-wave radar. IEEE Trans. Instrum. Meas. **75**, 1–15 (2026)
6. Choi, J., Oh, K., Kwon, O., Kwon, J., Kim, J., Yoo, S.: Non-contact respiration rate measurement from thermal images using multi-resolution window and phase-sensitive processing. IEEE Access **11**, 112706–112718 (2023)
7. Alves, R., van Meulen, F., Overeem, S., Zinger, S., Stuijk, S.: Thermal cameras for continuous and contactless respiration monitoring. Sensors **24**(8118), 1–20 (2024)
8. Analia, R., Forster, A., Xie, S.-Q., Zhang, Z.: Adaptive thermal imaging signal analysis for real-time non-invasive respiratory rate monitoring. Sensors **26**(278), 1–32 (2026)
9. Abbas, A.K., Heimann, K., Jergus, K., Orlikowsky, T., Leonhardt, S.: Neonatal non-contact respiratory monitoring based on real-time infrared thermography. Biomed. Eng. Online **10**, 93 (2011)
10. Lahiri, B.B., Bagavathiappan, S., Jayakumar, T., Philip, J.: Medical applications of infrared thermography: a review. Infrared Phys. Technol. **55**(4), 221–235 (2012)
11. Shu, S., Liang, H.-R., Zhang, Y., Zhang, Y., Yang, Z.: Non-contact measurement of human respiration using an infrared thermal camera and the deep learning method. Meas. Sci. Technol. **33**(7), 075202 (2022)
12. Maurya, L., Zwiggelaar, R., Chawla, D., Mahapatra, P.: Non-contact respiratory rate monitoring using thermal and visible imaging: a pilot study on neonates. J. Clin. Monit. Comput. **37**(3), 815–828 (2023)
13. Pereira, C.B., et al.: Noncontact monitoring of respiratory rate in newborn infants using thermal imaging. IEEE Trans. Biomed. Eng. **66**(4), 1105–1114 (2019)
14. Welch, P.D.: The use of fast Fourier transform for the estimation of power spectra. IEEE Trans. Audio Electroacoust. **15**(2), 70–73 (1967)

Artificial Intelligence for Reducing Alarm Fatigue in Hospitals: A Systematic Review

Milla Kosonen(✉)

Faculty of Medicine and Health Technology, Tampere University, 33100 Tampere, Finland
milla.kosonen@tuni.fi

Abstract. Frequent false alarms are a major problem in hospitals. The overwhelming number of alarms can cause alarm fatigue. Alarm fatigue is defined as the desensitization of clinicians to alarms, which can lead to delayed responses and to true instability. This systematic review aimed to explore the use of artificial intelligence (AI) to reduce alarm fatigue in hospitals. Four databases, PubMed, Scopus, IEEE Xplore and Web of Science, were searched to identify relevant studies. Studies that aimed to mitigate alarm fatigue using AI were included. Studies published before 2015 were excluded. The final review included 31 studies. Most of the studies focused on arrhythmia or vital sign threshold alarms. Some studies developed early warning scores to replace current threshold-based alarms. Overall, the most common machine learning (ML) model was random forest. The most common neural network model was the convolutional neural network (CNN). Neural networks were mostly used to reduce false arrhythmia alarms, and less often to reduce false threshold alarms. The reviewed studies provided evidence that AI and ML solutions are promising tools for improving the accuracy of patient monitoring and patient safety. However, many studies lacked proper external and clinical validation. In addition, small sample sizes and a lack of annotated data were major limitations. More rigorous performance evaluations are required before AI solutions can be applied in clinical practice.

Keywords: health informatics · patient monitoring · artificial intelligence · alarm fatigue · biomedical engineering

1 Introduction

Advanced multiparameter patient monitoring devices provide continuous surveillance of a patient's state in hospitals via measuring vital signs. A key functionality of patient monitors is the generation of alarms that notify clinical staff of sudden deterioration and other critical changes in a patient's condition. Performing a timely response to these critical alarms is essential to ensure patient safety.

Supplementary Information The online version contains supplementary material available at https://doi.org/10.1007/978-3-032-28819-6_37.

M. Säreströniemi et al. (Eds.): NCDHWS 2026, CCIS 3010, pp. 573–597, 2026.
https://doi.org/10.1007/978-3-032-28819-6_37

Accurate alarms are especially important in critical care, where patients are in an unstable state. However, multiple studies have shown that most of the alarms generated in hospitals are irrelevant, which means that they do not require the response of hospital personnel and have no clinical relevance [1–3]. In addition, as monitors become more advanced, more information about the patient is created through new parameters. Although this could improve care by providing a more detailed view of the patient's state, it can also create a flood of information that the already busy hospital staff cannot adequately handle. Together, these two factors contribute to a phenomenon often referred to as alarm fatigue. Alarm fatigue describes the desensitization to alarm sounds that causes a range of problems to both clinicians and patients. Alarm fatigue is one of the most difficult and significant problems in the health technology industry and a major patient safety concern. Frequent and mostly irrelevant alarms reduce nurses' trust in the monitoring system and interfere with their work [4]. In addition, alarm fatigue has been shown to be associated with burnout [5], increased perceived stress [6], and a greater tendency to make medical errors among critical care nurses [7]. An increase in the number of non-actionable alarms can also increase the response time to following alarms [8].

Typically, patient monitors generate alarms when physiological parameters, such as heart rate (HR), exceed some predefined limits. These alarms are known as threshold alarms. In addition to vital sign threshold alarms, the monitors generate arrhythmia alarms that indicate cardiac complications, and they are typically detected on the basis of an electrocardiogram (ECG). Currently, both threshold and arrhythmia alarms have low specificity and precision. Physiological alarms generated by patient monitors can be divided to clinically actionable and non-actionable alarms. Hravnak and colleagues [3] divide clinically non-actionable alarms into three categories: invalid alarms (technically incorrect), technically correct alarms that require awareness but not immediate action, and technically correct alarms that require neither action nor awareness.

Estimates on the proportion of non-actionable alarms out of the total number of alarms vary. According to Hravnak and colleagues [3] 72–99% of total alarm burden is caused by invalid alarms or valid alarms that do not require awareness or action from clinicians. Paine and colleagues [9] found that 74–99% of alarms were non-actionable (adult intensive care unit (ICU) 74% to >99%; pediatric ICU 87% to 97%; mixed adult and pediatric post-anesthesia care unit (PACU) 83%). Schmid and colleagues [1] evaluated threshold alarms of multiple parameters, including HR, pulse rate (PR), oxygen saturation (SpO2), central venous pressure (CVP), systolic, diastolic and mean arterial blood pressure (BP), and body temperature in an operating room during surgery. They inspected 4893 threshold alarms and 71.84% (3515) were annotated as clinically irrelevant. Drew and colleagues [2] characterized alarms of 461 patients in five ICUs over a period of 31 days and detected 1,154,201 arrhythmia alarms, 612,927 threshold alarms and 791,632 technical alarms. Here, technical alarms refer to artifacts and problems with sensors, probes or line connections (e.g., noisy ECG signal, ECG leads fail, SpO2 probe off) [2]. Drew and colleagues [2] further annotated 12,671 alarms from six arrhythmias, namely, asystole, ventricular fibrillation, ventricular tachycardia, accelerated ventricular rhythm, pause, and ventricular bradycardia, and found that 88.8% were false.

Earlier solutions to alarm fatigue include, among others, adding time delays before triggering an alarm [1,10], frequently changing ECG electrodes [11], using disposable ECG lead wires instead of reusable ones [12], and training clinicians on alarm management [13]. Disposable ECG lead wires and frequent electrode changes prevent noise and artifacts in ECG and therefore prevent technical alarms. Different adaptive alarm parameter adjustment strategies have also been proposed. These strategies include adding adaptive time delays that depend on the severity of the limit violation [1], increasing the upper limit of some alarms (HR, respiratory rate (RR) and temperature) after surgery, increasing the upper limit of HR and RR during daytime, and decreasing the lower limits at night, and triggering alarms based on vital sign trends calculated from linear regression slopes over a specified time window [14].

However, these methods have not been able to sufficiently reduce the alarm burden which is why more advanced solutions are still needed [15]. With increasing availability of rich data and computing resources, the low alarm accuracy problem can be addressed with new data-driven solutions. This systematic review aims to evaluate the current stage of using AI to reduce irrelevant alarms in hospitals, identify knowledge gaps, and provide a starting point for future research on intelligent alarms. More specifically, this systematic review attempts to answer the following research questions: 1) How is AI used to reduce alarm fatigue in hospitals? 2) What type of data are used to develop the methods, and how are the data processed? 3) How is the performance of the developed methods measured? 4) How is model explainability taken into account? 5) What should be focused on in the future?

AI refers to the ability of computers to perform tasks that typically require human intelligence. ML is a branch of AI that involves creating models that learn patterns from large amounts of data. These models can then be used to make predictions from new data. Currently, ML is the main focus of AI in many fields and is sometimes used interchangeably with the term AI. This review focuses on ML, but also considers other AI solutions and advanced signal processing methods. Studies addressing alarm fatigue often focus on ICUs and critical care units. In this review, we also include studies from general wards, given the typically large number of patient days spent in the ward in a common hospital setting.

Chromik and colleagues [16] have performed a systematic literature review on computational methods to mitigate alarm fatigue. They provide an overview of the topic and suggest that future research should focus on alarm actionability. Chromik and colleagues [16] evaluate computational methods, including those involving AI. However, their review does not comprehensively evaluate AI solutions or focus on details relevant to developing AI-based clinical decision support systems. To our knowledge, no systematic review exists that evaluates the use of AI to improve alarm accuracy. Other systematic reviews, including [17], have focused on describing the issue of low alarm accuracy and general solutions to it. Therefore, a systematic review of AI solutions is necessary.

This review is performed according to the Preferred Reporting Items for Systematic reviews and Meta-Analyses (PRISMA) guideline and is structured as follows. In Sect. 2, the eligibility criteria, information sources, search strategy and selection process are explained in detail. In Sect. 3, the characteristics of the selected studies are presented and subcategories are analyzed. Finally, Sect. 4 discusses the results and future directions and Sect. 5 concludes the review.

2 Methods

2.1 Eligibility Criteria

The general criteria for including a study in the review were formulated as follows.

1. The objective of the study is to mitigate alarm fatigue by reducing false alarms in hospitals.
2. Artificial intelligence is used to achieve the objective.

Furthermore, studies were excluded if they were not peer reviewed, were not available in English, or if the full-text article was not available.

2.2 Information Sources

Four databases, namely Scopus, Web of Science, PubMed and IEEE Xplore, were searched to find relevant literature as they give good coverage of both technological and medical publications. In addition, articles were identified from other sources by inspecting the reference lists of relevant articles. Articles published before 2015 were excluded to focus on recent advancements. The last search was done on the 2nd of July 2025.

2.3 Search Strategy

A set of keywords describing the research area was identified and formulated as search queries. The query for Web of Science, PubMed and IEEE Xplore was as follows: ("alarm fatigue" OR "alarm management") AND ("machine learning" OR "artificial intelligence" OR "deep learning" OR "signal processing") AND ("intensive care" OR "critical care" OR "post-anesthesia care unit" OR "intermediate care unit" OR "icu" OR "general ward"). A different query was used for Scopus because the search allowed only 8 boolean operators. The query used in Scopus was: ("alarm fatigue") AND ("machine learning" OR "artificial intelligence" OR "deep learning" OR "signal processing") AND ("intensive care" OR "general ward" OR "intermediate care unit" OR "post-anesthesia care unit").

2.4 Selection Process

First, the results from the searched databases were combined, and the duplicates were removed. Then, one reviewer screened the titles and abstracts, and excluded studies that did not meet the eligibility criteria. Studies for which inclusion could not be decided based on the title and abstract were moved to the next step for full-text review. Each study that passed the screening phase moved on to the full-text review stage, where the same reviewer assessed the eligibility criteria based on the complete article.

2.5 Data Items

After the full-text review, one reviewer extracted the following data items from each eligible article: publication year; data source; patient group characteristics; targeted alarms; description of the used data and features; dataset size; method, including the used ML model; how events were annotated; how model performance was evaluated; and whether explainability techniques were used.

3 Results

3.1 Study Selection

The study selection process is presented as a flow diagram in Fig. 1. The database search resulted in a total of 200 studies. After removing duplicates, 156 studies remained. Citation searching identified an additional 7 studies. Of the 156 studies obtained from the database search, 93 were excluded after screening the titles and abstracts. The remaining 63 records, along with the 7 records obtained through citation searching, were assessed for eligibility during the full-text review phase. Of the 63 records from the databases, 39 were excluded, and of the 7 records from citation searching, none were excluded. This resulted in 31 studies included in the review. Figure 2 shows the publication year distribution of the included studies.

3.2 Data Sources

Open-access databases were utilized in 17 studies and 2 studies [18,19] collected data prospectively in the study. Geographically, the datasets were obtained mostly from the USA, some from Europe, and one from Australia, Israel and Canada, each. Table 1 shows the data sources and their geographical location for each study.

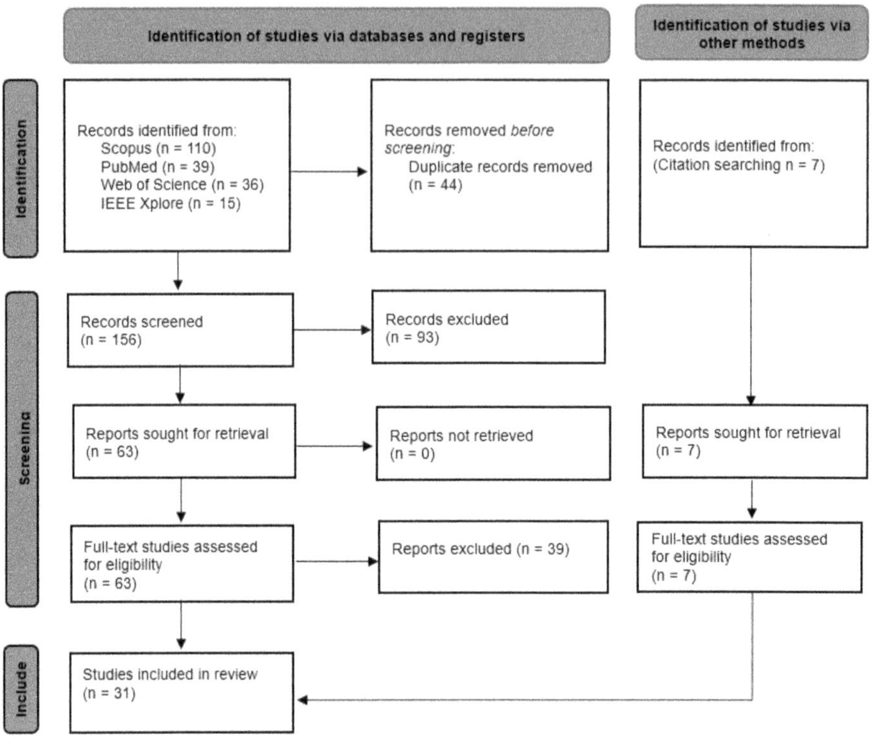

Fig. 1. PRISMA flow diagram.

Open-access databases included MIMIC-II [20], MIMIC-III [21], MIMIC-IV [22], HiRID [23], Preterm Infant Cardio-Respiratory Signals (PICS) [24], MIT-BIH Arrhythmia Database [25], CapnoBase [26], University of Queensland vital signs dataset [27], and the PhysioNet/Computing in Cardiology Challenges from 2011 and 2015 [28,29] (PhysioNet/CinC 2011 and 2015).

Some studies utilized more than one data source. For example, [30] used data collected at Massachusetts General Hospital to train and the PhysioNet/CinC 2015 data to validate the developed model, [31] used data collected at University of California San Francisco and PhysioNet/CinC 2011 data to train the model, and [32] used data collected at Michigan Medicine as the main data source and the CapnoBase database to compare the proposed model with previously developed methods. One study [23] utilized two open databases, HiRID for training and MIMIC-III for external validation of the developed model. One study [33]

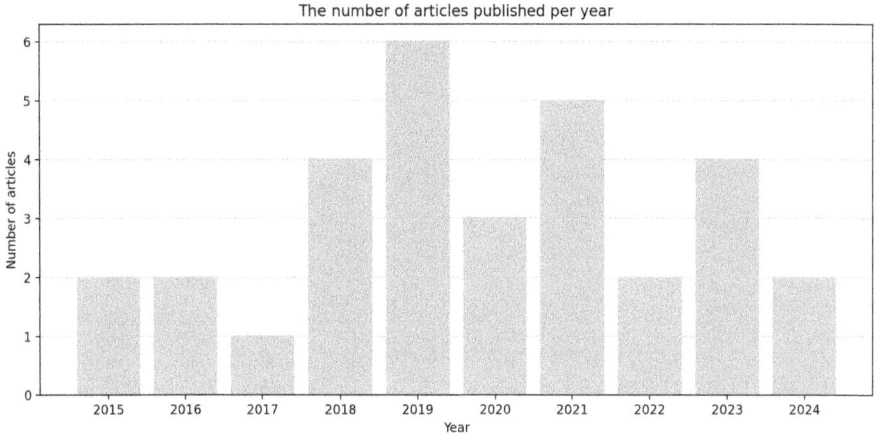

Fig. 2. Publication year distribution of the included articles.

used two open databases, PhysioNet/CinC 2011 for training and testing, MIT-BIH database for testing and the MIT-BIH noise stress test (NST) database to balance unacceptable and acceptable ECG segments in the training data.

3.3 Patient Groups

The studied patient groups include both adult and pediatric patients. The specific groups for adults include ICU and other critical care unit patients, ICU patients with cardiovascular and respiratory conditions, post-anesthesia care unit (PACU) patients, surgical-trauma step-down unit (SDU) patients, and patients with hematologic malignancies in the medical ward. Pediatric patient groups include ICU patients with congenital heart disease (CHD), neonates in ICU, preterm infants in ICU, and general pediatric patients from ICU and floor units. Data were also collected from surgical patients who underwent anesthesia (unspecified age). Table 2 shows the patient groups along with the studies. One study [33] did not specify information on the patient group.

The number of patients was specified in 15 studies [18,19,30,32,44–47,49,51–56]. The number of patients used in the studies ranges from 10 to 8507. Table 3 shows the number of patients by patient group.

Many studies (n = 16) did not specify the number of patients but rather the number of admissions, ICU stays, segments, alarms, events, monitoring hours, or records that were used for training, validation, and testing of the model [23,31,33–43,48,50,57]. The issue with this is that the number of patients is

Table 1. Data sources of the reviewed studies.

Type	Data source/Institution	Location	Study
Open-access	MIMIC-II	USA	[34–37]
	PhysioNet/CinC 2015	USA & Europe	[30,38–40]
	MIMIC-III	USA	[23,41,42]
	PhysioNet/CinC 2011	USA	[31,33]
	CapnoBase	Canada	[32]
	HiRID	Switzerland	[23]
	MIMIC-IV	USA	[43]
	MIT-BIH Arrhythmia Database	USA	[33]
	MIT-BIH NST	USA	[33]
	PICS	USA	[44]
	University of Queensland Vital Signs Dataset	Australia	[45]
Other	UCLA Ronald Reagan Medical Center	USA	[46–48]
	Level-1 Trauma Center (adult surgical-trauma SDU)	no info	[49,50]
	Máxima Medical Center (NICU)	Netherlands	[51,52]
	Texas Children's Hospital	USA	[53,54]
	Children's Hospital of Eastern Ontario	Canada	[19]
	Lucile Packard Children's Hospital	USA	[55]
	Massachusetts General Hospital (ICU)	USA	[30]
	Michigan Medicine	USA	[32]
	Rigshospitalet, University of Copenhagen (PACU)	Denmark	[18]
	Tel Aviv Medical Center (ICU)	Israel	[56]
	UCSF Helen Diller Medical Center	USA	[46]
	UCSF Alarm Study dataset	USA	[31]
	Unspecified large tertiary care hospital (critical care units)	no info	[57]

essential to evaluate the generalization ability of the model. In addition, if the dataset is divided into training and testing sets without ensuring that the two groups contain different patients, there is a possibility of data leakage. Data leakage from training to testing set can bias the results, and the performance estimate on the separate test data becomes overly optimistic. The number of alarms, events or segments are more difficult to compare to each other since the studies use different lengths of time segments and define alarm events differently. The number of ICU stays or admissions provide information on the scale of the dataset, but multiple stays or admissions can originate from the same patient.

Table 2. Patient groups in the reviewed studies.

Population	Ward/Group	Studies
Adult (n = 17 studies)	ICU/Critical care units	[23,31,32,34–37,41–43,46,47,56]
	PACU	[18]
	Surgical-trauma SDU	[49,50]
	Hematologic malignancies in medical ward	[48]
Pediatric (n = 7 studies)	ICU with CHD	[53,54]
	Neonatal ICU	[19,44]
	Preterm infants ICU	[51,52]
	Generic ICU and floor units	[55]
Unspecified (n = 7 studies)	ICU	[30,38–40]
	ICU and SDU	[57]
	Surgical cases under anesthesia	[45]
	Unspecified	[33]

3.4 Targeted Alarms

The included studies focused on arrhythmia (n = 13) [30,31,33–40,44,53,54] or threshold alarms (n = 11) [19,32,41,43,49–52,55–57]. The rest of the studies (n = 6) [18,23,42,46–48] use critical events as targets for prediction and aim to replace current single-parameter threshold alarms. In addition, one study [45] presents a reasoning mechanism to decide how to deliver alarms to caregivers. The study used HR as an example, but the method could be applied to any alarm type. In general, the idea of the method is to decide whether alarms of the same type occurring within a short time period should be delivered together as one notification or as separate ones. Most of the studies addressing false arrhythmia alarms include five arrhythmias, namely, asystole, extreme bradycardia (EB), extreme tachycardia (ET), ventricular fibrillation (VF), or flutter, and ventricular tachycardia (VT) events. The studies targeting threshold alarms mainly focus on HR, SpO2, RR, and non-invasive BP (NBP).

3.5 Data Types

The selected studies used various physiological signals collected in hospitals to develop models. These signals included vital signs (e.g., HR, SpO2, RR, BP, temperature), ECG, photoplethysmogram (PPG), arterial blood pressure (ABP), pulmonary arterial diastolic pressure (PAPD), fraction of inspired oxygen (FiO2), and CVP. Other used data types include laboratory values, treatment-related information (e.g., medications and ventilation mode), alarm occurrence patterns, time of day, time since administration to the unit and

Table 3. Number of patients in each group and study. The studies not shown in the table did not specify the number of patients.

Population	Ward/Group	Studies	# patients
Adult (46–7688 patients)	ICU/Critical care units	[56]	7688
		[46]	6899
		[47]	5018
		[42]	912
		[30]	410
		[32]	46
	PACU	[18]	178
	SDU	[49]	2153
Pediatric (10–8507 patients)	Neonatal ICU	[19,44]	10
	ICU with CHD	[53,54]	40
	Generic ICU and floor units	[55]	8507
	Preterm infants ICU	[51]	66
		[52]	55
Unspecified (32 patients)	Surgical cases under anesthesia	[45]	32

patient information such as age, sex, diagnosis, ethnicity, race, and hospital department. One study [19] combined physiological signals and motion-related data measured with a pressure sensitive mat.

Some studies (n = 9) made predictions based on a single physiological signal: PPG in [32], ECG in [31,33,44,53,54], HR in [45], and ABP in [35,36]. Other studies (n = 22) used a combination of physiological signals, patient demographics, laboratory values and treatment-related values, or used only alarm occurrence patterns [46,47]. Four studies included patient information [23,43,48,55]. Of these four studies, two also included laboratory results [23,48] and two included treatment-related values, medications in [43], medications and ventilator mode, among others, in [23]. Figure 3 shows the number of studies that utilized each physiological signal to develop the prediction model. The studies are shown in 3 groups: studies targeting arrhythmia or threshold alarms and studies developing EWSs. The figure shows that ECG, PPG, and ABP waveforms were used primarily in arrhythmia alarm studies, while EWSs and threshold alarm studies focused on HR, RR, and SpO2.

3.6 ML Models

Most of the studies used supervised ML in their methodology. Two studies used unsupervised learning, one with autoencoder models [44] and one with a diffusion model [34], one study used a weakly supervised approach [57] and one developed a rule-based logic without ML [45]. Two studies utilized contrastive learning [34,38].

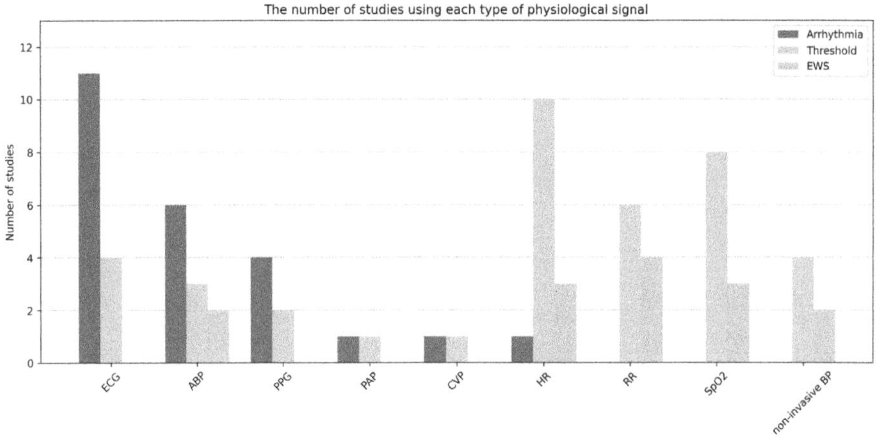

Fig. 3. The physiological signals used to make predictions shown in 3 groups based on the alarms that were targeted. The groups include studies targeting arrhythmia or threshold alarms, and studies developing EWSs.

The ML models used in the studies included neural networks, tree-based models, simple linear models including linear discriminant analysis (LDA) and logistic regression (LR), and other classifiers including support vector machine (SVM), k-nearest neighbors (KNN), and naive bayesian classifier (NBC). The neural network models include recurrent neural network (RNN), gated recurrent unit (GRU), long short-term memory (LSTM) network, convolutional neural network (CNN), multi layer perceptron (MLP), diffusion model and autoencoders with five different layer architectures: 1D-CNN, LSTM, RNN, GRU, and a combination of LSTM and CNN. The tree-based methods include random forest (RF), extreme gradient boosting (XGBoost), decision tree (DT), gradient-boosted ensembe of decision trees (lightGBM), categorical boosting (CatBoost), bagged decision trees (BDT) and extremely randomized trees (ERT).

Additionally, one study compared time series forecasting based on LSTM, RNN and GRU to statistical time series forecasting models, namely, autoregressive integrated moving average (ARIMA) and the extension including exogenous variables (ARIMAX) [41]. In 8 studies, more than one ML model was tested [23,35–37,41,42,44,50]. Table 4 shows which studies used each model. Random forest, logistic regression and CNN were the most frequently used models.

3.7 Feature Engineering

For traditional ML models, the physiological signals have to be transformed into features. In contrast, neural network models, e.g., LSTM and CNN, can automatically learn relevant information from the raw time series data without manual feature extraction. Studies that used raw physiological signals as input and extracted features automatically include [30,33,34,38,41,42,44,47,53] (n = 9). Some studies [30,38] (n = 2) combined learned features with handcrafted

Table 4. Studies using each ML model.

Category	Model	Studies
Neural networks (n = 11)	CNN	[30,33,38,42,53]
	LSTM	[23,41,42,47]
	MLP	[42,48]
	RNN	[41]
	GRU	[41]
	Diffusion model	[34]
	Autoencoder (LSTM, RNN, GRU, CNN, CNN + LSTM)	[44]
Tree-based models (n = 16)	Random forest	[18,35,36,39,40,49,50,55–57]
	Decision tree	[37,42]
	XGBoost	[19,52]
	LightGBM	[23]
	CatBoost	[43]
	Bagged decision tree	[37]
	Extremely randomized tree	[36]
Linear and other classifiers (n = 11)	Logistic regression	[23,42,46,50,51,54]
	SVM	[32,35–37,50]
	LDA	[31,50]
	KNN	[37,50]
	Naive bayesian	[50]

features. The rest of the studies that utilized physiological signals used only handcrafted features [19,31,32,35–37,39,40,43,49–52,54,57] (n = 15) or parameter values at a single time point [48,56] (n = 2). Handcrafted features from physiological signals included, among others, basic statistics (minimum, maximum, average, median, standard deviation, range, kurtosis, skewness, quartiles), slope-related features, morphological features, auto- and inter-correlation, periodicity, sharpness, and stability measures.

3.8 Event Annotation

Most studies used supervised ML. Supervised ML models require labeled training data. For this reason, it is important to examine how different studies have annotated events. In most cases, alarm events were labeled as either a true or false alarm [19,34–38,40,44,49,50,53,54,56,57]. In some cases, the target was signal quality (poor or good quality) [31–33]. In one study, the target was actionability [51]. In some studies, the predicted outcome was related to clinical deterioration, e.g., ICU transfer, cardiac arrest, or advisory alarm followed by critical alarm [18,23,42,46–48,52]. Two studies [43,55] used regression models and one study [41] developed a time series forecasting model.

In most of the studies, clinicians or other experts were asked to manually annotate the events [18,19,30–40,42,49,50,53,54]. In addition to manual annotation, some studies used automatic annotation methods, including rule-based [23,44,51,56,57] and event-based annotation [46–48,52]. In rule-based annotation, a set of rules was defined to determine whether an alarm was true or false. In event-based annotation, the occurrence of an event (e.g., code-blue event, ICU transfer) indicated clinical deterioration and was used to form the positive class.

3.9 Performance Evaluation

The studies evaluated the performance of the ML models with standard performance metrics, including area under the receiver operating characteristic curve (AUC), area under the precision-recall curve (AUPRC), mean absolute error (MAE), accuracy, sensitivity (recall, true positive rate), specificity (true negative rate), precision, positive predictive value (PPV) or precision, negative predictive value (NPV), F1-score and Youden's index. Some studies also used the reduction in the total number of alarms compared to the current alarm system. Some arrhythmia alarm studies [30,34,38,40] used the PhysioNet 2015 challenge score, which emphasizes the importance of high sensitivity by penalizing for false negatives. One study [41] used a different score that penalized for false positives instead of false negatives.

The quality of the performance evaluation varied among the studies. In general, ML models can be evaluated using internal and external validation. Typically, the available dataset is divided into train, validation, and test sets. The validation and test sets constitute internal validation. The validation set is typically involved in model development, hyperparameter tuning, and comparing different models. Instead of a single validation set, a cross-validation scheme can be used, in which the training data is split into equal-sized subsets. One subset at a time is used for validation, while the others are used for training. In addition, studies can perform external validation, in which the model is tested using a dataset from a different population that was not involved in the development of the model.

Most of the studies used cross-validation to evaluate internal performance and tune hyperparameters ($n = 21$) [19,30,31,33,35–42,44,46,49–52,54,56,57]. Some studies used a single validation set to tune hyperparameters or compare the performance of different models [47,48,53]. One study used a temporal split, in which admissions during the last year of a five-year period were used for validation and testing [23]. One study used out-of-bag error estimation instead of cross-validation [18] and one study randomly split the data into training and validation sets 100 times. [32]. Two studies did not mention a validation set or cross-validation, but used an internal held-out test set [34,55]. One study mentions using a grid search to tune hyperparameters and an internal held-out test set to evaluate performance [43].

An external test set was used in 4 studies [23,30,33,46]. In 15 studies, only an internal test set was used [19,31,34,38,40,42,43,47–50,52–55]. In 11 studies, performance evaluation was based solely on cross-validation, multiple random partitions, or out-of-bag error estimation, and neither an internal nor an external held-out test set was used [18,32,35–37,39,41,44,51,56,57].

3.10 Model Explainability

Model explainability or interpretability was explored in 13 studies [23,30,34,40, 43,46,50–54,56,57]. Methods for explaining predictions included Local Interpretable Model-Agnostic Explanations (LIME) [53], Gradient-weighted Class Activation Map (Grad-CAM) [30], SHapley Additive exPlanations (SHAP) [23,43], visualization of generated signals against true signals in a generative model [34] and by computing feature importance using Gini impurity [56,57], permutation importance [30,57] or univariate logistic regression [50]. Some studies (n = 4) [46,51,52,54] preferred to use interpretable features and simple ML models, such as logistic regression or decision trees, over deep learning and neural network models to ensure that the models' predictions can be easily explained. Other studies (n = 7) [33,38,41,42,44,47,48] used neural networks but did not attempt to explain the predictions.

3.11 Subgroup Summaries

In the previous sections, three distinct groups were identified: arrhythmia alarms, threshold alarms and EWSs. These groups were analyzed together in the previous sections. The following three sections present and discuss the characteristics and performance of each group in more detail.

Arrhythmia. Supplementary Table 1 shows a summary of studies developing methods to reduce false arrhythmia alarms. The summary shows the publication year, targeted alarms, patient group and size, dataset size, data source and used ML model. The table shows that the earlier arrhythmia alarm methods from 2015 to 2022 [31,35–37,39,40,54] have focused on expert-informed handcrafted features and traditional ML classification models, including SVM, KNN, LDA, random forest and decision tree. The studies published more recently during years 2022 to 2024 [30,33,34,38,44,53], in contrast, have focused more on using advanced deep learning techniques. These techniques include CNN and its variants including a deformable CNN architecture and an ensemble of CNNs, LSTM, diffusion model, autoencoders and contrastive learning.

Table 5 shows the performance scores of each study. The performance results for both deep learning and traditional ML models are promising. Based on the reviewed studies, it is unclear whether the use of more complex models results in significant performance improvements. Additionally, the models used different datasets and have different targets which makes it difficult to directly compare the results. Two studies experimented with hybrid approaches, in which automatically learned features are combined with handcrafted features [30,38]. Both of these studies found that the hybrid approach results in better performance than using only learned features.

Poor signal quality contributes to false arrhythmia alarms. In 2011, a PhysioNet/Computing in Cardiology challenge focused on predicting ECG signal quality. The dataset provided in the challenge was used in two reviewed studies focusing on signal quality [31,33]. In [33], a novel deformable 1D-CNN architecture was used, while in [31] a simple LDA classifier was developed. The 1D-CNN model performed better than the LDA classifier in all the metrics that were reported.

The reviewed studies can be compared to the current arrhythmia alarm system by using the estimated false alarm rates generated by the monitoring equipment. Drew and colleagues [2] annotated 12,671 arrhythmia alarms as true or false and discovered that 88.8% of them were false. This corresponds to a positive predictive value (PPV), or precision, of 11.2%. Four studies reported PPVs and all were higher than the estimated PPV in the current system. Two studies [30,39] compared the PPVs of their methods to those of the Philips bedside monitors used in the MIMIC-II study [58], the GE Healthcare bedside monitors used in the University of California, San Francisco (UCSF) alarm study [2], and the bedside monitors used to collect the PhysioNet 2015 data [28]. They found that the proposed methods outperformed current monitors in terms of PPV.

Threshold. Supplementary Table 2 shows a summary of studies attempting to reduce false threshold alarms. The table shows that HR and SpO2 alarms were addressed the most and that random forest and boosting techniques (CatBoost and XGBoost) were the most frequently used models, appearing in 8 out of the 11 studies that used an ML model. Only one study used neural networks, specifically RNN, GRU, and LSTM. Interestingly, CNN was not used in any study, despite being a popular method for reducing false arrhythmia alarms. In addition, unlike for arrhythmia alarm studies, there has been no increase in the use of deep learning models for threshold alarm studies in recent years, which could be a research gap. Waveform data were rarely used to form features in threshold alarm studies. However, one study [57] that did utilize waveform data found that waveforms improve performance for both RR and SpO2 alarms. A significant improvement was especially observed for SpO2 alarms.

Various approaches to reducing false threshold alarms were identified, such as threshold optimization, time series forecasting, weak supervision, pressure-sensitive mats, evaluating alarm actionability or relevance, assessing signal quality and modifying alarm presentation through alarm grouping. Table 6 summarizes the methods to reduce false threshold alarms. The table shows that most studies used classification models.

Table 5. Summary of performance of the studies targeting arrhythmia-related alarms. For reference the PPVs of MIMIC-II and PhysioNet 2015 were 46.1% and 39.6%, respectively, as reported in [30]. KLDK = Kullback-Leibler Divergence kernel, CV = cross-validation, ERT = extreme random trees, VT = ventricular tachycardia, VF = ventricular fibrillation, ASYS = asystole, ET = extreme tachycardia.

Study	Model	Acc.	Sens.	Spec.	PPV	Eval.
[53]	CNN (3-model ensemble)	-	85.2	95.0	-	internal test
[44]	RNN (with output correction)	-	97.0	91.4	56.0	CV
[33]	Deformable 1D-CNN	99.6	99.6	99.7	99.7	internal test
[34]	diffusion model	80.1 (VT), 90.0 (VF)	96.5 (VT), 91.7 (VF)	57.1 (VT), 88.8 (VF)	-	internal test
[38]	1D-CNN	-	96.0	86.0	-	internal test
[54]	logistic regression	-	90.0 (threshold 0.73)	83.0	-	internal test
[30]	CNN	93.9 (external)	93.5 (CV)	-	82.9 (CV)	CV and external test
[39]	random forest	74.7	81.5	-	66.1	CV
[35]	KLDK-SVM	96.9	100	93.8	-	CV
[40]	random forest	-	95.0	85.0	-	internal test
[31]	LDA	93.1	96.3	90.0	-	internal test
[36]	ERT	-	80.51 (VF)–99.46 (ET)	90.30 (ET)–99.66 (ASYS,VF)	-	CV
[37]	SVM	90.6	93.1	87.0	-	CV

Table 7 presents the performance scores of threshold alarm studies that used a classification model. Compared to current threshold-based alarms, three studies reported a reduction in the total number of alarms. The studies report reductions of 44.1%–50.5% [55], 80% [52] and 99% [45] in the total number of alarms.

Table 6. Short descriptions of approaches in studies targeting threshold alarms.

Study	Description
[43]	Personalize alarm limits by predicting suitable thresholds based on previously used values.
[57]	Classify alarms as real or artifact using weak supervision.
[41]	Use time series forecasting to predict if an alarm occurs within the following hour.
[19]	Classify alarms as real or artifact using motion-related data collected with a pressure sensitive mat.
[51]	Predict alarm actionability defined by caregiver responses, e.g., silencing, following an alarm.
[32]	Classify PPG segments as good or poor quality.
[45]	Develop a method to group alarms and decide how caregivers are notified.
[52]	Predict whether a red alarm follows a yellow alarm to identify critical cardiorespiratory alarms early.
[56]	Classify alarms as true or false by defining true alarms based on seven clinical conditions.
[55]	Personalize alarm limits.
[49]	Classify alarms as real or artifact using non-invasive vital sign data.
[50]	Classify alarms as real or artifact using non-invasive vital sign data.

Table 7. Summary of performance of studies targeting threshold alarms. CV = cross-validation.

Study	Model	AUC	Sens.	Spec.	PPV	Eval.
[57]	random forest	95.1 (RR), 94.0 (SpO2)	-	-	-	CV
[19]	XGBoost	-	80.0	50.0	-	CV, internal test
[51]	logistic regression	-	81.0	65.0	-	CV
[32]	SVM	-	93.0	92.0	-	internal test
[52]	XGBoost	89.0	33.0	98.0	-	internal test
[56]	random forest	-	97.0–99.0	98.0–99.0	98.0–99.0	CV
[55]	random forest	-	62.0	49.0	-	internal test
[49]	random forest	85.0 (RR), 77.0 (BP), 79.0 (SpO2)	-	-	-	internal test
[50]	random forest (RR), logistic regression (BP), naive bayes (SpO2)	94.0 (RR), 84.0 (BP), 72.0 (SpO2)	-	-	-	internal test

Early Warning Scores. Supplementary Table 3 shows a summary of EWS studies. The targeted outcomes include circulatory failure [23], respiratory distress [42], in-hospital code blue events [46,47], early signs of deterioration [18] and clinical deterioration defined by ICU transfer and cardiac arrest [48]. The studies used both traditional ML models, such as random forest, SVM and logistic regression, and neural networks, including LSTM, CNN and MLP. Two studies

[23,42] compared multiple models. In [23], gradient-boosted ensemble of decision trees was the best model compared to logistic regression and LSTM, while in [42] CNN was evaluated as the most suitable model over LSTM, decision tree and logistic regression.

Table 8 presents the performance scores for EWS studies. The goal of most EWS studies was to develop a new, continuous score that indicates patient deterioration and is more informative and accurate than single-variable threshold alarms. Many of the reviewed EWS studies reported improved performance and a reduction in false and total alarm rates compared to current systems. In [18], the number of false alarms decreased by 85% (from 147 to 22) and the number of missed critical events decreased by 73% (from 111 to 30) compared to current SpO2, systolic BP, HR and RR alarms used in the PACU. In [46], the alarm frequency reduction rate, i.e., the average hourly reduction in alarm frequency compared to current alarms, was reported to be over 90% for both internal and external tests. In [42] the proposed model resulted in a 99% reduction in alarms per patient per day for both RR and SpO2 alarms.

Table 8. Summary of performance of studies developing early warning scores.

Study	Model	Acc.	AUC	Sens.	Spec.	PPV	Eval.
[23]	lightGBM	-	94.0	90.0 (fixed)	-	30.0	internal test
[42]	CNN	92.0	96.0	90.0	93.0	-	internal test
[46]	logistic regression	-	86.0	81.8	78.9	53.5	internal test
[18]	random forest	92.2	96.9	90.6	93.0	-	OOB error
[47]	LSTM	79.4	85.5	85.8	72.6	-	internal test
[48]	MLP	-	-	93.3	96.9	77.6	internal test

4 Discussion

In this section, future directions for reducing alarm fatigue with AI are outlined based on the results. The limitations of this review are also discussed.

4.1 Future Directions

Alarm Threshold Optimization and Human-in-the-Loop Techniques. Two studies attempted to automatically adjust or provide AI-based suggestions for optimal alarm thresholds based on the patient's individual needs. These studies had some limitations. In [43], the prediction targets were the thresholds used in the actual measurements, which were manually set by clinicians. This assumes that these thresholds were optimal, which is not always the case. In [55], evaluating the predicted thresholds against the actual thresholds was difficult because no information on alarm relevance was available. The benefit of AI-assisted threshold adjustment is that clinicians would still make the final decision on how to adjust the thresholds, and no alarms would be replaced or automatically silenced. This method would be easier to implement in practice and likely encounter less resistance from clinicians. In general, more human-in-the-loop methods should be developed, as these types of solutions are largely missing.

Advanced Deep Neural Networks. Advanced deep neural networks were primarily used to reduce false arrhythmia alarms. In future work, these advanced models could also be used to reduce false threshold alarms. Furthermore, since studies addressing threshold alarms mainly use traditional ML models, they also tend to use handcrafted features. Additionally, only a few studies utilized waveform data (e.g., ECG and PPG) with threshold alarms. Only a few studies have used a hybrid approach combining expert knowledge encoded in handcrafted features with deep learning-derived features. This combined feature set could be tested in more applications, especially to reduce false threshold-based alarms. Using more advanced models could improve accuracy but reduce interpretability. There is usually a trade-off between performance and model interpretability. Simple models are easily explainable, but they achieve lower accuracy in complex prediction tasks. Techniques exist to explain predictions made by deep neural networks that could be applied more widely in healthcare applications to improve explainability. Examples of these techniques include Local Interpretable Model-agnostic Explanations (LIME), SHapley Additive exPlanations (SHAP), and Gradient-weighted Class Activation Mapping (Grad-CAM). Some studies have utilized these methods, but many still lack analysis of explainability and interpretation of predictions.

Data Availability and Annotation. More effort should be put towards rigorous performance evaluation, especially in areas such as practical use in hospitals and generalizability across different patient populations. A major constraint of practical ML applications, especially in healthcare, is the limited availability of high-quality training data. Patient monitoring is no exception, as was evident in the reviewed studies. Almost all of the reviewed studies identified poor data availability as a limitation of their research and an area for improvement in the future. More specifically, the lack of annotated data hinders the development of accurate prediction models. Future efforts should focus on creating structured methods for alarm annotation. Furthermore, there is a need for databases containing alarm information. With a structured annotation method and resources dedicated to expert annotation, a large-scale alarm database could be created. Structured annotations would also ensure that data shifts, i.e., changes in data properties over time, do not negatively affect model performance because models could be periodically evaluated and updated with new data more easily. For arrhythmia alarms and, in general, for processing biological waveform data, foundation models, transfer learning, and data augmentation could improve model performance when training data resources are limited. In addition, utilizing semi- and unsupervised ML techniques would be beneficial when annotated data resources are limited. Unsupervised models, such as autoencoders, were used in only a few studies. Besides data availability and external validation, regulatory concerns and technical aspects affecting practical implementation such as computational efficiency should be considered before clinical deployment of AI models. Detailed evaluation of the maturity level of the AI models is left for future research.

4.2 Limitations of This Study

From a methodological perspective, this study is limited in that one single reviewer screened and reviewed the articles. Incorporating two or more reviewers could have improved the reliability of the review process by ensuring that it did not rely on the opinion of one person. Comparing the performance of the reviewed studies was difficult because some studies had different prediction targets and used different datasets. In addition, the studies used different metrics to measure performance.

5 Conclusions

This systematic review aimed to explore the use of AI and ML methods to reduce alarm fatigue in hospitals. Alarm fatigue is a phenomenon in which healthcare staff become desensitized to alarms, which can delay responses to critical alarms. It is caused by an overwhelming number of alarms and the low accuracy of current patient monitoring systems, which trigger a large number of false alarms. Previous solutions to alarm fatigue have focused on behavioral changes, such as training staff to use monitors more effectively, frequently replacing ECG electrodes, and manually adjusting alarm parameters, such as time delays and high and low limits. AI and ML offer the possibility to develop more personalized solutions.

This review included studies whose objective was to mitigate alarm fatigue by reducing false alarms in hospitals using AI. Four databases, PubMed, Web of Science, IEEE Xplore and Scopus, were searched to find relevant articles. Studies published before 2015 were excluded. In addition, studies for which the full text was not available, and studies that were not peer-reviewed or written in English, were excluded. The search was extended by citation searching. One reviewer screened the titles and abstracts of the articles and evaluated the full texts. This review followed the Preferred Reporting Items for Systematic reviews and Meta-Analyses (PRISMA) guidelines.

A total of 31 studies were included in the review. These studies covered a variety of patient groups, including both pediatric and adult patients. The number of patients in the study population ranged from 10 to 8507. The most common method of data collection was extracting data retrospectively from monitors and electronic health records, or using data from open-access databases. The most commonly used open-access databases were MIMIC-II, MIMIC-III, and the 2015 PhysioNet/Computing in Cardiology challenge dataset. Most of the data came from the USA and Europe. Two categories were identified based on targeted alarms, namely threshold and arrhythmia alarms. In addition, a third group that developed early warning scores was identified. The most common ML models were random forest, logistic regression, SVM and CNN. However, the most common ML model varied among the three subgroups. CNN was the most common model for arrhythmia alarms, random forest for threshold alarms, and LSTM and logistic regression for EWS.

The proposed models achieved promising results, with many studies reporting a reduction in the number of false alarms and improved precision compared to current alarm systems. However, only four studies used an external test set. The absence of external validation limits the ability to evaluate model performance in patient populations other than the development set. Future efforts should focus on establishing more comprehensive performance evaluation methods. This should include the analysis of generalizability across different patient populations and the evaluation of performance in clinical settings. In addition, creating databases that include alarm data and relevance annotations is crucial. Finally, ensuring the explainability of models is essential for their reliability and usefulness.

Acknowledgments. This study was completed as part of doctoral studies in the Doctoral School of Industry Innovations (DSII). The doctoral project is a collaboration with Tampere University and GE Healthcare Finland.

Disclosure of Interests. The author has no competing interests to declare that are relevant to the content of this article.

References

1. Schmid, F., et al.: Reduction of clinically irrelevant alarms in patient monitoring by adaptive time delays. J. Clin. Monit. Comput. **31**, 213–219 (2017)
2. Drew, B.J., et al.: Insights into the problem of alarm fatigue with physiologic monitor devices: a comprehensive observational study of consecutive intensive care unit patients. PLoS ONE **9**, e110274 (2014)
3. Hravnak, M., et al.: A call to alarms: current state and future directions in the battle against alarm fatigue. J. Electrocardiol. **51**, S44–S48 (2018)
4. Lewandowska, K., Weisbrot, M., Cieloszyk, A., Mędrzycka-Dąbrowska, W., Krupa, S., Ozga, D.: Impact of alarm fatigue on the work of nurses in an intensive care environment—a systematic review. Int. J. Environ. Res. Public Health **17**, 8409 (2020)
5. Ding, S., et al.: The relationship between alarm fatigue and burnout among critical care nurses: a cross-sectional study. Nurs. Crit. Care **28**, 940–947 (2023)
6. Salameh, B., Abdallah, J., Alkubati, S.A., ALBashtawy, M.: Alarm fatigue and perceived stress among critical care nurses in the intensive care units: Palestinian perspectives. BMC Nurs. **23**, 261 (2024)
7. Gündoğan, G., Erdağı Oral, S.: The effects of alarm fatigue on the tendency to make medical errors in nurses working in intensive care units. Nurs. Crit. Care **28**, 996–1003 (2023)

8. Bonafide, C.P., et al.: Association between exposure to nonactionable physiologic monitor alarms and response time in a children's hospital. J. Hosp. Med. **10**, 345–351 (2015)
9. Paine, C.W., et al.: Systematic review of physiologic monitor alarm characteristics and pragmatic interventions to reduce alarm frequency. J. Hosp. Med. **11**, 136–144 (2016)
10. Yang, J.K., et al.: Mitigating alarm fatigue and improving the bedside experience by reducing nonactionable alarms. J. Pediatr. **276**, 114278 (2025)
11. Cvach, M.M., Biggs, M., Rothwell, K.J., Charles-Hudson, C.: Daily electrode change and effect on cardiac monitor alarms: an evidence-based practice approach. J. Nurs. Care Qual. **28**, 265–271 (2013)
12. Albert, N.M., et al.: Differences in alarm events between disposable and reusable electrocardiography lead wires. Am. J. Crit. Care **24**, 67–74 (2015)
13. Bi, J., et al.: Effects of monitor alarm management training on nurses' alarm fatigue: a randomised controlled trial. J. Clin. Nurs. **29**, 4203–4216 (2020)
14. Van Rossum, M.C., et al.: Adaptive threshold-based alarm strategies for continuous vital signs monitoring. J. Clin. Monit. Comput. **36**, 407–417 (2022)
15. Gul, G., Intepeler, S.S., Bektas, M.: The effect of interventions made in intensive care units to reduce alarms: a systematic review and meta-analysis study. Intensive Crit. Care Nurs. **75**, 103375 (2023)
16. Chromik, J., et al.: Computational approaches to alleviate alarm fatigue in intensive care medicine: a systematic literature review. Front. Digit. Health **4** (2022)
17. Winters, B.D., et al.: Technological distractions (part 2): a summary of approaches to manage clinical alarms with intent to reduce alarm fatigue. Crit. Care Med. **46**, 130–137 (2018)
18. Olsen, R.M., Aasvang, E.K., Meyhoff, C.S., Sorensen, H.B.D.: Towards an automated multimodal clinical decision support system at the post anesthesia care unit. Comput. Biol. Med. **101**, 15–21 (2018)
19. Kyrollos, D.G., Greenwood, K., Harrold, J., Green, J.R.: Detection of false alarms in the NICU using pressure sensitive mat. In: 2021 IEEE Sensors Applications Symposium (SAS), (Sundsvall, Sweden), pp. 1–5. IEEE (2021)
20. Saeed, M., et al.: Multiparameter intelligent monitoring in intensive care II: a public-access intensive care unit database*. Crit. Care Med. **39**, 952–960 (2011)
21. Johnson, A.E.W., et al.: MIMIC-III, a freely accessible critical care database. Sci. Data **3**, 160035 (2016)
22. Johnson, A.E.W., et al.: MIMIC-IV, a freely accessible electronic health record dataset. Sci. Data **10**, 1 (2023)
23. Hyland, S.L., et al.: Early prediction of circulatory failure in the intensive care unit using machine learning. Nat. Med. **26**, 364–373 (2020)
24. Gee, A.H., Barbieri, R., Paydarfar, D., Indic, P.: Predicting bradycardia in preterm infants using point process analysis of heart rate. IEEE Trans. Biomed. Eng. **64**, 2300–2308 (2017)
25. Moody, G.B., Mark, R.G.: The impact of the MIT-BIH arrhythmia database. IEEE Eng. Med. Biol. Mag. Q. Mag. Eng. Med. Biol. Soc. **20**(3), 45–50 (2001)
26. Karlen, W., Turner, M., Cooke, E., Dumont, G., Ansermino, J.M.: CapnoBase: signal database and tools to collect, share and annotate respiratory signals. In: 2010 Annual Meeting of the Society for Technology in Anesthesia (2010)
27. Liu, D., Görges, M., Jenkins, S.A.: University of Queensland vital signs dataset: development of an accessible repository of anesthesia patient monitoring data for research. Anesth. Analg. **114**, 584–589 (2012)

28. Clifford, G.D., et al.: The PhysioNet/computing in cardiology challenge 2015: reducing false arrhythmia alarms in the ICU. In: 2015 Computing in Cardiology Conference (CinC), (Nice, France), pp. 273–276. IEEE (2015)
29. Goldberger, A.L., et al.: Physiobank, physiotoolkit, and physionet: components of a new research resource for complex physiologic signals. Circulation **101**(23), e215–e220 (2000)
30. Bollepalli, S.C., et al.: Real-time arrhythmia detection using hybrid convolutional neural networks. J. Am. Heart Assoc. **10**, e023222 (2021)
31. Shahriari, Y., Fidler, R., Pelter, M.M., Bai, Y., Villaroman, A., Hu, X.: Electrocardiogram signal quality assessment based on structural image similarity metric. IEEE Trans. Biomed. Eng. **65**, 745–753 (2018)
32. Sabeti, E., Reamaroon, N., Mathis, M., Gryak, J., Sjoding, M., Najarian, K.: Signal quality measure for pulsatile physiological signals using morphological features: applications in reliability measure for pulse oximetry. Inform. Med. Unlocked **16**, 100222 (2019)
33. Allam, J.P., Samantray, S., Sahoo, S.P., Ari, S.: A deformable CNN architecture for predicting clinical acceptability of ECG signal. Biocybern. Biomed. Eng. **43**, 335–351 (2023)
34. Wu, F., Zhao, G., Qian, X., Lehman, L.-W.H.: A diffusion model with contrastive learning for ICU false arrhythmia alarm reduction. In: Proceedings of the Thirty-Second International Joint Conference on Artificial Intelligence, (Macau, SAR China), pp. 4912–4920, International Joint Conferences on Artificial Intelligence Organization (2023)
35. Chandar, V.R.K., Thangamani, M.: Suppression of noises using fast independent component analysis (FICA) and signal saturation using fuzzy adaptive histogram equalization (FAHE) for intensive care unit false alarms. Measurement **145**, 400–409 (2019)
36. Lameski, P., Zdravevski, E., Koceski, S., Kulakov, A., Trajkovik, V.: Suppression of intensive care unit false alarms based on the arterial blood pressure signal. IEEE Access **5**, 5829–5836 (2017)
37. Wang, X., Gao, Y., Lin, J., Rangwala, H., Mittu, R.: A machine learning approach to false alarm detection for critical arrhythmia alarms. In: 2015 IEEE 14th International Conference on Machine Learning and Applications (ICMLA), (Miami, FL, USA), pp. 202–207. IEEE (2015)
38. Zhou, Y., et al.: A contrastive learning approach for ICU false arrhythmia alarm reduction. Sci. Rep. **12**, 4689 (2022)
39. Au-Yeung, W.-T.M., et al.: Real-time machine learning-based intensive care unit alarm classification without prior knowledge of the underlying rhythm. Eur. Heart J. Digit. Health **2**, 437–445 (2021)
40. Au-Yeung, W.-T.M., Sahani, A.K., Isselbacher, E.M., Armoundas, A.A.: Reduction of false alarms in the intensive care unit using an optimized machine learning based approach. NPJ Digit. Med. **2**, 86 (2019)
41. Chromik, J., et al.: Forecasting thresholds alarms in medical patient monitors using time series models. In: Proceedings of the 15th International Joint Conference on Biomedical Engineering Systems and Technologies, pp. 26–34. SCITEPRESS - Science and Technology Publications (2022)
42. Pardasani, R., Chaudhuri, R., Awasthi, N., Goel, M.: Machine learning and deep learning approaches to quantify respiratory distress severity and predict critical alarms. In: 2020 IEEE International Conference on Healthcare Informatics (ICHI), (Oldenburg, Germany), pp. 1–11. IEEE (2020)

43. Schmidt, D., Chromik, J., Arnrich, B.: Recommender system for alarm thresholds in medical patient monitors. In: Proceedings of the 16th International Joint Conference on Biomedical Engineering Systems and Technologies (BIOSTEC 2023) - HEALTHINF, pp. 74–85. INSTICC, SciTePress (2023)
44. Rahman, J., Brankovic, A., Khanna, S.: Machine learning model with output correction: towards reliable bradycardia detection in neonates. Comput. Biol. Med. **177**, 108658 (2024)
45. Fernandes, C.O., Miles, S., Lucena, C.J.P.D., Cowan, D.: Artificial intelligence technologies for coping with alarm fatigue in hospital environments because of sensory overload: algorithm development and validation. J. Med. Internet Res. **21**, e15406 (2019)
46. Xiao, R., Do, D., Ding, C., Meisel, K., Lee, R.J., Hu, X.: Generalizability of Super-Alarm via cross-institutional performance evaluation. IEEE Access **8**, 132404–132412 (2020)
47. Xiao, R., King, J., Villaroman, A., Do, D.H., Boyle, N.G., Hu, X.: Predict in-hospital code blue events using monitor alarms through deep learning approach. In: 2018 40th Annual International Conference of the IEEE Engineering in Medicine and Biology Society (EMBC), (Honolulu, HI), pp. 3717–3720. IEEE (2018)
48. Hu, S.B., Wong, D.J.L., Correa, A., Li, N., Deng, J.C.: Prediction of clinical deterioration in hospitalized adult patients with hematologic malignancies using a neural network model. PLoS ONE **11**, e0161401 (2016)
49. Chen, L., et al.: Using supervised machine learning to classify real alerts and artifact in online multisignal vital sign monitoring data*. Crit. Care Med. **44**, e456–e463 (2016)
50. Hravnak, M., Chen, L., Dubrawski, A., Bose, E., Clermont, G., Pinsky, M.R.: Real alerts and artifact classification in archived multi-signal vital sign monitoring data: implications for mining big data. J. Clin. Monit. Comput. **30**, 875–888 (2016)
51. Cabrera-Quirós, L., et al.: Listen to the real experts: detecting need of caregiver response in a NICU using multimodal monitoring signals. In: Companion Publication of the 2021 International Conference on Multimodal Interaction, (Montreal QC Canada), pp. 344–352. ACM (2021)
52. Joshi, R., Peng, Z., Long, X., Feijs, L., Andriessen, P., Van Pul, C.: Predictive monitoring of critical cardiorespiratory alarms in neonates under intensive care. IEEE J. Transl. Eng. Health Med. **7**, 1–10 (2019)
53. Ju, Y., Waugh, J.L., Singh, S., Rusin, C.G., Patel, A.B., Jain, P.N.: A multimodal deep learning tool for detection of junctional ectopic tachycardia in children with congenital heart disease. Heart Rhythm O2 **5**, 452–459 (2024)
54. Waugh, J.L., Patel, R., Ju, Y., Patel, A.B., Rusin, C.G., Jain, P.N.: A novel automated junctional ectopic tachycardia detection tool for children with congenital heart disease. Heart Rhythm O2 **3**, 302–310 (2022)
55. Poole, S., Shah, N.: Addressing vital sign alarm fatigue using personalized alarm thresholds. In: Biocomputing 2018, (Kohala Coast, Hawaii, USA), pp. 472–483. WORLD SCIENTIFIC (2018)
56. Hever, G., Cohen, L., O'Connor, M.F., Matot, I., Lerner, B., Bitan, Y.: Machine learning applied to multi-sensor information to reduce false alarm rate in the ICU. J. Clin. Monit. Comput. **34**, 339–352 (2020)

57. Dey, A., et al.: Weakly supervised classification of vital sign alerts as real or artifact. In: AMIA ... Annual Symposium proceedings. AMIA Symposium, vol. 2022, pp. 405–414 (2022)
58. Aboukhalil, A., Nielsen, L., Saeed, M., Mark, R.G., Clifford, G.D.: Reducing false alarm rates for critical arrhythmias using the arterial blood pressure waveform. J. Biomed. Inform. **41**(3), 442–451 (2008)

Structured LLM-Generated Clinical Discharge Summaries for Nordic Healthcare Digitalization and Wireless Health Integration

Aleka Melese Ayalew(✉), MdRabiul Hasan, Tapio Seppänen, and Mourad Oussalah

Center for Machine Vision and Signal Analysis, University of Oulu, 90014 Oulu, Finland
{Aleka.Ayalew,MdRabiul.Hasan,Tapio.Seppanen,Mourad.Oussalah}@oulu.fi

Abstract. Nordic healthcare systems that implement universal electronic health records need interoperable clinical documentation to ensure seamless care coordination among hospital networks, primary care, and home healthcare services. Current discharge summaries lack structural standardization, contributing to 20% of patients experiencing preventable adverse events within 30 days of hospital discharge. While AI-assisted documentation offers automation potential for resource-constrained healthcare systems, clinical deployment remains limited by hallucination rates of 18–64%. We present **a hybrid LLM framework** combining parameter-efficient fine-tuning with retrieval-augmented generation to produce structured 11-section discharge summaries compatible with national EHR systems. Evaluation across six transformer architectures on MIMIC-IV clinical notes demonstrates that hybrid RAG augmentation reduces hallucination rates compared to fine-tuning alone, with improvements up to 12.4% points (Gemma: 36.3% to 23.9%). The best configuration (Llama-3.1-8B Hybrid) achieves 18.5% hallucination rate with ROUGE-1 of 0.466. The framework addresses critical requirements for Nordic digital health infrastructure: (1) structured output compatible with national EHR platforms; (2) reduced documentation burden supporting physician workforce sustainability; (3) improved patient comprehension for aging populations; and (4) potential for wireless health integration. Results demonstrate technical maturity for pilot testing in Nordic healthcare testbed environments, supporting care pathway digitalization and population health management initiatives.

Keywords: Digital Health · Large Language Model · Wireless Health Monitoring · Clinical Note Summarization · RAG · Parameter-Efficient Fine-Tuning

1 Introduction

Nordic healthcare systems have largely adopted electronic health records, establishing a digital framework for integrated care delivery throughout hospital net-

M. Säreströniemi et al. (Eds.): NCDHWS 2026, CCIS 3010, pp. 598–607, 2026.
https://doi.org/10.1007/978-3-032-28819-6_38

works, primary care, and home healthcare services [1]. Despite this technological foundation, clinical documentation remains inconsistent, limiting the potential for seamless health information exchange. Discharge summaries, which bridge hospital care and post-discharge management, exemplify this challenge. Patients comprehend fewer than 30% of discharge instructions, while clinicians spend 5–10 min reviewing individual summaries due to variable formatting [2]. Approximately 20% of discharged patients experience preventable adverse events within 30 days, many attributable to incomplete medication reconciliation. These quality gaps are particularly concerning for Nordic countries with aging populations requiring complex care coordination across multiple providers and wireless health monitoring systems.

Conventional narrative discharge summaries are unable to ensure that important elements like medication modifications, diagnostic reasoning, and follow-up requirements are systematically included [3]. Research shows that 25% of discharge summaries do not include pending laboratory findings, 15% do not explain post-discharge care obligations, and 40% do not have complete medication lists [4]. These shortcomings jeopardize the interoperability objectives at the heart of digital health projects, prevent smooth data flow between healthcare systems, and require receiving physicians to get clarification from discharging teams.

Large language models (LLMs) demonstrate capabilities for clinical natural language processing through their ability to capture long-range dependencies in clinical text [5]. Parameter-efficient fine-tuning methods, particularly QLoRA [6], enable adaptation of foundation models to clinical tasks. These methods reduce computational requirements by over 99% compared to full fine-tuning, making deployment feasible in resource-constrained healthcare settings. However, LLM-based clinical summarization systems face important limitations that must be addressed before integration into digital health workflows:

- **Factual Hallucination:** Generative models produce medically inaccurate information not present in source notes, with reported hallucination rates of 18–64% [7]. Fabricated content includes non-existent medications and incorrect dosages, posing patient safety risks that reduce trust in LLM-assisted healthcare.
- **Format Inconsistency:** Most systems produce unstructured narrative outputs, limiting integration with electronic health records and health information exchanges [8]. The absence of guaranteed structural completeness means key components may be omitted without detection, compromising data quality for downstream digital health applications.
- **Retrieval-Content Leakage:** While retrieval-augmented generation (RAG) can ground outputs in factual evidence [9], applying RAG to clinical summarization risks content leakage, where the model may inadvertently incorporate information from retrieved patient cases rather than extracting exclusively from the target patient's note, raising both accuracy and privacy concerns.

To address these gaps, we propose a hybrid framework combining parameter-efficient fine-tuning with retrieval-augmented generation for structured clinical discharge summarization for digital health integration. Our contributions include: (1) a Hybrid PEFT with RAG framework that uses retrieved cases as structural templates while preventing content leakage through explicit prompt engineering; (2) systematic comparison of six transformer architectures evaluating the impact of RAG augmentation on structured summarization quality and hallucination reduction; and (3) evidence that medical-domain RAG reduces hallucination rates by up to 34% compared to fine-tuning alone, enhancing the reliability required for clinical deployment in Nordic healthcare systems.

2 Materials and Methods

Our method addresses clinical summarization through a two-phase architecture that combines parameter-efficient adaptation with retrieval-augmented generation. Phase 1 fine-tunes transformer models using QLoRA for memory-efficient training, while Phase 2 integrates medical-domain retrieval to reduce hallucination. Figure 1 illustrates this framework. This study evaluates Phases 2–3; Phases 1 and 4 represent future integration directions.

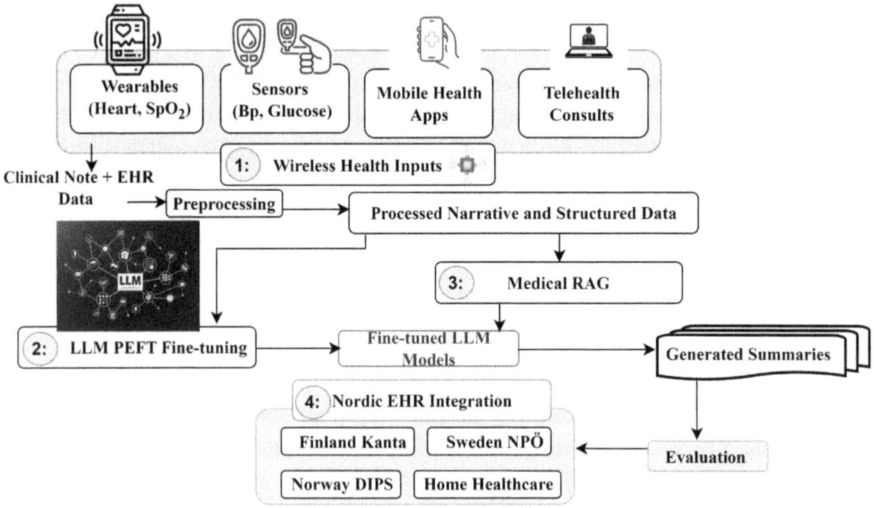

Fig. 1. Four-phase framework for structured clinical discharge summarization with Nordic healthcare integration. Phase 1: Wireless health inputs from wearables, sensors, mobile health apps, and telehealth. Phase 2: QLoRA fine-tuning of six transformer architectures. Phase 3: Medical-domain RAG with S-PubMedBERT and MedCPT reranking. Phase 4: Nordic EHR integration and home healthcare support.

2.1 Dataset and Preprocessing

We use the MIMIC-IV database [10], comprising clinical discharge records from Beth Israel Deaconess Medical Center. MIMIC-IV was selected as the largest publicly available English-language clinical discharge dataset with structured notes. Our preprocessing pipeline includes four stages: (1) medical-aware chunking that segments long clinical notes while preserving section boundaries; (2) tokenization and normalization; (3) clinical abbreviation expansion using regex patterns; and (4) structured format extraction into 11-section clinical sections: Case Type, Patient & Service, Chief Complaint, History of Present Illness, Past Medical/Surgical History, Medications, Physical Examination, Investigations/Labs/Imaging, Assessment/Impression, Discharge Condition, and Follow-Up & Recommendations. The 11-section structure was derived from MIMIC-IV clinical documentation patterns using rule-based extraction that reorganizes existing clinician-authored text without creating new medical facts, preserving factual content while presenting it in a uniform template. The dataset is split into 70% training, 15% validation, and 15% testing.

2.2 Phase 1: Parameter-Efficient Fine-Tuning

We implement QLoRA [6] with Unsloth optimization to fine-tune six transformer architectures: Mistral-7B-Instruct, Llama-3.1-8B-Instruct, Gemma-2-9B-IT, BioMistral-7B (domain-adapted), Phi-3-Medium-14B, and Qwen2.5-7B-Instruct. All models use 4-bit quantization with LoRA adapters (rank $r = 64$, $\alpha = 64$) targeting attention and feed-forward layers. Training uses identical hyperparameters across models: batch size 4 with gradient accumulation over 2 steps (effective batch size 8), learning rate 1×10^{-4} with linear warmup and decay, 3 epochs, and gradient checkpointing. Each model is trained to generate structured 11-section discharge summaries compatible with Nordic EHR systems. Training was conducted on NVIDIA A100 GPUs (40GB) with 4-bit quantization.

2.3 Phase 2: Hybrid PEFT with RAG

Phase 2 augments fine-tuned models with medical-domain RAG to reduce hallucination and maintain structural consistency. Our hybrid approach combines internalized knowledge from Phase 1 with external evidence from similar clinical cases.

RAG Corpus Construction. The retrieval corpus comprises training and validation sets (85% of data), with test set excluded to prevent data leakage:

$$\mathcal{C} = \mathcal{D}_{\text{train}} \cup \mathcal{D}_{\text{val}}, \quad \mathcal{C} \cap \mathcal{D}_{\text{test}} = \emptyset \tag{1}$$

where $\mathcal{C}$ is the retrieval corpus, $\mathcal{D}_{\text{train}}$, $\mathcal{D}_{\text{val}}$, and $\mathcal{D}_{\text{test}}$ are training, validation, and test sets respectively.

Dense Retrieval. We use S-PubMedBERT-MS-MARCO [11] for medical-domain embeddings. Given a query clinical note q with embedding $\mathbf{e}_q$, FAISS enables efficient similarity search selecting the top-k most semantically similar cases:

$$\text{Top-}k(q) = \underset{S \subseteq \mathcal{C}, |S|=k}{\arg\max} \sum_{d_i \in S} \text{sim}_{\cos}(\mathbf{e}_q, \mathbf{e}_i) \tag{2}$$

where $\mathbf{e}_q$ and $\mathbf{e}_i$ are embeddings of query and candidate documents, $\text{sim}_{\cos}$ is cosine similarity, and $k = 20$ for initial dense retrieval.

Structured Context Engineering. Retrieved cases serve as format/structure templates reinforcing the 11-section organization, while explicit prompt instructions constrain factual extraction to the target patient's note only. Retrieved cases are integrated into the generation prompt as format examples prepended to the input clinical note, with explicit instructions constraining factual extraction to the target note only while using retrieved cases as structural templates. The prompt instructs: *Extract ALL facts strictly from the Current Patient Note. Use retrieved cases ONLY as format/structure templates for structuring your output into 11 sections. Never copy patient-specific information from retrieved cases.* This design prevents content leakage while enabling format-consistent generation, which represents our key architectural insight that decouples structural guidance from content extraction.

2.4 Evaluation Metrics

We employ an evaluation framework spanning three dimensions. **Lexical Overlap Metrics:** ROUGE-1, ROUGE-2, and ROUGE-L measure unigram, bigram, and longest common subsequence overlap respectively; METEOR accounts for synonyms and stemming; BLEU evaluates n-gram precision with brevity penalty. **Semantic Similarity:** BERTScore computes precision, recall, and F1 using ClinicalBERT embeddings, capturing semantic equivalence beyond surface-level matching. **Hallucination Detection:** We measure factual accuracy through Coverage (proportion of generated content supported by source notes) and Hallucination Rate (proportion of unsupported content). Hallucination Rate is computed as the proportion of generated sentences where fewer than 30% of key terms (words longer than four characters) appear in the source clinical note. Lower hallucination rates indicate higher factual fidelity, for clinical safety.

3 Results and Discussion

We evaluated six transformer architectures using structured 11-section output format, comparing fine-tuning alone versus hybrid PEFT with RAG augmentation. Table 1 presents the comparison across all metrics. All method comparisons (Fine-tuned vs. Hybrid) are statistically significant (paired t-test, $p<0.001$). Paired t-tests are appropriate as samples are paired (same test set for both conditions), metrics exhibit approximately normal distributions across test cases, and sample size satisfies parametric test assumptions.

3.1 Key Findings

Impact of RAG Augmentation. As illustrated in Fig. 2, Hybrid PEFT with RAG improves performance over fine-tuning alone across all six models. The largest ROUGE-2 improvements are observed in Phi (+23.0%, from 0.235 to

Table 1. Structured Summarization Performance: Fine-tuned vs. Hybrid PEFT with RAG. FT = Fine-Tuned (baseline without RAG), Hybrid = Hybrid PEFT with RAG. All results use the structured 11-section format. R = ROUGE, MET = METEOR. P., Rec., F1 = BERTScore Precision, Recall, F1. Cov. = hallucination coverage, Rate = hallucination rate (lower is better).

Model	Method	R-1	R-2	R-L	MET	BLEU	P.	R.	F1	Cov.	Rate
Mistral	FT	.366	.221	.240	.241	.117	.852	.843	.848	.713	.287
	Hybrid	.376	.245	.263	.260	.133	.856	.844	.850	.727	**.272**
BioMistral	FT	.361	.224	.247	.237	.113	.851	.845	.848	.706	.294
	Hybrid	.384	.247	.267	.266	.134	.854	.845	.849	.712	**.288**
Phi	FT	.371	.235	.257	.247	.138	.854	.852	.853	.707	.293
	Hybrid	.408	.289	.294	.324	.173	.871	.857	.863	.776	**.224**
Qwen	FT	.409	.261	.274	.274	.146	.858	.849	.853	.716	.284
	Hybrid	.439	.334	.311	.311	.180	.867	.856	.861	.722	**.278**
Gemma	FT	.423	.308	.311	.292	.165	.871	.860	.866	.637	.363
	Hybrid	.428	.324	.328	.307	.175	.875	.868	.870	.761	**.239**
Llama	FT	.459	.324	.306	.323	.197	.873	.858	.865	.809	.191
	Hybrid	**.466**	**.334**	**.316**	**.330**	**.205**	**.873**	**.858**	**.865**	**.815**	**.185**

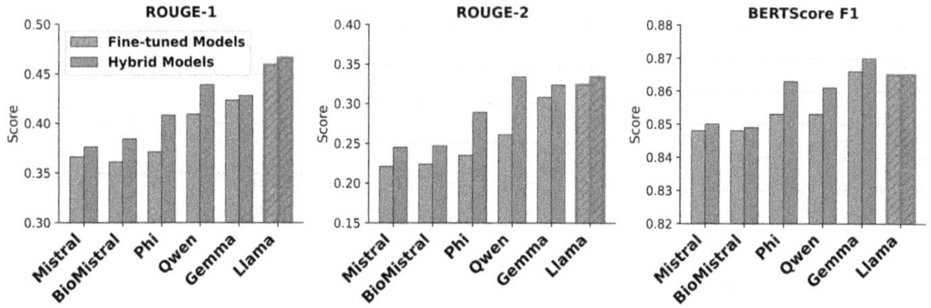

Fig. 2. Performance comparison across ROUGE-1, ROUGE-2, and BERTScore F1 metrics for Fine-tuned versus Hybrid PEFT with RAG using structured format. Hybrid augmentation (blue) improves over Fine-tuned baseline (orange) across all models. Llama-3.1-8B achieves the highest scores. (Color figure online)

0.289) and Qwen (+28.0%, from 0.261 to 0.334). On average, Hybrid augmentation achieves +4.9% higher ROUGE-1, +13.4% higher ROUGE-2, and +12.0% higher METEOR compared to fine-tuning alone.

Hallucination Reduction. Figure 3 shows that RAG augmentation reduces hallucination rates across all models. The largest improvement is observed in Gemma (-12.4% points, from 36.3% to 23.9%). Average hallucination rate decreases from 28.5% (Fine-tuned) to 24.8% (Hybrid), representing a 3.7% point improvement.

Best Performing Configuration. Llama-3.1-8B with hybrid RAG achieves the best overall performance (ROUGE-1: 0.466, ROUGE-2: 0.334) and the lowest hallucination rate (18.5%). This represents an effective balance between summarization quality and factual accuracy suitable for Nordic EHR deployment.

3.2 Discussion

Our results demonstrate that hybrid RAG augmentation enhances the reliability of structured discharge summaries for digital health integration. The consistent hallucination reduction across all six models (average 3.7% points, up to 12.4 pp for Gemma) confirms that retrieval-based grounding improves factual accuracy without sacrificing summarization quality. The best configuration (Llama Hybrid, 18.5% hallucination) approaches safety thresholds suitable for clinical decision support systems. Achieving 100% section completeness could enable automated extraction pipelines that map discharge summary sections to standardized EHR fields (medications, diagnoses, follow-up plans), supporting health information exchange protocols like HL7 FHIR and interoperability frameworks.

From a Nordic digital health deployment perspective, the structured format could address regional healthcare system requirements. Nordic countries with universal healthcare systems require scalable solutions that integrate across hospital districts, municipal primary care, and home healthcare services. The 11-section format aligns with Nordic clinical documentation standards, potentially enabling wireless health monitoring systems to automatically extract medication regimens and follow-up schedules for remote patient management. This standardization could benefit aging Nordic populations where post-discharge care increasingly relies on telehealth consultations and sensor-based monitoring. Structured outputs could reduce cognitive burden on receiving physicians who currently spend 5–10 min reviewing variable-format summaries, potentially addressing workforce sustainability concerns in countries facing physician shortages. Moreover, integration with national EHR platforms (Finland's Kanta, Sweden's NPÖ, Norway's DIPS) requires predictable section structures that could enable automated data mapping, supporting cross-border Nordic health information exchange initiatives.

Comparison with Prior Work. Our best configuration (Llama-3.1-8B, 18.5% hallucination) outperforms zero-shot GPT-4 approaches that report 42% hallucination rates [12]. Unlike existing methods that use retrieved content directly for answer generation, our framework introduces a distinct separation. Retrieved cases provide *structural templates* for the 11-section format while factual content is extracted exclusively from the source patient note. This decoupling prevents content leakage, an important concern in clinical settings where incorporating information from other patients' records poses safety and privacy risks. The structured format achieves comparable performance to full fine-tuning methods through QLoRA optimization.

Limitations. This study demonstrates technical feasibility using the MIMIC-IV clinical dataset. Direct transferability to Nordic healthcare systems requires val-

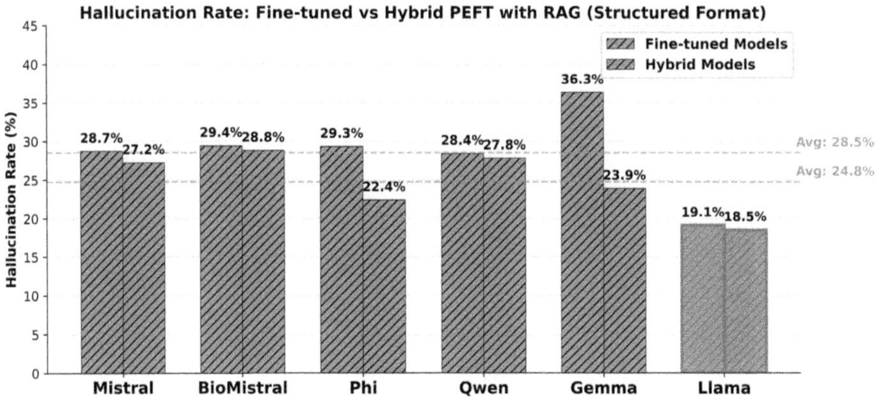

Fig. 3. Hallucination rate comparison between Fine-tuned and Hybrid PEFT with RAG using structured format. Hybrid augmentation (green) achieves lower hallucination rates than Fine-tuned baseline (orange) across all models. Llama-3.1-8B achieves the lowest rate at 18.5%. (Color figure online)

idation with European clinical data and workflows. The 11-section structure has not been validated with Nordic physicians or patients. Claims regarding physician burden reduction, patient comprehension, and wireless health integration represent anticipated benefits rather than empirically validated outcomes. The 18.5% hallucination rate reflects automated detection rather than clinical expert evaluation; acceptable thresholds for clinical use remain an open question requiring healthcare practitioner involvement. Future work must include prospective validation in Nordic healthcare settings, clinical evaluation, and integration testing with national EHR systems.

4 Conclusions

We demonstrated that hybrid RAG-augmented structured discharge summaries show technical feasibility and improved quality metrics, representing progress toward future integration into Nordic digital health infrastructure. Evaluation across six transformer architectures reveals that RAG augmentation consistently reduces hallucination rates (average 3.7 pp, up to 12.4 pp), with the best configuration (Llama-3.1-8B Hybrid) achieving 18.5% hallucination and 100% organizational completeness.

The framework demonstrates potential to address critical requirements for Nordic healthcare digitalization: (1) **National EHR Interoperability**: Structured output could enable direct mapping to platforms such as Finland's Kanta services and Sweden's NPÖ, supporting cross-organizational health information exchange; (2) **Workforce Sustainability**: Automated generation could reduce documentation time from 5–10 min to seconds, addressing physician shortages while maintaining quality; (3) **Aging Population Support**: Standardized formatting could improve patient comprehension beyond current 30% rates, critical for elderly populations managing multiple chronic conditions; (4) **Wireless Health Integration**: Structured sections (medications, follow-up plans) could provide foundation for interfacing with remote monitoring systems and mobile health applications deployed in home care; and (5) **Testbed Readiness**: Hybrid RAG achieves hallucination rates below 25% (best: 18.5%), approaching rates that may enable pilot testing in digital health testbed environments like Oulu.

The results demonstrate technical maturity for prospective evaluation in Nordic healthcare settings. Recommended next steps include: pilot testing with national EHR systems to validate section mapping; integration with wireless monitoring platforms for post-discharge care management; multi-lingual evaluation for Swedish, Norwegian, Danish, and Finnish clinical documentation; and longitudinal studies measuring impact on care coordination quality and patient outcomes across Nordic care pathways.

Acknowledgments. This work was partly supported by the Finnish Research Council Profi 7 Hybrid Intelligence and the University of Oulu Doctoral School fund.

Disclosure of Interests. The authors have no competing interests to declare.

References

1. Journal of Medical Internet Research - A Nordic Perspective on Patient Online Record Access and the European Health Data Space
2. Lee, C., Vogt, K.A., Kumar, S.: Prospects for AI clinical summarization to reduce the burden of patient chart review. Front. Digit. Health **6**, 1475092 (2024)
3. Chatterton, B., Chen, J., Schwarz, E.B., Karlin, J.: Primary care physicians' perspectives on high-quality discharge summaries. J. Gen. Int. Med. **39**(8), 1438–1443 (2024)
4. Ng, I.K., et al.: How to write a good discharge summary: a primer for junior physicians. Postgrad. Med. J. **101**(1198), 764–772 (2025)
5. Lin, C., Kuo, C.-F.: Roles and potential of Large language models in healthcare: a comprehensive review. Biomed. J. **48**(5), 100868 (2025)
6. Dettmers, T., Pagnoni, A., Holtzman, A., Zettlemoyer, L.: QLORA: efficient fine-tuning of quantized LLMs. In: Proceedings of the 37th International Conference on Neural Information Processing Systems, NIPS '23, pp. 10088–10115, Red Hook, NY, USA, 2023. Curran Associates Inc
7. Ji, Z., et al.: Survey of hallucination in natural language generation. ACM Comput. Surv. **55**(12), 248:1–248:38 (2023)
8. Jia, J., Nishi, H.: A flexible two-stage anonymization framework for narrative medical records adapting to various language models. Comput. Biol. Med. **195**, 110624 (2025)
9. Ahn, Y., Lee, S.-G., Shim, J., Park, J.: Retrieval-augmented response generation for knowledge-grounded conversation in the wild. IEEE Access **10**, 131374–131385 (2022)
10. Johnson, A.E.W., et al.: MIMIC-IV, a freely accessible electronic health record dataset. Scientific Data **10**(1), 1 (2023)

11. Gu, Y., et al.: Domain-specific language model pretraining for biomedical natural language processing. ACM Trans. Comput. Healthc. **3**(1), 2:1–2:23 (2021)
12. Christopher, Y.K., et al.: Evaluating large language models for drafting emergency department discharge summaries (2024)

Structured Multi-extraction Prompting Improves LLM-Based Biomedical Relation Extraction Without Fine-Tuning

Frederik Labonté(✉), Suraj Giri, Claudius Herbrik, and Lucie Flek

Universität Bonn/B-IT Bonn-Aachen Institute of Informatics, Bonn, Germany
flabonte@uni-bonn.de, flek@bit.uni-bonn.de

Abstract. Annotated text data is essential for structuring biomedical knowledge. State-of-the-art machine learning models achieve F1 scores >90% for named entity recognition (NER), but relation extraction (RE) remains challenging, with F1 scores of $\tilde{6}0\%$ (up to 75–80% on binary datasets using additional strategies). These models require fine-tuning on costly manually annotated datasets.

This paper investigates structured multi-extraction prompting as a technique for enabling Large Language Models (LLMs) such as Mistral and OpenAI models to perform biomedical relation extraction (RE) without fine-tuning, reducing manual annotation burdens. We evaluate this approach across zero-shot and few-shot settings and compare extracting relations individually versus in batches, assessing whether multi-extraction with structured generation can serve as a viable, cost-effective alternative to fine-tuned models.

Our results show that multi-extraction prompting with structured generation significantly boosts LLM performance on biomedical relation extraction (RE) tasks, roughly matching fine-tuned models on binary classification in zero-shot settings and approaching their performance on multi-class tasks with few-shot examples but the gap remains larger in those cases. By providing the model with a list of entities and leveraging structured, dynamic generation, we harness LLMs' in-context learning to enhance both efficiency and accuracy. This method improves performance by up to 19% while reducing token usage by up to 550%, lowering computational costs comparing it to a single extraction baseline.

In summary, structured multi-extraction prompting enables modern LLMs to perform binary RE tasks without fine-tuning, matching or approaching the performance of small specialised models, while substantially reducing token usage and computational cost—making them viable annotators for low-resource scenarios where little to no training data exists.

Keywords: Large Language Models · Relation Extraction · Biomedical Texts · Text Mining

M. Säreströniemi et al. (Eds.): NCDHWS 2026, CCIS 3010, pp. 608–643, 2026.
https://doi.org/10.1007/978-3-032-28819-6_39

1 Introduction

1.1 Background and Motivation

Biomedical articles contain large amounts of knowledge. Extracting that knowledge is valuable to enable scientists to easily find structured overviews of existing knowledge, driving further research. Relation extraction from free-form text is normally a task that requires human experts, which makes it slow and expensive. Therefore, interest exists to use machines to automate this task. However, small specialised models depend on existing annotated texts for a given task to work. Large Language Models are known for being efficient at working with just descriptions of tasks (zero-shot) [1] or a handful of examples (few-shot) [2]. Additionally, the capabilities of Large Language Models (LLMs), such as OpenAI's ChatGPT, are steadily reported to increase [3], with model providers claiming graduate level understanding of natural sciences. Some papers have looked at the question of how well LLMs do as biomedical annotators [4,5], but none, to our knowledge, have tested differently structured prompts and multiple models across two different tasks to evaluate the efficacy of the idea more systematically, especially in conjunction with structured generations.

To this end, we test annotation performance of different models of the GPT family, Mistral as the cheaper European competitor and a handful of smaller, self-hostable open source LLMs. The comprehensive list can be found in Sect. 2.2. We test them on two biomedical datasets, BioRED [6] and CDR [7], for the task of relation extraction (RE). BioRED is a multi-class labeling dataset focusing on gene-gene and gene-disease interactions, while CDR focuses on chemically-induced diseases (CID). We propose multi-extraction prompting with structured generation as the core technique under investigation: rather than querying the model for each entity pair individually, we present the model with a full list of entities and extract all relations in a single structured prompt. We evaluate this approach against a single-extraction baseline and across zero-shot and few-shot settings, using the labels "single" (one question per prompt) and "multi" (multiple questions per prompt) to distinguish the two extraction modes throughout.

1.2 Research Questions

1. Does multi-extraction prompting with structured generation boost performance over single-extraction prompting, and does it reduce computational cost?
2. To what extent can modern LLMs approach the performance of small, fine-tuned models on biomedical relation extraction (RE) tasks without fine-tuning?
3. How do the capabilities scale across binary and multi-class classification tasks?

1.3 Related Work

Specialised Extraction Models. Biomedical relation extraction has evolved from rule-based systems and feature-engineered methods [7,8] to neural approaches using Long Short Term Memory networks (LSTMs) and attention mechanisms [9]. The introduction of domain-specific pre-trained models marked a significant advance: BioBERT [10], PubMedBERT [11] and later BioGPT [6]—all based on the Bidirectional Encoder Representations from Transformers (BERT) architecture—demonstrated that biomedical pre-training substantially improves named entity recognition (NER) and RE performance, which can be boosted further with fine-tuning. For NER tasks, models like BioBERT achieve a performance of around 94% F1 in the detection of diseases and chemicals. Yet, they only reach about 60% F1 in the related RE task [12], showing that RE is in fact a harder task to overcome.

LLMs as Extraction Models. There has been general interest in using LLMs as relation extraction tools. Earlier work showed that LLMs can perform near state-of-the-art (SOTA) fine-tuned extraction models on general extraction tasks, such as extracting relations from New York Times articles, particularly when exact matching criteria are relaxed [13]. Building on this, a 2024 study published in *Nature* explored the use of LLMs specifically for relation extraction in materials science, leveraging structured generation output [14].

LLMs as Biomedical Extraction Models. Recent work has explored general-purpose LLMs for biomedical tasks as well. Chen et al. [4] benchmarked LLMs across biomedical Natural Language Processing (NLP) tasks, finding variable performance across domains. Agrawal et al. [15] showed that GPT-3 performs well at zero-/few-shot clinical information extraction, while Hu et al. [5] demonstrated that prompt engineering substantially enhances LLM extraction quality. Gilardi et al. [16] found that ChatGPT outperforms crowd-workers for annotation tasks, though LLM outputs exhibit inherent non-determinism [17] and hallucination risks.

Datasets and Current State-of-the-Art Performance. On our target datasets, the BioRED dataset, the best extraction models achieved F1 scores of 77.17% for relation pair identification and 58.95% for relation type classification during the recent BioCreative VIII Challenge [18]. Lai et al. [19] showed that fine-tuned LLMs clearly outperform their none fine-tuned counterparts on BioRED, raising the performance of Llama 3.2 11B from 29% to 75% for relation pair identification and 10% to 56% for multi-class relation labeling. This result demonstrates that fine-tuning LLMs can be just as effective as fine-tuning smaller specialised models. For CDR, the Multi-view Merge Representation (MMR) model [20] achieved a SOTA 78.95% F1 score. Despite these advances, systematic evaluation of LLM families across model sizes and prompting strategies for biomedical RE remains limited; a gap our work addresses by evaluating zero-

and few-shot prompting across multiple models and datasets, and by introducing multi-extraction prompting with structured generation as a technique to jointly improve performance and reduce computational cost.

2 Materials and Methods

Here we introduce the data, prompting structure, and model parameters used in our experiments. We focus on three groups of models: OpenAI models, selected for their leading performance, Mistral models, included as a cost-effective alternative, and a set of smaller 3-8B parameter models from the Llama, Ministral, and Qwen families. Together, these allow us to study performance across different model sizes, architectures, and computational budgets.

2.1 Datasets

We evaluate our approach on two biomedical relation extraction datasets, namely BioRED [6] and CDR [7]. These datasets present different challenges: BioRED features multi-class relations across diverse entity types, while CDR focuses on binary chemical-disease causality. Table 1 summarizes their key characteristics.

Table 1. Whole Dataset Comparison and Key Statistics.

Dataset	Documents	Relations	Entity Types	Relation Types	Task
BioRED	500	5341	6	9	Multi-class
CDR	1500	3111	2	2	Binary

BioRED. BioRED [6] is a comprehensive biomedical relation extraction dataset containing PubMed abstracts annotated for six entity types and eight original relation types, we add the negative, "No_Relation" label making it nine relation types. the methodology is discussed in the paragraph titled Negative Example Generation. The corpus consists of 400 training and 100 test documents with 4,178 and 1,163 annotated relations respectively. Table 2 presents detailed corpus statistics.

Entity and Relation Types. The six entity types represent key biomedical concepts: GeneOrGeneProduct, DiseaseOrPhenotypicFeature, ChemicalEntity, SequenceVariant, OrganismTaxon, and CellLine. Eight relation types capture diverse biomedical interactions, exhibiting significant class imbalance as shown in Table 3.

Three relation types (Association, Positive Correlation, Negative Correlation) account for 96.9% of training relations and 97.3% of test relations, while five minority classes (Bind, Co-Treatment, Comparison, Drug Interaction, Conversion) represent only 3.1% and 2.7% respectively. This severe class imbalance

Table 2. BioRED Corpus Statistics for Training and Test Sets.

Metric	Train	Test
Documents	400	100
Total Entities	13,351	3,535
Total Relations	4,178	1,163
Entities per Document (mean)	33.4	35.4
Relations per Document (mean)	10.4	11.6

Table 3. BioRED Relation Type Distribution Showing Strong Class Imbalance.

Relation Type	Train	Test
Association	2,192 (52.5%)	635 (54.6%)
Positive Correlation	1,089 (26.1%)	325 (28.0%)
Negative Correlation	763 (18.3%)	171 (14.7%)
Bind	61 (1.5%)	9 (0.8%)
Co-Treatment	31 (0.7%)	14 (1.2%)
Comparison	28 (0.7%)	6 (0.5%)
Drug Interaction	11 (0.3%)	2 (0.2%)
Conversion	3 (0.1%)	1 (0.1%)
Total	**4,178**	**1,163**

poses a significant challenge for multi-class relation classification, particularly for minority classes with fewer than 50 training examples.

Negative Example Generation. Since BioRED only annotates positive relations, we generated negative examples to create a balanced dataset. First, we analyzed the proximity patterns of positive relations and found that 98.6% occur within a 3-sentence window. Based on this, we generated negative candidates by pairing all co-occurring entities within the same passage that are at most three sentences apart and do not have an annotated relation. We then filtered these candidates to retain only entity pair types that appear in positive examples (e.g., GeneOrGeneProduct - GeneOrGeneProduct, ChemicalEntity - DiseaseOrPhenotypicFeature), ensuring biological plausibility. This process yielded a final training set of 8,356 examples (4,178 positive + 4,178 negative) with a balanced 1:1 ratio.

CDR. The CDR (Chemical-Disease Relations) corpus [7] from BioCreative V focuses on binary classification of Chemical-Induced Disease (CID) relations in PubMed abstracts. Unlike BioRED's multi-class, multi-entity scenario, CDR addresses a focused task: identifying whether a chemical substance causally induces a disease or phenotypic feature, creating a positive and a negative label.

Corpus Characteristics. CDR provides explicit negative annotations, eliminating the need for negative example generation. The corpus contains 1,500 documents split equally into training, development and test sets (500 each) with 16,498 total entity pairs. Table 4 presents detailed statistics.

Table 4. CDR Corpus Statistics across Train, Development, and Test Sets.

Metric	Train	Dev	Test
Documents	500	500	500
Total Entity Pairs	5,585	5,395	5,518
Positive (CID)	1,037 (18.6%)	1,010 (18.7%)	1,064 (19.3%)
Negative (No Relation)	4,548 (81.4%)	4,385 (81.3%)	4,454 (80.7%)
Unique Chemicals	665	661	677
Unique Diseases	715	652	683
Avg. Words per Document	207.8	207.8	207.8

Entity Types and Task Definition. CDR annotates only two entity types, both standardized with Medical Subject Headings (MeSH) identifiers:

- **Chemical:** Chemical compounds and substances (e.g., D008750 for alpha-methyldopa)
- **Disease:** Disease names and phenotypic features (e.g., D007022 for hypotensive conditions)

The task is binary classification: given a Chemical-Disease entity pair, determine whether the chemical induces the disease (CID) or not (No_Relation). Example positive relation: Desferrioxamine (D003676) induces pigmentary retinal deposits (D012164). Example negative: Naloxone (D009270) does not induce hypertensive conditions (D006973).

Class Distribution and Imbalance. The dataset exhibits a consistent 4.7:1 negative-to-positive ratio (19% positive class) across all splits, representing realistic class imbalance encountered in pharmacovigilance applications where most chemical-disease co-mentions do not represent causal relationships. This consistent imbalance across training, development and test sets enables reproducible evaluation of model robustness to class imbalance.

Complementary Benchmark Value. CDR serves as a complementary benchmark to BioRED in several ways:

(1) **Task complexity:** Binary vs. multi-class classification tests a model's performance across different granularities.
(2) **Entity diversity:** 2 vs. 6 entity types evaluate generalization to varying entity type combinations.
(3) **Negative examples:** Explicit vs. generated negatives validates negative generation quality.

2.2 Models

In this study, we evaluated a selection of advanced language models from OpenAI and Mistral. The models were chosen to provide a spectrum of capabilities, from high-performance cutting-edge systems to efficient, cost-effective alternatives suitable for large-scale experimentation. Specifically, we considered the following:

- **GPT-4.1-2025-04-14** [21]: A full-scale GPT-4.1 model released in April 2025, designed for advanced natural language understanding, reasoning, and generation. It is widely used in tasks requiring nuanced comprehension and coherent long-form outputs.
- **GPT-4.1-mini-2025-04-14** [22]: A smaller, lower-latency variant of GPT-4.1 released simultaneously. While slightly less capable than the full GPT-4.1, it maintains strong performance on conversational and text completion tasks, making it suitable for faster experimentation.
- **GPT-5-mini-2025-08-07-medium** [23]: A medium-sized version of the latest GPT-5-mini series, released in August 2025. It incorporates efficiency improvements and updated training data, offering a balance between performance and computational cost for a wide range of NLP tasks.
- **GPT-5-mini-2025-08-07-low** [24]: A smaller, low-resource variant of GPT-5-mini designed to minimize computing and memory usage while still providing reasonable text generation and reasoning abilities, ideal for cost-sensitive applications.
- **Mistral-large-2512** [25]: A large, open-weight Mistral model released in December 2025. It provides competitive language modeling capabilities at a significantly lower cost than proprietary models, making it suitable for research requiring scalable inference.
- **Mistral-medium-2508** [26]: A medium-sized Mistral variant from August 2025, offering a compromise between computational efficiency and predictive performance. It is effective for experimentation on moderately sized datasets or tasks.
- **Mistral-small-2506** [27]: A small, highly efficient Mistral model released in June 2025, optimized for rapid prototyping, lightweight deployment, and situations with limited computational resources.
- **Llama 3 Family** [28]: A state-of-the-art family of open-weight language models developed by Meta, covering multiple parameter scales and instruction tuned variants. In this study, we evaluated Llama-3.1-8B, Llama-3.1-8B-Instruct, Llama-3.2-3B-Instruct, and the domain-specialized language model Llama3-OpenBioLLM-8B, which is adapted for biomedical and life sciences tasks.
- **Mistral and Ministral Families** [29]: A collection of open-weight models from Mistral AI designed to balance performance and efficiency across a range of deployment scenarios. The evaluated models include BioMistral-7B, Ministral-3-3B-Instruct-2512, and Ministral-3-8B-Instruct-2512, spanning domain-specialized and instruction-tuned configurations.

- **Qwen 3 Family** [30]: A family of open-weight large language models developed by Alibaba, emphasizing multilingual capabilities and computational efficiency. We considered Qwen3-4B-Instruct-2507, Qwen3-8B, and the quantized Qwen3-8B-FP8 variant, which is optimized for reduced memory footprint and faster inference.

2.3 Model Parameters

All models were run at temperature 0 if possible. Temperature controls the randomness with which the next token is predicted - a higher temperature increases the number of words the next token can be selected from. By setting the temperature to 0, we achieve the least fluctuation in performance. On self-hosted models, 0-temperature sets the model to deterministic behaviour, whereas in API use (where models are accessed remotely via a standardised interface, provided by the AI companies) the effects of batching leads to only reducing non-determinism. The newer GPT-5 models exclusively support temperature 1 and are subsequently run at that temperature. The max_tokens parameter was set to 10,000 for non-reasoning and 20,000 for reasoning models, controlling how many tokens the model is allowed to produce in response to a given prompt. Some models use reasoning tokens, which effectively makes the model "think out loud" before producing its final output. The reasoning effort controls roughly how much compute is used on this thinking step, and is indicated behind the model names - if nothing is indicated, the model was run in non-reasoning mode.

2.4 Prompt Design

To standardize the prompting we used prompt templates that contain a task description, the possible labels with a short description and a set of critical instructions. Additionally, we included the possibility to contain an example and, finally, the case the model is supposed to answer. Examples of this can be seen in Fig. 1 and 2. PromptID was used for debugging purposes and set to none for the experiments. To generate prompts without examples, none was simply passed to the template, leaving the examples empty. When examples were included, they were formatted first and then entered at the position of the example place holder in the template. Examples consist of one abstract with all of its annotation for each possible label, so that each label was represented at least once in the examples.

Since we wanted to test if passing multiple questions at once works just as well as passing one question at a time, there are two prompt templates. The reason for this is that if multiple questions perform the same or better, a lot of compute and money can be saved. The difference between the two templates is that, in one case, a single relationship is passed to the model to evaluate, while in the other case a list of relations is passed. In both cases the model is tasked with deciding on the label for the relations based on the given abstract.

```
You are a biomedical relation extraction expert.
Prompt_ID:{prompt_id}
Task: Identify if the realtion between two specified entities is chemically inducing a disease or
symptoms of a disease.

Valid relation types (respond with EXACTLY ONE of these words):
- CID: stands for Chemically induced Disease, give this label if the two enteties are a chemical
and a disease where the chemical induces the disease or its symptoms.
- No_Relation: The two enteties are according to the text not involved in chemically inducing a
Disease.

CRITICAL INSTRUCTIONS:
1. Only annotate EXPLICIT relations stated in the text
2. If entities co-occur WITHOUT a clear relationship → respond with "No_Relation"
3. Do NOT infer or assume relationships not explicitly stated
4. When uncertain → respond with "No_Relation"
{examples}
---

Analyze this case:
Text: {text}
Entity1: {e1} ({entity_type1}), Entity2: {e2} ({entity_type2})

Respond in the following format:
Reasoning: [Explanaiton why]
Relation: [one word from the list above]
```

Fig. 1. Here we show the prompt structure for the CDR dataset and the single-question case.

```
You are a biomedical relation extraction expert.
Prompt_ID:{prompt_id}
Task: Identify if the realtion between two specified entities is chemically inducing a disease or
symptoms of a disease.

Valid relation types (respond with EXACTLY ONE of these words):
- CID: stands for Chemically induced Disease, give this label if the two enteties are a chemical
and a disease where the chemical induces the disease or its symptoms.
- No_Relation: The two enteties are according to the text not involved in chemically inducing a
Disease.

CRITICAL INSTRUCTIONS:
1. Only annotate EXPLICIT relations stated in the text
2. If entities co-occur WITHOUT a clear relationship → respond with "No_Relation"
3. Do NOT infer or assume relationships not explicitly stated
4. When uncertain → respond with "No_Relation"
{examples}
---

Analyze this case:
Text: {text}
Entities:
{entity_list}

Respond in the following format:
Reasoning: [one sentence explaining why]
Relation: [a numbered list of all entetiy pairs and their relations]
```

Fig. 2. Here we show the prompt structure for the CDR dataset and the multi-question case.

2.5 Inference

We ran each model with each set of prompts five times since the model provider APIs have an inherent level of non-determinism [17,31]. Then, average and standard deviation where calculated. A limiting factor to the amount of runs is simply the cost of using API services.

Structured Generation. To make the model evaluation as consistent as possible, we employed structured generations, meaning that the model is expected to return a valid JSON format. Another problem for our multi-extraction approach, where we present the model with a list of relations to label, is that if the model forgets or skips an entry, the whole evaluation of a list becomes invalid. Therefore, we need to enforce a structure that makes it impossible for the model to skip over an entry. To achieve this, we extracted the question from the original prompt and forced the model to repeat it back to us. This way, it repeats the original list and then fills out the fields in the list that we leave open for it. We accomplished this by using the Pydantic library and designing a schema dynamically for each prompt. In short, this approach ensures the following:

- **Dynamic Literal Types**: Each entity pair gets its own `Literal` type constraint, ensuring exact string matching for entity names.
- **Enforced Completeness**: By making each `relation_i` field required (using `...` as the default), the model cannot return a valid response without classifying all entity pairs.
- **Type Safety**: The `relation` field uses `Literal[*possible_answers]` to restrict outputs to predefined categories, preventing hallucinated or invalid relationship types.
- **Scalability**: The function adapts to any number of entity pairs through dynamic model creation, avoiding hardcoded schemas.

2.6 Data Selection

Due to budget limitations it is not possible to test the full dataset. We sampled 20 abstracts at random and made sure to add at least one abstract for each class. This resulted in 23 abstracts for BioRED with 474 relations, while the CDR sampling resulted in 20 abstracts with 190 relations. The same sampled subset was used consistently across all models and prompting configurations, ensuring that all comparisons are made on identical data (Table 5).

To validate the smaller test set as a valid proxy for the full dataset, we performed a complete experimental run using Mistral small on both the sampled subset and the full test set. A paired t-test across all metrics showed no statistically significant difference between the two, with the exception of a small precision difference on CDR ($p = 0.03$), which slightly favoured the reduced set—indicating that the subset does not inflate performance estimates. Full results of this comparison are shown in Table 19 in the Appendix. This gives us confidence that comparisons against state-of-the-art baselines reported in the literature, while not a perfect one-to-one comparison since those baselines were obtained on the full datasets, remain meaningful and that any performance difference introduced by the subsampling is likely to be small.

Table 5. Counts of Unique Classes for each Subsample and Baseline F1 Scores

Category	BioRED Subsample	CDR Subsample	BioRED Subsample
No_Relation	213	159	213
Relation	-	-	262
Association	115	-	-
Positive Correlation	70	-	-
Positive Correlation	69	-	-
Bind	4	-	-
Co-Treatment	1	-	-
Drug Interaction	1	-	-
Comparison	1	-	-
Conversion	1	-	-
CID	-	32	-
F1 Macro Majority Class	0.0536	0.4543	0.3555
F1 Macro Random	0.0718	0.4379	0.4987

3 Results

The discussion of the results will be split into three parts. First, we will show the overall performance across prompt types, models and datasets. Next, we will investigate the differences between prompt types and look at the impact of zero-shot vs. few-shot prompting and the effect of multi- vs. single-question extraction. Lastly, we will take a look at possible explanations for the observed behaviour.

3.1 Label Explanations and Methodology Recap

This section summarizes the labels and methodology used throughout the subsequent sections and graphs. All models and prompting configurations were evaluated on the same sampled subset of abstracts, ensuring that all reported comparisons reflect differences in model and prompting behaviour rather than differences in evaluation data.

Error Calculation. Since the use of models provided by Mistral and OpenAI does introduce a level of non-determinism, we ran each experiment five times. We report the mean and the standard deviation as error bars.

The Four Prompt Types. Our experimental design evaluates four distinct prompting strategies, which vary along two dimensions: **how we ask the prompt (single or multi)** and **if we provide examples or not (examples or zero)**.

- **Multi**: The model receives all entity pairs from an abstract simultaneously in a single prompt and annotates them collectively. This results in one prompt per abstract.
- **Single**: The model receives one entity pair at a time, with each pair presented in a separate prompt. This results in one prompt per entity pair.
- **Zero**: Zero-shot prompting with no examples provided to the model.
- **Examples**: Few-shot prompting where the model receives one example per relation class. Each example consists of an abstract, a question, and the corresponding annotations, formatted consistently with the target prompt style.

The Four Prompt Configurations. Combining these two dimensions yields four experimental conditions, as can be seen in Table 6.

Table 6. Overview of the four prompt type configurations. n denotes the number of entity pairs in an abstract.

Configuration	Aggregation	Examples	Prompts/Abstract
Multi-Zero	All pairs per prompt	None	1
Multi-Examples	All pairs per prompt	One per class	1
Single-Zero	One pair per prompt	None	n
Single-Examples	One pair per prompt	One per class	n

These configurations allow us to systematically evaluate the impact of multi- and single-extraction while also enabling us to examine the effect of providing examples on overall RE performance.

3.2 State-of-the-Art Models

All graphs contain a red line indicating the current state-of-the-art performance reported on the given task, taken from reported scores in the literature. All the models reported here are using a combination of a pre-trained small transformer model and some additional layer and/or specific fine-tuning to improve performance. For example, the Multi-view Merge Representation (MMR) model introduced by Yi Zhang et. all. achieves an F1 score of 78.95% on the CDR dataset [20]. This was accomplished by using a combination of a transformer model base with a U-Net layer and Graph Convolution Network layer. However, the model does still require fine-tuning. Alternatively, the BioREx paper uses an unmodified BERT model but makes use of additional related datasets to effectively increase the training pool for the fine-tuning, increasing performance to a state-of-the-art level [32].

3.3 Performance Across the CDR and BioRED Dataset

When comparing the two datasets, it is important to note that BioRED is a multi-class classification task while the CDR dataset is a binary classification task. However, for the BioRED dataset, if one looks at the task of relation detection it can also be turned into a binary task of relation or no relation labeling. The comparison of those can be seen in Fig. 3.

On the BioRED multi-class classification task in Fig. 3(a), the best performing model was GPT-5-mini with medium reasoning and the multi-examples prompt, followed by Mistral medium. All other prompt types performed worse across models with the exception of single-examples for GPT-4.1 and GPT-5-mini-low. None of the models reach the reported best performance of 58.95% macro F1 [18], with the best performing model reaching a macro F1 of 51%. On the CDR dataset, the following performance was observed: as can be seen in Fig. 3(b), Mistral large was the best performing model in three out of four cases, only losing to GPT-4.1 in the single-zero test case, performing best in multi-examples and multi-zero. It scored up to 74.8% macro F1, approaching the SOTA performance on the CDR dataset [20] with an F1 score of 78.95%.

We can compare this to the performance of relation detection on the BioRED dataset, treating it like a binary classification by simply differentiating if an entity pair has a relation or not. This is shown in Fig. 3(c). Here, Mistral medium is the best performing model with the multi-example prompting strategy. By providing a list of relations to extract in one prompt and examples, it exceeds the reported best performance of F1 77.17% [18] and reaches F1 80.54%. All of the models clearly beat both the random and the majority class baseline in all three datasets.

3.4 Effect of Prompting Strategies

Figure 4 shows the macro F1 score on the y axis and the different test cases we described (single-zero, multi-zero, single-examples, multi-examples) on the x axis. The graphic showcases the effects of adding few-shot examples, as well as the effect of making the model answer multiple questions at once instead of individual prompts. Surprisingly, few-shot examples did not help performance and were observed to harm it in many cases, regarding binary classification tasks, while providing examples did increase performance on the more complex multi-classification task. Additionally, we can see that specifically the Mistral small and medium models benefit the most from providing a list of entity pairs to extract instead of a one-prompt-one-pair approach. Although the GPT models show more moderate gains for the binary classification cases, they still profit similarly to Mistral large, which was a bit more responsive than the OpenAI models.

When analysing the multi-class case, we can see that nearly all models, especially in the multi-extraction case, profit from the given examples. Furthermore, GPT and Mistral models benefit equally from the multi-extraction prompting

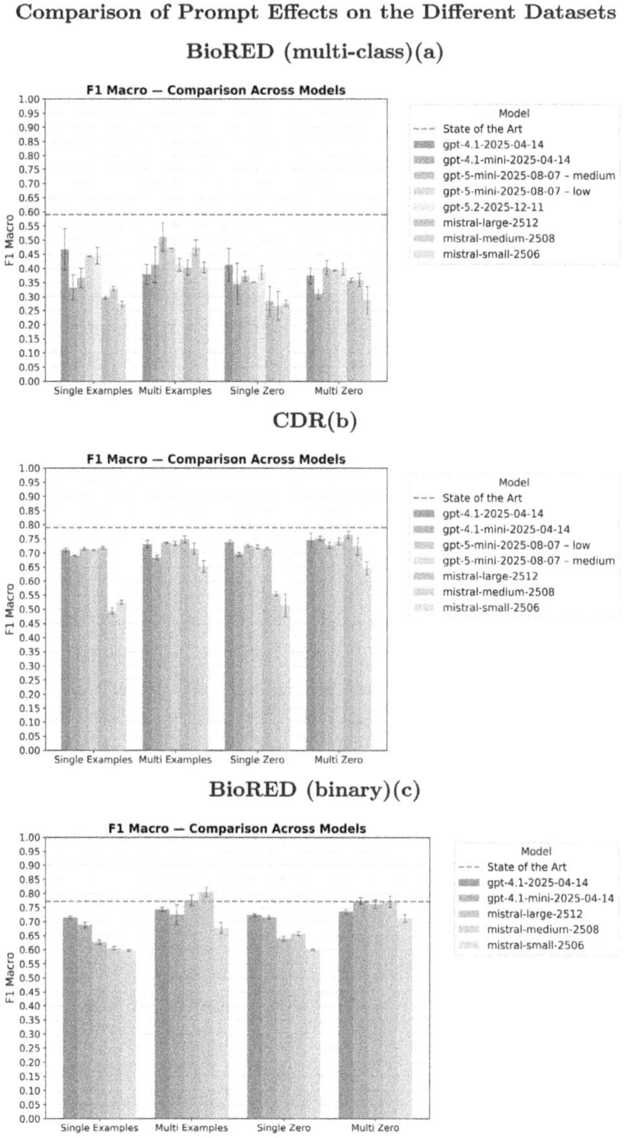

Fig. 3. Performance across models for three relation labeling tasks: **BioRED multi-class (a)**, **CDR (b)**, and **BioRED binary (c)**. For CDR and BioRED binary, the **red line** marks current SOTA. Prompt types indicate whether the model extracted one relation per prompt (**single**) or all relations from one abstract at once (**multi**); **zero** denotes zero-shot prompting (see Table 6). CDR and BioRED binary are binary labeling tasks; BioRED multi-class is a multi-classification task.

vs. single-extraction prompting. There is one exception: GPT 4.1, which performed best on its single-examples run. This, of course, leads to these questions: Why do these models prefer extracting multiple relations in one prompt instead of one per prompt? Do they learn from their previous generations, which they can't in the one-prompt-per-relation pair case?

Normalising for the Amount of Examples. Since in the prior experiment we choose to normalise by providing the same amount of examples per class, two for the binary case and nine for the multi-class case, the observation could also be due to the binary cases having less examples.

To ensure that the differences between binary and multi-class classification performance, as well as the preferences for certain prompting types are not due to example count, we conducted an additional experiment by taking the BioRED dataset and using the examples taken for the multi-class case with their labels binarized. The outcome can be seen in Fig. 5. From these results, we can observe that the same pattern holds true as with two examples, although the performance penalties for using examples slightly increases, indicating that adding more examples harms performance. This can also be supported by the fact that the performance of Mistral medium dropped from 80.54% to 74.4% F1 macro.

3.5 Open Self-hosted Models

Besides the previously named models, we looked at a group of small, self-hosted models to assess their performance and to determine whether the trends observed previously remained consistent as well. These models are particularly noteworthy because they can be run by small research groups without massive compute budgets. In Table 7, we show the performance on the CRD dataset, where Qwen and Mistral models performed best. The trends observed in the larger models persisted, with two exceptions: the Qwen models benefited more from the provided examples, while the older Llama and Mistral 7B models did not benefit as much from the multi-extraction pattern. The overall best performance achieved was F1 65% by Mistral 3 8B Instruct, which is on par with Mistral small, a 24B model. However, as expected, the overall performance did not reach the best score of the larger models (F1 74.8%). Additionally, we ran experiments on the BioRED dataset. On the Binary set, the best performance was achieved by Qwen3 4B Instruct with F1 70%, closely followed by Mistral 8B at F1 68%, again roughly matching Mistral small. The older models, however, did not benefit as much from the multi-extraction approach. Finally, for multi-classification on the BioRED dataset, the best-performing models were Mistral 8B and Qwen 4B, both achieving F1 34% with multi-extraction prompting. Once more, the older models benefited less from multi-extraction prompting, and only the combination of examples and multi-extraction prompting showed a positive impact. Moreover, we observed no clear benefit of OpenBioLLM over the other Llama models.

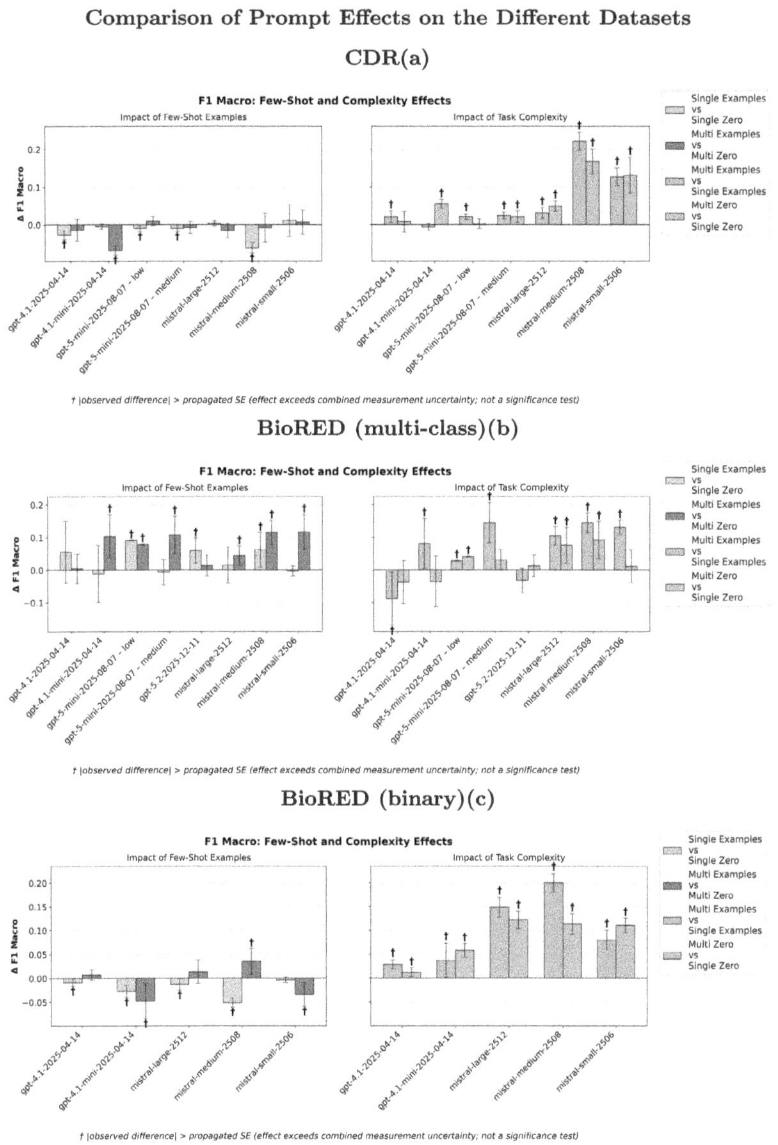

Fig. 4. Effects of few-shot examples (left) and multi-relation prompting (right) on three relation labeling tasks: CDR (a), BioRED multi-class (b), and BioRED binary relation pair detection (c). **Single-examples** and **single-zero** use one prompt per entity pair; **zero** denotes zero-shot single prompting; **multi** provides a list of relations in one prompt (see Table 6). A † marks effects exceeding the mean squared error. Left: positive values indicate that examples improve performance; blue = single-prompting, brown = multi-prompting. Right: positive values indicate that list-based prompting outperforms single-pair prompting; green = few-shot, grey = zero-shot. (Color figure online)

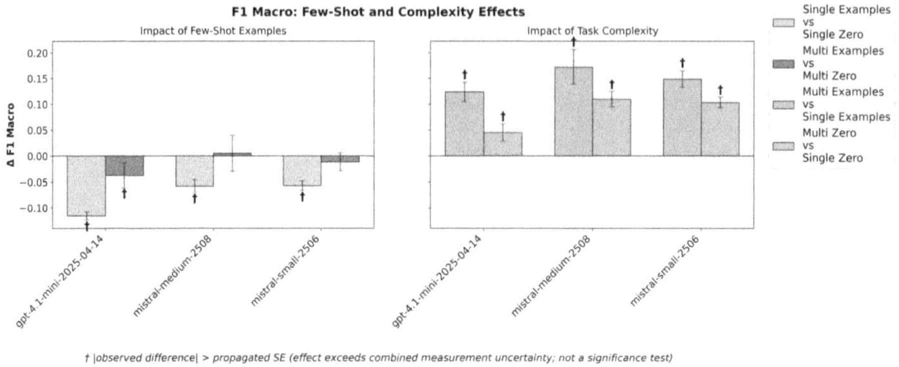

Fig. 5. In this figure, the effect of examples (left) and extracting multiple relations at once instead of one per prompt (right) are shown. The blue bars signify the difference between single-extraction with and without examples. Brown shows the same for multi-extraction. Green indicates the difference between multi-extraction with examples and single-extraction with examples. Lastly, grey shows the difference between multi- and single-extraction with no examples. All of this refers to the binarized BioRED dataset using the same examples as in the multi-class case, nine in total. (Color figure online)

Table 7. Performance on the CRD Dataset This table shows the F1-macro scores for a group of small LLMs that can be hosted on a single 24GB VRAM GPU. The best score in each column is highlighted in bold. The prompt types indicate if the model received one prompt to extract one relation (single) or one prompt to extract all relations from one abstract (multi). Zero indicates that no examples were given. The current SOTA performance is 77%. For more details, see Table 6.

Model	single-examples	single-zero	multi-zero	multi-examples
BioMistral-7B	0.192	0.126	0.175	0.314
Llama-3.1-8B	0.177	0.107	0.241	0.319
Llama-3.1-8B-Instruct	0.366	0.345	0.412	0.434
Llama-3.2-3B-Instruct	0.123	0.122	0.184	0.265
Llama3-OpenBioLLM-8B	0.225	0.241	0.275	0.294
Ministral-3-3B-Instruct-2512	**0.575**	**0.563**	0.598	0.587
Ministral-3-8B-Instruct-2512	0.115	0.143	**0.655**	0.629
Qwen3-4B-Instruct-2507	0.558	0.564	0.377	**0.632**

3.6 Summary Model Performance and Prompt Effects

In Table 8 we summarise the average performance across the prompt types and display the highest score achieved. A notable observation is that larger models perform better on average with zero-shot prompting than smaller models. Furthermore, some models, such as Mistral medium, strongly benefit from the provided examples. This leads to the conclusion that while the average performance on the binary datasets benefits from zero-shot prompting the most when using larger models, the best performing models are mostly observed with the multi-example prompting strategy.

Table 8. Prompt strategy comparison. Values are mean (max) F1 macro as decimal numbers. **Bold** indicates the best value per row for mean and max separately.

Dataset	Single-Zero	Single-Ex	Multi-Zero	Multi-Ex
CDR	0.667 (0.738)	0.652 (0.718)	**0.729** (**0.764**)	0.715 (0.748)
BioRED	0.338 (0.413)	0.364 (0.468)	0.360 (0.404)	**0.438** (**0.511**)
BioRED Binary	0.668 (0.724)	0.647 (0.715)	**0.751** (0.774)	0.745 (**0.805**)
BioRED Binary 9ex	0.664 (0.720)	0.587 (0.605)	**0.750** (0.772)	0.735 (**0.777**)
open models CDR	0.277 (0.564)	0.291 (0.575)	0.365 (**0.655**)	**0.434** (0.632)
open models BioRED	0.140 (0.219)	0.137 (0.238)	0.142 (0.319)	**0.184** (**0.338**)
open models BioRED Binary	0.449 (0.688)	**0.490** (0.661)	0.422 (0.641)	0.458 (**0.697**)

3.7 Prompt Robustness

To evaluate whether the multi-extraction prompt template is robust to arbitrary wording changes while preserving its structure, three LLMs (Claude, Mistral, and Gemini) were each asked to reword the original template. Five experimental runs of zero-shot multi-extraction were then conducted across all four prompt versions and two models, with mean macro F1 reported in Table 9. For Mistral Medium 2508, macro F1 ranged from 0.746 to 0.774, and for Mistral Small 2506 from 0.727 to 0.752, yielding maximum pairwise deltas of 0.028 and 0.025 respectively. In both cases, all pairwise differences remain well within the standard deviation of each distribution (0.013–0.028), indicating that performance is robust to prompt wording and that no version offers a practically meaningful advantage over the others.

3.8 Learning from Previous Generations?

To test the hypothesis that in the multi-case the models learn from their generations, we did a full experimental run on the CRD dataset with the Mistral small model. We used multi-extraction prompting, providing the model with lists for extraction. Then, we traced for each index position, which is the order in which the model works through the annotation task, F1, precision, recall, accuracy and the per class accuracy. We expected the latter indices to show a better performance compared to early ones due to in-context learning [33].

To ensure that performance increases across indices were due to model-learning and not a shift in the true distribution of labels at a given position, we plotted these distributions and calculated the relative difference between predicted and ground truth labels at each interval. Additionally, we re-ran the

Table 9. Prompt version comparison. Values are mean (std) F1 macro as decimal numbers. **Bold** indicates the best mean value per model.

Model	reworded_0	reworded_1	reworded_2	reworded_3
Mistral Medium 2508	**0.774** (0.021)	0.746 (0.028)	0.763 (0.022)	0.755 (0.020)
Mistral Small 2506	0.747 (0.013)	0.727 (0.020)	0.732 (0.021)	**0.752** (0.022)

experiment with a cut-down version of the dataset that ensures that the class distribution is even across intervals. The results can be seen in the upper plot in Fig. 6. As is shown, the model starts with over-predicting the CID (Chemically Induced Disease label). This behaviour then moves closer to the real distribution as index increases up to position 19. At the same time, performance metrics also increase across the board, with the exception of the CID accuracy, which decreases slightly up to position 11. However, the accuracy gains on the other class still increase the total score.

If we look at the lower plot in Fig. 6 with even distribution, we see a different behaviour. Scores also increase compared to the first position, however, they reach their maximum around index 6–7. A few things should be mentioned here: the data only goes up to position 15, since after filtering for equal distribution across index positions, the amount of total data was decreased. Secondly, it is not possible to create an even distribution across index positions without shuffling the index positions. The fact that we still see an improvement up to position seven indicates that this is evidence for in-context learning as an explanation for the improved performance in the multi-extraction prompting.

3.9 Token Efficiency

Next, we will examine the overall token use for the different prompting types across the prompting types and the CRD and BioRED datasets. In Table 10 and Table 11 we can see that across the two datasets, multi-extraction prompting performs best. As reported above, in the multi-class case examples help while in the binary CDR dataset they hinder the performance. Notably, on the BioRED dataset the inclusion of examples combined with multi-extraction amplified the effectiveness of both. Furthermore, from the table we can see that multi-extraction prompting decreases output tokens by around 40%, while giving examples increases the input tokens by around 49% compared to the single-zero baseline and 139% against the multi-zero case. However, compared to providing the single-examples case, the multi-prompting uses around 550% less input tokens.

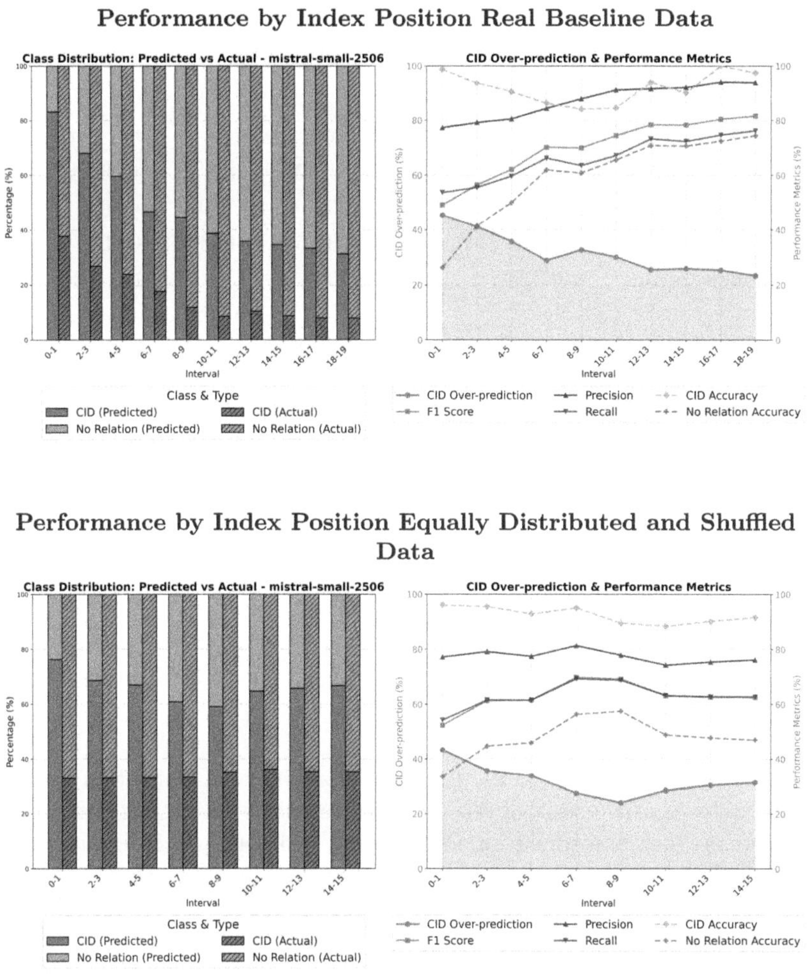

Fig. 6. On the left, the predicted labels of the model for an interval of two index positions is shown next to the true distribution. On the right, the percentage of over-prediction of the CID label (red) is shown in addition to precision (blue), recall (purple), and F1 score (green) for the full **CRD** dataset run with Mistral small. In addition, we also show the accuracy as dotted lines for the two labels. All of this was shown for index positions with at least 100 entries. (Color figure online)

Table 10. Token usage and performance comparison for the BioRED dataset, total tokens used for a complete run and the % differences compared with the zero-single case, which we use as a baseline.

Prompt Type	Completion Tokens	Prompt Tokens	F1 Score
Multi-Examples	137,041 (−43.1%)	2,641,620 (+48.9%)	**+28.6%**
Multi-Zero	142,216 (−40.9%)	183,265 (−89.7%)	+7.0%
Single-Examples	245,878 (+2.1%)	12,532,520 (+606.5%)	+9.6%
Single-Zero	240,823	1,773,770	0

Table 11. Token usage and performance comparison for the CRD dataset, total tokens used for a complete run and the % differences compared with the zero-single case, which we use as a baseline.

Prompt Type	Completion Tokens	Prompt Tokens	F1 Score
Multi-Examples	56,166 (−41.6%)	265,545 (−52.1%)	+7.2%
Multi-Zero	58,507 (−39.2%)	80,145 (−85.5%)	**+9.3%**
Single-Examples	96,941 (+0.8%)	1,220,175 (+120.0%)	−2.2%
Single-Zero	96,184	554,540	0

4 Discussion

From all of this we can derive the following: for binary classification tasks, like the CDR dataset or the task of relation pair detection on the BioRED dataset, LLMs that are not fine-tuned for this specific task can be configured through prompting alone to approach, and in some cases match, the performance of specialized fine-tuned extraction models, though results vary across datasets and fine tuned baselines are not consistently beaten (c.f. Fig. 3), like the fine-tuned BERT model used by BioREx [32]. For those binary tasks, when using multi-extraction prompting, the performance difference between models is relatively small and reasoning or none-reasoning models perform on the same level. It should be noted that our evaluation of reasoning models was limited in scope—only a small number of configurations were tested—and the observations reported here should be interpreted as preliminary rather than conclusive. For multi-class classification tasks the models benefit more from examples. The effect of providing multiple examples and all entities as a list instead of one by one in separate prompts strongly affects all models; here we can observe performance gains of up to 10 points F1 macro. The only model that did not profit from it was GPT-4.1. Here, reasoning seems to matter as GPT-5-mini is the best performing model. Yet, for gpt-5-mini the reasoning effort does not seem to matter much for this task. A potential explanation, could be that reasoning models tend to work better with longer context and the fact that they, in particular, are trained to learn from their generations generally helping in this task. These reasoning models are not specifically trained for biomedical RE which might lead to the fact that extra reasoning tokens due not further improve performance. This would explain why performance is increased between reasoning and none-reasoning models while the level of reasoning has little impact.

It is important to note that the performance of F1 macro on the multi-class case is strongly affected by a few entries since the data distribution is very unbalanced. When we only look at the four most prominent categories (association, positive correlation, negative correlation and no relation) we see an F1 macro score of 58.6 for GPT-5-mini medium reasoning, taking it to the same level of performance as the fine-tuned models. The LLMs tend to over-predict the minority classes, leading to good recall and bad precision.

We find a potential explanation for the performance improvements observed through multi-extraction vs single-extraction. From Fig. 6 we can come to the conclusion that the models learn from their previous generations. It seems that, for example, the model behaviour to over-predict a single class decreases when a few cases were answered with the other label. This indicates that models might start with a bias but after encountering a case in which the other label clearly was the correct choice, the bias decreases. The true distribution changing can be attributed to the fact that abstracts tend to mention the most important finding in the beginning, which will often be the reported connection and we queried the model about entity pairs in the order of them appearing in the text. When we present the model with the new test set where we balanced the distribution across indices we cannot avoid to also shuffle the order in which we ask the questions, which leads to the order of questions asked and the position of entity pairs in the text not aligning anymore. This seems to counteract the effect of learning to some degree. We still clearly observe the performance rising up to position 7 but afterwards, it declines again. However, it still stays above the performance of the first few positions. This indicates that the model does profit from being asked to label entity pairs in order of the text as well.

Lastly, we observed that providing examples harms performance on simpler tasks while improving performance on more complex ones. Although no conclusive evidence conclusion can be drawn here, we suspect that the reason for the observed behaviour might be a bias towards the positive label [34]. In Fig. 5, we can observe that after the amount of examples is increased, the negative effect of the few-shot examples increases, especially in the single-extraction case. The reason for this could be that they are not well-balanced since, in the single case, we provide one example each, meaning that we provide the model with eight positive labels and one negative label. While we always provide full tables in the multi-extraction case, making the class-split more balanced since "No Relation" is the most common label. This further points towards label bias playing a role here as other papers have reported that few-shot prompting can increase label biases [35]. The general bias towards positive labels might be increased through providing examples. This bias decreases in the multi-class case where we have multiple positive labels. Nevertheless, all of this is simply an educated guess and not experimentally proven.

5 Conclusion

Returning to the questions set in the beginning:

1. Does multi-extraction prompting with structured generation boost performance over single-extraction prompting, and does it reduce computational cost?
2. To what extent can modern LLMs approach the performance of small, fine-tuned models on biomedical RE tasks without fine-tuning?
3. How do the capabilities scale across binary and multi-class classification tasks?

We can now answer these questions.

5.1 Performance of Current LLMs on Biomedical RE

The performance of current LLMs provided by Mistral and OpenAI: for binary classification tasks all of the tested LLMs, with the exception of Mistral small and to a lesser extent GPT4.1-mini, either slightly beat current specialized models on the relation detection task on the BioRED dataset (F1 80.54% vs 77.17%) or underperform on the CDR dataset (F1 74.8% vs 78.95%) by around 4%. This is achieved without any fine-tuning on the task. When examining the multi-extraction task, the best models reached an F1 score of 51% while the current best is 58.95%. From these results, we can conclude that LLMs represent a promising and competitive approach for binary classification tasks as annotators, particularly in low-resource settings where fine-tuning data is scarce, though they do not consistently outperform fine-tuned baselines. This could be used to generate pre-annotations for human annotators, speeding up the annotation process [36]. Sadly, small local models are not yet on the same level of performance, although it is promising to see that even small 4B and 8B models are matching the performance of 24B models of mid-2025, if they are sufficiently modern. This turns them into a promising target for fine-tuning, as it may lead to a state-of-the-art zero- or few-shot prompting performance on biomedical extraction tasks. Notably, even the small models manage to beat the baselines of GPT-4 which were established in the BioRED (Biomedical Relation Extraction Dataset) track at BioCreative VIII [18]. GPT-4 reached an F1 score of 42.93% for the binary entity pair recognition task and 20.85% for the multi-class labeling task, while the smaller models achieved 70% and 34% respectively. This demonstrates the impact of multi-extraction prompting with structured generation, even when applied to models not specifically optimised for biomedical RE.

5.2 Effects of Prompting Strategies and Their Influence on Binary and Multi-class Classification

Regarding our second and third goal, we have shown that multi-extraction, i.e. presenting the model with multiple extraction tasks in one prompt and using structured generations to enforce correct list outputs, significantly increases model performance for all Mistral models, leading to them outperforming OpenAI's models in the binary classification tasks. It also offers small benefits to all GPT models in binary classification but harms performance of GPT-4.1 in the multi-class case. The reasoning models from OpenAI benefited strongly from the multi-extraction approach in the multi-class classification task as well. Yet, providing few-shot examples only helped in the multi-class case. Furthermore, we show that the improvement is likely due to in-context learning. We recommend the use of zero-shot multi-extraction for binary classification and few-shot multi-extraction for multi-class RE. Additionally, we recommend the use of Mistral large, Mistral medium or GPT-5-mini with these prompting patterns for best performance, while also being cost effective based on the performance observed. If highest accuracy is not the goal but cheapest inference for binary classification tasks, the Qwen 4B and Ministral 3 family seem promising. When using small models, the few-shot multi-extraction provided the most consistency, most likely due to small models needing the examples to follow the format properly. Additionally, we show that multi-extraction prompting not only increases performance but, when comparing zero-shot token usage, it also needs 40% less input tokens and 85% to 90% less output tokens. If we compare multi-extraction to single-extraction within few-shot prompts, we see a 40% decrease in output tokens and a 170% to 550% decrease in input tokens. These results clearly show that multi-extraction prompting with structured generation simultaneously improves performance and reduces computational cost, making it the recommended approach for LLM-based biomedical RE without fine-tuning, in most cases.

6 Limitations and Outlook

Due to budget and time limitations, all model evaluations were performed on a sampled subset rather than the full datasets. While the subset was statistically validated as a reliable proxy, the SOTA baselines reported throughout are taken from the literature and were obtained on the full datasets, meaning a small level of incomparability remains. For the same reasons, the testing of reasoning models was cursory. Follow-up work could dive more into the effect and potential performance of reasoning models, especially true frontier models with high reasoning [37]. Additionally, the effect of examples could be investigated more in-depth. There is a chance that the performance differences observed are due to the selection of exact examples which was not further explored here. Although, this seems unlikely since the trend is the same between the two datasets and changing the amount of examples did increase the observed trend. An in-depth paper on the effects of quality and number of examples on the performance of extraction tasks will be the focus of some of our followup work.

Moreover, it has to be said that two datasets only provide a general idea of model performance across the variety of existing tasks. We would encourage interested readers to submit links to datasets they think are of interest through the following Google survey: https://forms.gle/u32QeAzEVKZ8Lqpq9.

This way, we hope to collect and build a benchmark suite that reflects the interests of the biomedical community. Lastly, since reasoning models performed best in the more complex multi-class case, we plan to investigate reinforcement learning for LLM's reasoning for biomedical annotation tasks, such as the ones investigated here.

Acknowledgments. The BioRED dataset was developed by Luo et al. and released as part of BioCreative VII. We thank the annotators and organizers for providing this valuable resource to the biomedical NLP community. This work has been additionally supported by TRA Modeling at the University of Bonn and the Lamarr Institute.

Data Availability. The BioRED and CRD datasets are openly available. Processing code is available at github.com/caisa-lab/Structured-Multi-Extraction-Prompting-for-Biomedical-Relation-Extraction.

Disclosure of Interests. There are no conflicts of interest in the creation of this work.

A Appendix

A.1 CDR Dataset Results

See Table 12.

Table 12. LLM Benchmark Results: CDR Dataset.

Model	Prompt	F1-macro	F1-micro	Precision	Recall	Accuracy
GPT-4.1	Multi-Zero	0.746 ± 0.025	0.816 ± 0.025	0.721 ± 0.020	0.834 ± 0.015	0.816 ± 0.025
GPT-4.1	Single-Zero	0.738 ± 0.008	0.797 ± 0.007	0.720 ± 0.006	0.863 ± 0.009	0.797 ± 0.007
GPT-4.1	Multi-Ex	0.731 ± 0.013	0.798 ± 0.012	0.711 ± 0.010	0.836 ± 0.012	0.798 ± 0.012
GPT-4.1	Single-Ex	0.711 ± 0.007	0.768 ± 0.007	0.704 ± 0.004	0.848 ± 0.004	0.768 ± 0.007
GPT-4.1-mini	Multi-Zero	0.752 ± 0.008	0.816 ± 0.006	0.727 ± 0.007	0.857 ± 0.013	0.816 ± 0.006
GPT-4.1-mini	Single-Zero	0.696 ± 0.006	0.761 ± 0.005	0.687 ± 0.005	0.812 ± 0.008	0.761 ± 0.005
GPT-4.1-mini	Single-Ex	0.691 ± 0.002	0.748 ± 0.002	0.690 ± 0.002	0.828 ± 0.005	0.748 ± 0.002
GPT-4.1-mini	Multi-Ex	0.684 ± 0.008	0.777 ± 0.009	0.667 ± 0.006	0.746 ± 0.006	0.777 ± 0.009
GPT-5-mini (L)	Multi-Ex	0.737 ± 0.002	0.801 ± 0.003	0.717 ± 0.002	0.848 ± 0.008	0.801 ± 0.003
GPT-5-mini (L)	Multi-Zero	0.728 ± 0.011	0.795 ± 0.008	0.709 ± 0.009	0.834 ± 0.017	0.795 ± 0.008
GPT-5-mini (L)	Single-Zero	0.726 ± 0.004	0.782 ± 0.003	0.715 ± 0.005	0.864 ± 0.011	0.782 ± 0.003
GPT-5-mini (L)	Single-Ex	0.716 ± 0.005	0.770 ± 0.006	0.711 ± 0.003	0.862 ± 0.003	0.770 ± 0.006
GPT-5-mini (M)	Multi-Zero	0.742 ± 0.013	0.807 ± 0.015	0.720 ± 0.009	0.847 ± 0.006	0.807 ± 0.015
GPT-5-mini (M)	Multi-Ex	0.734 ± 0.008	0.799 ± 0.009	0.714 ± 0.005	0.844 ± 0.005	0.799 ± 0.009
GPT-5-mini (M)	Single-Zero	0.721 ± 0.007	0.779 ± 0.004	0.710 ± 0.007	0.855 ± 0.015	0.779 ± 0.004
GPT-5-mini (M)	Single-Ex	0.711 ± 0.002	0.765 ± 0.004	0.706 ± 0.001	0.854 ± 0.004	0.765 ± 0.004
Mistral-L	Multi-Zero	0.764 ± 0.013	0.829 ± 0.014	0.737 ± 0.010	0.860 ± 0.015	0.829 ± 0.014
Mistral-L	Multi-Ex	0.748 ± 0.013	0.812 ± 0.011	0.725 ± 0.010	0.857 ± 0.014	0.812 ± 0.011
Mistral-L	Single-Ex	0.718 ± 0.005	0.772 ± 0.005	0.712 ± 0.003	0.863 ± 0.003	0.772 ± 0.005
Mistral-L	Single-Zero	0.715 ± 0.003	0.770 ± 0.003	0.709 ± 0.003	0.859 ± 0.005	0.770 ± 0.003
Mistral-M	Multi-Zero	0.724 ± 0.031	0.795 ± 0.034	0.705 ± 0.022	0.817 ± 0.017	0.795 ± 0.034
Mistral-M	Multi-Ex	0.716 ± 0.020	0.782 ± 0.019	0.700 ± 0.015	0.824 ± 0.020	0.782 ± 0.019
Mistral-M	Single-Zero	0.556 ± 0.007	0.587 ± 0.008	0.633 ± 0.005	0.735 ± 0.010	0.587 ± 0.008
Mistral-M	Single-Ex	0.494 ± 0.011	0.510 ± 0.013	0.627 ± 0.003	0.706 ± 0.008	0.510 ± 0.013
Mistral-S	Multi-Ex	0.653 ± 0.021	0.709 ± 0.022	0.666 ± 0.014	0.790 ± 0.024	0.709 ± 0.022
Mistral-S	Multi-Zero	0.646 ± 0.024	0.705 ± 0.033	0.660 ± 0.010	0.778 ± 0.018	0.705 ± 0.033
Mistral-S	Single-Ex	0.525 ± 0.008	0.547 ± 0.009	0.635 ± 0.002	0.728 ± 0.005	0.547 ± 0.009
Mistral-S	Single-Zero	0.515 ± 0.040	0.539 ± 0.037	0.616 ± 0.042	0.698 ± 0.072	0.539 ± 0.037

A.2 BioRED Dataset Results

See Table 13.

Table 13. LLM Benchmark Results: BioRED. Complete evaluation across all models and prompt types.

Model	Prompt	F1-macro	F1-micro	Precision	Recall	Accuracy
GPT-4.1	Single-Ex	0.468 ± 0.073	0.481 ± 0.075	0.446 ± 0.078	0.681 ± 0.104	0.481 ± 0.075
GPT-4.1	Single-Zero	0.413 ± 0.059	0.523 ± 0.007	0.389 ± 0.053	0.629 ± 0.063	0.523 ± 0.007
GPT-4.1	Multi-Ex	0.379 ± 0.035	0.530 ± 0.010	0.373 ± 0.022	0.509 ± 0.050	0.530 ± 0.010
GPT-4.1	Multi-Zero	0.375 ± 0.027	0.536 ± 0.015	0.364 ± 0.031	0.544 ± 0.015	0.536 ± 0.015
GPT-4.1-mini	Multi-Ex	0.413 ± 0.063	0.426 ± 0.022	0.453 ± 0.066	0.502 ± 0.054	0.426 ± 0.022
GPT-4.1-mini	Single-Zero	0.345 ± 0.074	0.482 ± 0.090	0.314 ± 0.069	0.564 ± 0.111	0.482 ± 0.090
GPT-4.1-mini	Single-Ex	0.333 ± 0.044	0.409 ± 0.003	0.322 ± 0.045	0.624 ± 0.044	0.409 ± 0.003
GPT-4.1-mini	Multi-Zero	0.310 ± 0.019	0.497 ± 0.015	0.345 ± 0.022	0.376 ± 0.050	0.497 ± 0.015
GPT-5-mini (L)	Multi-Ex	0.510 ± 0.032	0.595 ± 0.017	0.449 ± 0.042	0.735 ± 0.040	0.595 ± 0.017
GPT-5-mini (L)	Single-Ex	0.394 ± 0.033	0.492 ± 0.003	0.344 ± 0.023	0.708 ± 0.052	0.492 ± 0.003
GPT-5-mini (L)	Multi-Zero	0.384 ± 0.017	0.558 ± 0.007	0.354 ± 0.011	0.532 ± 0.028	0.558 ± 0.007
GPT-5-mini (L)	Single-Zero	0.357 ± 0.005	0.503 ± 0.006	0.321 ± 0.004	0.636 ± 0.003	0.503 ± 0.006
GPT-5-mini (M)	Multi-Ex	0.511 ± 0.051	0.595 ± 0.015	0.443 ± 0.047	0.740 ± 0.065	0.595 ± 0.015
GPT-5-mini (M)	Multi-Zero	0.404 ± 0.025	0.563 ± 0.013	0.371 ± 0.018	0.562 ± 0.048	0.563 ± 0.013
GPT-5-mini (M)	Single-Zero	0.373 ± 0.018	0.509 ± 0.008	0.332 ± 0.013	0.677 ± 0.039	0.509 ± 0.008
GPT-5-mini (M)	Single-Ex	0.367 ± 0.034	0.489 ± 0.005	0.323 ± 0.023	0.653 ± 0.090	0.489 ± 0.005
GPT-5.2	Single-Ex	0.446 ± 0.029	0.509 ± 0.008	0.408 ± 0.037	0.725 ± 0.012	0.509 ± 0.008
GPT-5.2	Multi-Ex	0.413 ± 0.022	0.555 ± 0.016	0.400 ± 0.019	0.601 ± 0.025	0.555 ± 0.016
GPT-5.2	Multi-Zero	0.399 ± 0.022	0.547 ± 0.012	0.393 ± 0.023	0.605 ± 0.030	0.547 ± 0.012
GPT-5.2	Single-Zero	0.386 ± 0.023	0.520 ± 0.006	0.357 ± 0.017	0.633 ± 0.050	0.520 ± 0.006
Mistral-L	Multi-Ex	0.403 ± 0.027	0.573 ± 0.019	0.363 ± 0.019	0.658 ± 0.024	0.573 ± 0.019
Mistral-L	Multi-Zero	0.359 ± 0.008	0.539 ± 0.014	0.331 ± 0.011	0.626 ± 0.007	0.539 ± 0.014
Mistral-L	Single-Ex	0.298 ± 0.006	0.365 ± 0.004	0.294 ± 0.005	0.720 ± 0.002	0.365 ± 0.004
Mistral-L	Single-Zero	0.284 ± 0.054	0.370 ± 0.058	0.283 ± 0.061	0.608 ± 0.124	0.370 ± 0.058
Mistral-M	Multi-Ex	0.474 ± 0.028	0.596 ± 0.029	0.434 ± 0.021	0.690 ± 0.053	0.596 ± 0.029
Mistral-M	Multi-Zero	0.360 ± 0.023	0.541 ± 0.030	0.339 ± 0.017	0.572 ± 0.057	0.541 ± 0.030
Mistral-M	Single-Ex	0.329 ± 0.008	0.427 ± 0.013	0.316 ± 0.005	0.688 ± 0.054	0.427 ± 0.013
Mistral-M	Single-Zero	0.268 ± 0.052	0.403 ± 0.071	0.261 ± 0.055	0.639 ± 0.089	0.403 ± 0.071
Mistral-S	Multi-Ex	0.404 ± 0.019	0.494 ± 0.033	0.403 ± 0.011	0.606 ± 0.017	0.494 ± 0.033
Mistral-S	Multi-Zero	0.288 ± 0.049	0.452 ± 0.068	0.284 ± 0.058	0.483 ± 0.076	0.452 ± 0.068
Mistral-S	Single-Zero	0.277 ± 0.011	0.411 ± 0.005	0.298 ± 0.011	0.525 ± 0.055	0.411 ± 0.005
Mistral-S	Single-Ex	0.273 ± 0.010	0.360 ± 0.008	0.275 ± 0.007	0.679 ± 0.040	0.360 ± 0.008

A.3 Binary Classification Results

See Table 14.

Table 14. LLM Benchmark Results: Binary Classification. Evaluation on binary classification tasks.

Model	Prompt	F1-macro	F1-micro	Precision	Recall	Accuracy
GPT-4.1	Multi-Ex	0.743 ± 0.007	0.746 ± 0.007	0.744 ± 0.007	0.744 ± 0.007	0.746 ± 0.007
GPT-4.1	Multi-Zero	0.736 ± 0.007	0.739 ± 0.007	0.736 ± 0.007	0.736 ± 0.007	0.739 ± 0.007
GPT-4.1	Single-Zero	0.724 ± 0.005	0.727 ± 0.004	0.724 ± 0.004	0.724 ± 0.005	0.727 ± 0.004
GPT-4.1	Single-Ex	0.715 ± 0.005	0.720 ± 0.004	0.717 ± 0.005	0.714 ± 0.005	0.720 ± 0.004
GPT-4.1-mini	Multi-Zero	0.774 ± 0.011	0.784 ± 0.011	0.801 ± 0.015	0.770 ± 0.011	0.784 ± 0.011
GPT-4.1-mini	Multi-Ex	0.725 ± 0.034	0.749 ± 0.024	0.794 ± 0.025	0.728 ± 0.028	0.749 ± 0.024
GPT-4.1-mini	Single-Zero	0.716 ± 0.007	0.739 ± 0.006	0.773 ± 0.006	0.717 ± 0.006	0.739 ± 0.006
GPT-4.1-mini	Single-Ex	0.688 ± 0.010	0.715 ± 0.008	0.745 ± 0.008	0.692 ± 0.009	0.715 ± 0.008
Mistral-L	Multi-Ex	0.775 ± 0.018	0.782 ± 0.018	0.788 ± 0.021	0.772 ± 0.017	0.782 ± 0.018
Mistral-L	Multi-Zero	0.762 ± 0.015	0.768 ± 0.015	0.770 ± 0.016	0.760 ± 0.015	0.768 ± 0.015
Mistral-L	Single-Zero	0.640 ± 0.008	0.685 ± 0.006	0.743 ± 0.009	0.655 ± 0.007	0.685 ± 0.006
Mistral-L	Single-Ex	0.627 ± 0.008	0.685 ± 0.007	0.780 ± 0.012	0.651 ± 0.007	0.685 ± 0.007
Mistral-M	Multi-Ex	0.805 ± 0.017	0.811 ± 0.016	0.818 ± 0.017	0.802 ± 0.017	0.811 ± 0.016
Mistral-M	Multi-Zero	0.771 ± 0.020	0.780 ± 0.018	0.792 ± 0.020	0.767 ± 0.019	0.780 ± 0.018
Mistral-M	Single-Zero	0.657 ± 0.006	0.697 ± 0.004	0.753 ± 0.005	0.669 ± 0.005	0.697 ± 0.004
Mistral-M	Single-Ex	0.605 ± 0.006	0.664 ± 0.005	0.736 ± 0.008	0.631 ± 0.005	0.664 ± 0.005
Mistral-S	Multi-Zero	0.712 ± 0.014	0.729 ± 0.012	0.744 ± 0.012	0.712 ± 0.013	0.729 ± 0.012
Mistral-S	Multi-Ex	0.678 ± 0.019	0.703 ± 0.017	0.726 ± 0.022	0.681 ± 0.018	0.703 ± 0.017
Mistral-S	Single-Zero	0.602 ± 0.004	0.666 ± 0.002	0.756 ± 0.002	0.631 ± 0.002	0.666 ± 0.002
Mistral-S	Single-Ex	0.598 ± 0.003	0.661 ± 0.002	0.742 ± 0.003	0.627 ± 0.002	0.661 ± 0.002

A.4 Binary Classification (9 Examples) Results

See Table 15.

Table 15. LLM Benchmark Results: Binary Classification (9 Examples). Binary classification with 9-shot prompting.

Model	Type	F1-macro	F1-micro	Precision	Recall	Accuracy
gpt-4.1-mini	single_ex	0.604 ± 0.002	0.659 ± 0.002	0.711 ± 0.002	0.627 ± 0.002	0.659 ± 0.002
gpt-4.1-mini	multi_ex	0.728 ± 0.017	0.757 ± 0.013	0.827 ± 0.010	0.731 ± 0.015	0.757 ± 0.013
mistral-M	single_ex	0.605 ± 0.009	0.667 ± 0.005	0.753 ± 0.004	0.633 ± 0.006	0.667 ± 0.005
mistral-M	multi_ex	0.777 ± 0.031	0.789 ± 0.023	0.809 ± 0.006	0.775 ± 0.029	0.789 ± 0.023
mistral-S	single_ex	0.552 ± 0.006	0.639 ± 0.004	0.750 ± 0.009	0.600 ± 0.004	0.639 ± 0.004
mistral-S	multi_ex	0.701 ± 0.014	0.736 ± 0.012	0.812 ± 0.027	0.708 ± 0.012	0.736 ± 0.012

B Open Models Performance

B.1 BioRED

See Table 16.

Table 16. LLM Benchmark Results: open models BioRED dataset, no standard deviation because runs are deterministic

Model	Type	F1-macro	F1-micro	Precision	Recall	Accuracy
BioMistral-7B	single-examples	0.075	0.162	0.125	0.317	0.162
BioMistral-7B	single-zero	0.085	0.261	0.129	0.123	0.261
BioMistral-7B	multi-zero	0.087	0.154	0.080	0.107	0.154
BioMistral-7B	multi-examples	0.058	0.095	0.136	0.057	0.095
Llama-3.1-8B	single-examples	0.116	0.099	0.168	0.376	0.099
Llama-3.1-8B	single-zero	0.095	0.213	0.184	0.140	0.213
Llama-3.1-8B	multi-examples	0.107	0.204	0.182	0.130	0.204
Llama-3.1-8B	multi-zero	0.066	0.112	0.135	0.078	0.112
Llama-3.1-8B-Instruct	single-examples	0.141	0.244	0.173	0.433	0.244
Llama-3.1-8B-Instruct	multi-examples	0.161	0.291	0.196	0.447	0.291
Llama-3.1-8B-Instruct	multi-zero	0.140	0.244	0.207	0.330	0.244
Llama-3.1-8B-Instruct	single-zero	0.128	0.257	0.186	0.233	0.257
Llama-3.2-3B-Instruct	multi-examples	0.230	0.267	0.294	0.269	0.267
Llama-3.2-3B-Instruct	single-zero	0.159	0.265	0.190	0.455	0.265
Llama-3.2-3B-Instruct	multi-zero	0.063	0.164	0.117	0.162	0.164
Llama-3.2-3B-Instruct	single-examples	0.115	0.198	0.151	0.284	0.198
Llama3-OpenBioLLM-8B	multi-examples	0.000	0.000	0.000	0.000	0.000
Llama3-OpenBioLLM-8B	single-zero	0.134	0.246	0.169	0.282	0.246
Llama3-OpenBioLLM-8B	single-examples	0.067	0.084	0.149	0.337	0.084
Llama3-OpenBioLLM-8B	multi-zero	0.044	0.059	0.205	0.029	0.059
Ministral-3-3B-Instruct-2512	single-zero	0.186	0.425	0.205	0.420	0.425
Ministral-3-3B-Instruct-2512	single-examples	0.170	0.375	0.198	0.467	0.375
Ministral-3-3B-Instruct-2512	multi-examples	0.242	0.461	0.249	0.539	0.461
Ministral-3-3B-Instruct-2512	multi-zero	0.191	0.421	0.204	0.379	0.421
Ministral-3-8B-Instruct-2512	multi-zero	0.319	0.522	0.294	0.615	0.522
Ministral-3-8B-Instruct-2512	single-zero	0.219	0.497	0.211	0.302	0.497
Ministral-3-8B-Instruct-2512	single-examples	0.178	0.444	0.179	0.290	0.444
Ministral-3-8B-Instruct-2512	multi-examples	0.338	0.528	0.301	0.651	0.528
Qwen 4B Instruct	multi-zero	0.223	0.463	0.229	0.392	0.463
Qwen 4B Instruct	single-examples	0.238	0.286	0.253	0.360	0.286
Qwen 4B Instruct	multi-examples	0.336	0.423	0.292	0.604	0.423
Qwen 4B Instruct	single-zero	0.116	0.349	0.125	0.177	0.349

B.2 BioRED Binary Relation Pair Detection

See Table 17.

Table 17. LLM Benchmark Results: Open models BioRED Binary Classification, no standard deviation because runs are deterministic

Model	Type	F1-macro	F1-micro	Precision	Recall	Accuracy
BioMistral-7B	single-examples	0.456	0.564	0.562	0.524	0.564
BioMistral-7B	multi-zero	0.280	0.474	0.370	0.295	0.474
BioMistral-7B	single-zero	0.268	0.566	0.444	0.345	0.566
BioMistral-7B	multi-examples	0.217	0.438	0.259	0.266	0.438
Llama-3.1-8B	single-zero	0.455	0.585	0.670	0.541	0.585
Llama-3.1-8B	single-examples	0.448	0.568	0.583	0.526	0.568
Llama-3.1-8B	multi-zero	0.411	0.564	0.605	0.517	0.564
Llama-3.1-8B	multi-examples	0.215	0.425	0.436	0.258	0.425
Llama-3.1-8B-Instruct	single-zero	0.526	0.613	0.670	0.575	0.613
Llama-3.1-8B-Instruct	single-examples	0.616	0.665	0.714	0.635	0.665
Llama-3.1-8B-Instruct	multi-zero	0.537	0.634	0.768	0.593	0.634
Llama-3.1-8B-Instruct	multi-examples	0.539	0.634	0.759	0.593	0.634
Llama-3.2-3B-Instruct	single-zero	0.423	0.573	0.657	0.526	0.573
Llama-3.2-3B-Instruct	multi-zero	0.340	0.549	0.420	0.346	0.549
Llama-3.2-3B-Instruct	single-examples	0.465	0.596	0.734	0.551	0.596
Llama-3.2-3B-Instruct	multi-examples	0.246	0.509	0.394	0.309	0.509
Ministral-3-3B-Instruct-2512	multi-examples	0.662	0.663	0.681	0.675	0.663
Ministral-3-3B-Instruct-2512	single-zero	0.688	0.691	0.688	0.689	0.691
Ministral-3-3B-Instruct-2512	multi-zero	0.420	0.623	0.462	0.429	0.623
Ministral-3-3B-Instruct-2512	single-examples	0.661	0.661	0.674	0.671	0.661
Ministral-3-8B-Instruct-2512	multi-zero	0.641	0.642	0.642	0.644	0.642
Ministral-3-8B-Instruct-2512	multi-examples	0.688	0.688	0.692	0.693	0.688
Ministral-3-8B-Instruct-2512	single-zero	0.298	0.579	0.450	0.356	0.579
Ministral-3-8B-Instruct-2512	single-examples	0.276	0.556	0.418	0.340	0.556
Qwen3-4B-Instruct-2507	single-zero	0.665	0.665	0.667	0.669	0.665
Qwen3-4B-Instruct-2507	multi-examples	0.697	0.709	0.713	0.696	0.709
Qwen3-4B-Instruct-2507	single-examples	0.487	0.733	0.492	0.484	0.733
Qwen3-4B-Instruct-2507	multi-zero	0.363	0.554	0.394	0.383	0.554
Qwen3-8B	multi-zero	0.316	0.568	0.395	0.353	0.568
Qwen3-8B	single-examples	0.491	0.598	0.666	0.556	0.598
Qwen3-8B	multi-examples	0.396	0.547	0.505	0.501	0.547
Qwen3-8B	single-zero	0.354	0.606	0.467	0.380	0.606
Qwen3-8B-FP8	multi-zero	0.493	0.608	0.736	0.565	0.608
Qwen3-8B-FP8	single-examples	0.515	0.600	0.635	0.563	0.600
Qwen3-8B-FP8	multi-examples	0.464	0.581	0.624	0.539	0.581
Qwen3-8B-FP8	single-zero	0.365	0.613	0.488	0.385	0.613

B.3 CDR Dataset

See Tables 18.

Table 18. Open models LLM Benchmark Results: CDR dataset, no standard deviation because runs are deterministic

Model	Type	F1-macro	F1-micro	Precision	Recall	Accuracy
BioMistral-7B	single-examples	0.192	0.204	0.530	0.510	0.204
BioMistral-7B	single-zero	0.126	0.199	0.393	0.346	0.199
BioMistral-7B	multi-zero	0.175	0.188	0.457	0.488	0.188
BioMistral-7B	multi-examples	0.314	0.314	0.598	0.588	0.314
Llama-3.1-8B	single-examples	0.177	0.194	0.586	0.516	0.194
Llama-3.1-8B	single-zero	0.107	0.178	0.306	0.329	0.178
Llama-3.1-8B	multi-examples	0.319	0.319	0.565	0.566	0.319
Llama-3.1-8B	multi-zero	0.241	0.241	0.452	0.457	0.241
Llama-3.1-8B-Instruct	single-examples	0.366	0.366	0.605	0.619	0.366
Llama-3.1-8B-Instruct	multi-examples	0.434	0.450	0.567	0.607	0.450
Llama-3.1-8B-Instruct	multi-zero	0.412	0.424	0.560	0.592	0.424
Llama-3.1-8B-Instruct	single-zero	0.345	0.346	0.586	0.594	0.346
Llama-3.2-3B-Instruct	multi-examples	0.265	0.398	0.383	0.392	0.398
Llama-3.2-3B-Instruct	single-zero	0.122	0.194	0.391	0.335	0.194
Llama-3.2-3B-Instruct	multi-zero	0.184	0.272	0.381	0.359	0.272
Llama-3.2-3B-Instruct	single-examples	0.123	0.199	0.391	0.346	0.199
Llama3-OpenBioLLM-8B	multi-examples	0.294	0.445	0.376	0.361	0.445
Llama3-OpenBioLLM-8B	single-zero	0.241	0.246	0.560	0.535	0.246
Llama3-OpenBioLLM-8B	single-examples	0.225	0.230	0.523	0.513	0.230
Llama3-OpenBioLLM-8B	multi-zero	0.275	0.346	0.375	0.305	0.346
Ministral-3-3B-Instruct-2512	single-zero	0.563	0.602	0.625	0.724	0.602
Ministral-3-3B-Instruct-2512	single-examples	0.575	0.644	0.599	0.674	0.644
Ministral-3-3B-Instruct-2512	multi-examples	0.587	0.691	0.588	0.640	0.691
Ministral-3-3B-Instruct-2512	multi-zero	0.598	0.691	0.601	0.665	0.691
Ministral-3-8B-Instruct-2512	multi-zero	0.655	0.717	0.662	0.780	0.717
Ministral-3-8B-Instruct-2512	single-zero	0.143	0.168	0.084	0.500	0.168
Ministral-3-8B-Instruct-2512	single-examples	0.115	0.188	0.391	0.342	0.188
Ministral-3-8B-Instruct-2512	multi-examples	0.629	0.686	0.648	0.761	0.686
Qwen3-4B-Instruct-2507	multi-zero	0.377	0.607	0.411	0.460	0.607
Qwen3-4B-Instruct-2507	single-examples	0.558	0.607	0.606	0.689	0.607
Qwen3-4B-Instruct-2507	multi-examples	0.632	0.686	0.654	0.774	0.686
Qwen3-4B-Instruct-2507	single-zero	0.564	0.607	0.620	0.714	0.607

Table 19. Paired t-test comparison between the sampled subset and the full test set, based on a complete run with Mistral small. This comparison was used to validate that the subset used for all model evaluations serves as a representative proxy for the full dataset. A negative difference indicates the reduced set underperforms the full set. Significance level $\alpha = 0.05$. Note that p-values of $p < 0.05$ are marked with * and Δ = Reduced – Full.

Dataset	Metric	Reduced	Full	Δ	p-value
CDR	F1 Macro	0.4003	0.4290	−0.0287	0.228
	F1 Micro	0.4842	0.5388	−0.0546	0.178
	Accuracy	0.4842	0.5388	−0.0546	0.178
	Precision	0.3999	0.3825	+0.0174	0.032*
	Recall	0.6145	0.6549	−0.0403	0.090
BioRED	F1 Macro	0.6119	0.6528	−0.0409	0.101
	F1 Micro	0.6476	0.7086	−0.0609	0.062
	Accuracy	0.6476	0.7086	−0.0609	0.062
	Precision	0.6546	0.6666	−0.0120	0.279
	Recall	0.7555	0.7917	−0.0362	0.089

The reduced test set yields comparable or lower performance than the full test set across the majority of metrics and datasets. The one statistically significant difference detected (CDR, Precision, p = 0.03) showed the reduced set slightly outperforming the full set by a small margin (+0.017), indicating that deviations from the full set do not result in inflated performance estimates. We therefore treat the reduced test set as a valid proxy for evaluation.

Dynamic Literal Creation for Structured Output Validation

Overview. This implementation shown below ensures that language models return complete structured outputs by dynamically creating type-constrained models using Pydantic. By leveraging Python's `Literal` types, the function guarantees that every expected entity pair receives a classification, preventing the model from omitting required answers.

Listing 1.1. Dynamic Structured Output Builder with Literal Types

```
def build_structured_output_for_prompt(prompt: str):
"""
Constructs a Pydantic model that enforces complete responses
for all entity pairs extracted from the input prompt.

Args:
prompt: Input text containing entity pairs to classify

Returns:
A dynamically created Pydantic model class with required
```

```
fields for each entity pair
"""

# Extract entity pairs from the prompt that need classification
entity_pairs = extract_entity_pairs_for_literals(prompt)

# Define the finite set of possible relationship classifications
# Using a simplified binary classification for demonstration
possible_answers = ["No_Relation", "CID"]

# Alternative multi-class configurations (commented):
# Full relation set for biomedical entity relationships:
# possible_answers = ['Association', 'Positive_Correlation',
#                     'Negative_Correlation', 'No_Relation',
#                     'Cotreatment', 'Drug_Interaction',
#                     'Bind', 'Comparison', 'Conversion']

# Create individual Pydantic models for each entity pair
entry_models = []

for i, (entity1, entity2) in enumerate(entity_pairs):
# Define fields with Literal types to constrain values
fields = {
        # Entity1 must exactly match the first entity string
        'Entity1': (Literal[entity1], ...),

        # Entity2 must exactly match the second entity string
        'Entity2': (Literal[entity2], ...),

        # Free-text explanation for the classification
        'reason': (str, ...),

        # Relation must be one of the predefined categories
        # The * operator unpacks possible_answers into Literal
        'relation': (Literal[*possible_answers], ...)
}

# Dynamically create a uniquely named model for this pair
entry_model = create_model(
f'RelationEntry_{i}',  # Unique class name
**fields                # Unpack field definitions
)

entry_models.append(entry_model)

# Construct the final container model with required fields
# for each entity pair, preventing partial responses
relation_fields = {}

for i, model in enumerate(entry_models):
# Each relation field is required (denoted by ...)
# ensuring the model cannot omit any entity pair
relation_fields[f'relation_{i}'] = (model, ...)

# Create the top-level model that enforces completeness
RelationDict = create_model('RelationDict', **relation_fields)

return RelationDict
```

References

1. Ohse, J., et al.: Zero-shot strike: testing the generalisation capabilities of out-of-the-box LLM models for depression detection. Comput. Speech Lang. **88**, 101663 (2024). https://doi.org/10.1016/j.csl.2024.101663. https://www.sciencedirect.com/science/article/pii/S0885230824000469
2. Cahyawijaya, S., Lovenia, H., Fung, P.: LLMs are few-shot in-context low-resource language learners (2024). https://arxiv.org/abs/2403.16512
3. Zhao, W.X., et al.: A survey of large language models (2025). https://arxiv.org/abs/2303.18223
4. Chen, Q., et al.: Benchmarking large language models for biomedical natural language processing applications and recommendations. Nat. Commun. **16**(1) (2025). https://doi.org/10.1038/s41467-025-56989-2
5. Hu, Y., et al.: Improving large language models for clinical named entity recognition via prompt engineering (2024). https://arxiv.org/abs/2303.16416
6. Luo, L., Lai, P.T., Wei, C.H., Arighi, C.N., Lu, Z.: Biored: a rich biomedical relation extraction dataset. Briefings Bioinform. **23**(5) (2022). https://doi.org/10.1093/bib/bbac282
7. Li, J., et al.: Biocreative V CDR task corpus: a resource for chemical disease relation extraction. Database **2016**, baw068 (2016). https://doi.org/10.1093/database/baw068
8. Peng, Y., Yan, S., Lu, Z.: Transfer learning in biomedical natural language processing: an evaluation of BERT and ELMO on ten benchmarking datasets (2019). https://arxiv.org/abs/1906.05474
9. Verga, P., Strubell, E., McCallum, A.: Simultaneously self-attending to all mentions for full-abstract biological relation extraction (2018). https://arxiv.org/abs/1802.10569
10. Lee, J., et al.: Biobert: a pre-trained biomedical language representation model for biomedical text mining. Bioinformatics **36**(4), 1234–1240 (2019). https://doi.org/10.1093/bioinformatics/btz682
11. Gu, Y., et al.: Domain-specific language model pretraining for biomedical natural language processing. ACM Trans. Comput. Healthc. **3**(1), 1–23 (2021). https://doi.org/10.1145/3458754
12. Kanjirangat, V., Rinaldi, F.: Enhancing biomedical relation extraction with transformer models using shortest dependency path features and triplet information. J. Biomed. Inform. **122**, 103893 (2021). https://doi.org/10.1016/j.jbi.2021.103893. https://www.sciencedirect.com/science/article/pii/S1532046421002227
13. Wadhwa, S., Amir, S., Wallace, B.: Revisiting relation extraction in the era of large language models. In: Proceedings of the Annual Meeting of the Association for Computational Linguistics, vol. 2023, pp. 15566–15589 (2023). https://doi.org/10.18653/v1/2023.acl-long.868
14. Dagdelen, J., et al.: Structured information extraction from scientific text with large language models. Nat. Commun. **15**(1), 1418 (2024). https://doi.org/10.1038/s41467-024-45563-x
15. Agrawal, M., Hegselmann, S., Lang, H., Kim, Y., Sontag, D.: Large language models are few-shot clinical information extractors (2022). https://arxiv.org/abs/2205.12689
16. Gilardi, F., Alizadeh, M., Kubli, M.: Chatgpt outperforms crowd workers for text-annotation tasks. Proc. Natl. Acad. Sci. **120**(30) (2023). https://doi.org/10.1073/pnas.2305016120

17. Atil, B., et al.: Non-determinism of "deterministic" LLM settings (2025). https://arxiv.org/abs/2408.04667
18. Islamaj, R., et al.: The overview of the biored (biomedical relation extraction dataset) track at biocreative VIII. Database **2024**, baae069 (2024). https://doi.org/10.1093/database/baae069
19. Lai, P.T., Wei, C.H., Tian, S., Leaman, R., Lu, Z.: Enhancing biomedical relation extraction with directionality. Bioinformatics **41**(Suppl. 1), i68–i76 (2025). https://doi.org/10.1093/bioinformatics/btaf226
20. Zhang, Y., Peng, J., Cheng, B., Liu, Y., Jiang, C.: MMR: a multi-view merge representation model for chemical-disease relation extraction. Comput. Biol. Chem. **110**, 108063 (2024). https://doi.org/10.1016/j.compbiolchem.2024.108063. https://www.sciencedirect.com/science/article/pii/S1476927124000513
21. OpenAI: GPT-4.1 technical report (2025), version 2025-04-14. https://platform.openai.com/docs/models/gpt-4.1
22. OpenAI: GPT-4.1-mini technical report (2025), version 2025-04-14. https://platform.openai.com/docs/models/gpt-4.1-mini
23. OpenAI: GPT-5-mini technical report (medium) (2025), version 2025-08-07. https://platform.openai.com/docs/models/gpt-5-mini
24. OpenAI: GPT-5-mini technical report (low) (2025), version 2025-08-07. https://platform.openai.com/docs/models/gpt-5-mini
25. Mistral AI: Mistral large model release (2025), version 2512. https://docs.mistral.ai/models/mistral-large-3-25-12
26. Mistral AI: Mistral medium model release (2025), version 2508. https://docs.mistral.ai/models/mistral-medium-3-1-25-08
27. Mistral AI: Mistral small model release (2025), version 2506. https://docs.mistral.ai/models/mistral-small-3-2-25-06
28. Llama 3 model releases (2025), version 2506. https://www.llama.com/models/llama-3/
29. Mistral AI: Mistral small model release (2025), version 2506. https://docs.mistral.ai/models
30. Qwen-3: Qwen-3 model release (2025), version 2506. https://qwen-3.com/en
31. He, H., Lab, T.M.: Defeating nondeterminism in LLM inference. Thinking Machines Lab: Connectionism (2025). https://doi.org/10.64434/tml.20250910. https://thinkingmachines.ai/blog/defeating-nondeterminism-in-llm-inference/
32. Lai, P.T., Wei, C.H., Luo, L., Chen, Q., Lu, Z.: Biorex: improving biomedical relation extraction by leveraging heterogeneous datasets (2023). https://arxiv.org/abs/2306.11189
33. Coda-Forno, J., Binz, M., Akata, Z., Botvinick, M., Wang, J., Schulz, E.: Meta-in-context learning in large language models. In: Oh, A., Naumann, T., Globerson, A., Saenko, K., Hardt, M., Levine, S. (eds.) Advances in Neural Information Processing Systems, vol. 36, pp. 65189–65201. Curran Associates, Inc. (2023). https://proceedings.neurips.cc/paper_files/paper/2023/file/cda04d7ea67ea1376bf8c6962d8541e0-Paper-Conference.pdf
34. Reif, Y., Schwartz, R.: Beyond performance: quantifying and mitigating label bias in LLMs (2024). https://arxiv.org/abs/2405.02743
35. Ma, H., et al.: Fairness-guided few-shot prompting for large language models. In: Oh, A., Naumann, T., Globerson, A., Saenko, K., Hardt, M., Levine, S. (eds.) Advances in Neural Information Processing Systems, vol. 36, pp. 43136–43155. Curran Associates, Inc. (2023). https://proceedings.neurips.cc/paper_files/paper/2023/file/8678da90126aa58326b2fc0254b33a8c-Paper-Conference.pdf

36. Goel, A., et al.: LLMs accelerate annotation for medical information extraction. In: Hegselmann, S., et al. (eds.) Proceedings of the 3rd Machine Learning for Health Symposium. Proceedings of Machine Learning Research, vol. 225, pp. 82–100. PMLR (2023). https://proceedings.mlr.press/v225/goel23a.html
37. OpenAI: GPT-5.2 technical report (2025), version 2025-12-11. https://openai.com/index/introducing-gpt-5-2/

AI-Assisted Documentation in Social Welfare Services: Insights from a Pilot Conducted in the Wellbeing Services County of North Ostrobothnia

Niko Korhonen[1(✉)], Jarmo Reponen[2], Timo Alalääkkölä[1], Aappo Keränen[1], Jaana Kokko[1], Roni Huhta[3], Joonas Haataja[1], Tenho Moilanen[1], Miika T. Nieminen[1,2], Mikko Reinikka[1], and Heikki Mikkonen[1]

[1] Wellbeing Services County of North Ostrobothnia, Oulu, Finland
niko.korhonen@pohde.fi
[2] Research Unit of Health Sciences and Technology, University of Oulu, Oulu, Finland
[3] ESKO Systems Ltd, Oulu, Finland

Abstract. Artificial intelligence (AI) and large language models (LLMs) are increasingly explored as tools to reduce administrative burden in health and social care. In Finland, wellbeing services counties carry extensive responsibilities for organizing social welfare and healthcare services, including documentation practices that are often time-consuming, complex, and essential for service quality. While LLM applications have progressed rapidly in healthcare settings, experimentation within social welfare work remains limited. This paper reports findings from a pilot conducted in the wellbeing services county of North Ostrobothnia, where a generative AI–based documentation tool was tested by social welfare professionals. The results indicate improvements in documentation efficiency, uniformity, and interaction quality, but also highlight ethical, legal, and sociotechnical challenges concerning data protection, transparency, professional accountability, and contextual applicability. The pilot suggests that LLMs can support social welfare practice when implemented responsibly, with strong professional oversight and attention to contextual factors.

Keywords: Social welfare · Artificial intelligence · Large language models · Documentation · Digitalization

1 Introduction

The use of artificial intelligence in health and social care has expanded rapidly, and new application areas are continuously being explored. In healthcare, large language models have been used to structure clinical text and streamline workflows, often following an "augmented intelligence" principle in which professionals retain decision-making authority [1]. In social welfare, comparable initiatives remain limited, even though documentation is a core element of client work and directly influences service safety. Studies

M. Särestöniemi et al. (Eds.): NCDHWS 2026, CCIS 3010, pp. 644–647, 2026.
https://doi.org/10.1007/978-3-032-28819-6_40

have identified shortcomings in social welfare documentation [2], and national assessments have noted the potential of AI applications to support social welfare professionals [3]. Sociotechnical systems theory, which conceptualizes social and technical elements as an integrated whole, provides a useful framework for examining technological solutions in social welfare [4]. High-quality knowledge production in social work relies on professional expertise and its integration with technological systems [5].

Following the 2023 social and healthcare reform in Finland, wellbeing services counties became responsible for organizing both social and healthcare services. This shared responsibility also entails a unified digital environment in which documentation practices and technological solutions span both sectors. The AI-assisted documentation pilot is situated within this broader context, where integration enables consistent development pathways.

The aim of the pilot was to investigate *how an AI-assisted documentation tool can support social workers' documentation practices and what limitations may arise in client-facing work.*

2 Materials and Methods

The pilot was conducted iteratively and collaboratively together with social welfare professionals and experts in digital solutions in May 2025 until February 2026. In total, 33 professionals from various social welfare service areas used the AI-assisted documentation tool in several dozen real client encounters. The tool records the encounter, generates a transcript using speech-to-text technology, and produces a structured draft through a large language model guided by predefined prompts. The draft is reviewed and edited by professional before being manually transferred into the client information system.

Some professionals used the tool in nearly all encounters, while others tested it only a few times. The participating professionals met monthly to discuss their experiences and further refine the prompts. During this period, seven co-development workshops were organized, in which users shared experiences and reflected on the use of the AI-assisted documentation tool. No separate survey instruments were used; instead, feedback was collected through facilitated discussions in these workshops. These meetings provided a forum for open dialogue between social workers using the application and the professionals responsible for its development.

During the development meetings, social welfare professionals simulated realistic client situations, and the AI-assisted documentation tool was used to produce high-quality simulated encounter records. The role of social welfare professionals was essential, as they were best positioned to evaluate which prompts produced documentation that met social welfare requirements. The development meetings collected user experiences and information about challenges encountered during the pilot. The developers received crucial information about system malfunctions and were able to improve the application based on user feedback. The development meetings provided a comprehensive overview of both the opportunities and challenges associated with using the AI-assisted documentation tool.

3 Results

The pilot demonstrated clear gains in documentation efficiency and quality. Professionals reported that the AI-assisted tool significantly reduced the time required for record-keeping and produced more consistent and structurally uniform documents across service areas. The reduced need for manual note-taking also improved the quality of client interaction, with both workers and clients describing encounters as more natural and focused. The tool was particularly beneficial in multidisciplinary child welfare meetings, where it helped capture complex discussions more comprehensively than simultaneous manual documentation.

Alongside these benefits, several limitations emerged. The desktop-only availability restricted usability in mobile work environments, and intermittent technical malfunctions occasionally disrupted documentation. Some professionals began to rely heavily on the tool after repeated successful uses, raising concerns about reduced critical oversight of AI-generated text. A small number of clients expressed ideological opposition to AI use, leading to the tool being omitted in those encounters.

Use of the tool varied between participants, reflecting differences in work contexts and personal preferences. Despite this variation, the accumulated number of AI-assisted encounters reached several dozen during the pilot period. Feedback discussed in the workshops consistently highlighted reduced documentation effort and improved focus on interaction, while technical limitations were identified as key challenges. Overall, the pilot suggests that AI-assisted documentation can enhance workflow efficiency and interaction quality in social welfare services, if issues related to technical stability, mobility, professional oversight, and client acceptability are adequately addressed.

4 Discussion

Based on the pilot, AI-assisted documentation can support the quality of social welfare records and reduce the workload associated with documentation. Co-development proved essential, as collaboration between professionals and technology specialists produced solutions that were both practical for everyday work and preserved professional accountability.

Key issues for further development include integration with client information systems, usability and reliability of the application, and enabling mobile use. This aligns with previous research indicating that the implementation of digital solutions is influenced by the technical maturity of the system and the characteristics of the operational environment [6]. Ethically sustainable implementation requires transparency, traceability, and human oversight—principles, also widely recognized in international guidelines [7, 8]. Because social welfare work often involves clients in vulnerable positions, it is crucial to ensure that the use of AI is conducted ethically, transparently,

and with full respect for clients' rights. At the same time, it is essential that deployed technologies are sufficiently mature to ensure smooth use and to meaningfully support the work of professionals.

This study has several limitations. The pilot relied on qualitative feedback collected during co-development workshops, and no structured questionnaires or time measurements were applied at this stage. In addition, usage intensity varied substantially between participants. Future phases of the project will address these limitations by incorporating structured user surveys and quantitative measures of documentation time and workload.

5 Disclosure of Interests.

The authors have no competing interests to declare that are relevant to the content of this article.

References

Matheny, M., Thadaney Israni, S., Whicher, D., Ahmed, M.: AI and human intelligence: augmented intelligence. In: Matheny, M., et al. (eds.) Artificial Intelligence in Health Care, pp. 17–18. National Academy of Medicine (2022).https://ehealthresearch.no/files/documents/Rapporter/Andre/2019-12-AI-in-Health-Care.pdf

Kääriäinen, A.: Dokumentointi osana asiakasturvallisuutta. Janus **30**(4), 392–406 (2022). https://doi.org/10.30668/janus.114678

Heinäsenaho, M., Virtanen, T., Hyttinen, H.: Sosiaali- ja terveydenhuollon digitalisaation pitkän aikavälin mahdollisuudet: Työryhmän loppuraportti. Sosiaali- ja terveysministeriö (2025). https://urn.fi/URN:ISBN:978-952-00-4245-5

Trist, E.L., Bamforth, K.W.: Some social and psychological consequences of the longwall method of coal getting. Human Relat. **4**(1), 3–38 (1951)

Salovaara, S.: Tietojärjestelmät osana sosiaalityön tiedonmuodostusta. Acta electronica Universitatis Lapponiensis **383** (2024). https://urn.fi/URN:ISBN:978-952-337-436-2

Haverinen, J., Keränen, N., Tuovinen, T., Ruotanen, R., Reponen, J.: National development and regional differences in eHealth maturity in Finnish public health care: Survey study. JMIR Med. Inf. **10**(8), e356 (2022). https://pubmed.ncbi.nlm.nih.gov/35969462/

Euroopan parlamentti ja neuvosto. Regulation (EU) 2024/1689 (AI Act) (2024). https://eur-lex.europa.eu/eli/reg/2024/1689

World Health Organization. Ethics and governance of artificial intelligence for health (2021). https://www.who.int/publications/i/item/9789240029200

Self-adaptive AI in Clinical Decision Support: A Systematic Review

Kavishwa Wendakoon(✉) and Nirnaya Tripathi

University of Oulu, P.O. Box 123, 90014 Oulu, Northern Ostrobothnia, Finland
{Kavishwa.WendakoonMudiyanselage,Nirnaya.Tripathi}@oulu.fi

Abstract. Clinical decision support and other medical software increasingly embed adaptive AI capabilities to personalize recommendations, manage uncertainty, and respond to changing clinical contexts. However, safety-critical deployment requires more than algorithmic performance: adaptive behavior must remain governable, auditable, and aligned with clinical workflows and regulatory expectations. This paper presents a systematic literature review of self-adaptive AI in medical software, synthesizing techniques, challenges, and socio-technical implications through a digital health systems lens. Following PRISMA and established software engineering guidance for evidence-based reviews, we screened 423 records and included 20 peer-reviewed studies. We categorize adaptation approaches (e.g., parameter tuning, model updating, context-aware policies, and human-in-the-loop mechanisms) and analyze how systems address key deployment concerns such as workflow fit, transparency, accountability, safety assurance, and post-deployment monitoring. Our synthesis highlights recurring gaps: limited reporting of governance controls for updates, insufficient operationalization of safety constraints during adaptation, and inconsistent treatment of auditability and clinician override. We conclude with a deployment-oriented research agenda for trustworthy self-adaptive medical AI, emphasizing constraint-aware adaptation, evidence/provenance practices, and socio-technical evaluation in real clinical pathways.

Keywords: Self-Adaptive Systems · Clinical Decision Support Systems · Digital Health Systems · Socio-Technical Systems · Trustworthy Medical AI

1 Introduction

Digital health combines software-intensive technologies such as mobile health (mHealth), telemedicine, remote monitoring, and data-driven decision support to improve healthcare delivery and efficiency [2]. In parallel, regulators have increasingly emphasized *medical software*, including Software as a Medical Device (SaMD) and Mobile Medical Applications, where software performs medical functions independently of dedicated hardware [1]. This shift reflects the expanding scope and impact of medical software on care pathways, clinical operations, and population health [2,25].

M. Särestöniemi et al. (Eds.): NCDHWS 2026, CCIS 3010, pp. 648–668, 2026.
https://doi.org/10.1007/978-3-032-28819-6_41

Within this landscape, self-adaptive artificial intelligence (AI) is attracting growing attention for clinical decision support [8]. Unlike static models that are trained once and deployed unchanged, self-adaptive AI is designed to operate under evolving clinical context and streaming data, where patient state, data quality, and workflow conditions can change rapidly [5]. In principle, these properties can make healthcare software more resilient and context-aware; in practice, however, safety-critical deployment raises hard software engineering questions about integration, assurance, and governance (Fig. 1).

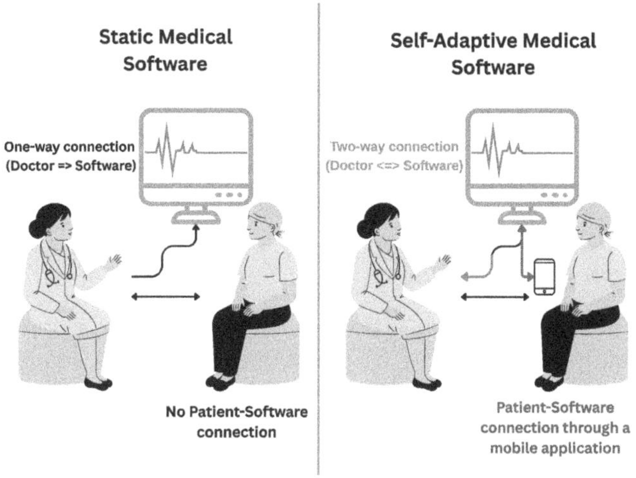

Fig. 1. Comparison between static and self-adaptive medical software.

1.1 Research Problem and Objectives

Despite rapid progress, deploying self-adaptive AI in real clinical environments remains challenging. Medical software must satisfy demanding requirements for security, privacy, and regulatory compliance, while operating within heterogeneous healthcare IT ecosystems [26]. Trust and adoption are further constrained by limited transparency, interpretability, and fairness assurances, especially when adaptive behavior changes system outputs over time [34]. In addition, adaptive capabilities must align with existing regulatory and assurance expectations for medical AI, including how updates are validated and governed across the product lifecycle [19]. Many clinical AI systems today remain effectively static in deployment, motivating continual monitoring and updating practices to maintain reliability as clinical conditions and data distributions shift [14]. Taken together, these issues highlight a core software engineering gap: how to engineer adaptive medical software that remains effective in dynamic settings while remaining trustworthy, auditable, and deployable within clinical workflows.

Accordingly, the objectives of this study are:

- To examine the evidence on self-adaptive AI techniques applied in medical software systems reported in the literature.

- To synthesize key technical, socio-technical, ethical, and regulatory challenges that hinder integration of adaptive AI into clinical workflows.
- To analyze reported benefits and impacts of self-adaptive AI in medical software across clinical, operational, and socio-technical dimensions.

1.2 Research Process

To address the study objectives, we formulated three research questions (Table 1) and conducted a protocol-driven systematic literature review (Sect. 3). The review searched six databases, Scopus, ACM Digital Library, IEEE Xplore, Web of Science, SpringerLink, and PubMed, and screened records using predefined eligibility criteria (Table 2), and synthesized evidence on adaptation techniques, deployment constraints, and reported outcomes. Backward and forward snowballing via Google Scholar complemented the database search. The final collection comprised 20 primary studies (Table 3).

1.3 Research Contribution

This review provides an engineering-oriented synthesis of self-adaptive AI in medical software. Specifically, it (i) characterizes the main adaptation mechanisms and software-engineering approaches reported in the literature, (ii) synthesizes the technical, socio-technical, ethical, and regulatory challenges affecting deployment and sustained use, and (iii) summarizes reported clinical, operational, and socio-technical impacts. The main contribution is a deployment-oriented perspective that emphasizes workflow integration, post-deployment assurance, and governance of adaptive behavior in safety-critical clinical settings.

2 Background Literature

Digital health has increasingly shifted care delivery toward software-intensive services such as remote monitoring, telemedicine, and data-driven clinical decision support [2]. In this context, medical software is no longer limited to supporting documentation and administration; it increasingly performs medical functions and influences clinical decision-making, including within SaMD and mobile medical applications [1]. As the clinical role of software expands, so do the engineering demands placed on these systems, particularly around reliability, safety, security, and lifecycle governance [2,25].

2.1 Self-adaptive Systems and Medical Software as a Dynamic Socio-technical Environment

Self-adaptive systems were originally studied to help software remain dependable under changing environments by embedding feedback loops that monitor system state, analyze conditions, plan adaptation, and execute changes at runtime [7, 23]. When applied to medical software, the "environment" is both technical and socio-technical: patient physiology evolves, data streams vary in quality and completeness, and clinical workflows differ across units, institutions, and contexts of care [5]. Consequently, adaptation in healthcare often concerns not only algorithmic updates but also the alignment of system behavior with clinical processes and human oversight.

A defining characteristic of self-adaptive AI in medical software is that adaptation occurs *during operation* in response to contextual changes rather than solely through offline development cycles [23]. This perspective is particularly relevant to digital health systems operating in dynamic settings (e.g., remote monitoring and telemedicine), where continuous data flows and evolving operational conditions can cause static models to degrade or become mismatched to clinical practice [5,14]. From a software engineering standpoint, this raises new questions about how to represent adaptation goals, bound permissible changes, and ensure that runtime updates remain safe, traceable, and clinically meaningful.

2.2 Self-adaptive AI Techniques in Digital Health

Clinical AI systems increasingly rely on machine learning and deep learning to support tasks such as risk prediction, triage, and patient monitoring, as mentioned before [8]. However, many deployed models remain effectively static after release, which can limit robustness when patient populations, measurement devices, or documentation practices change [14]. Self-adaptive AI seeks to address these limitations by enabling systems to adjust to new conditions through mechanisms such as continual tuning, context-aware reconfiguration, or adaptive optimization under operational constraints [5].

Importantly, self-adaptation in medical AI is not only a modeling choice; it is a *system design choice*. Adaptive behavior can be realized through a spectrum of strategies: from conservative adjustments (e.g., calibration or threshold adaptation) to more substantial updates (e.g., periodic model updates triggered by operational signals). In digital health deployments, these strategies must be engineered with explicit consideration of the surrounding clinical workflow, the availability and quality of data, and the practical realities of integration into healthcare IT ecosystems [26]. Thus, the literature motivates studying self-adaptive AI not merely as algorithms but as part of end-to-end medical software systems that must operate reliably in real-world clinical environments.

2.3 Trust, Assurance, and Regulation for Adaptive Medical AI

Because medical AI is safety-critical, adaptation introduces additional assurance challenges compared to static software. Clinicians and patients may be reluctant to rely on systems that behave as opaque "black boxes", especially if model behavior changes over time and conflicts with clinical judgment [34]. Beyond interpretability, concerns about fairness and transparency can hinder adoption when the consequences of errors or unequal performance are clinically significant [34]. These issues are amplified for adaptive systems because the basis for decisions may evolve, complicating accountability and oversight.

Regulatory and governance considerations further shape what types of adaptation are feasible in practice. Adaptive behavior must be aligned with applicable regulatory expectations and assurance standards, including how updates are validated, documented, and controlled across the software lifecycle [19]. At the same time, engineering constraints such as security and privacy requirements can limit how data is collected, shared, and used for adaptation, and integration complexity can obstruct the deployment of adaptive capabilities in real care settings [26]. Collectively, these factors motivate a software-engineering-centered view of adaptive medical AI: successful translation depends on the co-design of learning components and the surrounding mechanisms for monitoring, validation, and change management.

3 Methodology

We conducted a systematic literature review (SLR) to synthesize peer-reviewed evidence on *self-adaptive AI in medical software* and to examine how such systems are designed, deployed, evaluated, and governed in safety-critical healthcare contexts. The review followed PRISMA for transparent reporting [24] and Kitchenham's guidance for evidence-based software engineering reviews [22]. The process comprised planning, study selection, data extraction, synthesis, and validity assessment.

3.1 Planning

Scope and Operational Definition. The review focused on medical software systems that implement explicit *self-adaptive* or *autonomous* AI capabilities. To reduce construct ambiguity across disciplines, a study was considered eligible only if it reported a defined adaptation mechanism that changed system behaviour during operation or across deployment, such as recalibration, model switching, continual or online updating, or federated aggregation. Studies describing only offline retraining without an explicit adaptation loop were excluded. This conservative definition helped distinguish self-adaptive systems from periodically retrained static models [22].

Three research questions (RQs), shown in Table 1, guided the review and structured data extraction and synthesis.

Information Sources and Search Strategy. Searches were conducted in Scopus, ACM Digital Library, IEEE Xplore, Web of Science, SpringerLink, and PubMed to cover software engineering, computing, and health informatics literature. PubMed was included to strengthen biomedical and clinical informatics coverage.

Table 1. Research questions formulated in the study

Research Questions (RQs)
RQ1: What self-adaptive AI techniques and software engineering approaches have been applied in medical software systems?
RQ2: What technical, ethical, and regulatory challenges arise when integrating self-adaptive AI into safety-critical medical environments?
RQ3: What reported benefits and impacts of self-adaptive AI have been observed across clinical, operational, and socio-technical dimensions of healthcare delivery?

Search terms were derived from the RQs and refined iteratively through a scoping pass. The query was anchored primarily in RQ1 and combined self-adaptation terms, AI terms, healthcare or medical software context terms, and explicit update-pathway terms. A representative base query is shown below:

> ("self-adapt*" OR "self-manag*" OR "adaptive AI" OR "autonomous AI" OR "adaptive system*") AND ("artificial intelligence" OR "machine learning" OR "deep learning") AND (healthcare OR clinical OR "medical software" OR "clinical decision support" OR "patient monitoring" OR EHR) AND (recalibrat* OR "model switch*" OR "continual update*" OR "online update*" OR "runtime adaptation" OR "adaptive optimization" OR "federated aggregation")

Database-specific syntax and field restrictions were adapted per platform while preserving the same conceptual structure. Broad challenge- and benefit-oriented terms were not emphasized in the main query because these dimensions were addressed during screening and synthesis rather than primary retrieval.

Eligibility Criteria. Eligibility was defined using a PICO-inspired structure aligned with healthcare and software engineering review practice [22]. Table 2 reports the final inclusion and exclusion criteria.

Quality Appraisal. Given heterogeneity in clinical domains and evaluation designs, we applied a lightweight quality appraisal to contextualize the evidence [22]. Each included study was scored 0 or 1 on five criteria: clarity of the adaptation mechanism, clarity of the clinical setting and dataset, evaluation rigor, evidence of external validity, and reporting of deployment or assurance considerations. Total scores therefore ranged from 0 to 5. These scores were used to support interpretation rather than exclusion.

3.2 Conducting

Study Selection Procedure. The selection process followed the PRISMA 2020 stages of identification, screening, eligibility, and inclusion [24]. Screening

Table 2. Inclusion and Exclusion Criteria for Study Selection

Category and Criteria
Population/Setting
I1. Studies conducted in clinical or healthcare settings involving software-based solutions.
I2. Studies involving healthcare providers, patients, or healthcare software users.
Intervention/System Characteristics
I3. AI-based systems with explicit self-adaptation or autonomous behaviour via a defined update/adaptation pathway (e.g., recalibration, model switching, continual/online updates, federated aggregation).
I4. Adaptive AI systems implemented as medical software (e.g., decision support, monitoring, workflow support) or clearly positioned for clinical deployment.
Study Types
I5. Peer-reviewed journal articles, conference proceedings, or book chapters.
I6. English-language studies.
I7. Publications from 2019–2025.
Exclusion Criteria
E1. No AI/ML component.
E2. No explicit adaptive/autonomous mechanism as defined above.
E3. Grey literature (e.g., technical reports, theses, editorials).
E4. Full text could not be retrieved after reasonable attempts.
E5. Wrong population or setting.
E6. Non-English language.
E7. Wrong study design (e.g., review article, editorial, commentary, conceptual or perspective paper, or other non-primary study).

management, duplicate removal, and decision tracking were supported using Covidence systematic review software [31].

The database search returned 423 records in total. Covidence identified 134 duplicates automatically, and 3 additional duplicates were removed manually, resulting in 286 unique records for title and abstract screening. Screening and full-text eligibility assessment were conducted primarily by the first author using the predefined criteria and were checked by the supervisor. Borderline cases were resolved through discussion until consensus was reached.

After title and abstract screening, 28 reports were retained for full-text assessment and 258 were excluded. At the full-text stage, 16 reports were excluded for documented reasons: 10 were unrelated to self-adaptive AI in medical software, 3 had an ineligible study design, 2 could not be retrieved in full text, and 1 had the wrong population or setting. This yielded 12 studies from the database search.

To improve recall, backward and forward snowballing was then performed in Google Scholar on the included studies and key seed papers using the same eligibility criteria. Snowballing added 8 eligible studies, producing a final set of 20 primary studies. Following PRISMA 2020 terminology, records whose full text could not be obtained were treated as reports not retrieved [24]. Figure 2 summarizes the study selection process.

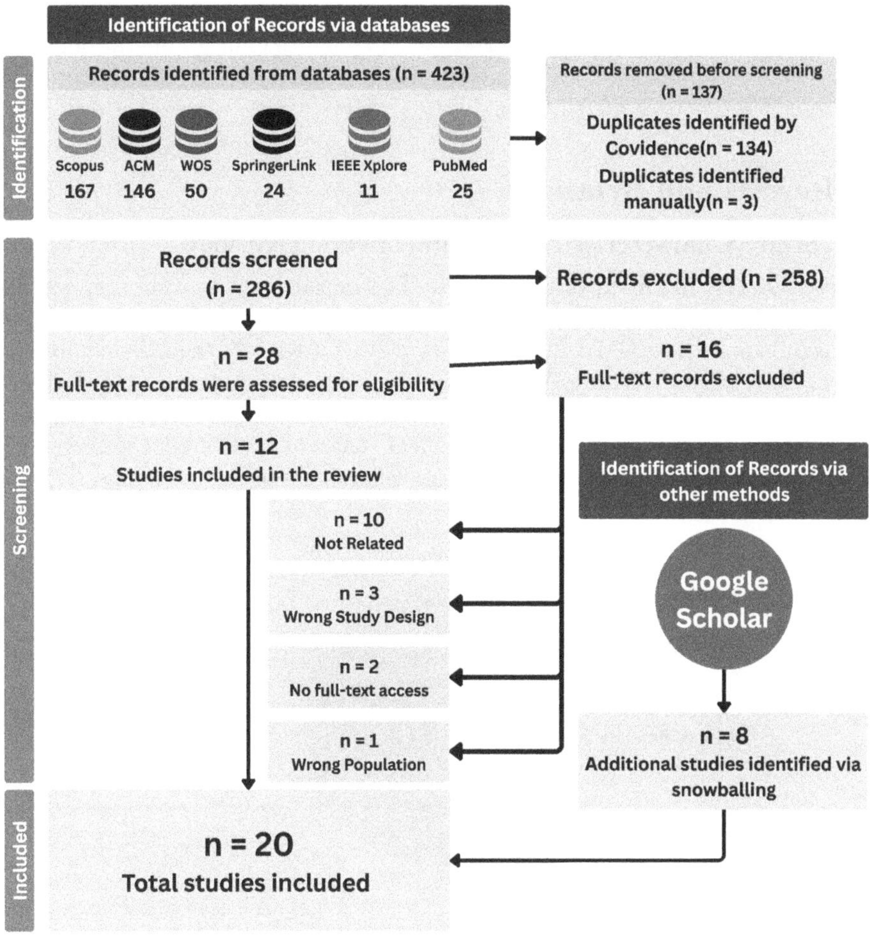

Fig. 2. PRISMA flow diagram of study selection.

Data Extraction. Data extraction was conducted primarily by the first author using a structured form aligned with the research questions. The form captured bibliographic information, clinical domain, adaptation mechanism, AI technique, deployment context, evaluation design, and the reported challenges and benefits. The form was piloted on a subset of studies and refined before full extraction. Extracted data were checked by the supervisor, and any uncertainties were resolved through discussion until consensus was reached.

3.3 Data Analysis and Reporting

We performed quantitative and qualitative synthesis following Kitchenham's guidance [22]. Quantitative synthesis summarized frequencies of technique families, evaluation settings, and challenge categories to characterize trends and evidence gaps. Qualitative synthesis used thematic coding aligned with RQ1-RQ3 to consolidate adaptation patterns and implementation approaches, integration and assurance challenges, and reported benefits across clinical, operational, and socio-technical dimensions. Bibliometric charts (Figs. 3 and 4) visualize publication trends and source distribution.

4 Results and Synthesis

4.1 Study Characteristics and Bibliometric Overview

Source Distribution and Retrieval. The initial identification step yielded 423 records from six indexing databases. As shown in Fig. 3, Scopus contributed 167 records and the ACM Digital Library contributed 146, together comprising 74% of all retrieved records. Web of Science (50), SpringerLink (24), PubMed (25) and IEEE Xplore (11) contributed the remainder. This distribution suggests that research on self-adaptive AI in medical software is strongly represented in computing and multidisciplinary venues, reflecting the software-intensive and cross-disciplinary nature of the topic.

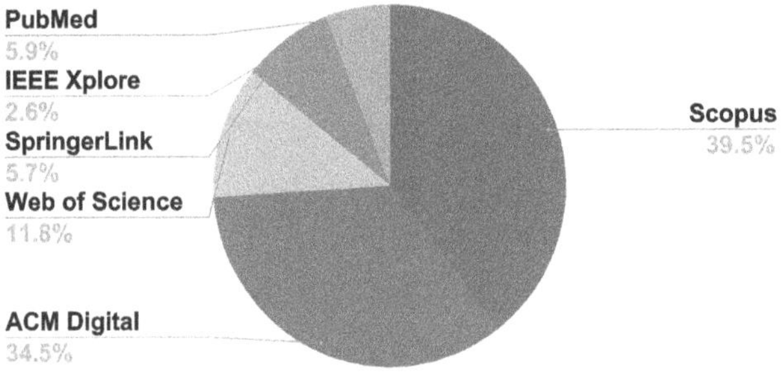

Fig. 3. Distribution of retrieved records by database during identification.

4.2 RQ1: Self-adaptive AI Techniques and Deployment Patterns

To support a deployment-oriented synthesis, the evidence was grouped by *adaptation pathway*, that is, by how and where behaviour changes are introduced into the medical software system. For concision, the reviewed studies are synthesized into three broad patterns: (i) autonomous AI services, (ii) federated learning and secure distributed adaptation, and (iii) optimization- and robustness-oriented adaptation strategies.

Table 3. Overview of Primary Studies

ID	Ref	Year	Source	ID	Ref	Year	Source
P1	[4]	2024	Scopus	P11	[3]	2023	Scopus
P2	[6]	2024	Scopus	P12	[9]	2021	Scopus
P3	[13]	2025	Scopus	P13	[17]	2023	WOS
P4	[18]	2020	Scopus	P14	[20]	2024	WOS
P5	[21]	2023	Scopus	P15	[30]	2023	Scopus
P6	[32]	2024	Scopus	P16	[37]	2020	Scopus
P7	[26]	2024	GScholar	P17	[27]	2024	GScholar
P8	[33]	2025	GScholar	P18	[34]	2024	GScholar
P9	[19]	2019	GScholar	P19	[12]	2024	GScholar
P10	[10]	2025	GScholar	P20	[11]	2020	GScholar

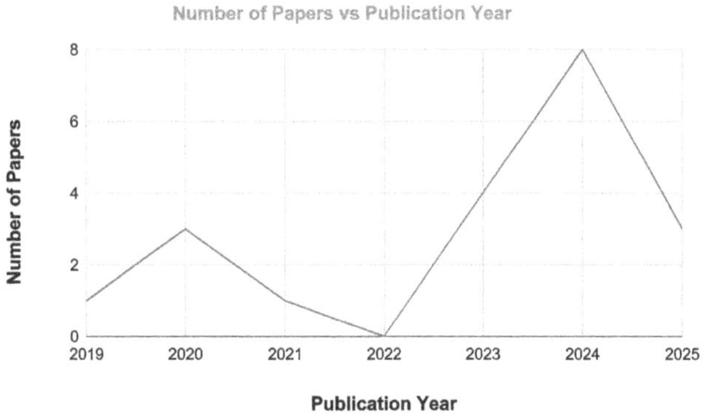

Fig. 4. Distribution of included studies by publication year (2019–2025).

Autonomous AI Services. The most mature and deployment-relevant evidence concerned autonomous AI services embedded into clinical workflows, particularly in diabetic eye disease screening [3,4,9,13,17,20]. These studies show an engineering pattern in which adaptation is bounded at the service boundary through mechanisms such as input-quality handling, workflow-specific decision rules, and implementation practices that support safe use in real clinical pathways. In this cluster, adaptation is not merely a model property; it is tightly coupled to deployment readiness, staffing, and operational integration.

Federated Learning and Secure Distributed Adaptation. A second cluster used federated learning to support cross-site model improvement without centralizing raw patient data [27,33]. Here, adaptation occurs across institutions rather than at a single point of care. The main contribution is therefore not only improved predictive performance, but also a distributed update mechanism that can preserve privacy while allowing learning across heterogeneous sites. Otoum et al.

further extend this pathway with blockchain-based integrity and provenance support, highlighting how distributed adaptation quickly becomes a governance problem as well as a learning problem [27].

Optimization- and Robustness-Oriented Adaptation Strategies. A smaller but technically diverse set of studies used reinforcement learning, self-aware optimisation, transfer learning, and self-learning or ensemble-based methods to sustain performance under constraints, domain shift, or non-stationary physiological signals [10,11,18,30,37]. Although these approaches differ in implementation, they share a common goal: adapting model behaviour when inputs, acquisition conditions, or operational contexts change. Reinforcement-learning-based work framed adaptation as iterative optimisation under constraints; transfer learning emphasized portability across imaging settings; and self-learning approaches focused on robustness through re-weighting, filtering, or ongoing parameter adjustment. Compared with autonomous AI services and federated learning, these studies are less directly tied to mature workflow deployment, but they broaden the range of adaptive strategies currently explored in medical software.

Overall, RQ1 indicates that self-adaptive AI in healthcare is not dominated by a single technique family. Instead, the literature suggests a continuum from tightly bounded workflow-embedded services to distributed and optimization-oriented forms of adaptation. The more directly adaptation affects clinical operation, the more important bounded change, monitoring, and implementation controls become.

4.3 RQ2: Integration, Assurance, and Governance Challenges

Across the included studies, the most persistent barriers were concentrated around deployment and lifecycle assurance rather than isolated performance deficits. For concision, these challenges are synthesized into four broader themes.

Data Quality, Heterogeneity, and Distribution Shift. Clinical data remain noisy, incomplete, and heterogeneous across sites and contexts, which makes adaptation difficult to stabilize in practice [11,12,33,37]. In self-adaptive systems, update pathways can amplify instability when incoming data are not comparable or when drift is poorly characterized. This is especially visible in federated settings with cross-site heterogeneity and in continuous monitoring scenarios where transient noise may be mistaken for meaningful change.

Operational Integration and Deployment Constraints. Several studies indicate that technically promising systems may still fail in practice if they do not fit clinical workflows and information infrastructures [17,21,26,32]. For self-adaptive AI, integration is more demanding than for static AI because downstream actors must cope not only with outputs, but also with the possibility that system behaviour evolves over time. Additional burdens such as model tuning, monitoring infrastructure, runtime complexity, and maintainability further increase deployment risk in healthcare environments where latency, uptime, and operational simplicity matter [10,30].

Assurance, Trust, and Governance of Change. Trust remains fragile when clinicians cannot understand how recommendations are generated or how they may change across updates [21,34]. In adaptive systems, accountability extends beyond initial model validation to questions of what changed, why it changed, and who approved or monitored the change. Several studies therefore emphasize governance issues around material change, re-validation, clinician oversight, and post-deployment accountability, all of which are especially important in safety-critical clinical settings [6,21,34].

Security, Privacy, and Fairness over Time. Privacy-preserving adaptation does not eliminate broader governance risk. Federated learning reduces the need to centralize raw patient data, but introduces new attack surfaces, coordination problems, and integrity trade-offs, particularly when augmented with mechanisms such as blockchain [27,33]. At the same time, fairness is not a one-time pre-deployment property in adaptive AI. Evidence from autonomous retinal screening shows that demographic variability and deployment conditions can affect equitable performance, motivating continuous subgroup monitoring and mitigation rather than one-off fairness claims [4,20].

Taken together, RQ2 indicates that the main bottlenecks are socio-technical and lifecycle-oriented. The challenge is not only to design an adaptive model, but to engineer adaptive medical software whose behaviour remains safe, interpretable, auditable, and operationally manageable over time.

4.4 RQ3: Reported Benefits and Impacts

The reported benefits of self-adaptive AI clustered into four main categories: clinical robustness, operational efficiency, privacy-preserving collaboration, and socio-technical benefits related to access, equity, and trust.

Clinical Robustness Under Heterogeneous Conditions. Several studies reported that adaptive mechanisms helped sustain or improve performance under variability, drift, or heterogeneous acquisition conditions [11,33,37]. In these studies, the key promise of adaptation was resilience: rather than assuming a static deployment environment, the systems attempted to remain usable when datasets, devices, or physiological signals changed.

Operational Efficiency and Deployability. The strongest operational evidence came from autonomous screening systems in diabetic eye care, where AI services supported increased throughput and reduced dependence on specialist availability [3,13,17,20]. In optimisation-oriented work, adaptation was also associated with improved efficiency or reduced computational overhead while maintaining acceptable predictive performance [10].

Privacy-Preserving Collaboration and Secure Distributed Learning. Federated learning studies reported benefits in enabling model development across institutions without centralising patient data, thereby supporting collaboration in settings where privacy constraints would otherwise limit adaptation [27,33]. Where secure provenance mechanisms were added, the literature also suggested potential benefits for integrity and auditability, although these came with additional complexity [27].

Access, Equity, and Trustworthy Operation. Autonomous diabetic eye disease screening studies reported expanded access to care, including in settings with limited specialist resources [3,13,20]. In parallel, work on bias mitigation and ethics assurance suggested that adaptive systems may support more equitable and trustworthy operation when transparency, clinician oversight, and monitoring are treated as part of the deployment architecture rather than as afterthoughts [4,21].

At the same time, the evidence base remains uneven. Some benefit claims are grounded in real-world or clinic-scale deployment, whereas others rely on narrower datasets, shorter evaluation horizons, or more constrained experimental conditions [10,30,37]. As a result, the most defensible conclusion is that self-adaptive AI shows clear promise, but sustained benefit depends on the presence of explicit governance, monitoring, and workflow integration mechanisms.

4.5 Cross-RQ Synthesis

A central finding across RQ1-RQ3 is that technique choice, reported benefit, and deployment challenge are tightly coupled. Table 4 summarizes this cross-RQ relationship. Autonomous AI services offer the clearest path to operational impact, but they also place the greatest pressure on workflow integration, fairness monitoring, and accountable oversight. Federated learning offers privacy-preserving collaboration, but turns adaptation into a multi-party governance problem. Optimisation-oriented, transfer-based, and self-learning approaches offer robustness and flexibility, but their practical value depends on whether safe update triggers, validation boundaries, and monitoring mechanisms are explicitly engineered.

In summary, the included evidence suggests that self-adaptive AI becomes clinically meaningful not simply when adaptation is technically possible, but when adaptive behaviour is *bounded, monitored, auditable, and reversible.* This is the key software-engineering implication of the review: the real challenge is not only to engineer adaptive models, but to engineer adaptive medical software systems that remain governable in practice.

Table 4. Cross-RQ synthesis linking technique clusters, benefits, challenges, and governance needs.

Technique cluster	Main reported benefits	Main deployment challenges	Governance needs
Autonomous AI services	Workflow efficiency, scalable screening, improved access, potential equity gains [3,13,20]	Workflow/EHR integration, fairness drift, clinician trust, accountable change management [4,17,34]	Bounded decision scope, audit trails, subgroup monitoring, explicit override and rollback pathways [6,21]
Federated learning and secure distributed adaptation	Privacy-preserving multi-site learning, cross-institution collaboration [27,33]	Site heterogeneity, coordination complexity, security and integrity risks [27,33]	Update authorisation, provenance, integrity controls, site-level monitoring, incident response [6,27]
Reinforcement-learning-based optimisation	Adaptive optimisation under constraints, potential efficiency gains [10,18]	Limited assurance of learned behaviour, computational burden, validation difficulty [10]	Validation gates, monitored promotion of updates, documented optimisation boundaries [6,34]
Transfer learning and self-learning robustness	Portability across settings, robustness under shift and non-stationarity [11,30,37]	Hidden domain shift, noisy updates, version-control burden, uncertain external validity [11,30,37]	Shift detection, re-validation triggers, versioning, safe fallback modes, continuous monitoring [21,34]

5 Discussion

This systematic literature review synthesized evidence on self-adaptive AI in medical software across 20 peer-reviewed studies, guided by three research questions: **RQ1** (techniques and engineering approaches), **RQ2** (integration, assurance, and governance challenges), and **RQ3** (reported benefits and impacts). Overall, the literature indicates growing technical maturity-including autonomous clinical AI services, federated learning for privacy-preserving collaboration, reinforcement learning for optimization, and transfer/self-learning strategies for robustness-alongside persistent barriers to real-world translation. Importantly, many barriers are not purely algorithmic; they are *software engineering and digital health implementation* problems involving clinical workflow fit, interoperability, post-deployment assurance, and accountable change management in safety-critical environments [7,21,23,34].

5.1 Key Findings and Implications for Digital Health and Medical Software Engineering

From Model-Centric Innovation to System-Level Deployment. The reviewed literature indicates a shift from retrospective model development toward deployment-oriented adaptive systems. Autonomous AI in diabetic eye care shows how adaptive software can be embedded into clinical pathways to improve throughput and reduce dependence on specialist availability [3,13,20]. Federated learning extends this shift to cross-site settings, where privacy and heterogeneity become first-order operational constraints rather than secondary implementation issues [27,33]. Together, these studies suggest that the key challenge is no longer only model performance, but sustainable deployment in real clinical ecosystems.

Integration and Post-deployment Assurance Remain First-Order Barriers. Across the review, the most persistent barriers concern workflow fit, interoperability, and assurance of changing behaviour. Studies on deployment and ethics show that adaptive systems must integrate with existing workflows, support traceable updates, and provide mechanisms for monitoring, verification, and rollback when performance degrades or conditions change [6,17,21,32,34]. Yet concrete governance mechanisms for post-deployment updates remain underspecified in much of the evidence base.

Trustworthiness is a Socio-technical Requirement. Explainability alone is insufficient to sustain trust in adaptive medical AI. The reviewed studies suggest that trustworthy deployment depends on clinician oversight, accountable governance, and continuous monitoring of subgroup performance as systems evolve [4,21,34]. This is especially important where adaptive behaviour may alter outputs over time and where fairness risks emerge across populations.

Privacy-Preserving Adaptation Creates New Governance Trade-Offs. Federated learning can reduce the need to centralize patient data, but it also introduces new security, coordination, and governance burdens. Cross-site heterogeneity can affect performance, while integrity-enhancing mechanisms such as blockchain improve provenance at the cost of added complexity [27,33]. Privacy-preserving adaptation should therefore be treated as a system-level design problem requiring explicit security controls and operational governance, rather than as a purely technical solution.

5.2 Study Limitations and Threats to Validity

Scope and Selection Bias. Our search focused on peer-reviewed literature in English (2019–2025) and excluded grey literature and non-English studies by design (Table 2). Despite multi-database searching and snowballing, selection bias may remain [22,24]. Additionally, included studies are concentrated in certain domains (notably ophthalmology and pediatric monitoring), which may under-represent other clinically important areas.

Construct Validity. Self-adaptive AI is inconsistently defined across communities. Some studies focus on architectural/runtime adaptation (e.g., federated learning under non-IID data), whereas others emphasize workflow or organizational adaptation. This heterogeneity blurs boundaries between self-adaptive systems and periodically retrained models [7,23,36]. We mitigated this risk using explicit eligibility criteria (Table 2) and protocol-driven coding aligned with Kitchenham's SLR guidance [22].

Internal Validity. Screening and coding involve judgment and the primary studies vary widely in design, datasets, and metrics, limiting direct comparability and increasing the risk of misclassification. Many studies report retrospective or single-site evaluation, reducing inference strength about generalizability and robustness [9,13,15]. We documented decisions and followed PRISMA to support transparent selection and reproducible reporting [24].

External Validity. Limited multi-site and prospective evaluations constrain generalizability, particularly in federated learning where non-IID data and infrastructure constraints complicate transfer to new sites [33,36]. Evidence of demographic performance variability further motivates caution when transferring autonomous imaging pipelines across populations [4].

Conclusion Validity. Heterogeneity of outcomes (e.g., AUC, sensitivity/specificity, workflow throughput) and study designs precluded meta-analysis; therefore, we relied on qualitative synthesis [22,24]. Publication bias is also possible, as negative results are less frequently reported.

5.3 Related Work

Prior surveys on self-adaptive systems provide cross-domain foundations. Wong et al. map how self-adaptive systems (SAS) research evolved across domains and quality attributes, and Gheibi et al. synthesize how machine learning can be embedded into Monitor-Analyze-Plan-Execute over a shared Knowledge base (MAPE-K) feedback loops (including online and reinforcement learning), emphasizing engineering concerns when coupling learning with adaptation [16,35]. These surveys are valuable but intentionally abstract away domain-specific constraints such as clinical workflow integration, regulated assurance practices, and data governance under protected health information.

A complementary line of work addresses definitional clarity and assurance. Petrovska et al. highlight the lack of consensus definition for self-adaptive systems and propose requirements toward such a definition, while Pekaric et al. review safety and security for SAS, emphasizing that adaptation mechanisms can introduce new hazards and attack surfaces [28,29]. Our review extends these threads by grounding synthesis in medical software and digital health translation: we connect adaptation mechanisms to clinical workflow fit, privacy/security constraints, fairness and trust, and lifecycle governance for updates-dimensions that are central to safety-critical deployment but peripheral in cross-domain surveys [21,34].

5.4 Implications for Practice and Future Research

The evidence suggests that progress in self-adaptive medical AI will depend less on isolated algorithmic gains than on system-level engineering of integration, assurance, and governance. We therefore distill four priorities for both practitioners and researchers:

1. **Design for workflow fit and bounded change.** Adaptive behavior should be integrated with clinical workflows from the outset and constrained to defined triggers, permissible update actions, and fallback states, rather than treated as an open-ended modeling feature [6,17,32].
2. **Make monitoring, oversight, and auditability first-class requirements.** Post-deployment monitoring of drift, data quality, and subgroup performance, together with audit trails, clinician override, and rollback mechanisms, should be engineered as core deployment controls rather than added after release [4,21,34].
3. **Engineer privacy together with security and governance.** Privacy-preserving adaptation, especially in federated settings, should be accompanied by explicit integrity controls, provenance, and site-level governance to manage heterogeneity and distributed risk [27,33].
4. **Strengthen the evidence base with longitudinal, multi-site evaluation.** The field now needs more prospective and multi-site studies with consistent reporting, subgroup analyses, and deployment-relevant outcomes to establish generalizability, fairness, and resilience across settings [3,4,20,33].

Overall, the review suggests that self-adaptive AI becomes clinically valuable when adaptive behaviour is bounded, monitored, and governable in practice, not merely when model updating is technically feasible [21,34].

6 Conclusion

This systematic literature review synthesized 20 peer-reviewed studies on self-adaptive AI in medical software and shows a transition from conceptual discussion toward early deployment-oriented systems. Across the reviewed evidence, self-adaptation is most clearly realized through bounded autonomous clinical services, privacy-preserving distributed learning, and robustness-oriented update strategies, with reported benefits including improved resilience under shift, greater workflow efficiency, and expanded access in selected settings [3,11,13,20,27,33,37].

At the same time, the main barriers to clinical translation remain engineering- and socio-technical rather than purely algorithmic. Recurrent challenges concern workflow integration, external validation, post-deployment monitoring, fairness oversight, and governance of model change in heterogeneous clinical environments [4,17,21,27,34]. Overall, the review suggests that self-adaptive AI becomes clinically meaningful when adaptive behaviour is bounded, monitored, auditable, and aligned with clinical accountability structures. The key implication is therefore not simply to make medical AI adaptive, but to engineer adaptive medical software that remains trustworthy, governable, and deployable over time [21,34].

Acknowledgments. This research is supported by FAST (Finnish Software Engineering Doctoral Research Network), funded by the Finnish Ministry of Education and Culture, and conducted as part of the doctoral program at the University of Oulu in close collaboration with academic and industrial partners.

Disclosure of Interests. The authors have no competing interests to declare that are relevant to the content of this article.

References

1. Digital health center of excellence | FDA. https://www.fda.gov/medical-devices/digital-health-center-excellence/software-medical-device-samd. Accessed 14 Oct 2025
2. What is digital health | U.S. food and drug administration (FDA). https://www.fda.gov/medical-devices/digital-health-center-excellence/what-digital-health. Accessed 14 Oct 2025
3. Abramoff, M.D., et al.: Autonomous artificial intelligence increases real-world specialist clinic productivity in a cluster-randomized trial. NPJ Digit. Med. **6**(1), 184 (2023). https://doi.org/10.1038/s41746-023-00931-7
4. Abràmoff, M.D., et al.: Mitigation of AI adoption bias through an improved autonomous AI system for diabetic retinal disease. NPJ Digit. Med. **7**(1), 369 (2024). https://doi.org/10.1038/s41746-024-01389-x. https://www.nature.com/articles/s41746-024-01389-x
5. Ahmed, Z., Pandey, A., Sharma, A., Tandon, A., Teena, Kumar, S.: Optimizing real-time medical diagnostics with adaptive ai algorithm. In: 2024 7th International Conference on Contemporary Computing and Informatics (IC3I), vol. 7, pp. 974–979 (2024). https://doi.org/10.1109/IC3I61595.2024.10828588
6. Aquino, Y.S.J., et al.: Defining change: exploring expert views about the regulatory challenges in adaptive artificial intelligence for healthcare. Health Policy Technol. **13**(3), 100892 (2024)
7. Bucchiarone, A., Mongiello, M.: Ten years of self-adaptive systems: from dynamic ensembles to collective adaptive systems. In: From Software Engineering to Formal Methods and Tools, and Back (2019). https://api.semanticscholar.org/CorpusID:203978721
8. Carrasco Ramírez, J.: AI in healthcare: revolutionizing patient care with predictive analytics and decision support systems. J. Artif. Intell. Gen. Sci. (JAIGS) **1**, 31–37 (2024). https://doi.org/10.60087/jaigs.v1i1.p37. ISSN: 3006-4023

9. Channa, R., Wolf, R., Abramoff, M.D.: Autonomous artificial intelligence in diabetic retinopathy: from algorithm to clinical application. J. Diabetes Sci. Technol. **15**(3), 695–698 (2021). https://doi.org/10.1177/1932296820909900
10. Chaudhari, P.A., Khot, S.S.: Alzheimer's disease prediction using CAdam optimized reinforcement learning-based deep convolutional neural network model. Biomed. Signal Process. Control **108**, 107968 (2025). https://doi.org/10.1016/j.bspc.2025.107968. https://www.sciencedirect.com/science/article/pii/S1746809425004793
11. Czako, Z., Sebestyen, G., Hangan, A.: Colorectal image classification with transfer learning and auto-adaptive artificial intelligence platform. In: Rocha, Á., Adeli, H., Reis, L.P., Costanzo, S., Orovic, I., Moreira, F. (eds.) WorldCIST 2020. AISC, vol. 1160, pp. 534–543. Springer, Cham (2020). https://doi.org/10.1007/978-3-030-45691-7_50
12. Desani, N.R., Jabbireddy, S.: Data engineering challenges in ai for healthcare. Int. J. Sci. Res. (IJSR) **11**, 1647–1652 (2024). https://doi.org/10.21275/ES22106103914
13. Esmaeilkhanian, H., Gutierrez, K.G., Myung, D., Fisher, A.C.: Detection rate of diabetic retinopathy before and after implementation of autonomous AI-based fundus photograph analysis in a resource-limited area in belize. Clin. Ophthalmol. **19**, 993–1006 (2025). https://doi.org/10.2147/OPTH.S490473
14. Feng, J., et al.: Clinical artificial intelligence quality improvement: towards continual monitoring and updating of ai algorithms in healthcare. NPJ Digit. Med. **5**(1), 66 (2022). https://doi.org/10.1038/s41746-022-00611-y
15. Gahane, S., Khode, P., Verma, P.: Adaptive AI algorithms for real-time monitoring and intervention in pediatric healthcare systems. In: 2024 5th International Conference on Data Intelligence and Cognitive Informatics (ICDICI), pp. 864–869 (2024). https://doi.org/10.1109/ICDICI62993.2024.10810812
16. Gheibi, O., Weyns, D., Quin, F.: Applying machine learning in self-adaptive systems: a systematic literature review. arXiv preprint arXiv:2103.04112 (2021). https://arxiv.org/abs/2103.04112
17. Goldstein, J., Weitzman, D., Lemerond, M., Jones, A.: Determinants for scalable adoption of autonomous AI in the detection of diabetic eye disease in diverse practice types: key best practices learned through collection of real-world data. Front. Digit. Health **5** (2023).https://doi.org/10.3389/fdgth.2023.1004130. https://www.frontiersin.org/journals/digital-health/articles/10.3389/fdgth.2023.1004130/full
18. Greenwood, N., Sundaram, B., Muirhead, A., Copperthwaite, J.: Awareness without neural networks: achieving self-aware AI via evolutionary and adversarial processes. In: 2020 IEEE International Conference on Autonomic Computing and Self-Organizing Systems Companion (ACSOS-C), pp. 147–153 (2020). https://doi.org/10.1109/ACSOS-C51401.2020.00047. https://ieeexplore.ieee.org/document/9196426
19. He, J., Baxter, S.L., Xu, J., Xu, J., Zhou, X., Zhang, K.: The practical implementation of artificial intelligence technologies in medicine. Nat. Med. **25**, 30–36 (2019)
20. Huang, J.J., et al.: Autonomous artificial intelligence for diabetic eye disease increases access and health equity in underserved populations. NPJ Digit. Med. **7**, 196 (2024). https://doi.org/10.1038/s41746-024-01197-3
21. Kaas, M.H.L., Porter, Z., Lim, E., Higham, A., Khavandi, S., Habli, I.: Ethics in conversation: building an ethics assurance case for autonomous AI-enabled voice agents in healthcare. In: Proceedings of the First International Symposium on

Trustworthy Autonomous Systems, TAS 2023, pp. 1–13. Association for Computing Machinery, New York, NY, USA (2023). https://doi.org/10.1145/3597512.3599713. https://dl.acm.org/doi/10.1145/3597512.3599713

22. Kitchenham, B., Charters, S.: Guidelines for performing systematic literature reviews in software engineering, vol. 2 (2007)
23. Krupitzer, C., Roth, F.M., VanSyckel, S., Schiele, G., Becker, C.: A survey on engineering approaches for self-adaptive systems. Pervasive Mob. Comput. **17**, 184–206 (2015). https://doi.org/10.1016/j.pmcj.2014.09.009. https://www.sciencedirect.com/science/article/pii/S157411921400162X
24. Liberati, A., et al.: The prisma statement for reporting systematic reviews and meta-analyses of studies that evaluate health care interventions: explanation and elaboration. PLOS Med. **6**(7), 1–28 (2009). https://doi.org/10.1371/journal.pmed.1000100
25. Majchrowski, B.: Medical software's increasing impact on healthcare and technology management. Biomed. Instrum. Technol. **44 1**, 70–4 (2010). https://api.semanticscholar.org/CorpusID:23675627
26. Maleki Varnosfaderani, S., Forouzanfar, M.: The role of ai in hospitals and clinics: transforming healthcare in the 21st century. Bioengineering **11**(4) (2024). https://doi.org/10.3390/bioengineering11040337. https://www.mdpi.com/2306-5354/11/4/337
27. Otoum, Y., Hu, C., Said, E.H., Nayak, A.: Enhancing heart disease prediction with federated learning and blockchain integration. Future Internet **16**(10) (2024). https://doi.org/10.3390/fi16100372. https://www.mdpi.com/1999-5903/16/10/372
28. Pekaric, I., et al.: A systematic review on security and safety of self-adaptive systems. J. Syst. Softw. **203**, 111716 (2023). https://doi.org/10.1016/j.jss.2023.111716
29. Petrovska, A., Erjiage, G., Kugele, S.: Defining self-adaptive systems: a systematic literature review. arXiv preprint arXiv:2505.17798 (2025). https://arxiv.org/abs/2505.17798
30. Vadsaria, A.S., Raza, A., Hammad, M., Shahid, M.F.: Self-aware AI-enabled medical system. In: 2023 20th International Bhurban Conference on Applied Sciences and Technology (IBCAST), pp. 1–6 (2023). https://doi.org/10.1109/IBCAST59916.2023.10712990. https://ieeexplore.ieee.org/document/10712990/. ISSN: 2151-1411
31. Veritas Health Innovation: Covidence systematic review software. https://www.covidence.org
32. Vidal-Alaball, J., Panadés Zafra, R., Escalé-Besa, A., Martinez-Millana, A.: The artificial intelligence revolution in primary care: challenges, dilemmas and opportunities. Atención Primaria **56**(2), 102820 (2024). https://doi.org/10.1016/j.aprim.2023.102820. https://www.sciencedirect.com/science/article/pii/S0212656723002536
33. Vieira, P., Maia, E., Praça, I.: Acute pancreatitis mortality prediction with federated learning. In: Progress in Artificial Intelligence, pp. 98–109. Springer, Cham (2025)
34. Weiner, E.B., Dankwa-Mullan, I., Nelson, W.A., Hassanpour, S.: Ethical challenges and evolving strategies in the integration of artificial intelligence into clinical practice. arXiv abs/2412.03576 (2024). https://api.semanticscholar.org/CorpusID:274514568
35. Wong, T., Wagner, M., Treude, C.: Self-adaptive systems: a systematic literature review across categories and domains. arXiv preprint arXiv:2101.00125 (2021). https://arxiv.org/abs/2101.00125

36. Xia, Y., Chen, S.: Dual aggregated federated learning with depthwise separable convolution for smart healthcare. In: ICC 2023 - IEEE International Conference on Communications, pp. 154–159 (2023). https://doi.org/10.1109/ICC45041.2023.10278978
37. Zhao, J., Zhao, D., Shi, L., Kuang, Z., Jing, W., Wang, H.: Multilayer weighted integrated self-learning algorithm for automatic diagnosis of epileptic electroencephalogram signals. Comput. Intell. **38** (2020). https://doi.org/10.1111/coin.12414

From Guideline to Gameplay: A Pilot Study on AI Simulation in Medical and Physiotherapy Training

Maija Paukkunen[1(✉)], Elina Rintamäki[1], Kari Sinivuori[1], Eveliina Heikkala[1,2], Juhani Määttä[1,3], and Jaro Karppinen[1]

[1] Research Unit of Health Sciences and Technology, University of Oulu, Oulu, Finland
maija.paukkunen@oulu.fi
[2] Wellbeing Services County of Lapland, Oulu, Finland
[3] Wellbeing Services County of Northern-Ostrobothnia, Oulu, Finland

Abstract. Background: We designed an educational simulation, 'MediCampus AI', using a large language model with Retrieval-Augmented Generation to replicate realistic clinical scenarios aligned with evidence-based Current Care Guideline (CCG). We piloted the simulation to assess its usability for supporting clinical reasoning, patient interaction, and CCG implementation in medical and physiotherapy education. Methods: We used Educational Design Research method to develop artificial intelligence (AI)-based simulation prototype. Medical and physiotherapy students ($n = 11$) were randomized into simulation (SG) and traditional case-based learning groups (TG). User experiences and implementation determinants were measured with study-specific questions, the Determinants of Implementation Behavior Questionnaire (DIBQ-mp) rated using a 7-point Likert scale, and game-generated data. Results were reported as change in median scores before and after educational interventions. Open-ended questions were analysed using inductive content analysis. Results: A change in median scores in the DIBQ-mp items was observed in "knowledge" (+2 in SG vs. +1 in TG); "skills" (+3 vs. +1.5); "beliefs about capabilities" (+4 vs. +0.5); "beliefs about consequences" (+2 vs. +0.5); "social influences" (+1 vs. +0); "organization" (+3 vs. +1); "behavioral regulation" (+2 vs. +1); "intentions" (+0 vs. +0.5) and "innovation" (+0 vs. +1), "patient" (+1 vs. +1) and "innovation strategy" (+1 vs. +1). Four categories were identified from qualitative data: A) individually supportive game design; B) safe, scalable environment for future needs; C) content enhancements and D) usability/accessibility development needs. Conclusions: Virtual simulation seemed feasible for embedding CCGs into education. Compared with traditional case-based learning, the AI-based simulation showed greater improvements in most implementation determinants and supported competence and guideline-concordant behaviors.

Keywords: Clinical Reasoning · Education · Gamification · Generative artificial intelligence · Large language models · Practice guideline

M. Säreströniemi et al. (Eds.): NCDHWS 2026, CCIS 3010, pp. 669–686, 2026.
https://doi.org/10.1007/978-3-032-28819-6_42

1 Introduction

Clinical guidelines, such as the Finnish Current Care Guidelines (CCG), are important for enhancing quality of care. However, the mere existence of a guideline seldom changes treatment practices [1]. Moreover, guidelines rarely explain how to apply recommendations to individual cases through clinical reasoning and shared decision making with the patient, and these skills are still insufficiently practiced in professional training. When developing solutions for practical and complex educational problems, educational design research (EDR) is widely utilized [2].

Clinical reasoning is a core competence for healthcare professionals and essential for solving patient-specific problems [3]. This process can be described in distinct stages: assessing the patient's situation, collecting information, processing data, understanding the problem and establishing a diagnosis, setting goals, implementing interventions, evaluating outcomes, and reflecting and learning from the entire process. Learning games can be used effectively to practice clinical reasoning skills in medical education, and they are increasingly utilised to support such learning [3]. A single gameplay session has nearly doubled diagnostic accuracy among medical students and practicing physicians, with sustained improvements at three months [4].

Learning outcomes achieved with virtual simulation have been shown to transfer to patient cases involving similar problems [5] and increase learner satisfaction [6–8]. Large language models (LLMs) enable integration of a natural-language interface, dialogue, and interaction into learning games. However, existing educational games have largely overlooked the interpersonal interaction dimension [9], failing to provide tools for training communication and patient encountering.

This study aimed to design a simulation 'MediCampus AI' for teaching clinical reasoning and patient interaction, and to evaluate its usability both in medical and physiotherapy training as clinical reasoning is approached differently in these professions. Specifically, we aimed 1) to generate knowledge about user experiences to guide further development, and 2) to identify the determinants (e.g. knowledge, skills, intentions) of implementing CCG to improve educational value.

2 Materials and Methods

We describe an EDR process comprising: (i) orientation and design phase (collaborative designing of new utilizations of emerging artificial intelligence (AI)-based technologies and description of the software platform prototype); (ii) development phase (pilot trial with user groups); and (iii) retrospective phase (evaluation of learning outcomes and CCG implementation determinants with associated strategies to enhance with educational gaming). EDR was chosen for its pragmatic orientation and its aims to generate usable knowledge for improving educational practice. The evaluation was grounded in behavioral change theories, specifically Theoretical Domains Framework (TDF) [10] that is used to identify determinants to CCG implementation, linked to Behavior change wheel [11] to guide the selection of appropriate implementation strategies. The description of EDR is presented in Table 1.

Table 1. Educational design research applied in the study

Heading	Content
Problem context	Society-level: Globally, health systems face substantial problems with diagnostics and low-value care. A large proportion of patients' complaints concern the interaction during the clinical encounter Professional-level: Use of non-evidence-based practices Patient-level: Variable treatment outcomes Educational problems: Limited resources and opportunities for individualized feedback through traditional learning methods
Primary focus	Develop an innovative simulation to support clinical reasoning, patient interaction, diagnostic accuracy, and person-centered treatment decisions for medical and physiotherapy training
Intervention	'MediCampus AI' (educational simulation)
Knowledge created	Determinants of guideline implementation to inform strategies that enhance behavior change via educational gaming
Methods	Questionnaires; Learning analytics from gameplay
Scope	2024–2025, partial funding from Oulu University Innovation Centre
Practical contribution	An educational simulation for medical and physiotherapy teaching, comprising authentic clinical tasks aligned with clinical guidelines

2.1 Phase One: Orientation and Design Phase

Design Narrative. A multidisciplinary team including researchers, clinicians (physicians and physiotherapists) and software developers started the development project in 2024. The objective was to design an educational simulation using LLM (Open AI GPT-4o) and Retrieval-Augmented Generation (RAG) technology to replicate realistic clinical scenarios aligned with evidence-based recommendations. Following a review of existing simulations, we prioritized authenticity and alignment with clinical guidelines. The goal was to integrate problem-based learning elements into patient cases to create a context-rich learning environment (Supplementary Fig. 1).

The simulation was designed to foster clinical reasoning skills, including assessment, diagnostics, and treatment planning focusing specifically on 'Hand and forearm strain disorders' CCG [12], which was used as source data for simulation. Learners interact with diverse virtual patients including varying characteristics and personality types, each accompanied by structured assessment data and individualized treatment plans. The simulation allows learners to navigate cases independently or with the aid of pre-configured options, including the possibility of selecting unnecessary diagnostic tests to prompt reflection on low-value care, and thereby reinforcing critical thinking. The simulation provides case-specific feedback on patient–practitioner communication, diagnostic reasoning, and the appropriateness of treatment plans. AI generates varied responses on each playthrough, enhancing authenticity and replayability. 'MediCampus AI' virtual consultation flow: Patient intake → History taking → Physical examination → Investigations (if needed) → Diagnostics (+ differential diagnosis) → Management plan (patient education, treatment plan) → Feedback & reflection on above mentioned stages and patient encountering.

2.2 Phase Two: Development Phase

Data Collection. Recruitment took place via emails and posters between 5.-18.11.2024 for voluntary medical students at the University of Oulu and physiotherapy students at Oulu University of Applied Sciences. One week prior to the intervention, participants received instructions via email to familiarize themselves with the CCG together with a link to a pre-training Microsoft Forms questionnaire. This included background questions, study-specific items, and the modified Determinants of Implementation Behavior Questionnaire - multiprofessional version (DIBQ-mp) [13]. Sixteen DIBQ-mp items covering 11 TDF domains (Knowledge, Skills, Beliefs about capabilities, Beliefs about consequences, Intentions, Innovation, Organization, Patient, Innovation strategies, Social influences and Behavioral regulation) were rated using a 7-point Likert scale (1 = strongly disagree; 7 = strongly agree) at pre- and post-intervention. Feedback on the learning environments was also collected with three open-ended questions. Participants were randomly allocated to a simulation group (SG) or a traditional case-based learning group (TG). The SG was given two hours to complete simulations of four patient cases in smaller groups. The TG worked through four corresponding patient case scenarios over 1.5 h, followed by a 30-min feedback session led by an associate professor in physiatry, who gave a review of the correct diagnoses and the examinations that would have been appropriate in each situation. Training was free of charge. Participation was voluntary, written informed consent was obtained, and participants could withdraw at any state of the study. Research permits for this study were obtained from both the University of Oulu and Oulu University of Applied Sciences.

2.3 Phase Three: Retrospective Phase

Regarding quantitative analysis and statistical methods, demographic outcomes were summarized as medians and interquartile ranges. Within-group median changes from pre- to post-intervention were analyzed separately for each group, and P-values reported using the Wilcoxon Signed-Rank test. This non-parametric test was chosen due to non-normal distribution of the data. Analyses were conducted using SPSS statistics, version 29 (IBM Corporation, USA). For qualitive analysis and mixed methods, an inductive content analysis approach was applied to analyze the responses to open-ended questions [14]. The original expressions were extracted and open coded, named and grouped into subcategories based on content similarity and combined into generic categories, which were finally abstracted into main categories. Drawing on quantitative and qualitative findings, established elements of game-based learning, theory-informed knowledge, we explored how these components could be integrated to enhance the educational use of 'MediCampus AI'.

3 Results and Discussion

3.1 Quantitative Results

Of the participants, three (27.2%) were fifth-year and six (54.5%) sixth-year medical students, and two (18.2%) were fourth-year physiotherapy students (Supplementary Table 1). Simulation showed advantages in feedback supported learning, enjoyment and motivation, and was perceived as applicable for guideline-aligned training. Motivation to study was similar across groups. Students in SG reported that the visual design, game progression were clear, and rules easy to follow (Supplementary Table 2).

In SG, teams spend an average of 17 min solving a single patient case (range 8–24 min). The average mean overall rating provided by the game's feedback system was 3.4 out of 5 (range 3–4). The average cost of investigations conducted during the virtual consultation was €4.20 (range: €0–€42). Players arrived at the correct diagnosis in 70% of cases. The game provided feedback on: (i) communication (e.g., clarity and depth, experience of being heard, empathy and reflection); (ii) the accuracy and relevance of the diagnosis, (iii) concreteness and details of the treatment plan, (iv) the comprehensiveness of the patient guidance, and (v) support for treatment adherence. The feedback delivered by the game was appropriate and, in terms of content, consistent with the pre-specified design.

At baseline, the medians across the DIBQ-mp items were similar, with differences of no more than one scale point (data not shown). Eight of the 11 TDF domains showed greater median change in SG compared to the TG. These included: knowledge (+2 vs. +1); skills (+3 vs. +1.5); beliefs about capabilities (+4 vs. +0.5); beliefs about consequences (+2 vs. +0.5); social influences (+1 vs. +0); organization (+3 vs. +1) and behavioral regulation (+2 vs. +1). Conversely, greater median change was observed in the TG, compared to SG, in the following domains: intentions (+0 vs. +0.5) and innovation (+0 vs. +1). Results were equally good between groups for the subscales related to patient and innovation strategy (Table 2).

Table 2. Determinants of implementation behavior for Current Care guideline implementation. Bolded P-values denote statistically significant within-group differences between pre- and post-intervention.

Domain and construct	Simulation-based learning group (SG)		Traditional case-based learning group (TG)	
	Median change	P-value[1]	Median change	P-value[1]
Knowledge	**+ 2**	**0.034**	**+ 1**	**0.039**
Knowledge	+ 1	0.059	+ 0.5	0.096
Role clarity	+ 1		+ 0.5	
Skills	**+ 3**	0.102	**+ 1.5**	0.102
Skills	+ 1	0.102	+ 0.5	**0.025**
Skills	+ 2		+ 1	
Beliefs about capabilities	**+ 4**	0.066	**+ 0.5**	0.129
Self-efficacy	+ 1	0.059	+ 0.5	0.059
Perceived behavioral control	+ 3		0	

(continued)

Table 2. (*continued*)

Domain and construct	Simulation-based learning group (SG)		Traditional case-based learning group (TG)	
	Median change	P-value[1]	Median change	P-value[1]
Beliefs about consequences	**+ 2**	0.157	**+ 0.5**	1
Attitude	+ 1	0.180	0	0.655
Outcome expectancies	+ 1		+ 0.5	
Intentions	**+ 0**	0.317	**+ 0.5**	0.157
Intentions	0		+ 0.5	
Innovation	**+ 0**	1	**+ 1**	**0.046**
Innovation characteristics	0	0.317	+ 1	0.109
Innovation characteristics	0		0	
Organization	**+ 3**	0.276	**+ 1**	0.197
Organizational resources and support	+ 2	0.577	0	0.180
Organizational resources and support	+ 1		+ 1	
Patient	**+ 1**	0.783	**+ 1**	0.564
Patient characteristics	0	0.102	0	**0.046**
Patient characteristics	+ 1		+ 1	
Innovation strategy	**+ 1**	0.180	**+ 1**	0.059
Innovation strategies	0	0.194	+ 1	0.564
Innovation strategies	+ 1		0	
Social influences	**+ 1**	0.564	**0**	0.157
Descriptive norm	0	0.257	0	0.083
Social support	+ 1		0	
Behavioral regulation	**+ 2**	0.066	**+ 1**	0.024
Action planning	+ 2		+ 1	

[1] Wilcoxon signed ranks test

3.2 Qualitative Results

Four main categories were identified: AI simulation strengths were A) a game structure that supports the learning process individually, and B) a safe and scalable learning environment aligned with future needs (Supplementary Fig. 1). The development areas consisted of C) content-related enhancements, and D) usability and accessibility improvements (Supplementary Fig. 2). Students experienced interaction with virtual patients as credible and natural, encouraging learning communication skills. Simulation elements were perceived to support clinical reasoning with immediate responses to diagnostic questions, and evaluation and treatment of typical patient cases became familiar through repeated gameplay. The simulation was seen as suitable for novice professionals, also broader potential for use across various learner groups was recognized. AI simulation was described as a useful learning environment where practicing was realistic and safe. To better support learning, students recommended expanding the available examinations to allow for greater variety in clinical decision-making, and more complex patient cases. Usability and accessibility improvements included functionality, clarity of the user interface, and guidance.

3.3 Mixed Methods

To increase the ecological validity of edr-based knowledge and the likelihood that educational innovations will be used to transform educational practice, add pedagogical value and successful CCG Implementation, we present a description of future directions in educational simulation development that is based on our quantitative and qualitative results and behavioral change theories [10, 11] (Table 3).

Table 3. Mapping behavioral change techniques [11] matched with game features

Feature	Pedagogical value: Behavioral change and gamification techniques
1 Goals and planning	1.1 Problem solving: Challenges are proposed in various clinical cases 1.4 Action planning: Planning actions according to patient profile
2 Feedback & monitoring	2.1 Problem solving: Providing feedback based on clinical behaviors 2.4 Action planning: Monitoring and prompting clinical actions
3 Social support	3.2 Social support (practical): Opportunity for collaborative playing to support collaboration and knowledge building
4 Shaping knowledge	4.1 Instruction on how to perform the behavior: Evidence-based medical knowledge is demonstrated at the end of simulation 4.4 Behavioral experiments: Encouraging players to do experiments with virtual patients and to note whether the patients are grateful or annoyed
5 Natural consequences	5.1 Information about health consequences: Providing information about health consequences after performing clinical behaviors 5.6 Information about emotional consequences: Providing information about emotional consequences after performing various clinical behaviors
6 Comparison of behavior	6.1 Demonstration of behavior: Providing an example of the best practices that players can compare to the solutions
7 Associations	7.1 Prompts and cues: Immersion in the real world by enabling navigation within the appointment room, where the player can explore disorder-specific information and available assessment tools relevant to the patient's condition. Hints that are provided on request 7.7 Exposure: Enabling surprising events to unfold to enhance engagement through confrontation with a feared stimulus (hurry, lack of resources)

(*continued*)

Table 3. (*continued*)

Feature	Pedagogical value: Behavioral change and gamification techniques
8 Repetition and substitution	8.1 Behavioral practice/rehearsal: Allowing players to encounter pedagogically valuable and locally adapted hypothetical situations 8.7 Graded tasks: Presenting different game levels
9 Comparison of outcomes	9.1 Credible source: Receiving information by interviewing. Patient characters are distributed in the form of text, graphics, and audio
10 Reward and threat	10.10 Reward (outcome): Rewards are given at the end, depending on the accuracy and/or progress of the answers given
11 Regulation	11.3 Conserving mental resources: Providing pre-given options for patient history taking, assessment and treatment planning
12 Antecedents	12.1 Restructuring the physical environment: Using location awareness by putting simulation to the healthcare environment (visual observations)
13 Identity	13.3 Incompatible beliefs: Drawing attention to discrepancies between current behavior and evidence-based medical practice
14 Scheduled consequences	14.1 Behavior cost: Healthcare resource use triggers a reduction of virtual funds, simulating real-world cost implications of clinical decisions 14.2 Punishment: If a player selects unnecessary diagnostic tests or low-value care, the game may respond with a reduction in patient satisfaction score or a penalty in the performance rating 14.3 Remove reward: Removing rewards as a consequence of unwanted behavior, such as the use of non-evidence-based methods

3.4 Discussion

We developed and piloted an AI simulation that creates realistic patient scenarios for training clinical reasoning, decision-making, and patient–practitioner interaction. This is important because medicine requires not only technical proficiency but also human interaction and empathy [15]. In our pilot, the simulation was considered usable for medical and physiotherapy education, delivered personalized and immediate feedback, and supported guideline-aligned practice.

Our findings align with prior research showing that learning games can effectively support clinical reasoning and are generally motivating and acceptable to learners [3, 5–8]. Recent trial evidence suggesting that even a single gameplay session can substantially improve diagnostic accuracy [4] parallels our observation that simulation can target both cognitive and interpersonal skills. Extending these insights, our study demonstrates how

LLM–driven simulation can provide richer dialogue, context-sensitive feedback, and guideline-concordant prompts.

The simulation environment enables risk-free practice and iterative learning from error, with potential to replace resource-intensive physical setups and to discourage low-value investigations in real clinics. A need for risk-free training is evident to prepare students for real-world settings where enhancing patient safety is a priority. Additionally, AI-generated analytics can identify learning gaps to inform curriculum development, while aggregated de-identified usage data can reveal implementation barriers and guide theory-informed behavior-change strategies. To date, only a small minority of prior studies have based on the selection of game design elements on underlying theories, which has been suggested as a limitation in effectiveness assessments [16].

We situated this project within EDR pragmatic approach that iterates design, development, testing, and refinement to generate usable knowledge for improving educational practice. EDR is not a single method; it uses quantitative, qualitative, and mixed methods designs and requires the same transparency and evidential standards as other scientific research [2, 17]. Previous literature has presented 12 strategies to make gamification work in medical education [8]. 'MediCampus AI' meets most of them, including making learning fun, improving motivation, using experiential learning, feedback and technology, providing opportunities for repetition, ensuring sustainability and diversity. These elements support its usability also in larger transnational contexts and for the whole musculoskeletal field.

Strengths of this study include a multidisciplinary co-design and a pilot group involving both graduate-stage medical and physiotherapy students. The strength of the simulation is explicit mapping to guideline content. In addition, integration of behavior-change theory to link feedback to determinants such as knowledge, skills, beliefs about capabilities and consequences, has not been done before in the context of educational gaming. Limitations of this study include small sample size which limits precision and power. We also identified potential ceiling effects on DIBQ-mp domains in the SG. We did not assess long-term retention or transfer to clinical performance, nor did we evaluate cost-effectiveness. However, our primary aim was to evaluate usability.

4 Conclusions

AI-based simulation is a promising tool for teaching and training clinical reasoning and patient interaction while reinforcing guideline-concordant practice. Its updatability, personalized feedback, and potential for safe, scalable, and culturally adapted training make it a viable adjunct to traditional case-based teaching. It can be a feasible way to implement CCGs into education. A greater change was observed in most implementation determinants in the SG. It seemed to support students' competence and guideline-concordant implementation behaviors at least as well as traditional case-based teaching. However, further multi-site evaluations are needed to assess its value at scale.

Acknowledgements. We thank Mikael Karppinen, Eetu Huhtamäki and Jaakko Kujala for your invaluable technical expertise, all study participants, and the Finnish Medical Society Duodecim for permission to use the clinical guideline in this study.

Appendix/Supplementary Material

(See Supplementary Tables 1, 2, 6 and Supplementary Fig. 3).

Supplementary Table 1. Demographic characteristics

Characteristics	Simulation-based learning group (SG)[1] (n = 5)	Traditional case-based learning group (TG)[1] (n = 6)
Sex (female)	40% (2)	83.3% (5)
Educational field Medical student Physiotherapy student	80% (4) 20% (1)	83.3% (5) 16.7% (1)
Education level 4th year student 5th year student 6th year student	20% (1) 0% (0) 80% (4)	16,7% (1) 50% (3) 33.3% (2)
Time spent familiarizing with CCG less than 15 min 15–30 min 31–60 min more than 60 min	0% (0) 40% (2) 20% (1) 40% (2)	33,3% (2) 16.7% (1) 50% (3) 0% (0)

[1]Percentage (frequency); CCG = Current Care Guideline

Supplementary Table 2. Students' experiences on the learning environments

Question	Agree/Strongly agree % (n)	
	Simulation-based learning group (SG)[1] (n = 5)	Traditional case-based learning group (TG)[1] (n = 6)
This learning environment increased my motivation to practice assessment and treatment in line with the Finnish Current Care guideline (Käypä hoito) for ´Hand and forearm strain disorders´	80 (4)	66.6 (4)
The feedback I received supported my learning	80 (4)	50 (3)
I believe the learning environment prepared me well for real patient-counselling situations	80 (4)	100 (6)

(continued)

Supplementary Table 2. (*continued*)

Question	Agree/Strongly agree % (n)	
	Simulation-based learning group (SG)[1] (n = 5)	Traditional case-based learning group (TG)[1] (n = 6)
This learning environment was suitable for practicing the assessment and treatment of hand and forearm strain disorders	80 (4)	66.6% (4)
Studying in this learning environment was fun	60 (3)	33.3 (2)
I prefer to practice in this learning environment rather than with other methods	40 (2)	33.3 (2)
The learning environment motivated me to study	80 (4)	83.3 (5)
I would recommend this learning environment to my colleagues[1]	8.2	8.3
Game-specific items (simulation only)		
The game rules were clear and easy to understand	80 (4)	
The game's visual design was clear	100 (5)	
The simulated patients described their symptoms and answered my questions naturally	100 (5)	
This game was appropriately challenging for me	40 (2)	
Progression through the game was clear to me	100 (5)	
The game's visual design was clear	80 (4)	

[1] Percentage (frequency); [2] Mean

Supplementary Table 3. Determinants of implementation behavior (facilitators and barriers) for Current Care guideline implementation. Bolded P-values denote for statistically significant within-group difference between pre- and post-intervention.

Domain and construct	Question	Simulation-based learning group (SG)			Traditional case-based learning group (TG)		
		Post-intervention median (IQR)	Median change	P-value[1]	Post-intervention median (IQR)	Median change	P-value[1]
KnowledgeKnowledge Role clarity	I know how to deliver guideline-based intervention Objectives of guideline-based intervention and my role in this are clearly defined for me	6 (6–7) 7 (6–7)	**+ 2** + 1 + 1	**0.034** 0.059	6 (6–7) 6 (6–7)	**+ 1** + 0.5 + 0.5	**0.039** 0.096
Skills Skills Skills	I have been trained in delivering guideline-based intervention I have the skills to deliver guideline-based intervention	6 (6–6.5) 7 (6–7)	**+ 3** + 1 + 2	0.102 0.102	6 (5.8–7) 6 (5.8–7)	**+ 1.5** + 0.5 + 1	0.102 **0.025**
Beliefs about capabilities Self-efficacy Perceived behavioral control	I am confident that I can deliver guideline-based intervention For me, delivering guideline-based intervention is (very difficult – very easy)	6 (5.5–6.5) 6 (5–6)	**+ 4** + 1 + 3	0.066 0.059	5 (5–6) 5 (5–6)	**+ 0.5** + 0.5 0	0.129 0.059
Beliefs about consequences Attitude Outcome expectancies	For me, delivering guideline-based intervention is (not useful at all – very useful) If I deliver guideline-based intervention following the guidelines, this will strengthen the collaboration with professionals with whom I deliver guideline-based intervention	7 (6.5–7) 7 (5–7)	**+ 2** + 1 + 1	0.157 0.180	6.5 (6–7) 7 (6–7)	**+ 0.5** 0 + 0.5	1 0.655

(continued)

Supplementary Table 3. *(continued)*

Domain and construct	Question	Simulation-based learning group (SG)			Traditional case-based learning group (TG)		
		Post-intervention median (IQR)	Median change	P-value[1]	Post-intervention median (IQR)	Median change	P-value[1]
Intentions Intentions	How strong is your intention to deliver guideline-based intervention in the next three months? (not strong – very strong)	7 (7)	**0** 0	0.317	7 (6.75–7)	**+ 0.5** + 0.5	0.157
InnovationInnovation characteristics Innovation characteristics	It is possible to tailor guideline-based intervention to patients' needs? Guideline-based intervention is compatible with daily practice	7 (6–7) 7 (6.5–7)	**+ 0** 0 0	1 0.317	6 (5.8–6.3) 6 (6–7)	**+ 1** + 1 0	**0.046** 0.109
Organization Organizational resources and support Organizational resources and support	I expect that in the organization I will work, all necessary resources will be available to deliver guideline-based intervention I expect that I can count on support from the management of the organization I will work in, when things get tough around delivering guideline-based intervention	7 (4.5–7) 5 (4.5–6)	+ 3 + 2 + 1	0.276 0.577	6 (5–6.3) 6 (5–6.3)	+ 1 0 + 1	0.197 0.180
Patient Patient characteristics Patient characteristics	Patients consider participation in guideline-based intervention meaningful Patients of guideline-based intervention are positive about guideline-based intervention	6 (5–7) 6 (5–7)	**+ 1** 0 + 1	0.783 0.102	6 (5.3–6.3) 6 (5.3–6.3)	**+ 1** 0 + 1	0.564 **0.046**

(continued)

Supplementary Table 3. *(continued)*

Domain and construct	Question	Simulation-based learning group (SG)			Traditional case-based learning group (TG)		
		Post-intervention median (IQR)	Median change	P-value[1]	Post-intervention median (IQR)	Median change	P-value[1]
Innovation strategy Innovation strategies Innovation strategies	My study program provides training to deliver guideline-based intervention CCG provides sufficient intervention instructions and materials	6 (5.5–6.5) 7 (6.5–7)	**+1** 0 +1	0.180 0.194	6 (4.5–6.3) 6 (5.75–7)	**+1** +1 0	0.059 0.564
Social influences Descriptive norm Social support	Professionals with whom I deliver guideline-based intervention deliver guideline-based intervention following the guidelines I can count on support from professionals with whom I deliver guideline-based intervention when things get tough around delivering guideline-based intervention	6 (6–6.5) 6 (6–6.5)	**+1** 0 +1	0.564 0.257	6.5 (6–7) 6 (6–7)	**0** 0 0	0.157 0.083
Behavioral regulation Action planning	I have a clear plan of how I will deliver guideline-based intervention	6 (6–7)	**+2** +2	0.066	5.5 (5–7)	**+1** +1	0.024

[1] Wilcoxon signed ranks test; NS = non-significant; CCG = Current Care guideline

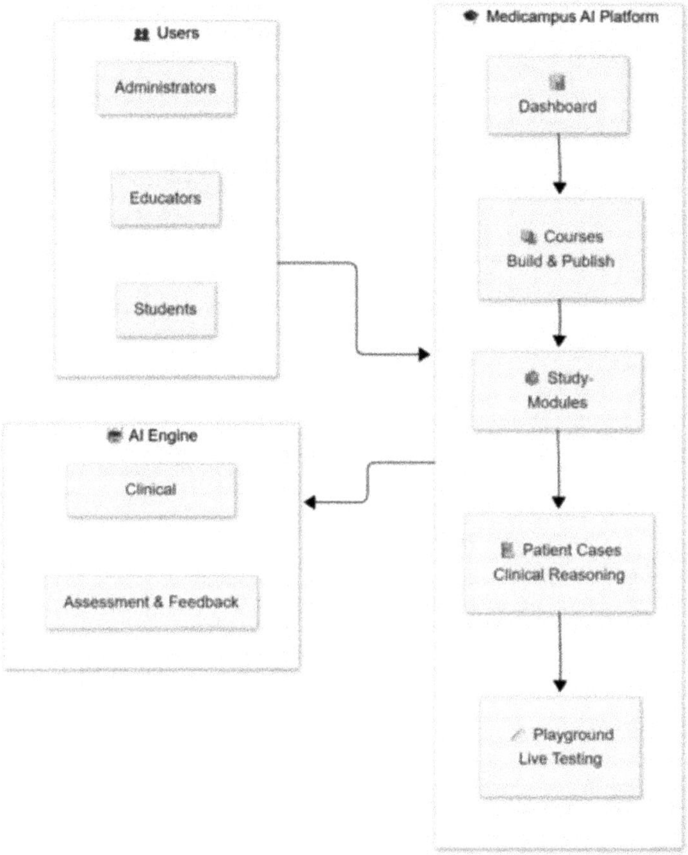

Supplementary Fig. 1. 'MediCampus AI' platform for AI-based education and learning

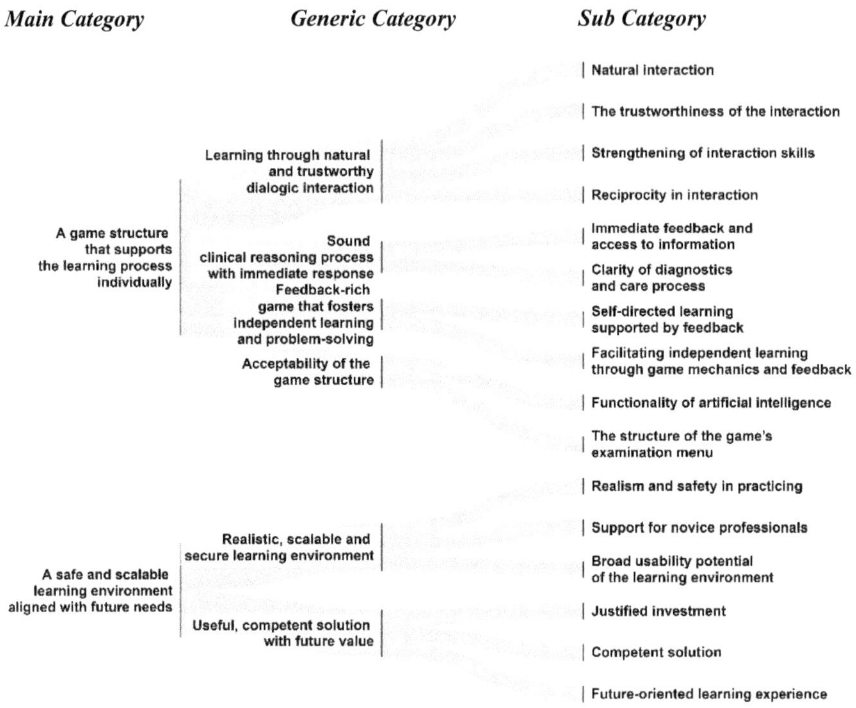

Supplementary Fig. 2. Strengths of the 'MediCampus AI' learning environment

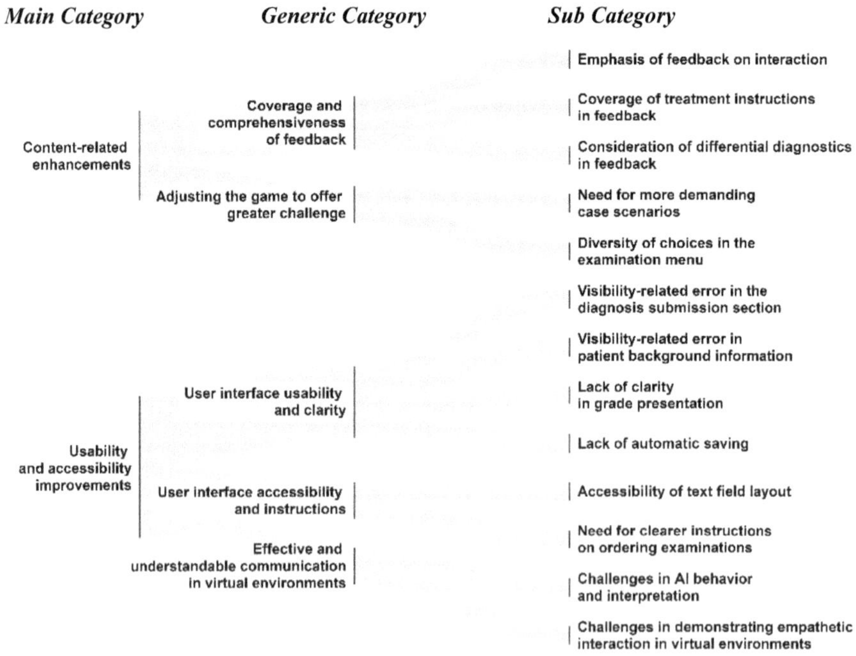

Supplementary Fig. 3. User experience–driven categories for further development of the 'MediCampus AI' learning environment

References

1. Reho, T., Paukkunen, M., Jokihaara, J., et al.: Käypä hoito käyttöön – etä- ja lähikoulutuksella yhtä hyviä tuloksia. (Implementing clinical guidelines – equally effective results with remote and in-person training.) Suom Lääkäril **80**, e44946 (2025)
2. McKenney, S., Reeves, T. Conducting Educational Design Research. Routledge, Abingdon (2018)
3. Koelewijn, G., et al.: Games to support teaching clinical reasoning in health professions education: a scoping review. Med. Educ. Online **29**, 2316971 (2024)
4. Morgan, D.J., Scherer, L., Pineles, L., et al.: Game-based learning to improve diagnostic accuracy: a pilot randomized-controlled trial. Diagnosis **11**(2), 136–141 (2024)
5. Middeke, A., Anders, S., Raupach, T., et al.: Transfer of clinical reasoning trained with a serious game to comparable clinical problems: a prospective randomized study. Simul. Healthcare **15**(2), 75–81 (2020)
6. Blanié, A., Amorim, M.A., Meffert, A., et al.: Assessing validity evidence for a serious game dedicated to patient clinical deterioration and communication. Adv. Simul. **5**(1), 4 (2020)
7. Alyami, H., Alawami, M., Lyndon, M., et al.: Impact of using a 3D visual metaphor serious game to teach history-taking content to medical students: longitudinal mixed methods pilot study. JMIR Ser. Games **7**(3), e13748 (2019)
8. Westera, W.: Why and how serious games can become far more effective: accommodating productive learning experiences, learner motivation and the monitoring of learning gains. J. Educ. Technol. Soc. **22**(1), 59–69 (2019)
9. Krishnamurthy, K., Selvaraj, N., Gupta, P., et al.: Benefits of gamification in medical education. Clin. Anat. **35**(6), 795–807 (2022)
10. Cane, J., O'Connor, D., Michie, S.: Validation of the theoretical domains framework for use in behaviour change and implementation research. Implement. Sci. **7**(1), 1–17 (2012)
11. Michie, S., Richardson, M., Johnston, M., et al.: The behavior change technique taxonomy (v1) of 93 hierarchically clustered techniques: building an international consensus for the reporting of behavior change interventions. Ann. Behav. Med. **46**(1), 81–95 (2013)
12. Käden ja kyynärvarren rasitussairaudet. Käypä hoito -suositus (Hand and forearm strain disorders Current Care Guideline). Suomalaisen Lääkäriseuran Duodecimin ja Suomen Työterveyslääkäriyhdistyksen asettama työryhmä. Helsinki: Suomalainen Lääkäriseura Duodecim (2024)
13. Paukkunen, M., Ala.Mursula, L., Öberg, B., et al.: Measuring the determinants of implementation behavior in multiprofessional rehabilitation. Eur. J. Phys. Rehabil. Med. 59(4), 488 (2023)
14. Elo, S., Kyngäs, H.: The qualitative content analysis process. J. Adv. Nurs. **62**(1), 107–115 (2008)
15. Nembhard, I.M., David, G., Ezzeddine, I., et al.: A systematic review of research on empathy in health care. Health Serv. Res. **58**(2), 250–263 (2023)
16. Aster, A., Laupichler, M.C., Zimmer, S., et al.: Game design elements of serious games in the education of medical and healthcare professions: a mixed-methods systematic review of underlying theories and teaching effectiveness. Adv. Health Sci. Educ. Theory Pract. **29**(5), 1825–1848 (2024)
17. Shavelson, R.J., Phillips, D.C., Towne, L., et al.: On the science of education design studies. Educ. Res. **32**(1), 25–28 (2003)

An Evaluation of PQC Placement as Feature Extractor and Classifier in Hybrid Quantum CNN and ViT Models on CIFAR-10

Khadija Amadoun[1(✉)], Chaïmaâ Kissi[2], Amlan Chakrabarti[3], and Tarik Boujiha[1]

[1] Engineering Science Laboratory, National School of Applied Sciences, Ibn Tofail University, Kenitra, Morocco
{khadija.amadoun,tarik.boujiha}@uit.ac.ma

[2] Advanced Systems Engineering Laboratory, National School of Applied Sciences, Ibn Tofail University, Kenitra, Morocco
chaimaa.kissi@uit.ac.ma

[3] A.K. Choudhury School of Information Technology, University of Calcutta, Kolkata, India
acakcs@caluniv.ac.in

Abstract. Hybrid Quantum-Classical (HQC) models have been shown to offer a promising strategy for leveraging near-term quantum computing resources for machine learning tasks. While initial studies have shown promise on small datasets, it remains uncertain how HQC models would scale and what their architectures would look like for a more complex problem, such as CIFAR-10. This paper poses a fundamental question with regard to the emplacement of a Parameterized Quantum Circuit (PQC) in a deep learning architecture to ensure most effectiveness in a deep learning architecture. In this experiment, a comprehensive evaluation of HQC models using four different architectures has been done, where a PQC has been used either as a front-end feature extractor or a back-end classifier. Our findings show a striking point where models using a PQC as a classifier always outperform models using a PQC as a feature extractor, which are computationally expensive and create information bottlenecks. Notably, our proposed HQC-ViT model, which combines a classical ViT with a quantum classifier, outperforms a purely classical ViT model, proposing a valuable architectural blueprint for hybrid models under NISQ constraints. Ultimately, optimizing PQC placement in vision models provides important architectural guidelines for deploying resource-efficient, quantum-assisted diagnostic tools in future digital health and medical imaging applications.

Keywords: Hybrid Quantum-Classical Models · Image Classification · Parameterized Quantum Circuit (PQC) · Convolutional Neural Networks (CNN) · Vision Transformer (ViT) · CIFAR-10

M. Särestöniemi et al. (Eds.): NCDHWS 2026, CCIS 3010, pp. 687–705, 2026.
https://doi.org/10.1007/978-3-032-28819-6_43

1 Introduction

Deep learning has transformed the field of computer vision by making it possible to do tasks like image classification and semantic segmentation better than ever before. Convolutional Neural Networks (CNNs) have been the most widely used architecture for many years. They use hierarchical layers of convolutions to learn spatial features well [1,2]. Even though these basic models are still very useful, the field is always changing, and more advanced architectures are showing better performance [3]. More recently, Vision Transformers (ViTs) have emerged as a powerful alternative, adapting the self-attention mechanisms that were transformative in natural language processing to vision tasks [4]. By treating an image as a sequence of patches, ViTs excel at capturing long-range, global dependencies, spawning a wide array of subsequent models and setting new state-of-the-art benchmarks [5].

At the same time, Quantum Machine Learning (QML) represents a new concept that has the potential to solve some computational challenges that can hardly be solved by classical computers [6]. Quantum circuits, by using quantum mechanical features like superposition and entanglement, can basically work in an exponentially large Hilbert space. This, in theory, opens the doors for developing models with drastically higher expressiveness. Most of the recent interest has focused on Variational Quantum Algorithms (VQAs), which aim to tackle complex problems by trying to find the best parameter setting for a quantum circuit [7].

However, the practical use of QML is presently limited by the restrictions of the quantum hardware. Currently, we are in the Noisy Intermediate-Scale Quantum (NISQ) era, which means the quantum devices are limited by the number of qubits, short coherence times, and high noise levels [8]. A pragmatic and hopeful way to proceed, therefore, is in Hybrid Quantum-Classical (HQC) models. These models establish a synergistic framework in which classical computers perform data processing and optimization, while a quantum co-processor is instructed to execute specific subroutines. The hybrid approach has been intensified as the main focus of the NISQ-era algorithm development. Thus, it represents the most feasible strategy to develop effective algorithms within NISQ constraints [9].

Rizvi et al. [10] introduced this hybrid strategy in computer vision by outlining two major architectures: the Hybrid Quantum-Classical Convolutional Neural Network (HQC-CNN) and the Hybrid Quantum-Classical Vision Transformer (HQC-ViT). Their work demonstrated the potential of these models on the MNIST handwritten digit dataset, showing competitive performance against classical counterparts.

While this foundational work is significant, its evaluation on MNIST leaves two critical questions unanswered. First, can these architectures scale effectively to more complex, multi-channel color image datasets? Second, and more fundamentally, where in a deep learning pipeline is a quantum component most effective? It is unclear whether a Parameterized Quantum Circuit (PQC) provides more benefit as a front-end feature extractor or as a back-end classifier.

Furthermore, CIFAR-10 will serve as a standardized benchmark for complex, multi-channel image classification, with the architectural insights provided being of tremendous relevance to digital health and medical imaging. The advancement of AI in healthcare largely relies on the development of efficient feature extraction and classification systems, which are capable of processing extremely complex health data with stringent computational constraints. The delineation of the most efficient placement of quantum components in a deep learning system will provide a fundamental architectural blueprint for future quantum-aided decision support systems. The translation of these hybrid systems from general computer vision benchmarks to specific health care tasks will enable the creation of extremely expressive, efficient systems for health care professionals.

This paper addresses both of these gaps. We extend the work of Rizvi et al. by migrating their architectures to the more challenging CIFAR-10 dataset. Furthermore, we introduce two novel "reversed" architectures, a CNN-QNN and a QNN-ViT, to conduct a systematic comparison of different quantum integration strategies. Our primary contributions are as follows:

- A systematic investigation of four distinct hybrid quantum-classical paradigms, comparing the use of a PQC as a front-end feature extractor versus a back-end classifier for both CNN and ViT backbones.
- A rigorous performance comparison of all four hybrid models against their equivalent, purely classical baselines to isolate and measure the impact of the quantum components.
- A comprehensive analysis of the trade-offs between model accuracy, the number of trainable parameters, and the computational cost of training for each paradigm.

This paper is organized as follows: In Sect. 2, we review related work in classical and quantum vision models. In Sect. 3, we describe our model architectures and experimental methodology. In Sect. 4, we present our findings. In Sect. 5, we offer a detailed discussion of these findings. In Sect. 6, we conclude our paper and propose future work.

2 Background and Related Work

This section provides an overview of the classical and quantum machine learning concepts that form the foundation of our work. First, we reviewed the core principles of Convolutional Neural Networks and Vision Transformers. Second, we introduced the necessary concepts from quantum computing for hybrid models, and situate our research within the existing literature on hybrid quantum-classical vision architectures.

2.1 Classical Vision Models

Convolutional Neural Networks (CNNs) represent a group of deep neural networks commonly used for image processing and analysis. The structural characteristics of CNNs are motivated by the human brain's visual cortex and have been designed to learn spatial hierarchies of features in an automatic and adaptive way. The main unit of a CNN is the convolutional layer, which processes an input image using a set of filters to automatically and adaptively produce an output representation. These filters are small matrices that can represent basic patterns such as edges, colors, and textures. Higher layers combine basic patterns to automatically and adaptively detect more complex patterns, such as shapes and components of shapes or objects. Pooling layers are regularly placed between layers to gradually lessen the spatial dimensionality, which is instrumental in reducing the number of parameters and producing an invariant feature representation [1,2].

Vision Transformers (ViTs) denote a newer architectural model that has been a serious contender to the traditional CNNs' supremacy [4]. ViTs do not apply sliding-window convolutions to the images. Instead, the image is viewed as a series of non-overlapping, fixed-size patches. Each of these patches is then flattened and linearly projected into an embedding vector. To incorporate the spatial information, a learnable position embedding is added to each patch embedding. The series of vectors is then passed through a regular Transformer encoder, defined by a series of Multi-Head Self-Attention blocks. The self-attention mechanism allows the model to determine which other patches are most relevant to the one it represents, thereby helping the model to learn complex, long-range global dependencies within an image. This power is very effective, especially on large-scale datasets [5].

2.2 Quantum Machine Learning Concepts

Parameterized Quantum Circuits (PQCs) or Variational Quantum Circuits (VQCs) are essentially the quantum equivalent of a classical neural network layer. A PQC is defined as a quantum circuit consisting of a series of quantum gates, some of which are parameterized by classical variables, θ. In most cases, these gates would be single-qubit rotation gates ($R_X(\theta_i)$, $R_Y(\theta_j)$) alongside a fixed two-qubit entangling gate (CNOT). A Variational Quantum Algorithm aims to achieve this by training the parameters, θ, so that the quantum circuit represents the unitary transformation $\mathrm{U}(\theta)$ that solves the task at hand. Usually, the training is carried out by a classical optimizer that iteratively updates θ by utilizing the gradient of the cost function, which is derived from the circuit output [7].

Data encoding represents an essential procedure for transferring conventional data into a quantum state. As quantum algorithms work with quantum states, a mapping needs to be established to indicate how classical feature vectors are represented in the high-dimensional Hilbert space. One way, which is also the work here, is Angle Embedding, whereby every classical feature x_i is utilized to geometrically define the rotation of a gate, for instance, $R_X(\pi x_i)$. The selection of the data encoding method is the cornerstone of a QML model design, and it greatly determines the model's performance and expressive power [11].

Measurement is the process of measuring classical data from the quantum state following the execution of the circuit. One of the methods of measuring classical data is to compute the expectation value of an observable for each qubit, like the Pauli-Z operator (σ_z), and then measure it. The result for each qubit is a classical number within the range $[-1, 1]$, which makes up the classical output vector and can be further processed by the next layers of a hybrid model.

2.3 Hybrid Quantum-Classical Vision Architectures

Hybrid architectural patterns have emerged as a result of the integration of PQCs into classical deep learning pipelines. Our paper is directed towards two of the most influential approaches in computer vision: quantum convolution and quantum classification.

Quantum Convolutional Layers: The concept of a Quantum Convolutional Neural Network (QCNN) basically means substituting a classical convolutional filter with a PQC. The fundamental ideas in the literature have been the first to demonstrate this concept by applying a small PQC to local patches of an input image, like a classical filter's receptive field [12,13]. The quantum circuit in this case, due to its potential to realize extremely complex and non-linear transformations, can be seen as a trainable feature extractor. The output pixels of the new feature map are formed by the measured results of the PQC, corresponding to each image patch. The original papers not only laid down the theoretical framework, but they were also mostly verified on toy or quantum-native datasets.

Building upon the foundational architectures proposed by Rizvi et al. [10], our research addresses their viability on the more complex, multi-channel CIFAR-10 dataset. Our primary contribution is a systematic investigation into a fundamental design question they left open: the optimal placement of the quantum component. We evaluate whether a PQC provides greater benefit as a front-end feature extractor or as a back-end classifier, providing a crucial analysis for designing effective hybrid models.

Quantum Classifiers: Another hybrid strategy is a robust classical CNN to extract features and a PQC as the final classification head. In such a setting, a classical CNN takes the input image and produces a compact, low-dimensional feature vector. This vector is subsequently used to encode a PQC that carries out the final classification task. The idea behind this is that the quantum circuit can embed classical features in a high-dimensional Hilbert space; thus, the quantum circuit can locate intricate correlations and decision boundaries in the data that are unattainable for a normal fully-connected layer [14]. They have been extensively studied for a myriad of applications, such as medical image analysis and transfer learning [15]. We have implemented this model as a focal reference to the quantum convolution model. This comparison enables us to locate the position of the deep learning pipeline where integration of a quantum component might bring the most advantage for CIFAR-10 classification.

2.4 Comparison to Prior Work

The landscape for CIFAR-10 is characterized by several key paradigms. Traditional methods, such as the specific CNNs examined in the study by Pant et

Table 1. Comparison of Related Work on CIFAR-10 and Positioning of Our Contribution.

Reference	Model Type	Specific Architecture	Key Finding/Focus on CIFAR-10	Gap Addressed by Our Work
Pant et al. [16]	Classical	Multiple CNN Architectures	Compared various classical CNN designs to identify the best-performing architecture specifically for CIFAR-10.	Provides a pure classical CNN baseline, but contains no quantum or Transformer components.
Tan [17]	Classical	Lightweight Vision Transformer (ViT)	Demonstrated that a lightweight ViT can outperform CNNs on CIFAR-10 without massive pre-training.	Establishes a strong, relevant classical ViT baseline, but does not explore hybrid quantum integration.
Henderson et al. [13]	Quantum Feature Extractor	Quanvolutional Neural Network (QNN)	introduced the "Quanvolutional" layer as a quantum feature extractor and demonstrated its potential on the MNIST dataset.	Represents the foundational proof-of-concept, but did not publish results on more complex datasets like CIFAR-10.
Trochun & Gordienko [18]	Hybrid Quantum	Quanvolutional NN & Hidden-Layer Replacement	Directly compared two different HQC designs on CIFAR-10, analyzing the trade-offs between them.	Investigated two hybrid paradigms, but did not include ViT-based models or quantum patch encoding.
This Work	**Hybrid Quantum**	**HQC-CNN, CNN-QNN, HQC-ViT, QNN-ViT**	**Systematic evaluation and comparison of multiple HQC designs on the full CIFAR-10 dataset.**	**Extends the Rizvi et al. models to CIFAR-10 and systematically compares four different HQC architectures (convolution, classifier, patch encoding) across both CNN and ViT backbones to identify the most effective integration strategy.**

al. [16] and the light Vision Transformer put forward by Tan [17], have thus formed a stable benchmark. At the same time, quantum and hybrid strategies have also been explored, from basic ideas such as "Quanvolutional" layers [13] to comparative studies of different hybrids implemented on CIFAR-10 datasets in [18].

Our work is primarily driven by the architectures proposed by Rizvi et al. [10]. They first explored the viability of HQC-CNN and HQC-ViT models on the MNIST dataset. However, it remains unclear whether they perform effectively on more complex real-world datasets, such as CIFAR-10, which includes color details and class complexity.

Thus, the current study makes a two-fold contribution to the literature: first, it generalizes the Rizvi et al. models to the more difficult CIFAR-10 dataset, and second, it conducts a more comprehensive comparison than existing work by testing four different paradigms of HQC models based on two architectures: CNN and ViT. Table 1 clearly localizes this contribution within the current state-of-the-art and the specific gap filled in the current work.

3 Methodology

In this section, we define the experimental setup used to test various Hybrid Quantum-Classical (HQC) vision models on the CIFAR-10 dataset. We detail the data preprocessing steps and the specific neural network architectures for the four models under investigation. Additionally, this section outlines the design of the parameterized quantum circuits as well as the overall training.

3.1 Dataset and Preprocessing

In all experiments, the CIFAR-10 dataset [19] was used. It consists of 60,000 color images, each with a size of 32×32 pixels, and is evenly distributed among ten mutually exclusive categories, such as "airplane," "automobile," and "bird". The CIFAR-10 dataset is divided into a training set with 50,000 images and a test set with 10,000 images. CIFAR-10 serves as an excellent proxy for real-world visual complexity, such as the complex, high-dimensional patterns found in multi-modal health data and medical imaging, due to its high intra-class variance and multi-channel (RGB) format. This presents a significantly harder, yet more realistic, challenge than the simple grayscale MNIST dataset used in prior foundational works [10]. To ensure a fair comparison and robust model training, the following preprocessing and augmentation steps were applied:

1. Preprocessing for HQC-CNN: We needed to ensure compatibility with the architecture initially employed by Rizvi et al. [10] on 28×28 grayscale images from MNIST datasets. The preprocessing for this model, therefore, included converting all images to grayscale form. Then, the images were resized to 28×28 pixels.
2. Preprocessing for all other models: For the CNN-QNN and the two ViT models, the images were kept unchanged and remained with 3 channels (RGB colors). However, for the two ViT models, the image dimensions were changed from 32×32 to 28×28. This specific resizing was strictly necessary to allow the image dimensions to be evenly divided by the 16 non-overlapping 7×7 patches without altering the core transformer logic or limiting classical capacity. Additionally, all pixel intensities were scaled between 0 and 1.
3. Data Augmentation: To prevent overfitting and promote generalization, standard data augmentation methods were employed while training all models. The process included randomized horizontal flips, randomized rotations (less than $10°$), and slight adjustments to the image width and height.

3.2 Model Architectures

We have implemented and tested four different HQC architectures along with classical baselines for comparison (where the quantum layer is replaced with a classical counterpart).

1. HQC-CNN (Quantum Convolutional Layer): This architecture, illustrated in Fig. 1, positions the quantum component at the beginning of the network. An input grayscale image is first processed by the QuantumConvLayer, which utilizes a 4-qubit parameterized quantum circuit (PQC) as a 2×2 convolution filter with a stride of 2. The resulting quantum feature map is then passed to a classical backend composed of two Conv2D blocks with batch normalization and dropout, followed by a GlobalAveragePooling2D layer and a final dense classifier.

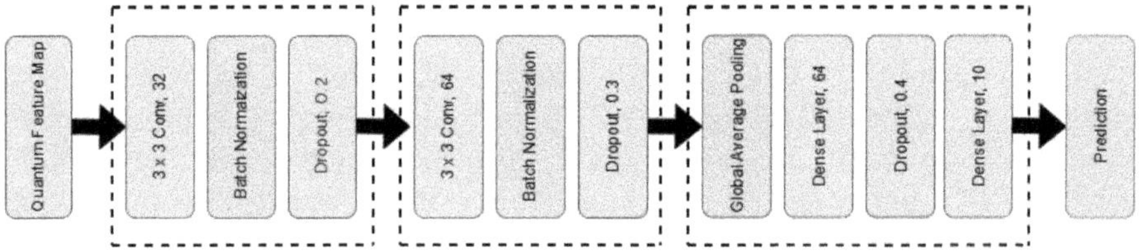

Fig. 1. The Hybrid Quantum-Classical CNN (HQC-CNN) Architecture. [Source: Rizvi et al., Mathematics, 2025], [10]

2. CNN-QNN (Quantum Classifier): In this model, illustrated in Fig. 2, a PQC is used as a back-end classifier. A classical CNN frontend, containing two convolution blocks (Conv2D + MaxPooling2D), first extracts spatial features from the 32×32 color images. The resulting feature map is flattened and passed through a dense layer, which reduces its dimensionality to match the number of qubits (4). This compact feature vector will then be encoded by the Quantum-Classifier Layer, and the outcomes of the parameterized quantum circuit will be used for a concluding dense layer for classification purposes with a softmax activation function.
3. HQC-ViT (Quantum Classifier Backend): This model, depicted in Fig. 3, couples a classical Vision Transformer (ViT) front-end with a PQC back-end. The

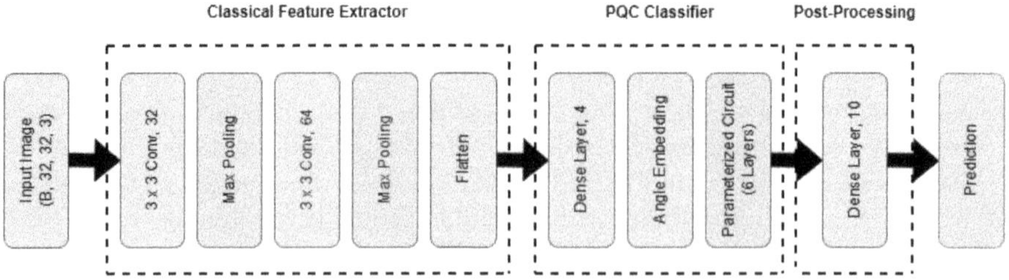

Fig. 2. The Hybrid CNN with a Quantum Classifier (CNN-QNN) Architecture.

ViT processes 28×28 color images by splitting them into 16 non-overlapping 7×7 patches and feeding them through a 4-layer Transformer encoder. The resulting [CLS] token embedding is projected into a 10-dimensional classical feature vector. This vector is then passed to a 10-qubit PQC to generate quantum features. Following the architecture of Rizvi et al. [10], a skip connection concatenates the original classical vector with the quantum feature vector, and a final linear layer performs classification on this combined result.

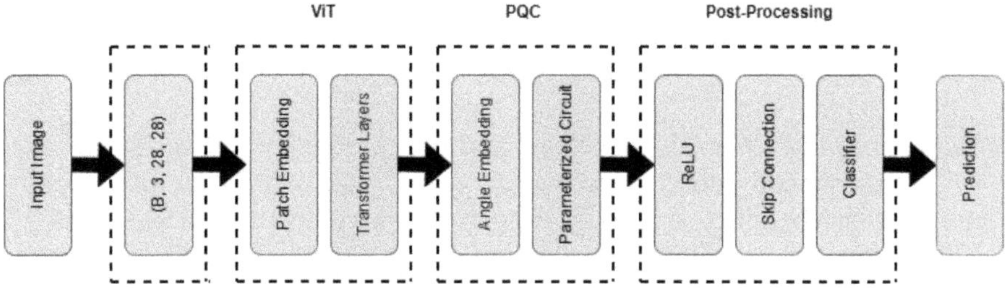

Fig. 3. The Hybrid Quantum-Classical Vision Transformer (HQC-ViT) Architecture. [Source: Rizvi et al., Mathematics, 2025], [10]

4. QNN-ViT (Quantum Patch Encoder): This final architecture, shown in Fig. 4, reverses the design of the HQC-ViT by using a PQC for feature extraction at the patch level. The input image is divided into 16 non-overlapping 7×7 patches. Each patch is then processed by a hybrid quantum-classical module: it is flattened, linearly projected to a 4-dimensional vector, and then encoded into a 4-qubit PQC. The measurement results from this quantum circuit are projected to the Transformer's embedding dimension (128), creating a sequence of quantum-enhanced patch embeddings. This sequence is then passed to a standard 4-layer Transformer backend for final classification based on the [CLS] token.

3.3 Quantum Circuit Design

The key building block for each hybrid model consists of a Parameterized Quantum Circuit (PQC). Despite variations in parameters, the common architecture includes data encoding and a trainable variational ansatz.

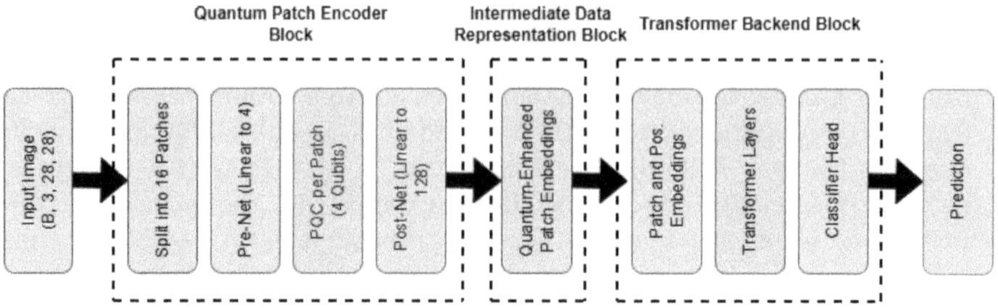

Fig. 4. The Quantum Patch Encoder Vision Transformer (QNN-ViT) Architecture.

- Data Encoding: For HQC-CNNs, qml.RX(np.pi*x_i, ...) gates are used to represent conventional values of each 2×2 patch. In other cases, qml.AngleEmbedding is used for encoding classical feature vectors.
- Variational Ansatz: The trainable part of the circuit aims to perform complex correlations. The HQC-CNN and CNN-QNN architectures use a series of single-qubit qml.RY gates followed by a string of entangling CNOT gates. This serves as their variational ansatz. The other models with a vision transformer architecture use qml.BasicEntanglerLayers for their variational ansatz. Details regarding qubit numbers for each architecture appear below in Table 2.

The number of quantum layers, or circuit depth, along with the precise count of trainable parameters for each PQC according to their use of variational ansatz (the single-qubit rotations and entangling gates) must be accurately tracked since they also contribute to the expressivity of the quantum components. The variational ansatz is repeated in the quantum circuit to form the full 'circuit depth'. For example, a CNN-QNN would have a circuit depth of 6 with respect to an execution on 4 qubits (resulting in 24 trainable parameters). On the other hand, the best performing HQC-ViT has a circuit depth of 5 on 10 qubits (resulting in 50 trainable parameters). This illustrates the parameter-efficient nature of quantum classifiers, in comparison to a classical dense layer (i.e., future comparisons can be drawn between the two methods). The complete architectural designs have been included in Table 2 below.

3.4 Experimental Setup

Both of the models were implemented using the Python programming language, which utilized the PennyLane library for the quantum components and TensorFlow, Keras, and PyTorch for the classical elements. The quantum circuits were run on the default qubit simulator. Training was done on a typical workstation computer, with the critical hyperparameters listed in Table 2. To enable a fair comparison and impose a time constraint on the training process, the EarlyStopping function was used with a patience of 10 epochs to monitor the validation loss. The best model was then selected for evaluation on the test set.

Table 2. Hyperparameter and Architectural Details.

Model	Framework	Optimizer	LR	Scheduler	Batch	Qubits	Q Layers	PQC Params
HQC-CNN	TF	Adam	1e-3	–	16	4	1	4
CNN-QNN	TF	Adam	1e-3	–	32	4	6	24
HQC-ViT	PyTorch	AdamW	3e-4	Cosine	64	10	5	50
QNN-ViT	PyTorch	AdamW	3e-4	Cosine	64	4	2	8

4 Results

This section provides the empirical results of the comparison study. In this study, the model was trained using the CIFAR-10 dataset until convergence. Early stopping on the validation loss was used to assess convergence. The three essential criteria used for model comparison are the test accuracy on the last epoch, the number of trainable parameters, and the average training time per epoch.

4.1 Overall Model Performance

The performance of the four hybrid schemes, along with their respective classical schemes, is given below in Table 3. There is a hierarchy of performance, where the approach of combining the quantum piece and the choice of the classical scheme are the controlling parameters.

It is interesting to note that the architectures that make use of the quantum circuit as a back-end classifier perform better than those that use it as a front-end feature extractor. Additionally, the HQC-ViT model, which uses a Vision Transformer along with a quantum classifier, performed the best, registering a test accuracy of 67.68%, which is considerably better than the results of the CNN-based approaches.

4.2 Analysis of Convolutional Architectures

The two CNN models illustrate the essential trade-off between accuracy and computation intensity (Fig. 5). The HQC-CNN model setup, which used a PQC for the extraction of features on grayscale images, recorded a total accuracy of 57.39% but involved heavy computation, with the average time per epoch taking close to 90 min. This is because of the large overhead involved in the simulation of the quantum circuit for every 2×2 patch of images.

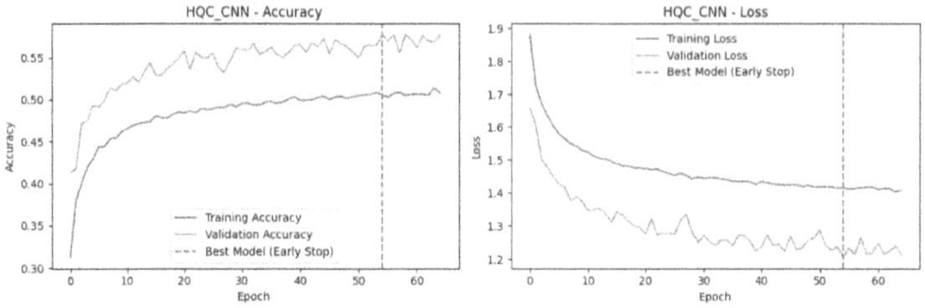

(a) HQC-CNN (Quantum Feature Extractor)

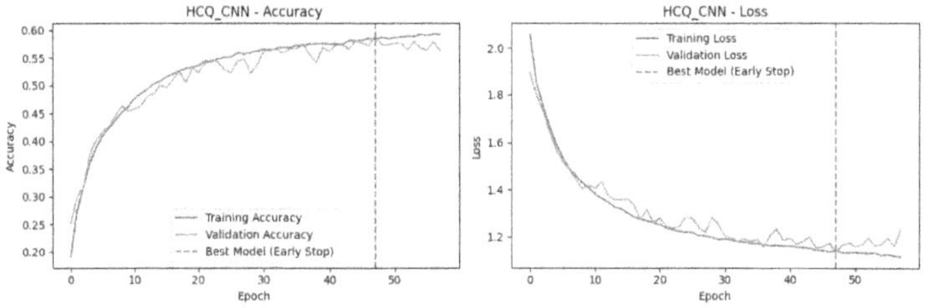

(b) CNN-QNN (Quantum Classifier)

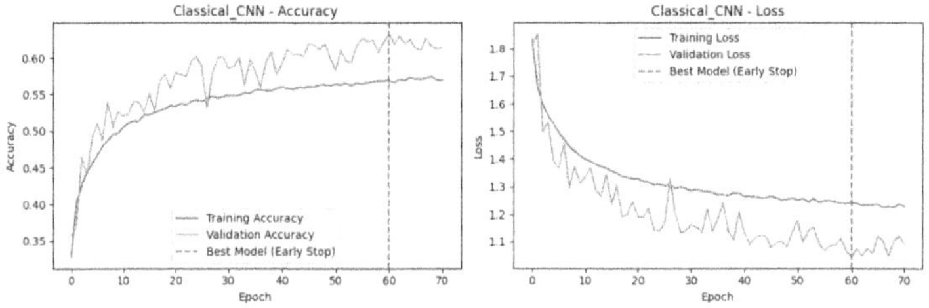

(c) Classical CNN (Grayscale)

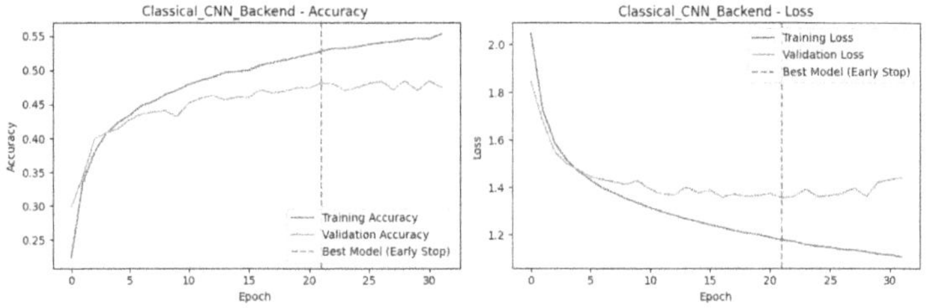

(d) Classical CNN (RGB))

Fig. 5. Training and validation dynamics for the convolutional architectures. The hybrid models (a, b) and their respective classical baselines (c, d) are shown.

By contrast, the CNN-QNN setup, where the PQC is used as the last classifier on the features extracted from the RGB images, reported a slightly better accuracy of 58.03%. Significantly, the training time of 48 s per epoch indicated that

Table 3. Overall Performance Comparison of HQC and Classical Models on the CIFAR-10 Test Set.

Model	Quantum Layer	Test Acc. (%)	Params (Trainable)	Train Time (s/epoch)
Convolutional Architectures (Grayscale 28×28)				
Classical-CNN	**No**	**62.38**	**24,702**	**≈34**
HQC-CNN	Yes (Feature Extractor)	57.39	24,686	≈5300
Convolutional Architectures (RGB 32×32)				
Classical-CNN	No	46.90	28,682	≈31
CNN-QNN	**Yes (Classifier)**	**58.03**	28,662	**≈48**
Transformer Architectures (RGB 28×28)				
Classical-ViT	No	63.68	552,568	≈189
HQC-ViT	**Yes (Classifier)**	**67.68**	**552,718**	**≈597**
QNN-ViT	Yes (Feature Extractor)	55.87	534,754	≈229

the HQC-CNN was surpassed by the CNN-QNN approach by over two orders of magnitude. Taken together, these findings make it clear that for CNN-based hybrid setups, the use of a quantum classifier at the tail end of the system is a much more viable and efficient approach.

The substantial training time for HQC-CNN is due to the per-batch quantum circuit invocations required for every sliding window of the convolution. Expectation values were computed analytically via the statevector simulator.

4.3 Analysis of Vision Transformer Architectures

The results for ViT-based models had the highest level of variation, thus demonstrating the effects of quantum placement on the stronger classical baseline (Fig. 6).

The HQC-ViT model, where a classical ViT feature extractor is integrated with a 10-qubit quantum classifier, showed the best performance. It was observed that the model was able to achieve a test accuracy of 67.68%, outperforming the classical model's accuracy of 63.68%. This result suggests a potential quantum benefit, where replacing a linear classifier with a parameterized quantum circuit (PQC) not only does not harm but rather improves model performance despite a comparable number of parameters, as well as a slight increase in training time.

On the other hand, with a 4-qubit PQC to encode every image patch in the QNN-ViT model, the lowest performance was seen with a test accuracy of 55.87%. This shows that the information bottleneck caused by the limited qubits in the quantum circuit did not result in expressive embeddings for every patch, like those that were obtained in a classical linear projection. This result further supports that using a PQC as a front-end feature extractor for raw images in a complex classification problem like CIFAR-10 was suboptimal.

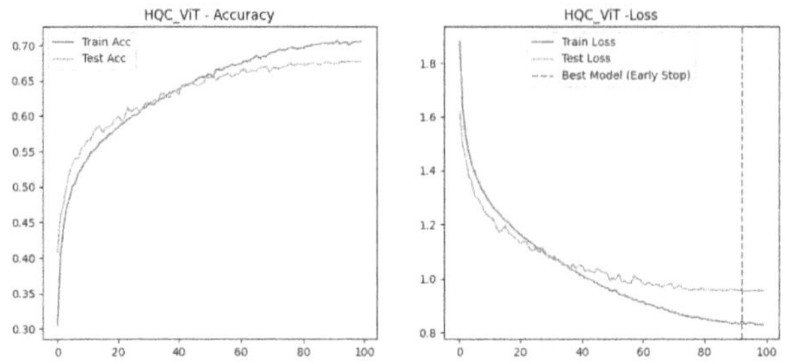

(a) HQC-ViT (Quantum Classifier)

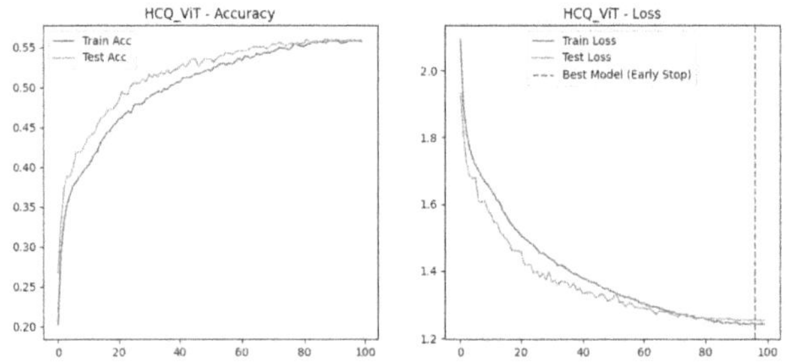

(b) QNN-ViT (Quantum Feature Extractor)

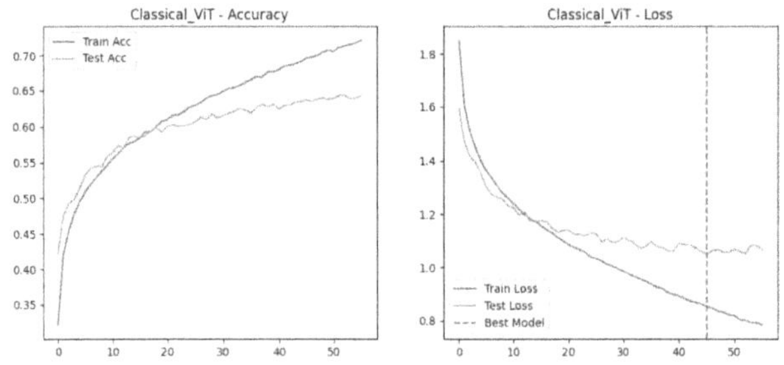

(c) Classical ViT Baseline

Fig. 6. Training and validation dynamics for the Vision Transformer architectures. The hybrid models (a, b) and their classical baseline (c) are shown.

5 Discussion

This paper contributes to the construction of Hybrid Quantum-Classical models by investigating the best position of the Parameterized Quantum Circuit (PQC). Indeed, in this rapidly growing area, there are broadly speaking two paradigms considered at the present stage. The first is to consider the PQC as a front-end feature extractor inspired by ideas involving the notion of 'quanvolutional' layers [13], while the second involves the PQC as a back-end classifier for the processed features in the classical domain [14,18]. The following experimental results confirm convincingly that the second approach strongly surpasses the first in the case of complex real-world datasets, such as CIFAR-10.

5.1 Key Findings Analysis

Our primary finding is that the architectural role of the Parameterized Quantum Circuit is the dominant factor for success in the models for the CNN as well as the ViT architecture.

Architectures featuring a PQC at the input stage, such as the HQC-CNN and the newly introduced QNN-ViT by the authors, are inherently not suited to such levels of model and/or data complexity. This assessment points to two significant problems that are probably inherent to such models. First, it would be prohibitively expensive to train such a model. Applying a PQC convolutionally, as in the HQC-CNN, resulted in a training time over 150 times longer than its classical counterpart. Moreover, these small PQCs act as a severe information bottleneck. This was demonstrated by the substantial degradation introduced in HQC-CNN's (57.39%) and QNN-ViT's (55.87%) performance compared to their baselines, indicating early "quanvolutional" methods' limitations for real-world-level vision tasks.

In the case of architectures employing a PQC as a back-end classifier, the effectiveness and feasibility become clear. This complementary combination, as incorporated in the CNN-QNN and HQC-ViT architectures, allows for the optimal performance of each component for its intended purpose. The classical part of the model is efficient in its capability to encapsulate high-dimensional images into a short, highly semantic feature vector, which is in turn appropriately processed by the PQC as a highly expressive classifier. This combination is computationally viable, incurring just a small overhead in terms of training time over the classical benchmarks. Much more significantly, it highlights the superior mathematical expressivity of quantum classifiers. The HQC-ViT model recorded 67.68%, which is an improvement over its robust classical baseline of 63.68%. Notably, the CNN-QNN model recorded 58.03%, which is an 11-point improvement over its classical model's 46.90% performance. We hypothesize that the presence of the PQC, projecting classical features into a high-dimensional Hilbert space, can identify intricate correlations and decision boundaries that are inaccessible to a simple classical dense layer.

5.2 Current Challenges and Limitations

The results presented in this paper provide architectural insights that need to be contextualized within the current quantum computing paradigm. It is noteworthy that the experiments carried out in this research were conducted using classical simulators to provide a clean environment without errors. As such, the performance improvements reported in this paper are purely a result of increased mathematical expressiveness rather than actual quantum speedup. The practical realization of the architectural models presented in this research would be heavily influenced by various hardware-related aspects of the NISQ processors. Furthermore, the number of qubits utilized in the proposed architectural models is relatively low (between 4 and 10), implying that the full expressiveness of these architectures may not be realized until more sophisticated quantum computing architectures are developed.

In addition to this, due to the computational complexity of quantum convolutions carried out using classical simulators (which takes approximately 5300 s per epoch for the HQC-CNN), the evaluation of the proposed architectural models is carried out using fixed random seeds for reproducibility. Future work will focus on statistical validation of the results reported in this research, including the computation of the mean and standard deviation for multiple runs of the experiment.

It is noteworthy that the quantum circuits and data encoding schemes utilized in this research are relatively simple. Future work will focus on exploring more complex ansatz circuits to more efficiently map classical information onto quantum bits. A potentially valuable extension of the work presented in this research is to utilize the successful realization of the HQC-ViT architecture for more complex tasks related to medical imaging and digital health.

5.3 Applications to Digital Health and Medical Imaging

One of the most important outcomes of this benchmarking study is the direct applicability to the future of digital health and medical image analysis, which is in line with the growing need to develop sophisticated, data-driven decision support systems in healthcare settings. In fact, machine learning problems in medical image analysis, like histopathological image analysis, MRI analysis, and anomaly detection in radiographs, are extremely challenging due to the high dimensionality of the data and the complex correlations needed to make accurate diagnoses.

The key outcome of this study, which is the marked effectiveness and computational feasibility of Parameterized Quantum Circuits (PQCs) when used as back-end classifiers, rather than front-end feature extractors, offers a practical roadmap to the incorporation of Quantum Machine Learning in AI in healthcare settings. In fact, in medical image analysis, front-end quantum convolutions, or "quanvolutional" layers, have been shown to have computationally intractable costs when processing large, high-resolution medical images in a healthcare setting. In this regard, the Hybrid Quantum-Classical Vision Transformer (HQC-ViT) framework, which has been shown in this study, is the optimal solution to this problem. In this workflow, a classical neural network is used to map high-resolution medical images into dense, semantic feature representations, which are subsequently encoded by the PQC, which is used exclusively in the classification stage. The PQC maps patient features to a high-dimensional Hilbert space, where complex, non-linear decision boundaries may be identified, which may enable the distinction between malignant and benign disease.

Accordingly, the architectural guidelines outlined in this study provide a foundation upon which future, next-generation diagnostic tools may be developed, with future work building upon this foundation by incorporating the optimized HQC-ViT and CNN-QNN architectures on specific medical image datasets, like MedMNIST or ISIC melanoma datasets, to validate the utility of quantum classifiers in providing sophisticated, model-based decision support to medical professionals.

6 Conclusion

In our research, we conduct a comprehensive analysis of the optimal integration approaches for Parameterized Quantum Circuits (PQCs) in both Convolutional Neural Networks (CNNs) and Vision Transformers (ViTs) for CIFAR-10 classification. Through our experiment of four different hybrid approaches with their classical counterparts, we aim to find where in a deep learning pipeline a quantum part provides superior improvement.

The above analysis provides a distinct and conclusive finding: using a PQC as a back-end classifier clearly outperforms it as a front-end feature extractor in terms of both performance and computational efficiency. Front-end quantum layers, when directly used on image patches, are severe information bottlenecks and are computationally utterly impractical for this size of data, with consistent subpar performance compared to their classical counterparts.

On the other hand, HQC-ViT, which uses a classical ViT for feature extraction and a PQC for classification, not only remains computationally feasible but also displays the highest test accuracy among all models. It shows a subtle yet noticeable performance improvement over the classical model, which demonstrates that replacing a classical classifier with a PQC can improve expressivity and model performance, offering valuable architectural guidance for hybrid design in the NISQ era.

Our results offer a strong recommendation for researchers and practitioners in the NISQ era. The most promising and practical approach for hybrid quantum-classical vision is to focus on architectures where PQCs are used as powerful, expressive classifiers for classically processed data. Future work should therefore investigate more advanced data encoding strategies and benchmark these architectures on real quantum hardware to evaluate their performance under realistic noise conditions. Furthermore, applying the HQC-ViT paradigm to other challenging domains like medical imaging and exploring co-design strategies for hardware-efficient quantum circuits are valuable next steps.

Applying this HQC-ViT paradigm to challenging healthcare domains, such as medical imaging and patient data analysis, represents a highly promising direction for future quantum-enhanced decision support systems.

Acknowledgements. We acknowledge our University for providing the hardware and software resources required to conduct the simulations for this study.

Conflict of Interest. The authors declare no conflict of interest.

References

1. LeCun, Y., Bottou, L., Bengio, Y., Haffner, P.: Gradient-based learning applied to document recognition. Proc. IEEE **86**(11), 2278–2324 (2002)
2. Krizhevsky, A., Sutskever, I., Hinton, G.E.: Imagenet classification with deep convolutional neural networks. In: Advances in Neural Information Processing Systems, p. 25 (2012)
3. Khan, A., Sohail, A., Zahoora, U., Qureshi, A.S.: A survey of the recent architectures of deep convolutional neural networks. Artif. Intell. Rev. **53**(8), 5455–5516 (2020)
4. Dosovitskiy, A.: An image is worth 16x16 words: transformers for image recognition at scale. arXiv preprint arXiv:2010.11929 (2020)
5. Han, K., et al.: A survey on vision transformer. IEEE Trans. Pattern Anal. Mach. Intell. **45**(1), 87–110 (2022)
6. Biamonte, J., Wittek, P., Pancotti, N., Rebentrost, P., Wiebe, N., Lloyd, S.: Quantum machine learning. Nature **549**(7671), 195–202 (2017)
7. Cerezo, M., et al.: Variational quantum algorithms. Nat. Rev. Phys. **3**(9), 625–644 (2021)
8. Preskill, J.: Quantum computing in the NISQ era and beyond. Quantum **2**, 79 (2018)
9. Bharti, K., et al.: Noisy intermediate-scale quantum algorithms. Rev. Mod. Phys. **94**(1), 015004 (2022)
10. Rizvi, S.M.A., Paracha, U.I., Khalid, U., Lee, K., Shin, H.: Quantum machine learning: towards hybrid quantum-classical vision models. Mathematics **13**(16), 2645 (2025)
11. Schuld, M.: Supervised quantum machine learning models are kernel methods. arXiv preprint arXiv:2101.11020 (2021)
12. Cong, I., Choi, S., Lukin, M.D.: Quantum convolutional neural networks. Nat. Phys. **15**(12), 1273–1278 (2019)
13. Henderson, M., Shakya, S., Pradhan, S., Cook, T.: Quanvolutional neural networks: powering image recognition with quantum circuits. Quantum Mach. Intell. **2**(1), 2 (2020)
14. Zhang, S.-X., Wan, Z.-Q., Lee, C.-K., Hsieh, C.-Y., Zhang, S., Yao, H.: Variational quantum-neural hybrid eigensolver. Phys. Rev. Lett. **128**(12), 120502 (2022)
15. Wang, A., Li, X., Li, L., Li, T.: QC-Net: a hybrid quantum-classical neural network model for medical image segmentation: A. Wang et al. Quantum Inf. Process. **24**(10), 340 (2025)
16. Pant, Y., Shah, G., Ojha, R., Thapa, R., Bhatta, B.: Comparison of CNN architecture of image classification using CIFAR10 datasets. Int. J. Eng. Technol. **1**(1), 37–52 (2023)
17. Tan, J.H.: Pre-training of lightweight vision transformers on small datasets with minimally scaled images. arXiv preprint arXiv:2402.03752 (2024)
18. Trochun, Y., Gordienko, Y.: Effectiveness of hybrid quantum-classical and quanvolutional neural networks for image classification. Inf. Comput. Intell. Syst. **5**, 68–79 (2024)
19. Krizhevsky, A., Hinton, G.: Learning multiple layers of features from tiny images. Technical report, University of Toronto (2009)

MEG-QA: Medical Evidence-Grounded Question Abbreviation for Consumer Health Queries via Retrieval-Augmented Generation and Knowledge Graph Constraints in Digital Health

Md Rabiul Hasan, Aleka Melese Ayalew(✉), and Mourad Oussalah

Center for Machine Vision and Signal Processing, University of Oulu, 90014 Oulu, Finland
{MdRabiul.Hasan,Aleka.Ayalew,Mourad.Oussalah}@oulu.fi

Abstract. Medical question abbreviation aims to condense long, consumer-facing medical questions into concise forms while preserving clinical intent and meaning. Despite recent progress with large language models, existing approaches frequently introduce unsupported medical concepts, omit critical qualifiers, or subtly alter the original information need, errors that are poorly captured by standard lexical and semantic evaluation metrics. This paper focuses on the MeQSum benchmark, where verbose consumer health questions are abbreviated into concise professional forms, a task-critical for digital health platforms enabling remote consultations.

We propose **MEG-QA (Medical Evidence-Grounded Question Abbreviation)**, a framework that aligns generation to both retrieved evidence and structured medical knowledge. MEG-QA integrates retrieval-augmented generation with knowledge graph grounding to guide abbreviations toward conceptually faithful and evidence-supported outputs. Instead of relying solely on prompt design or fine-tuning, MEG-QA constrains generation through alignment with normalized medical concepts and their relationships.

To evaluate faithfulness beyond surface similarity, we introduce the **CQA-Align Score**, a concept-qualifier-attribution alignment metric that measures whether the generated questions preserve medical concepts, maintain critical qualifiers, and avoid unsupported additions.

Experiments on the MedQSum dataset show that MEG-QA consistently improves faithfulness and intent preservation across models and adaptation paradigms, with substantial gains in CQA-Align that are not reflected by conventional metrics. These results highlight the importance of evidence-aligned and knowledge-generation for reliable medical question abbreviations.

Keywords: Medical Question Abbreviation · RAG · Knowledge Graph · Faithfulness · LLMs · Digital Health

M. Särestöniemi et al. (Eds.): NCDHWS 2026, CCIS 3010, pp. 706–726, 2026.
https://doi.org/10.1007/978-3-032-28819-6_44

1 Introduction

Medical question abbreviation seeks to condense long, consumer-facing medical questions into concise forms while preserving the original clinical intent and meaning. This task plays an important role in downstream applications such as medical question answering [1], retrieval and triage [2], where overly verbose inputs can reduce system efficiency or introduce ambiguity. Unlike generic summarization, medical question abbreviation is highly sensitive to semantic distortions: small changes in medical concepts, qualifiers, or scope can substantially alter the underlying information need [3].

Recent advances in large language models (LLMs) have led to strong performance on medical text generation tasks, including question rewriting and summarization [4]. Although LLM-based approaches produce fluent and concise outputs, it frequently exhibits failure modes that are particularly problematic in medical settings [5]. These include introducing unsupported medical concepts, omitting critical qualifiers (negation or temporality), and subtly shifting the intent of the original question [6]. These errors are often difficult to detect using standard evaluation metrics, which primarily measure surface-level similarity or embedding-based semantic overlap.

A growing body of work has explored retrieval-augmented generation (RAG) [7] and knowledge-grounded decoding to improve factual consistency in text generation [8]. Retrieval provides access to external evidence that can enrich model outputs, while structured medical knowledge offers constraints on plausible concept relations. However, existing approaches typically apply these techniques in isolation or evaluate them using metrics that remain insensitive to fine-grained medical faithfulness. As a result, improvements in lexical or semantic similarity do not necessarily translate to better preservation of medical meaning or intent [9].

In this work, we propose MEG-QA (Medical Evidence-Grounded Question Abbreviation), a framework that aligns medical question abbreviations with both retrieved evidence and structured medical knowledge. MEG-QA integrates retrieval-augmented generation with knowledge graph grounding to guide generation toward conceptually faithful and evidence-supported outputs. Rather than relying solely on prompt engineering or parameter adaptation, this framework explicitly aligns generation with normalized medical concepts and their relationships, discouraging unsupported additions and promoting consistency with the source question.

Beyond modeling, we argue that progress in medical question abbreviation requires evaluation methodologies that go beyond surface similarity [10]. To this end, we introduce *CQA-Align Score*, a concept-qualifier-attribution alignment metric designed to assess whether generated questions preserve core medical concepts, maintain critical qualifiers, and avoid unsupported assertions. By operating at the level of normalized concepts and their attributions, CQA-Align exposes faithfulness errors that are frequently missed by commonly used metrics such as ROUGE or BERTScore.

We evaluate MEG-QA on the MedQSum dataset across multiple model families and adaptation paradigms, including zero-shot, few-shot, and parameter-efficient fine-tuning settings. Our results show that MEG-QA consistently improves alignment-based faithfulness while maintaining strong lexical and semantic performance. Importantly, gains measured by CQA-Align reveal improvements in concept and intent preservation that are not reflected by conventional evaluation metrics alone.

More formally, this paper makes the following contributions:

1. We introduce MEG-QA, a retrieval- and knowledge-grounded framework for faithful medical question abbreviation.
2. We propose CQA-Align Score, a concept-qualifier-attribution alignment metric for evaluating faithfulness beyond surface similarity.
3. We provide a comprehensive empirical evaluation on the MedQSum dataset, including stepwise ablations that isolate the effects of retrieval and knowledge grounding.
4. We present qualitative analyses that illustrate how MEG-QA reduces common faithfulness errors in medical question abbreviation.

2 Related Work

2.1 Medical Question Summarization and Abbreviation

The field of medical question summarization and abbreviation aims to condense consumer health questions while preserving the underlying clinical intent. The MeQSum dataset formalized this task and remains the primary benchmark for medical question summarization research [11]. Early approaches relied on sequence-to-sequence models optimized for surface similarity, while more recent work has explored instruction-tuned large language models for medical question rewriting [12].

Recent studies show that LLMs can generate fluent and concise questions but frequently introduce semantic distortions, such as concept substitution or loss of critical qualifiers. Zhou *et al.* [13] and Li *et al.* [14] reported that instruction-tuning improves readability but does not reliably preserve clinical meaning. These findings highlight a gap between fluency-oriented optimization and faithful intent preservation, motivating approaches that explicitly constrain generation rather than relying solely on prompting or fine-tuning.

2.2 Retrieval-Augmented and Knowledge-Grounded Generation

Retrieval-augmented generation (RAG) is a widely used grounding mechanism that conditions generation on retrieved evidence [15]. More recent studies investigated *when* and *how* retrieval mechanisms should be invoked during generation [16]. A complementary direction post-edits or revises model outputs to improve attribution and reduce unsupported claims [17]. Additionally, recent work by Wu *et al.* [18] proposed monitoring mechanisms to detect unfaithful RAG outputs during decoding.

In biomedical generation specifically, knowledge graphs have been used to inject structured domain constraints [19]. These findings motivate our design choice to combine retrieval evidence with structured biomedical knowledge to better preserve concept-level intent and qualifiers in medical question abbreviations.

2.3 Evaluation Beyond Surface Similarity

Standard lexical and embedding-based metrics often fail to capture clinically consequential errors, such as qualifier loss and unsupported additions. Recent medical-domain work highlights the importance of faithfulness and hallucination mitigation in summarization pipelines. Related evaluation efforts emphasized factuality and robustness for health-related queries [20] and proposed domain-specific factuality benchmarks for medical evidence summarization. These recent works have motivated our *CQA-Align Score*, which evaluates faithfulness at the level of concepts, qualifiers, and attribution, complementing conventional similarity metrics.

3 MEG-QA Methodology

MEG-QA is a modular framework for faithful medical question abbreviation that aligns large language model (LLM) decoding with both retrieved medical evidence and structured biomedical knowledge. Given an input question x, MEG-QA combines sparse-dense retrieval, ontology-aware concept normalization, and knowledge-graph-guided alignment to discourage unsupported content while preserving clinical intent. An overview of the framework is shown in Fig. 1.

3.1 Problem Setup

Specifically, given an input medical question x, the goal of medical question abbreviation is to generate a shortened question $\hat{x}$ in such a way that preserves the original clinical information while reducing verbosity. Unlike generic summarization, abbreviations require strict semantic fidelity, and small distortions in medical concepts, qualifiers, or scope can substantially alter the intended meaning.

Formally, a faithful abbreviated question $\hat{x}$ must satisfy the following conditions:

1. **Concept Preservation**: Medically salient concepts expressed in x are retained in $\hat{x}$ without substitution or omission.
2. **Qualifier Consistency**: Critical modifiers associated with concepts like negation, temporality, uncertainty and conditionality remain unchanged.
3. **Intent Preservation**: The type and scope of the information requested in x are preserved in $\hat{x}$.
4. **No Unsupported Additions**: $\hat{x}$ does not introduce medical concepts or assertions that are not supported by the input question.

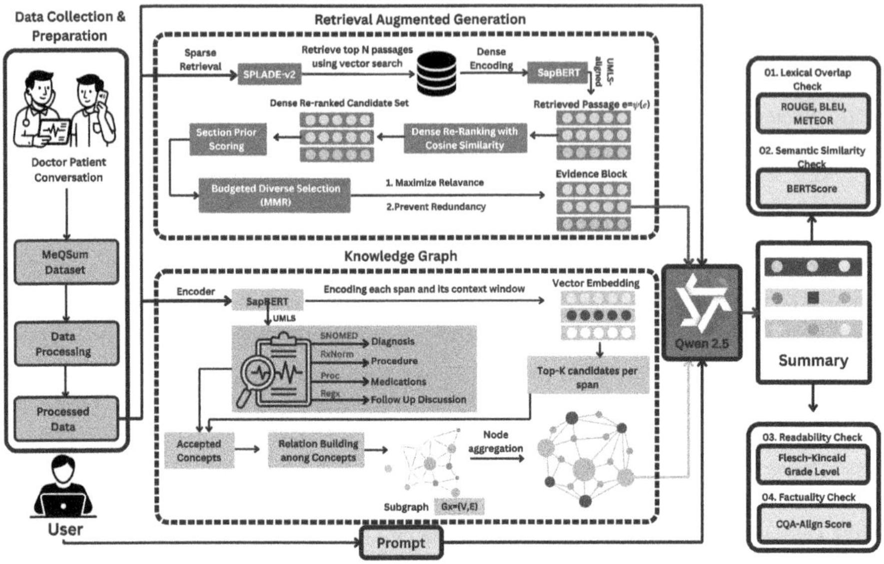

Fig. 1. Overview of the MEG-QA architecture integrating RAG-KG for evidence-grounded and knowledge-constrained medical question abbreviation.

MEG-QA approaches this task as an *alignment problem*, where generation must remain consistent with both evidence retrieved for the input question and structured medical knowledge derived from biomedical ontologies. Rather than relying solely on the parametric knowledge of the language model, MEG-QA explicitly incorporates external signals to guide generation toward minimal, and faithful abbreviations.

3.2 Evidence Retrieval

To ground generation in relevant medical context, MEG-QA employs retrieval-augmented generation that combines sparse lexical matching with dense semantic re-ranking. That is, given an input medical question x, we retrieve a set of candidate evidence passages $\mathcal{E} = \{e_1, \ldots, e_N\}$ from a medical corpus using a two-stage retrieval process.

Sparse Retrieval with SPLADE-v2: We first apply sparse retrieval using SPLADE-v2 [21], a neural bag-of-words retriever that expands queries into weighted lexical representations. Formally, let $\phi_{\text{splade}}(\cdot)$ denote the SPLADE-v2 encoder. The sparse relevance score between the input question x and a candidate passage e is computed as:

$$s_{\text{sparse}}(e \mid x) = \langle \phi_{\text{splade}}(x), \phi_{\text{splade}}(e) \rangle. \tag{1}$$

Sparse retrieval ensures coverage of clinically salient terms and supports exact or near-exact lexical matches that are critical in medical text.

Dense Re-ranking with SapBERT: To capture semantic similarity and handle medical synonymy, we re-rank retrieved passages using SapBERT [22], a biomedical sentence encoder trained to align synonymous concepts in UMLS. Let $\phi_{\text{SapBERT}}(\cdot)$ denote the SapBERT encoder. Dense semantic relevance is computed as:

$$s_{\text{dense}}(e \mid x) = \cos\left(\phi_{\text{SapBERT}}(x), \phi_{\text{SapBERT}}(e)\right). \tag{2}$$

This step mitigates limitations of purely lexical retrieval by aligning semantically equivalent medical expressions.

Combined Evidence Scoring: The final relevance score for each candidate passage integrates sparse relevance, dense similarity, and a section-prior signal as follows:

$$s(e \mid x) = s_{\text{dense}}(e \mid x) + \alpha\, s_{\text{sparse}}(e \mid x) + \beta\, s_{\text{prior}}(e), \tag{3}$$

where $s_{\text{prior}}(e)$ biases retrieval toward clinically informative sections (e.g., diagnosis or treatment), and α, β are tunable hyperparameters.

The resulting ranked candidate set serves as the input to a subsequent diversity-aware selection stage, ensuring that retrieved evidence is both relevant and non-redundant.

Budgeted Diverse Evidence Selection: Although dense re-ranking improves semantic relevance, the top-ranked passages are often highly repetitive. Including all of them is both inefficient and unnecessary. To form a compact evidence block that fits within the LLM context window, MEG-QA applies *budgeted diverse selection* using Maximal Marginal Relevance (MMR) [23].

Formally, starting from a ranked candidate set $\mathcal{E}$ and an empty selected set $\mathcal{S}$, passages are iteratively selected by optimizing:

$$\text{MMR}(e) = \lambda\, s(e \mid x) - (1 - \lambda) \max_{e' \in \mathcal{S}} \cos\left(\phi_{\text{SapBERT}}(e), \phi_{\text{SapBERT}}(e')\right) \tag{4}$$

where $s(e \mid x)$ is the combined relevance score from Sect. 3.2. The function $\phi_{\text{SapBERT}}(\cdot)$ maps passages to SapBERT embeddings, and $\lambda \in [0, 1]$ balances relevance and diversity.

This process continues until a predefined token budget B is reached. Enforcing this budget limits redundancy, prevents repeated evidence from dominating the prompt, and allows different facets of the medical question to be represented within the available context.

The resulting evidence block $\mathcal{S}$ is subsequently used for concept normalization and knowledge graph grounding.

3.3 Knowledge Graph Grounding

While retrieval provides external evidence, it does not explicitly encode structured medical semantics. To enforce semantic consistency and discourage unsupported content, MEG-QA incorporates a knowledge graph grounding component derived from biomedical ontologies.

Concept Normalization: Medical mentions in the input question x and selected evidence block $\mathcal{S}$ are normalized to standardized biomedical concepts using UMLS. Candidate concept spans are encoded with SapBERT, which is trained to align synonymous medical expressions. For each span c, a confidence score is computed as:

$$q(c) = \sigma(\mathbf{a}^\top \mathbf{u}_c + b), \tag{5}$$

where $\mathbf{u}_c$ denotes the SapBERT embedding of the span, $\mathbf{a}$ and b are learned parameters, and $\sigma(\cdot)$ is the sigmoid function. Only high-confidence concepts are retained for subsequent processing.

Normalized concepts are categorized into clinically relevant types, such as diagnoses, medications, procedures, and follow-up actions, using UMLS semantic types and linked terminologies including SNOMED CT and RxNorm.

Input-Conditioned Knowledge Graph Construction: From the accepted concepts, MEG-QA constructs an input-conditioned knowledge graph $G_x = (V, E)$, where nodes V correspond to UMLS concepts present in $x \cup \mathcal{S}$, and edges E represent semantic relations defined in biomedical ontologies (e.g., *treats*, *associated_with*, *causes*).

Relation plausibility between two concepts h and t is scored as:

$$s_{\text{rel}}(h, t) = \lambda_p \cdot \text{match}(h, t) + (1 - \lambda_p) \cos(\mathbf{z}_h, \mathbf{z}_t), \tag{6}$$

where $\mathbf{z}_h$ and $\mathbf{z}_t$ are concept embeddings, match$(\cdot)$ encodes ontology-defined relations, and λ_p balances symbolic and embedding-based signals.

Graph Representation: To encode local semantic structure, node-representations are refined via neighborhood aggregation over G_x. This representation captures clinically plausible concept configurations and serves as a structural prior during generation.

The resulting graph grounding provides explicit semantic constraints that complement retrieval-based evidence, enabling MEG-QA to reason over concept compatibility and reduce semantic drift during question abbreviation.

3.4 Alignment-Aware Generation

In MEG-QA, generation is guided by both retrieved textual evidence and signals from a structured medical knowledge graph. Rather than enforcing hard constraints, MEG-QA adopts an *alignment-aware generation* strategy that softly biases decoding toward outputs consistent with supported medical concepts and qualifiers.

Given the input question x, selected evidence block $\mathcal{S}$, and input-conditioned knowledge graph G_x, the base language model generates a candidate abbreviated question $\hat{x}$ in an autoregressive manner. At each decoding step, candidate tokens are scored not only by the model likelihood, but also by their consistency with the retrieved evidence and the knowledge graph.

Evidence Alignment: Tokens or spans that correspond to medical concepts observed in the retrieved evidence $\mathcal{S}$ are preferred. In contrast, tokens that introduce concepts not supported by the evidence are assigned lower scores. This encourages generation to remain grounded in external context rather than relying solely on the model's parametric knowledge.

Knowledge Graph Alignment: Knowledge graph grounding further constrains generation by discouraging concept combinations that are inconsistent with the structure of G_x. Candidate generations that introduce concepts not present in the graph, or violate plausible relations between concepts, receive a lower score during decoding. This mechanism helps prevent concept substitution, qualifier loss, and unsupported medical assertions.

Alignment-Aware Scoring. The score of a candidate generation $\hat{x}$ is computed as:

$$\mathcal{L}(\hat{x}) = \log P_{\text{LM}}(\hat{x} \mid x, \mathcal{S}) - \gamma \, \mathcal{L}_{\text{align}}(\hat{x}, G_x, \mathcal{S}), \tag{7}$$

where P_{LM} denotes the base language model probability, $\mathcal{L}_{\text{align}}$ penalizes misalignment with evidence and knowledge graph constraints, and γ controls the strength of alignment guidance.

This soft scoring formulation allows MEG-QA to trade off fluency and faithfulness, producing concise medical question abbreviations that remain clinically consistent without degrading readability.

Overall, alignment-aware generation acts as the integration point between retrieved evidence and structured medical knowledge, helping to reduce hallucinations and intent drift while remaining agnostic to the choice of the underlying language model.

4 Evaluation Metrics

We evaluate medical question abbreviation using a combination of standard automatic metrics and a task-specific metric designed to assess alignment. Conventional similarity-based metrics are useful for measuring surface overlap and general fluency, but they are limited in the medical setting, where even small semantic changes can shift the underlying clinical intent.

4.1 Standard Metrics

We report commonly used automatic metrics to assess surface quality and semantic similarity in medical question abbreviation. ROUGE-L measures lexical overlap via longest common subsequence, while BLEU and METEOR evaluate n-gram precision and alignment-based similarity, respectively. These metrics provide coarse indicators of content overlap and paraphrasing quality but remain largely token-centric [24].

To capture semantic similarity beyond lexical matching, we report BERTScore, which computes contextual embedding alignments between generated and reference questions. We additionally measure Flesch-Kincaid Grade

Level (FKGL) to assess readability, an important factor for consumer-facing medical text [25].

Despite their widespread use, these metrics do not explicitly evaluate medical faithfulness. High ROUGE, BLEU, METEOR, or BERTScore can be achieved even when clinically salient concepts are omitted, qualifiers such as negation or temporality are altered, or unsupported medical concepts are introduced. Such errors are particularly consequential in short-form medical question abbreviation, where compression amplifies semantic drift.

These limitations motivate the CQA-Align Score, which evaluates faithfulness at the level of medical concepts, associated qualifiers, and attribution to the source question, complementing standard similarity-based metrics.

4.2 CQA-Align Score

We propose *CQA-Align Score* (Concept-Qualifier-Attribution Alignment Score), a metric designed to evaluate faithfulness in medical question abbreviation. CQA-Align measures whether generated questions preserve clinically salient concepts, maintain critical qualifiers, and avoid unsupported medical assertions.

Concept Alignment (CQA-C): Medical concepts in the input question x and generated abbreviation $\hat{x}$ are normalized to UMLS concepts using SapBERT. Let $C(x)$ and $C(\hat{x})$ denote the resulting concept sets. Concept alignment is computed as:

$$\text{CQA-C} = \frac{2\,|C(x) \cap C(\hat{x})|}{|C(x)| + |C(\hat{x})|}. \tag{8}$$

Qualifier Alignment (CQA-Q): For each aligned concept, we verify whether associated qualifiers like negation or temporality are preserved. Specifically, qualifier alignment is defined as the average exact-match accuracy over shared concepts:

$$\text{CQA-Q} = \frac{1}{|C(x) \cap C(\hat{x})|} \sum_{c} \mathbb{I}\big(Q(c) = Q(\hat{c})\big). \tag{9}$$

Attribution Alignment (CQA-A): To penalize hallucinated content, we measure whether concepts introduced in $\hat{x}$ are supported by the input question:

$$\text{CQA-A} = 1 - \frac{|C(\hat{x}) \setminus C(x)|}{|C(\hat{x})|}. \tag{10}$$

Overall Score. Finally, the overall CQA-Align Score is computed as the unweighted average of the three components:

$$\text{CQA-Align} = \tfrac{1}{3}\big(\text{CQA-C} + \text{CQA-Q} + \text{CQA-A}\big). \tag{11}$$

Especially, CQA-Align enables fine-grained analysis of faithfulness errors that are not captured by similarity-based metrics.

5 Experimental Setup

5.1 Datasets and Baselines

We evaluate MEG-QA on the MeQSum dataset [11], which consists of 1,000 verbose consumer health questions (CHQs) reformulated into concise, professional medical questions. MeQSum is particularly relevant to Nordic digital health contexts, where short, accurate abbreviations of user queries in wireless telehealth apps, involving, e.g., remote populations in Finland and Sweden, can enhance accessibility and response efficiency. The dataset emphasizes paraphrase-style reformulation, preserving clinical intent, symptoms, and details in outputs averaging 15 to 25 words.

For preprocessing, we apply entity linking with SapBERT to normalize medical terms (e.g., "stomach pain" to "abdominal pain") and filter outliers with lengths exceeding 512 tokens. We use an 80%, 10%, and 10% for train, validation, and test split, with random seeding for reproducibility.

Baseline models include:

1. Zero-Shot and Few-Shot Prompting: Direct prompting of Mistral, Llama, and Qwen models with in-context examples (0 or 5 shots).
2. PEFT Variants: Parameter-efficient fine-tuning (QLoRA) on base models.
3. RAG: Retrieval-augmented generation using a sparse-dense pipeline for evidence selection.
4. Hybrid RAG and Knowledge Graph: RAG enhanced with knowledge graph grounding (UMLS-linked relations for plausibility checks).

All these baselines are evaluated under the same computational constraints to ensure a fair comparison.

Prompt Usage Across Paradigms. The MEG-QA prompt template is used during inference for all model variants. For ICL (zero-shot and few-shot) settings, the full template serves as the system prompt, with zero or five in-context exemplars inserted at the designated slot. For PEFT (QLoRA) models, the same template structure is used as both the training input format and the inference prompt, ensuring consistency between fine-tuning and evaluation conditions.

MEG-QA Prompt Template

```
Expertise: You are an expert medical professional specialized in
consumer health question reformulation.
Instruction: Abbreviate the verbose consumer health question into a
concise, professional medical question.
Guidance: Preserve all clinical entities (symptoms, conditions,
durations, medications), negation, uncertainty, and intent; avoid
unsupported claims.
Evidence:
«BEGIN EVIDENCE»
{e_1}
```

```
...
{e_k}
«END EVIDENCE»
(Optionally include m exemplars for few-shot ICL; omit for zero-shot
and PEFT.)
Input: {x}
MEG-QA Abbreviation: ...
```

5.2 Implementation Details

MEG-QA is implemented using PyTorch 2.9.1 on a Tesla V100 GPU with 32GB VRAM, ensuring compatibility with modest computational resources for digital health deployments, like edge devices for wireless telehealth. The generator uses Qwen-2.5, Mistral, or LLaMA as base models, adapted via parameter-efficient fine-tuning (PEFT) with LoRA (rank = 64, alpha = 32, dropout = 0.05, target modules: q_proj, k_proj, v_proj, o_proj, gate_proj, up_proj, down_proj).

Training hyperparameters include 4 epochs, a learning rate of 1e-4 with a cosine scheduler, a per-device batch size of 1 (gradient accumulation of 16 for an effective batch of 16), and FP16 precision. For retrieval, we employ a sparse-dense pipeline: SPLADE-v2 for high-recall term expansion and SapBERT for UMLS-aligned re-ranking, with a fixed 512-token evidence budget and Maximal Marginal Relevance (MMR, lambda = 0.7) for diversity.

The knowledge graph is induced using SapBERT for CUI linking and relation extraction (finding_of, treats), with plausibility checks via a minimal-revision objective (loss weighting 0.3 for unsupported triples). Generation uses beam search (beams = 6–8), max_new_tokens = 192, length_penalty = 1.1, and no_repeat_ngram_size = 3. For applicability, the framework's low-compute PEFT and KG constraints can enable integration with wireless health monitoring apps, where short consumer questions from wearable data require safe abbreviation.

6 Experimental Result and Error Analysis

6.1 Overall Performance

Table 1 summarizes the performances on the MeQSum dataset across three paradigms (zero-shot, few-shot) in-context learning and parameter-efficient fine-tuning via QLoRA across three backbones (Mistral, LLaMA, and Qwen), with staged variants that isolate the effects of retrieval (RAG) and RAG with knowledge graph grounding (RAG-KG). Overall, the results indicate that MEG-QA enhances lexical and semantic alignment while achieving substantial gains in concept-level faithfulness, with the largest improvements in CQA-Align score.

In absolute terms, MEG-QA (Qwen with QLoRA and RAG-KG) achieves the highest scores across all metrics, reaching ROUGE-1 0.54, ROUGE-L 0.51, Meteor 0.52, BERTScore 0.87, and CQA-Align 0.67, while maintaining strong readability (FKGL 9.3). Relative to the corresponding QLoRA Qwen baseline without grounding (ROUGE-1 0.52, CQA-Align 0.61), MEG-QA yields an increment of +0.02 in ROUGE-1 (4% relative improvement) and +0.06 in CQA-Align (10% relative improvement), indicating that the system enhances clinical faithfulness beyond stylistic changes in short consumer question abbreviation.

The staged results provide clear attribution of these gains. Under the QLoRA setting, introducing RAG increases ROUGE-1 from 0.52 to 0.53 (increment +0.01, approximately 2% relative) and CQA-Align from 0.61 to 0.65 (increment +0.04, approximately 7% relative), consistent with retrieval improving evidence coverage in short paraphrases. Adding knowledge graph grounding on top of RAG further increases CQA-Align to 0.67 (increment +0.02, approximately 3% relative), indicating that structured constraints reduce unsupported clinical concepts and stabilize entity-relation consistency beyond what retrieval alone can enforce. The same pattern is visible across backbones and ICL settings: adding RAG systematically raises overlap and semantic metrics, whereas adding knowledge graph grounding strengthens safety-oriented performance.

Across adaptation approaches, PEFT provides a clear advantage over ICL for the same backbone and system configuration. For example, the strongest ICL configuration (few-shot adaptation of Qwen with RAG-KG) reaches CQA-Align 0.65, whereas the PEFT full system reaches 0.67, an increment of +0.02 (approximately 3% relative). This suggests that parameter-efficient adaptation improves the model's ability to operationalize evidence and constraints during generation, particularly for short-form abbreviation, where compression pressure otherwise increases the likelihood of plausible but unsupported insertions in consumer queries.

These improvements are particularly relevant for digital health applications, where short, faithful reformulations in telehealth platforms minimize clinical risks and enhance user safety.

6.2 Ablation Studies

To isolate the contributions of retrieval augmentation (RAG) and knowledge graph grounding (RAG-KG), we conduct ablation studies on the MeQSum. Tables 2, 3, and 4 report absolute scores for the baseline (Base) within each paradigm, along with signed gains (Δ) for RAG and RAG-KG relative to the baseline. Higher values are better for ROUGE-1/2/L, Meteor, BLEU, BERTScore, and CQA-Align; lower values are better for FKGL.

Across all models (Fig. 2), RAG consistently improves lexical overlap (ROUGE-1/2/L) and semantic alignment (Meteor, BERTScore) by 0.02–0.05, reflecting better evidence coverage in short paraphrases. Adding knowledge graph grounding on top of RAG delivers the largest gains in faithfulness (CQA-Align +0.03–0.07) and readability (FKGL reduction of 0.1–0.3), demonstrating that structured constraints reduce unsupported concepts and stabilize entity-relation consistency beyond retrieval alone.

The Qwen backbone shows the strongest absolute performance and gains, with RAG-KG yielding +0.05 ROUGE-1 and +0.06 CQA-Align over base in the

Table 1. Overall performance on MeQSum medical question abbreviation. RAG improves evidence coverage, while KG grounding further improves alignment and readability (lower FKGL is better). R-1: Rouge 1, R-2: Rouge 2, R-L: Rouge L, M: Meteor, BS: BERTScore, CQA: Concept-Qualifier-Attribution Alignment Score

Method	Approach	Model	R-1	R-2	R-L	M	BLEU	BS	CQA	FKGL
ICL	Zero-shot	Mistral	0.44	0.22	0.39	0.40	0.17	0.76	0.51	10.4
		+ RAG	0.48	0.26	0.42	0.43	0.19	0.79	0.53	10.2
		+ RAG-KG	**0.50**	**0.28**	**0.44**	**0.45**	**0.20**	**0.82**	**0.56**	**10.1**
		Llama	0.43	0.21	0.38	0.39	0.16	0.71	0.46	10.5
		+ RAG	0.46	0.24	0.41	0.42	0.18	0.77	0.48	10.3
		+ RAG-KG	0.48	0.26	0.43	0.43	0.19	0.78	0.51	10.2
		Qwen	0.46	0.24	0.40	0.41	0.17	0.81	0.55	10.3
		+ RAG	0.49	0.26	0.43	0.44	0.19	0.83	0.57	10.1
		+ RAG-KG	**0.51**	**0.29**	**0.45**	**0.46**	**0.20**	**0.84**	**0.62**	**10.0**
	Few-shot	Mistral	0.47	0.25	0.41	0.42	0.19	0.79	0.50	10.2
		+ RAG	0.50	0.28	0.44	0.46	0.21	0.83	0.57	10.0
		+ RAG-KG	**0.52**	**0.30**	**0.46**	**0.48**	**0.22**	**0.84**	**0.63**	**9.9**
		Llama	0.45	0.24	0.41	0.40	0.18	0.76	0.58	10.3
		+ RAG	0.49	0.27	0.43	0.45	0.20	0.78	0.60	10.1
		+ RAG-KG	0.51	0.29	0.45	0.47	0.21	0.82	0.62	10.0
		Qwen	0.49	0.26	0.43	0.44	0.19	0.80	0.59	10.1
		+ RAG	0.51	0.30	0.45	0.47	0.21	0.83	0.64	9.9
		+ RAG-KG	**0.53**	**0.31**	**0.47**	**0.49**	**0.22**	**0.85**	**0.65**	**9.8**
PEFT	QLoRA	Mistral	0.49	0.28	0.44	0.47	0.21	0.82	0.60	9.8
		+ RAG	0.52	0.31	0.47	0.49	**0.23**	0.84	0.62	9.6
		+ RAG-KG	**0.53**	**0.32**	**0.48**	**0.50**	**0.23**	**0.84**	**0.66**	**9.5**
		Llama	0.48	0.27	0.43	0.46	0.20	0.81	0.58	9.9
		+ RAG	0.51	0.30	0.46	0.48	0.20	0.83	0.64	9.7
		+ RAG-KG	**0.52**	**0.31**	**0.47**	**0.49**	**0.22**	**0.85**	**0.67**	**9.6**
		Qwen	0.52	0.32	0.48	0.49	0.21	0.84	0.61	9.6
		+ RAG	0.53	0.34	0.50	0.51	0.24	0.87	0.65	9.4
		+ RAG-KG (MEG-QA)	**0.54**	**0.35**	**0.51**	**0.52**	**0.26**	**0.87**	**0.67**	**9.3**

PEFT paradigm. Mistral and Llama exhibit similar trends, with KG grounding providing the most pronounced safety improvements. These results underscore the complementary role of RAG (coverage) and KG (faithfulness) in reliable medical question abbreviation.

In digital health contexts, the ablation highlights the value of knowledge graph constraints for preventing clinical risks in short reformulations within telehealth platforms.

6.3 Error Analysis and Qualitative Insights

Aggregate metrics alone do not capture the clinical impact of abbreviation errors, as different failure modes carry different levels of risk in consumer health contexts. We therefore perform a detailed error analysis centered on concept-level correctness, examining diagnoses (Dx), medications (Rx), procedures (Proc), and follow-up instructions (Fup) as shown in Table 5.

In zero-shot and few-shot ICL, baseline models consistently show the weakest performance in Dx F1 (0.51–0.56), reflecting frequent omission or incomplete consolidation of diagnostic details in short paraphrases. Retrieval (RAG)

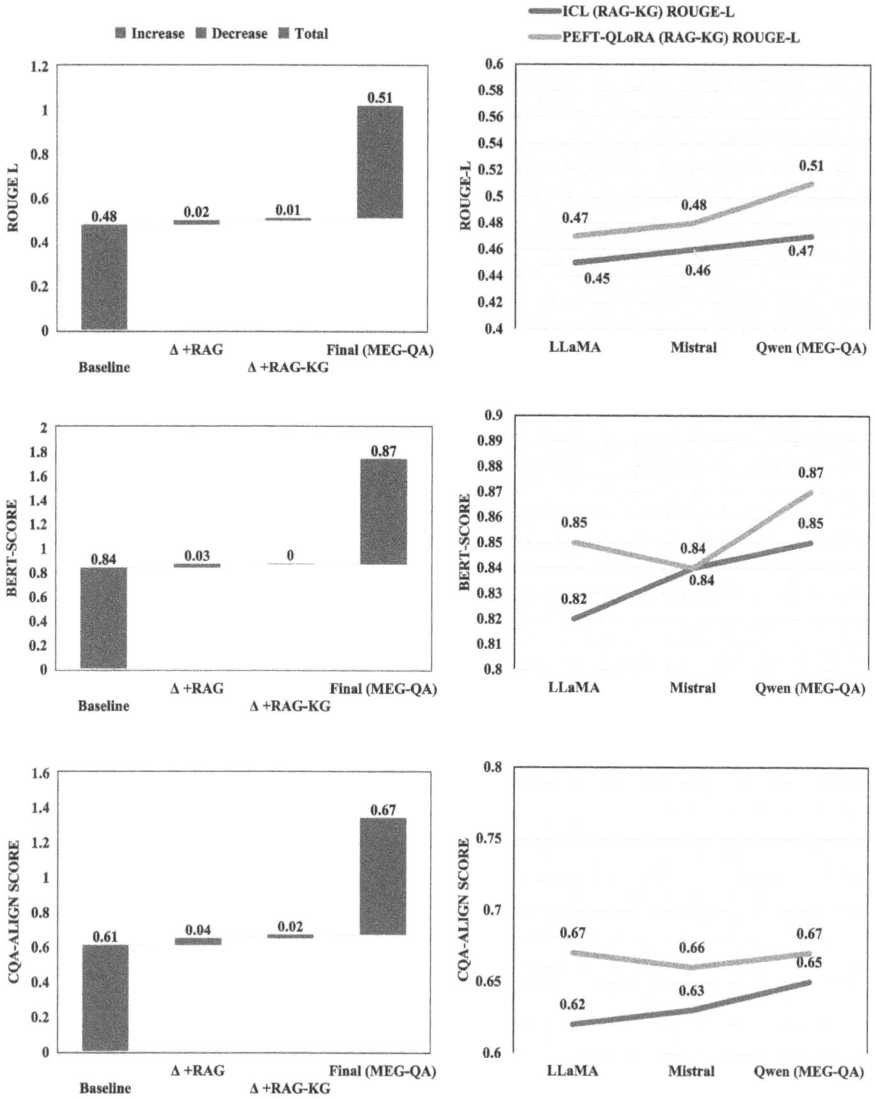

Fig. 2. (Left) Stepwise gains from RAG and RAG-KG and (Right) effect of ICL and PEFT adaptation approach of MEG-QA.

improves coverage across categories, but the most consistent gains occur when knowledge graph grounding (RAG-KG) is applied, particularly in Rx_F1 (medications) and Proc_F1 (procedures), where constraints reduce unsupported treatment or procedure inferences. PEFT baselines are stronger overall, yet still exhibit Dx as the weakest axis; MEG-QA shifts all variants to the high tier, achieving the highest Dx, Rx, Proc, and Fup F1 (0.64–0.75) and the lowest FKGL (9.3).

Table 2. Ablation study of Mistral on MeQSum.

Paradigm	Variant	R-L	Meteor	BLEU	BERTScore	CQA-Align	FKGL
Zero-shot	Base	**0.39**	**0.40**	**0.17**	**0.76**	**0.51**	**10.4**
	+RAG	+0.03	+0.03	+0.02	+0.03	+0.02	-0.2
	+RAG-KG (Ours)	+0.05	+0.05	+0.03	+0.06	+0.05	-0.3
Few-shot	Base	**0.41**	**0.42**	**0.19**	**0.79**	**0.50**	**10.2**
	+RAG	+0.03	+0.04	+0.02	+0.04	+0.07	-0.2
	+RAG-KG (Ours)	+0.05	+0.06	+0.03	+0.05	+0.13	-0.3
PEFT (QLoRA)	Base	**0.44**	**0.47**	**0.21**	**0.82**	**0.60**	**9.8**
	+RAG	+0.03	+0.02	+0.02	+0.02	+0.02	-0.2
	+RAG-KG (Ours)	+0.04	+0.03	+0.02	+0.02	+0.06	-0.3

Table 3. Ablation study of Llama on MeQSum.

Paradigm	Variant	R-L	Meteor	BLEU	BERTScore	CQA-Align	FKGL
Zero-shot	Base	**0.38**	**0.39**	**0.16**	**0.71**	**0.46**	**10.5**
	+RAG	+0.03	+0.03	+0.02	+0.06	+0.02	-0.2
	+RAG-KG (Ours)	+0.05	+0.04	+0.03	+0.07	+0.05	-0.3
Few-shot	Base	**0.41**	**0.40**	**0.18**	**0.76**	**0.58**	**10.3**
	+RAG	+0.02	+0.05	+0.02	+0.02	+0.02	-0.2
	+RAG-KG (Ours)	+0.04	+0.07	+0.03	+0.06	+0.04	-0.3
PEFT (QLoRA)	Base	**0.43**	**0.46**	**0.20**	**0.81**	**0.58**	**9.9**
	+RAG	+0.03	+0.02	+0.00	+0.02	+0.06	-0.2
	+RAG-KG (Ours)	+0.04	+0.03	+0.02	+0.04	+0.09	-0.3

Table 4. Ablation study of Qwen on MeQSum.

Paradigm	Variant	R-L	Meteor	BLEU	BERTScore	CQA-Align	FKGL
Zero-shot	Base	**0.40**	**0.41**	**0.17**	**0.81**	**0.55**	**10.3**
	+RAG	+0.03	+0.03	+0.02	+0.02	+0.02	-0.2
	+RAG-KG (Ours)	+0.05	+0.05	+0.03	+0.03	+0.07	-0.3
Few-shot	Base	**0.43**	**0.44**	**0.19**	**0.80**	**0.59**	**10.1**
	+RAG	+0.02	+0.03	+0.02	+0.03	+0.05	-0.2
	+RAG-KG (Ours)	+0.04	+0.05	+0.03	+0.05	+0.06	-0.3
PEFT (QLoRA)	Base	**0.48**	**0.49**	**0.21**	**0.84**	**0.61**	**9.6**
	+RAG	+0.02	+0.02	+0.03	+0.03	+0.04	-0.2
	+RAG-KG (MEG-QA)	+0.03	+0.03	+0.05	+0.03	+0.06	-0.3

7 Discussion

This section synthesizes the key findings from our evaluation of MEG-QA (Fig. 3) on the MeQSum dataset, highlights the framework's contributions to medical question abbreviation, and interprets the performance gains from a clinical perspective. We also address limitations and outline future directions.

7.1 Key Findings

Our experiments demonstrate that MEG-QA achieves the best performance among all evaluated configurations in consumer health question abbreviation, with consistent improvements in lexical overlap (ROUGE-1 up to 0.54), semantic alignment (Meteor 0.52, BERTScore 0.87), and faithfulness (CQA-Align 0.67). The staged variants reveal that RAG enhances evidence coverage, boosting ROUGE and BERTScore by 0.02–0.05, while KG grounding provides the largest gains in CQA-Align (0.03–0.07) by stabilizing entity-relation consistency in short paraphrases. Ablations confirm the complementary roles: RAG alone improves content recall, but combined RAG-KG reduces unsupported concepts, shifting faithfulness tiers from Low or Medium to High across paradigms. Category-wise breakdowns show Dx F1 as the persistent weakness in baselines (0.51–0.62), mitigated by MEG-QA's constraints (up to 0.64), underscoring its value for preserving clinical intent in concise outputs.

7.2 Contributions

MEG-QA's primary contribution is a novel, knowledge-aligned framework for reliable abbreviation of verbose consumer questions, integrating RAG with UMLS-grounded KG constraints to enforce conceptual fidelity without relying solely on prompt engineering or full fine-tuning. This dual-channel approach discourages unsupported claims and qualifier omissions, addressing gaps in prior MeQSum work. Additionally, CQA-Align introduces a UMLS-normalized metric that reveals error patterns hidden by standard scores, enabling safer evaluation in medical NLP.

7.3 Clinical Interpretation of Performance Gains

Clinically, MEG-QA's gains translate to improved safety and utility in consumer-facing platforms. The 0.08–0.13 increase in CQA-Align reflects better preservation of qualifiers like negation, uncertainty, and relations (symptom-cause), reducing the likelihood of misleading advice, which is critical in MeQSum's layperson queries, where omissions could lead to inappropriate self-diagnosis. For instance, baselines drop duration details, risking incomplete clinical context, while MEG-QA maintains them, enhancing interpretability for healthcare providers. Readability improvements (FKGL reduction to 9.3) ensure outputs remain accessible without sacrificing professionalism, supporting eHealth goals for equitable digital tools. In wireless scenarios, such as symptom reporting via mobile devices, MEG-QA minimizes hallucinations, potentially lowering unnecessary consultations in resource-limited regions.

7.4 Limitations

Despite strong performance, MEG-QA has limitations. The reliance on UMLS for KG grounding may introduce biases in non-English or underrepresented

Table 5. Category-wise CQA-Align breakdown on MeQSum, with Weakest Category (lowest F1 axis) and Faithfulness Tier (High ≥ 0.65, Medium 0.55–0.64, Low < 0.55). WC: Weakest Category, FT: Faithfulness Tier.

Paradigm	Model	Variant	CQA	Dx	Rx	Proc	Fup	FKGL	WC	FT
Zero-Shot ICL	Mistral	Base	0.51	0.52	0.64	0.55	0.53	10.4	Dx	Low
		+RAG	0.53	0.55	0.68	0.58	0.56	10.2	Dx	Low
		+RAG-KG	0.56	0.56	0.70	0.60	0.57	10.1	Dx	Medium
	Llama	Base	0.46	0.51	0.63	0.54	0.52	10.5	Dx	Low
		+RAG	0.48	0.54	0.67	0.56	0.55	10.3	Dx	Low
		+RAG-KG	0.51	0.55	0.69	0.58	0.56	10.2	Dx	Low
	Qwen	Base	0.55	0.53	0.66	0.56	0.55	10.3	Dx	Medium
		+RAG	0.57	0.57	0.70	0.59	0.58	10.1	Dx	Medium
		+RAG-KG	0.62	0.58	0.72	0.61	0.60	10.0	Dx	Medium
Few-Shot ICL	Mistral	Base	0.50	0.55	0.68	0.58	0.56	10.2	Dx	Low
		+RAG	0.57	0.58	0.72	0.61	0.59	10.0	Dx	Medium
		+RAG-KG	0.63	0.60	0.74	0.63	0.60	9.9	Dx	Medium
	Llama	Base	0.58	0.54	0.67	0.57	0.56	10.3	Dx	Medium
		+RAG	0.60	0.57	0.71	0.60	0.59	10.1	Dx	Medium
		+RAG-KG	0.62	0.59	0.73	0.62	0.61	10.0	Dx	Medium
	Qwen	Base	0.59	0.56	0.69	0.59	0.58	10.1	Dx	Medium
		+RAG	0.64	0.60	0.73	0.62	0.61	9.9	Dx	Medium
		+RAG-KG	**0.65**	**0.61**	**0.75**	**0.64**	**0.62**	**9.8**	**Dx**	**High**
PEFT (QLoRA)	Mistral	Base	0.60	0.59	0.73	0.62	0.60	9.8	Dx	Medium
		+RAG	0.62	0.61	0.76	0.64	0.62	9.6	Dx	Medium
		+RAG-KG	0.66	0.62	0.78	0.66	0.63	9.5	Dx	High
	Llama	Base	0.58	0.58	0.72	0.61	0.60	9.9	Dx	Medium
		+RAG	0.64	0.60	0.75	0.63	0.62	9.7	Dx	Medium
		+RAG-KG	**0.67**	**0.61**	**0.77**	**0.65**	**0.63**	**9.6**	**Dx**	**High**
	Qwen	Base	0.61	0.62	0.77	0.65	0.63	9.6	Dx	Medium
		+RAG	**0.65**	**0.63**	**0.80**	**0.68**	**0.65**	**9.4**	**Dx**	**High**
		+RAG-KG (MEG-QA)	**0.67**	**0.64**	**0.83**	**0.75**	**0.69**	**9.3**	**Dx**	**High**

medical terms. Short MeQSum inputs limit KG depth, potentially underutilizing relations in more verbose contexts. Computational overhead from RAG-KG (though modest with PEFT) may challenge edge deployment in low-power wireless devices. Finally, CQA-Align assumes perfect entity linking, which can falter on ambiguous layperson phrasing.

7.5 Future Work

Future extensions include multilingual adaptation for different languages, with local ontologies integration and incorporation of wireless sensor data into the KG for context-enriched abbreviation. We also plan to explore full fine-tuning for larger models and human evaluation in telehealth pilots to validate clinical utility.

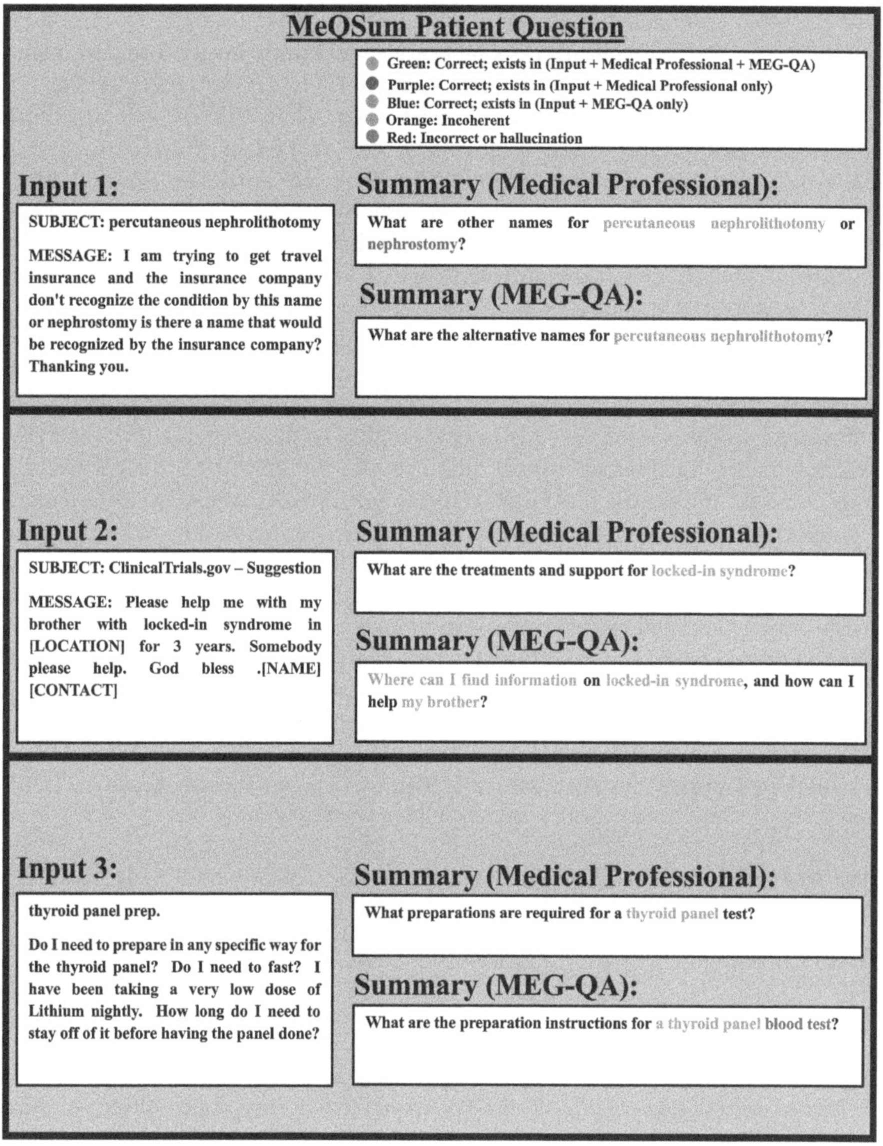

Fig. 3. MEG-QA medical question abbreviation from MeQSum dataset.

8 Conclusion

In this work, we presented MEG-QA, a new framework for medical evidence-grounded question abbreviation that combines retrieval-augmented generation with knowledge graph constraints to produce concise yet conceptually faithful reformulations of verbose consumer health questions. By grounding outputs in both retrieved evidence and structured medical knowledge, MEG-QA mitigates common issues in short paraphrase generation, including entity loss and unsupported assertions, which are especially problematic in digital health settings.

Experiments on the MeQSum dataset show that MEG-QA consistently outperforms prior approaches, achieving scores of 0.54 in ROUGE-1, 0.51 in ROUGE-L, and 0.67 in CQA-Align, outperforming both the original MeQSum seq2seq baseline [11] and recent instruction-tuned LLM results [12]. These improvements highlight the effectiveness of hybrid RAG-KG grounding, which not only boosts lexical and semantic similarity but also strengthens clinical faithfulness, as reflected in category-level F1 gains and shifts from low to high tiers. Moreover, the proposed CQA-Align metric offers a more fine-grained assessment of faithfulness beyond surface overlap, uncovering error patterns that traditional metrics often miss.

From a clinical perspective, MEG-QA's ability to preserve qualifiers and relations in concise outputs has direct implications for digital health ecosystems, where wireless telehealth platforms rely on accurate, trustworthy abbreviation to support remote consultations and reduce miscommunication risks in underserved areas.

Future work will explore extending MEG-QA to multilingual settings and incorporating wearable sensor information into the knowledge graph to enable richer contextual abbreviation. Overall, this framework contributes to the development of safe, evidence-aligned NLP for consumer health, supporting more accessible and dependable digital health applications.

Acknowledgments. This work was partly supported by the Finnish Research Council Profi 7 Hybrid Intelligence, which is gratefully acknowledged.

Disclosure of Interests. The authors have no competing interests to declare.

References

1. Singhal, K., et al.: Toward expert-level medical question answering with large language models. Nat. Med. **31**(3), 943–950 (2025)
2. Shi, Y., et al.: MKRAG: medical knowledge retrieval augmented generation for medical question answering. In: AMIA Annual Symposium Proceedings, vol. 2024, p. 1011 (2025)
3. Blašković, L., Tanković, N., Lorencin, I., Baressi Šegota, S.: Robust clinical querying with local LLMs: lexical challenges in NL2SQL and retrieval-augmented QA on EHRs. Big Data Cogn. Comput. **9**(10), 256 (2025)
4. Miao, Y., Zhao, Y., Luo, Y., Wang, H., Ying, W.: Improving large language model applications in the medical and nursing domains with retrieval-augmented generation: scoping review. J. Med. Internet Res. **27**, e80557 (2025)
5. Kim, J., Podlasek, A., Shidara, K., Liu, F., Alaa, A., Bernardo, D.: Limitations of large language models in clinical problem-solving arising from inflexible reasoning. Sci. Rep. **15**(1), 39426 (2025)
6. Genesis, J., Keane, F.: Integrating knowledge retrieval with generation: a comprehensive survey of rag models in NLP (2025)

7. Ajay Mukund, S., Easwarakumar, K.S.: Optimizing legal text summarization through dynamic retrieval-augmented generation and domain-specific adaptation. Symmetry **17**(5), 633 (2025)
8. Tran, H., Wang, J., Ting, Y., Yu, H., Huang, W., Chen, T.: Leaf: learning and evaluation augmented by fact-checking to improve factualness in large language models. In: Proceedings of the 2025 Conference on Empirical Methods in Natural Language Processing: Industry Track, pp. 338–363 (2025)
9. Joseph, S., et al.: Factpico: factuality evaluation for plain language summarization of medical evidence. In: Proceedings of the 62nd Annual Meeting of the Association for Computational Linguistics (Volume 1: Long Papers), pp. 8437–8464 (2024)
10. Schmidtová, P., et al.: Automatic metrics in natural language generation: a survey of current evaluation practices. arXiv preprint arXiv:2408.09169 (2024)
11. Abacha, A.B., Demner-Fushman, D.: On the summarization of consumer health questions. In: Proceedings of the 57th Annual Meeting of the Association for Computational Linguistics, pp. 2228–2234 (2019)
12. Jahan, I., Laskar, M.T.R., Peng, C., Huang, J.X.: A comprehensive evaluation of large language models on benchmark biomedical text processing tasks. Comput. Biol. Med. **171**, 108189 (2024)
13. Zhou, C., Liang, Y., Meng, F., Xu, J., Su, J., Zhou, J.: RC3: regularized contrastive cross-lingual cross-modal pre-training. arXiv preprint arXiv:2305.07927 (2023)
14. Li, S., Zhang, Y., Deng, C., Niu, Y., Zhao, H.: Better late than never: model-agnostic hallucination post-processing framework towards clinical text summarization. In: Findings of the Association for Computational Linguistics ACL 2024, pp. 995–1011 (2024)
15. Lewis, P., et al.: Retrieval-augmented generation for knowledge-intensive NLP tasks. Adv. Neural. Inf. Process. Syst. **33**, 9459–9474 (2020)
16. Jiang, Z., et al.: Active retrieval augmented generation. In: Proceedings of the 2023 Conference on Empirical Methods in Natural Language Processing, pp. 7969–7992 (2023)
17. Gao, L., et al.: RARR: researching and revising what language models say, using language models. In: Proceedings of the 61st Annual Meeting of the Association for Computational Linguistics (Volume 1: Long Papers), pp. 16477–16508 (2023)
18. Wu, D., Gu, J.-C., Yin, F., Peng, N., Chang, K.-W.: Synchronous faithfulness monitoring for trustworthy retrieval-augmented generation. arXiv preprint arXiv:2406.13692 (2024)
19. Goldsack, T., Zhang, Z., Tang, C., Scarton, C., Lin, C.: Enhancing biomedical lay summarisation with external knowledge graphs. arXiv preprint arXiv:2310.15702 (2023)
20. Kaur, N., Choudhury, M., Pruthi, D.: Evaluating large language models for health-related queries with presuppositions. In: Findings of the Association for Computational Linguistics: ACL 2024, pp. 14308–14331 (2024)
21. Formal, T., Lassance, C., Piwowarski, B., Clinchant, S.: Splade v2: sparse lexical and expansion model for information retrieval. arXiv preprint arXiv:2109.10086 (2021)
22. Liu, F., Shareghi, E., Meng, Z., Basaldella, M., Collier, N.: Self-alignment pretraining for biomedical entity representations. In: Proceedings of the 2021 Conference of the North American chapter of the Association for Computational Linguistics: Human Language Technologies, pp. 4228–4238 (2021)
23. Carbonell, J., Goldstein, J.: The use of MMR, diversity-based reranking for reordering documents and producing summaries. In: Proceedings of the 21st Annual Inter-

national ACM SIGIR Conference on Research and Development in Information Retrieval, pp. 335–336 (1998)
24. Junadhi, J., Agustin, A., Efrizoni, L., Okmayura, F., Habibie, D.R., Muslim, M.: Improving evaluation metrics for text summarization: a comparative study and proposal of a novel metric. J. Appl. Data Sci. **6**(2), 885–896 (2025)
25. Croxford, E., et al.: Current and future state of evaluation of large language models for medical summarization tasks. NPJ Health Syst. **2**(1), 6 (2025)

Abstracts

Evaluating Predictive Performance of Machine Learning Based Patient Selection for Spinal Cord Stimulation in Chronic Pain

Mohosina Akhter(✉) and Minna Isomursu

University of Oulu, Linnanmaa, Finland
mohosina.akhter@oulu.fi

Abstract. Chronic pain is a complex global health problem affecting approximately 20% of the adult population in developed countries. Spinal cord stimulation (SCS) is an established therapeutic option for selected patients with refractory chronic pain; however, identifying appropriate candidates remains challenging due to patient heterogeneity and the dependence on expert-driven decision-making. While machine learning (ML) approaches have gained interest as potential tools to support patient selection, their predictive performance and robustness under controlled conditions remain insufficiently explored. This study evaluates the predictive performance of multiple classical machine learning models for SCS appropriateness prediction using semi-synthetic datasets derived from a publicly available expert-informed framework of chronic pain scenarios. Linear and tree-based models were evaluated through a case-study research design, emphasizing model behavior, robustness, and interpretability rather than clinical deployment. Model performance was evaluated using a combination of regression-based and decision-oriented metrics, along with stress-testing on both the semi-synthetic evaluation data and additionally generated synthetic data covering unseen feature combinations, feature missingness, and label noise. Among the evaluated models, Random Forest achieved the lowest prediction error and highest explained variance, while showing consistent behavior under controlled missing data and label noise conditions. These findings suggest that machine learning models can learn structured relationships present in expert-defined clinical and psychosocial criteria. However, this study is limited by the use of synthetic data for model evaluation, and no claims regarding clinical effectiveness or real-world generalizability are made. This work provides a systematic evaluation of model performance and highlights directions for future validation using real-world clinical data.

Keywords: Spinal Cord Stimulation · Chronic Pain · Patient Selection · Predictive Modeling

M. Särestöniemi et al. (Eds.): NCDHWS 2026, CCIS 3010, pp. 729–731, 2026.
https://doi.org/10.1007/978-3-032-28819-6

Table 1 shows Model performance comparison (5-fold cross-validation mean scores).

Table 1. Model performance comparison (5-fold cross-validation mean scores)

Model	CV RMSE	CV R^2	CV Correctness
Linear Regression	1.345 ± 0.113	0.498 ± 0.100	0.283 ± 0.040
Decision Tree Regressor	1.513 ± 0.123	0.355 ± 0.187	0.442 ± 0.044
Random Forest Regressor	**1.162 ± 0.101**	**0.625 ± 0.077**	**0.473 ± 0.055**
Gradient Boosting Regressor	1.227 ± 0.086	0.577 ± 0.066	0.366 ± 0.016

Figure 1 shows true versus predicted values for the best-performing model.

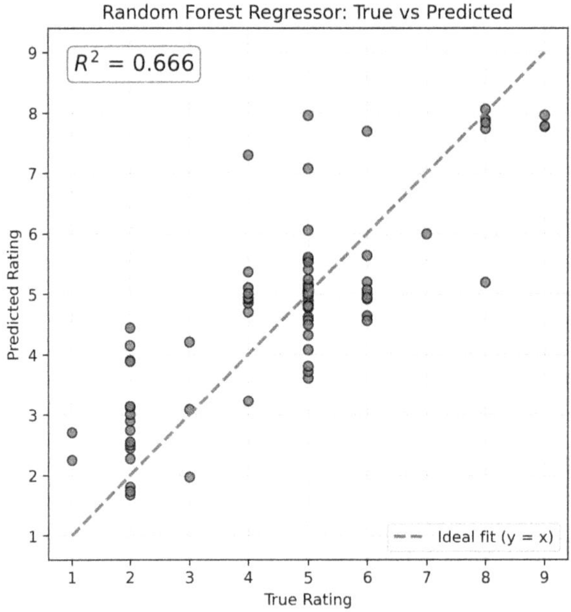

Fig. 1. True versus predicted values for the best-performing model.

Acknowledgments. This work has been co-funded by the European Union's Digital Europe Programme (DIGITAL) under grant agreement No. 101083544, and partly funded by Business Finland (No. 765/31/2023) and the University of Oulu.

References

1. Dahlhamer, J., Lucas, J., Zelaya, C., et al.: Prevalence of chronic pain and high-impact chronic pain among adults—United States, 2016. MMWR Morb. Mortal. Wkly Rep. **67**(36), 1001–1006 (2018)
2. Khadka, S.R., Karani, P., Gogineni, N., et al.: Advances in neurological pain management: bridging scientific innovations and clinical practice. Cureus **17**(3), e80447 (2025)
3. Thomson, S., Huygen, F., Prangnell, S., et al.: Appropriate referral and selection of patients with chronic pain for spinal cord stimulation: European consensus recommendations and e-health tool. Eur. J. Pain **24**(6), 1169–1181 (2020)
4. Gopal, J., Bao, J., Harland, T., et al.: Machine learning predicts spinal cord stimulation surgery outcomes and reveals novel neural markers for chronic pain. Sci. Rep. **15**, 9279 (2025)
5. Sahlin, U., Jiang, Y.: Monte Carlo simulation and Bayesian evidence synthesis. In: Safety and Reliability: Methodology and Applications, pp. 1589–1598. CRC Press (2014)
6. Dankar, F.K., Ibrahim, M.: Fake it till you make it: guidelines for effective synthetic data generation. Appl. Sci. **11**, 2158 (2021)
7. Pesado, P., Thomas, P. (eds.): Computer Science – CACIC 2024. Communications in Computer and Information Science, vol. 2520. Springer, Cham (2026)

Learning Health Systems as Enabler of Value-Based Care

Arild Faxvaag(✉)

Department of Neuromedicine and Movement Science, NTNU, Trondheim, Norway
arild.faxvaag@ntnu.no

Abstract. An important goal of any health system is to provide valuable care in a safe, effective and accountable manner. Yet, throughout the world, health systems struggle with accomplishing this. The Nordic countries rank among the world leaders in digitizing their health systems. Having EHRs, patient portals, health information exchange, health registries, laboratory and imaging systems in place, the Nordic health systems is also a unique arena for those who want to assess real-life impact and value of digital health tools. Has digitization of the Nordic health systems led to more effective, safer and valuable care? Are we now better at automating and at controlling the costs? Are we engaging and empowering the citizen in the best possible ways? The aim of this keynote is to present some of the budding insights and lessons learned, and to use these insights to sketch out an agenda for putting a learning health system at the center in the next rounds of architecture and information system designs.

Keywords: Learning health systems · Value-based care · Digital health

1 Introduction

We now have more that 30 years of experience with healthcare information systems in the Nordic countries [1]. There is a lot to learn from users' actual use and non-use of the systems, from their true positive effects, as well as from the effects that were planned for but that never materialized. We have learnt that healthcare information systems can empower clinicians, but also that clinicians that have learned how to use the systems effectively must invest a lot to develop the required information system skills. Finally, we have real-world evidence that healthcare information systems can cause system-level effects but also the opposite.

Institute of medicine describes a Learning health system (LHS) as 'a system in which science, informatics, incentives, and culture are aligned for continuous improvement and innovation, with best practices seamlessly embedded in the care process, patients and families as active participants in all elements, and new knowledge is captured as an integral by-product of the care experience' [2]. WHO describes a health system as all organizations, people and actions whose primary intent is to promote, restore or maintain health (WHO[1]). The backdrop of the LHS initiative is a healthcare sector that basically

[1] WHO Health system strengthening glossary: Available at https://cdn.who.int/media/docs/default-source/documents/health-systems-strengthening-glossary.pdf.

M. Särestöniemi et al. (Eds.): NCDHWS 2026, CCIS 3010, pp. 732–734, 2026.
https://doi.org/10.1007/978-3-032-28819-6

is awash with knowledges and competences but that lack the means of applying the right knowledges and competences in a sufficiently safe and accountable manner. According to Braithwaite et al., only 60% of the care that is provided is in line with guidelines, 30% is waste, duplicate or of low value, whereas 10% of patients are exposed to care that either is harmful or leads to adverse events [3]. Taken together, healthcare systems are in a situation that commands a new approach. The LHS initiative is an example of such a new approach.

2 Approach

Insights in the real-life value of true and tested healthcare information systems can be applied in health policy making as well as in healthcare information system design and engineering. High quality work within the healthcare system hinges on effective collaborations with the institutions that are responsible for educating the personnel and with institutions and enterprises responsible for the development of new knowledges medicines and medical devices.

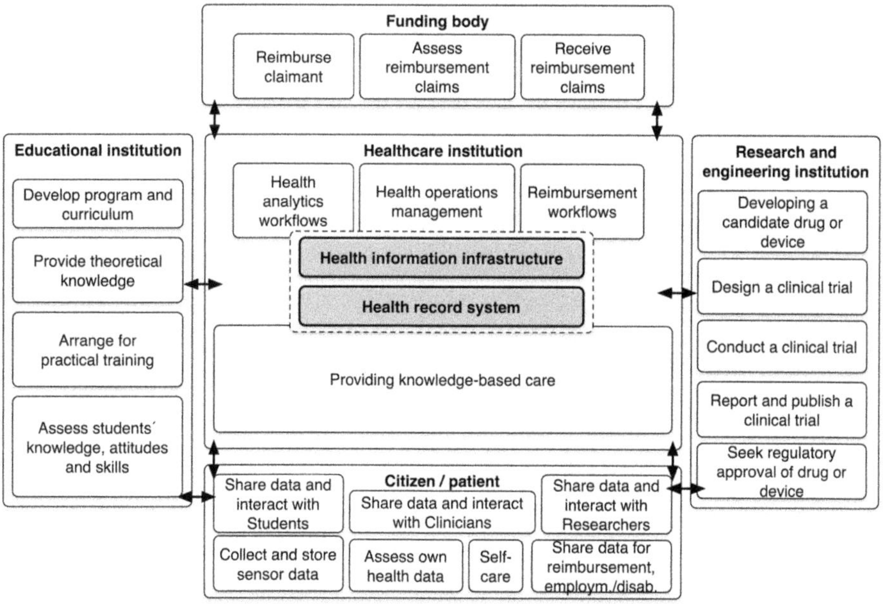

Fig. 1. Basic workflows, infrastructures and practices in a healthcare system and in the institutions that constitute the surrounding health ecosystem.

The keynote will ideate around the following questions: a) What are the most valuable insights from the nordic digital health experience? b) How can we enable clinicians, leaders, drug and medical device owners to learn from the true outcome of applying their skills or products? c) What are the possible designs of a health and healthcare information system architecture that eliminates today's digital barriers between healthcare systems and the surrounding ecosystem? d) What are the possible designs of EHR-systems that create a safer, more transparent and accountable healthcare system? and e) What are the possible designs of wellness information systems that fosters citizen-engagement in care, research as well as education?

Acknowledgments. This work is funded by NTNU.

Disclosure of Interests. The author has no competing interests to declare that are relevant to the content of this article.

References

1. Nordic Council of Ministers: The Nordic Region – towards being the most sustainable and integrated region in the world: Action Plan for 2021 to 2024 (2020). http://urn.kb.se/resolve?urn=urn:nbn:se:norden:org:diva-7139. Accessed 18 Nov 2022
2. Institute of Medicine. The Learning Healthcare System: Workshop Summary. The National Academies Press, Washington (2007)
3. J Braithwaite P Glasziou J Westbrook 2020 The three numbers you need to know about healthcare: the 60–30-10 Challenge BMC Med. 18 1 102

The Environmental Impacts of Artificial Intelligence in Decision-Making in Health and Social Care

Iina Latva-Teikari[1](✉), Elina Hyrkäs[2], and Outi Kanste[1]

[1] Research Unit of Health Sciences and Technology, University of Oulu, 90014 Oulu, Finland
iina.latva-teikari@oulu.fi

[2] Martti Ahtisaari Institute, University of Oulu, 90014 Oulu, Finland

Abstract. Rapid advances in artificial intelligence (AI) are transforming the health and social care sector. However, AI's environmental impacts remain an underexplored dimension. The aim of this study is to describe the perceptions held at decision-making levels in health and social care sector regarding the environmental impacts of AI, and to determine whether these impacts are reflected in AI related decision making and in the organisational culture of health and social care organisations.

Keywords: Artificial Intelligence · Decision-Making · Health and Social Care

1 Introduction

The health and social care industry is undergoing significant transformation due to the rapid development of artificial intelligence (AI) [1]. One potentially overlooked dimension of AI in the health and social care sector is its environmental impact, which is often overshadowed by its perceived benefits [2]. AI systems have been linked to high energy consumption [3, 4] and substantial amounts of carbon dioxide emissions [4]. As AI systems grow in complexity and usage, their energy requirements continue to rise [3]. Sustainable development is a key issue in health and social care [5], and all stakeholders should actively contribute to developing and implementing climate mitigation strategies [6]. According to the EU Artificial Intelligence Act [7], AI systems should be developed and used in ways that promote environmental sustainability and minimise their harmful impacts. The concrete consideration of environmental impacts in decision-making related to the deployment of AI has not been addressed in the reports or communications of the Ministry of Social Affairs and Health (Sosiaali- ja terveysministeriö, STM) or the Finnish Government.

It is crucial to acknowledge the hidden ecological costs and long-term environmental consequences of AI to fully understand its impact on the environment [3]. Given the complexity of environmental issues, evidence-based information is critically needed to inform environmental policy and decision-making [8]. The theory of evidence-informed

M. Säreströniemi et al. (Eds.): NCDHWS 2026, CCIS 3010, pp. 735–737, 2026.
https://doi.org/10.1007/978-3-032-28819-6

decision-making (EIDM) offers a comprehensive approach to sustainable decision-making and policy development by integrating scientific evidence into the decision-making process [9]. This enables an effective approach to addressing complex and layered environmental issues within the health and social care context.

According to previous research on the sustainable development and use of AI in healthcare, environmental considerations should be addressed alongside ethical dimensions [10]. The environmental impacts of data-driven AI-based health research [11] and the carbon footprint of digital health interventions, including AI [12], have been evaluated in previous scoping reviews. This study takes a step further by examining the perceptions held at the decision-making level in health and social care regarding the environmental impacts of AI and assessing whether these impacts are considered in decision-making.

2 Materials and Methods

This study consists of two phases: a qualitative descriptive study and a cross-sectional survey study. Phase one comprises a descriptive qualitative interview study involving decision-makers from STM, as well as from IT administration and top-level management in wellbeing services counties with university hospitals or active AI initiatives. The aim is to describe their perceptions of AI's environmental impacts. The data will be collected using in-depth qualitative interviews. The interview guide will be developed based on research literature on the environmental impacts of AI and Evidence-Informed Decision-Making (EIDM) theory. The data will be analysed using deductive-inductive content analysis. In phase two two cross-sectional surveys will be conducted with middle and operational level managers and professionals from wellbeing services counties with university hospitals or active AI initiatives. The instruments will be developed based on the insights gained from the initial interview study and the EIDM theory. The instruments will include items in which health and social care leaders evaluate how the environmental impacts of AI are considered in decision-making regarding its implementation. Health and social care professionals will evaluate the extent to which the environmental impacts of AI are reflected in the organisational culture and will also self-assess how they consider these impacts when making decisions about its use. The data will be analysed using descriptive and multi-method statistical methods.

3 Results and Discussion

The study is expected to reveal whether the environmental impacts of AI are considered in decision-making regarding its implementation and use in the Finnish health and social care sector. A preliminary assessment revealed variation among wellbeing services counties in AI utilisation and in the organisational location of AI-related decision-making, which predominantly occurs at the top management level, within IT administration, or in dedicated working groups. Benchmarking other Nordic healthcare systems show strong commitment to reducing emissions and promoting environmental responsibility; however, no evidence was identified indicating consideration of the environmental impacts associated with AI.

4 Conclusions

Sustainable development is a critical concern within the health and social care sector, and the environmental impacts of AI introduce a new dimension. The findings of this research will be utilised to support the development of health and social care practices and to inform decision-making processes, with consideration of environmental perspectives, thus contributing to the safety and well-being of both humans and the environment.

Disclosure of Interests. The authors have no competing interests to declare that are relevant to the content of this article.

References

1. Shaikh, M.I., Dsilva, J., Usmani, F.Z.A.: The influence of artificial intelligence on the healthcare industry in relation to sustainability. In: Singh, R., Shafik, W., Crowther, D., Kumar, V. (eds) Transforming Healthcare Sector Through Artificial Intelligence and Environmental Sustainability. Approaches to Global Sustainability, Markets, and Governance, pp. 89–104. Springer, Singapore (2024). https://doi.org/10.1007/978-981-97-9555-0_5
2. G Samuel C Richie 2022 Reimagining research ethics to include environmental sustainability: a principled approach, including a case study of data-driven health research J. Med. Ethics 49 6 428 433
3. A Zhuk 2023 Artificial intelligence impact on the environment: Hidden ecological costs and ethical-legal issues J. Digit. Technol. Law 1 4 932 950
4. Strubell, E., Ganesh, A., McCallum, A.: Energy and policy considerations for modern deep learning research. In: Proceedings of the AAAI Conference on Artificial Intelligence. vol. **34**(09), 13693–13696 (2020)
5. J Berniak-Woźny M Rataj 2023 Towards green and sustainable healthcare: a literature review and research agenda for green leadership in the healthcare sector Int. J. Environ. Res. Public Health 20 2 908
6. M Sergeant A Hategan 2023 What healthcare leadership can do in a climate crisis Healthc. Manage. Forum 36 4 190 194
7. EU Artificial Intelligence Act 13.6.2024/1689
8. DC Rose 2020 Policy windows for the environment: tips for improving the uptake of scientific knowledge Environ. Sci. Policy 113 47 54
9. World Health Organization WHO.: Evidence, policy, impact: WHO guide for evidence-informed decision-making. Geneva: World Health Organization; 2021. (2022)
10. C Richie 2022 Environmentally sustainable development and use of artificial intelligence in health care Bioethics 36 547 555
11. G Samuel AM Lucassen 2022 The environmental sustainability of data-driven health research: a scoping review Digit. Health 8 1 11
12. Z Lokmic-Tomkins 2022 Assessing the carbon footprint of digital health interventions: a scoping review J. Am. Med. Inform. Assoc. 29 12 2128 2139

Task-Dependent Central and Autonomic Responses to Sympathetic and Vagal Challenges

Runwei Lin(✉), Annemijn Hoff, and Ying Wang

Biomedical Signals and Systems, University of Twente, Enschede, the Netherlands
r.lin@utwente.nl

Abstract. The coordination of brain activity, heart rate variability (HRV) reflects the interplay between central and autonomic nervous system, yet the interpretation of these interactions are complex. In this study, we aim to explore the coupling pattern among electroencephalography (EEG) band power, HRV, and mean skin sympathetic nerve activity (SKNA) in different autonomic states. We collected these signals during two physiological challenges: isometric handgrip (IHG) and paced deep breathing (DB). Preliminary results reveal distinct responses, indicating task-dependent brain-heart dynamics. Following work will extend this framework using system-level multivariate analysis to investigate directed interactions between central and autonomic nervous systems.

Keywords: Brain-heart interplay · multimodal physiological signals

1 Introduction

The coordinated regulation of brain activity and cardiovascular function underlies adaptive physiological responses across a wide range of physiological contexts. Many previous studies of brainheart interaction (BHI) relied on electro encephalography (EEG) and heart rate variability (HRV) due to their non-invasive nature and high temporal resolution. However, interpretation of these interactions are often complicated, given HRV is influenced by multiple physiological processes and has limitations on representing sympathetic tone.

Consequently, how centralsympathetic regulation varies across distinct autonomic states remains insufficiently characterized. In this study, we collected multimodal recordings including EEG, electrocardiography (ECG), and skin sympathetic nervous activity (SKNA), which is a recently discovered non-invasive approach to measure sympathetic nervous activity [2], from healthy volunteers. The experiment included during two physiological challenges: isometric handgrip (IHG), primarily inducing sympathetic activation, and paced deep breathing (DB), enhancing parasympathetic modulation. To characterize state-dependent changes, we first examined task-dependent alterations in each signal separately to validate the effectiveness of the experimental paradigm. The preliminary results were summarized in this abstract.

M. Särestöniemi et al. (Eds.): NCDHWS 2026, CCIS 3010, pp. 738–740, 2026.
https://doi.org/10.1007/978-3-032-28819-6

2 Method

2.1 Data Collection and Preprocessing

The experiment was approved by the Ethics Committee Computer and Information Science of the University of Twente (reference number 250290). Data from eight healthy subjects were included in the analysis. Each subject completed three experimental conditions in the following order: a 5-min seated resting period, a 3-min isometric handgrip (IHG) task performed at 30% of the maximum voluntary contraction (MVC) (or until fatigue), and a 3-min paced deep-breathing (DB) task at a rate of six breaths per minute. The entire protocol was repeated three times for each subject.

EEG were analyzed with EEGLAB [1]. All EEG signals were band-pass filtered between 0.5 and 45 Hz, followed by bad-channel detection and removal. Independent component analysis was then applied to reject the artifacts. After signal reconstruction, all channels were re-referenced to the common average. Power spectral analysis was performed for four canonical EEG frequency bands: δ [1 Hz, 4 Hz], θ [4 Hz, 8 Hz], α [8 Hz, 13 Hz], β [13 Hz 30 Hz]. The R peaks were detected from the ECG using the Pan–Tompkins method, and the root mean square of successive differences (RMSSD) was calculated afterwards. SKNA is a non-invasive surrogate of sympathetic tone. In this study, it was extracted from the high frequency electrocardiography (ECG) by band-pass filtering using a fourth-order Butterworth filter with cutoff frequencies of 500 and 1000 Hz [2]. The filtered signal was then rectified and smoothed using a moving-average window of one second to obtain the average SKNA (aSKNA). Three EEG channels located over the central scalp regions (C3, C4, Cz) were selected for analysis as they are related to autonomic regulation. The EEG band power, RMSSD and mean aSKNA were averaged across the three repetitions. Consequently, differences among resting, DB and IHG were assessed separately for each marker using the Friedman test. Post-hoc comparisons were performed with Bonferroni correction to control for multiple comparisons across three conditions.

3 Results

Figure 1 presents the results of comparison among three tasks for EEG band power, mean aSKNA and RMSSD. Task-related power differences were observed only in the α-band. Specifically, α-band power was significantly reduced during IHG compared with rest across three channels, and a significant difference between DB and IHG was detected only at the C4 channel. No significant difference in α-band power was observed between DB and rest. In contrast, no task-related difference was found in the δ, θ, or β bands. RMSSD was significantly higher during DB than IHG, while no difference was observed between either task and rest. Mean aSKNA was elevated during IHG relative to rest, whereas no significant difference was found between DB and IHG or between DB and rest.

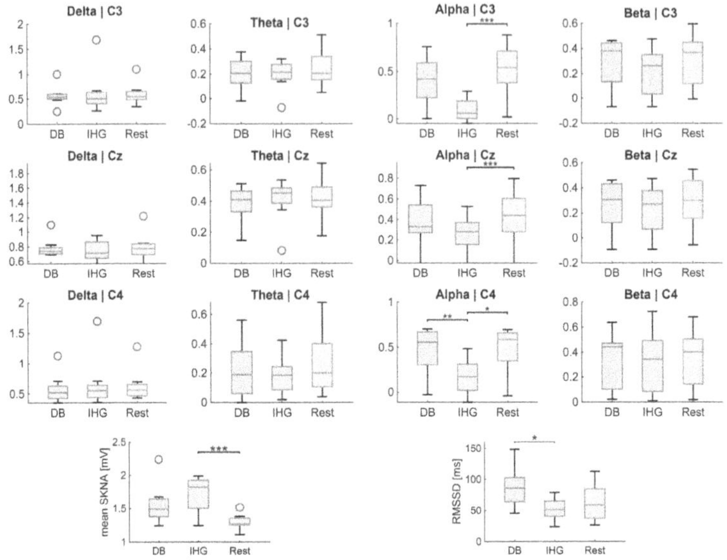

Fig. 1. Rows 1–3: EEG power in four frequency bands at channels C3, Cz and C4. Row 4: Mean aSKNA and RMSSD responses. Asterisks indicate statistical significance: *:$p < 0.05$; **:$p < 0.01$; ***:$p < 0.001$.

4 Discussion

The present findings indicate that IHG and paced DB elicit distinct central and autonomic responses: IHG triggers a decrease in α-band power in the central regions; meanwhile, it leads to a mean aSKNA increase (over rest) and HRV decrease (than DB). On the other hand, DB has weaker effects, but significantly increases HRV (over IHG). These results validates the existence of task-specific responses of central and autonomic nervous systems when probed with sympathetic versus vagal challenges. Future studies will extend this work using directional measures such as Granger causality. In particular, SKNA–EEG interactions are of special interest, as they provide a unique window into centralsympathetic nervous system coupling, which is largely underexplored.

References

1. Delorme, A., Makeig, S.: EEGLAB: an open source toolbox for analysis of single-trial EEG dynamics including independent component analysis. J. Neurosci. Methods **134**(1), 9–21 (2004)
2. Kusayama, T., et al.: Simultaneous noninvasive recording of electrocardiogram and skin sympathetic nerve activity (neuECG). Nat. Protoc. **15**, 1853–1877 (2020). https://doi.org/10.1038/s41596-020-0316-6

Measuring the Quality of AI-Generated Clinical Notes: A Systematic Review and Experimental Benchmark of Evaluation Methods

Alexandra Dahlberg[1,2(✉)], Tiila Käenniemi[3,4], Tiia Winther-Jensen[3], Olli Tapiola[1], Rami Luisto[5,6], Tuukka Puranen[1], Max Gordon[7], Enni Sanmark[1,8], and Ville Vartiainen[1,8]

[1] Clinicum, Faculty of Medicine, University of Helsinki, Helsinki, Finland
alexandra.dahlberg@harjunterveys.fi
[2] Mehiläinen, Helsinki, Finland
[3] Faculty of Arts, University of Helsinki, Helsinki, Finland
[4] Gofore Lead Oy, Helsinki, Finland
[5] Faculty of Information Technology, University of Jyväskylä, Jyväskylä, Finland
[6] Digital Workforce Services Plc, Helsinki, Finland
[7] Department of Clinical Sciences, Danderyd Hospital, Karolinska Institutet, Stockholm, Sweden
[8] Heart and Lung Center, Helsinki University Hospital, Helsinki, Finland

Abstract. High-quality clinical documentation is essential for safe and effective care, yet its production remains time consuming and prone to error. Large language models (LLMs) have shown potential for supporting clinical note generation, but their clinical adoption depends on how the quality of generated text is assessed, and current evaluation practices vary widely. We systematically searched Ovid Medline and Scopus on 10 April 2025 for peer-reviewed studies that used LLMs to generate clinical notes and reported an evaluation of text quality. Screening followed PRISMA guidelines, and the protocol was preregistered in PROSPERO. Evaluation metrics and outcome measures were synthesised narratively. Informed by these findings, we designed a controlled experimental setup using five synthetic clinical cases, with targeted perturbations to examine the behaviour of commonly used automated metrics and LLM-based evaluators. Thirty-seven studies met the inclusion criteria. Reported evaluations were dominated by lexical overlap metrics, primarily ROUGE and BLEU, whereas semantic similarity metrics such as BERTScore and BLEURT were less frequent. Human evaluation was common but heterogeneous in criteria and reporting, most often addressing correctness, fluency, and clinical acceptability. In the experimental analysis, lexical overlap metrics detected deletions and factual modifications but penalised meaning-preserving paraphrases. Semantic metrics and LLM-based evaluators were more tolerant of paraphrasing while remaining sensitive to clinically relevant changes, with performance varying by model and language. We conclude that lexical overlap metrics are insufficient as standalone proxies for clinical text quality and recommend a layered evaluation strategy combining semantic metrics, LLM-as-evaluator, and targeted human review to support scalable assessment.

T. Käenniemi and T. Winther-Jensen — Contributed equally.

M. Säreströniemi et al. (Eds.): NCDHWS 2026, CCIS 3010, pp. 741–742, 2026.
https://doi.org/10.1007/978-3-032-28819-6

Keywords: large language models · clinical text quality · clinical documentation · text quality · evaluation metrics · natural language processing · automated text evaluation · healthcare AI

Predicting Length of Stay in High Throughput Hospital Units

Lars Mattsson(✉) and Patrik Rydén

Department of Mathematics and Mathematical Statistics, Umeå University, Umeå, Sweden
{Lars.mattsson,Patrik.ryden}@umu.se

Abstract. Accurate prediction of patients' length of stay (LOS) in post-anesthesia care units (PACUs), is essential for efficient resource planning. LOS can be decomposed into a *care time* (CT) which is the time needed from arrival until medical treatment is completed, and a *waiting time* (WT) caused by operational constraints, such as limited capacity in downstream wards. CT is associated with patient data and therefore suitable for prediction. However, CT is not always observable, resulting in partially interval-censored data. This study evaluates different preprocessing-strategies for handling interval-censored observations when modelling LOS using machine learning (ML). The strategies were evaluated considering different ML-algorithms using real PACU data and 640 simulated datasets. Results show that applying a commonly used standard preprocessing strategy consistently yields the poorest performance. Overall, the findings highlight the necessity of selecting appropriate preprocessing strategies when applying ML to interval-censored clinical data.

Keywords: Interval censored data · Machine learning · Preprocessing strategies

1 Introduction

Patient length of stay (LOS) is a central driving factor for patient throughput across hospital units. To assure quality of care and to minimize resource blocking, LOS needs to be accurately estimated for effective day-to-day planning. This is especially important in high-throughput environments such as post-anesthesia care units (PACUs), where insufficient planning can create bottlenecks that block upstream surgeries [1] and ultimately compromise the quality of care.

The PACU at the University Hospital of Northern Sweden (UHNS) has historically relied on clinician expertise for planning; however, this approach does not leverage information available in clinical data and relies heavily on key personnel to maintain a functional patient flow. Machine learning (ML) that utilize patient admission data to predict LOS could allow for faster and more efficient planning. A patient's LOS can be decomposed in to *care time* (CT), defined as the time from arrival until fully medically treated, and consecutive *waiting time* (WT) that may be caused by organizational and capacity-related factors that are commonly not associated with the patient's admission data. This makes direct modeling of LOS inherently difficult [2] and suggests that CT

M. Säreströniemi et al. (Eds.): NCDHWS 2026, CCIS 3010, pp. 743–745, 2026.
https://doi.org/10.1007/978-3-032-28819-6

and WT should be modelled separately. A common challenge here is that CTs are not always observable, leading to partially interval-censored (IC) CT-observations [3].

In this study, we investigate preprocessing strategies (PSs) designed to handle IC-observations in ML tasks, using both real and simulated data.

2 Method

We consider a setting where a fraction of the CT-observations are IC, while the remaining observations are fully observed. Four PSs were considered: the *Midpoint* (MP), which replaces each censored observation with the midpoint of its interval; the *Endpoint* (EP), which replaces each censored observation with its upper bound; the *Remove-Censored* (RC), which treats censored observations as missing values; and the *Remove-Censored-Short* (RCS), which treats both censored observations and observations exceeding a prespecified threshold as missing values.

Each PS was evaluated on both real and simulated data using four different ML-methods: *Gradient Boosted Trees* [4], *Random Forest* [5], *Support Vector Machines* [6], and *Elastic Net Regression* [7]. Sixteen simulation designs were considered by varying the number of observations, variables and influential variables. For each design, 40 datasets were simulated, resulting in 640 datasets. Each data set was analyzed using 16 approaches, obtained by considering all combinations of PSs and ML-methods. The performance of the approaches was evaluated using a ranking score derived from the observed median absolute error (MeME), see Fig. 1.

The PACU data consists of 12,415 unique observations and >300 explanatory variables. Approximately 3% of the observations were recorded as interval censored; however, the true proportion of IC-observations is believed to be considerably higher. To reflect this, a subsampling procedure was applied, replacing a subset of uncensored observations with IC-observations, resulting in a data set with approximately 40% censored observations.

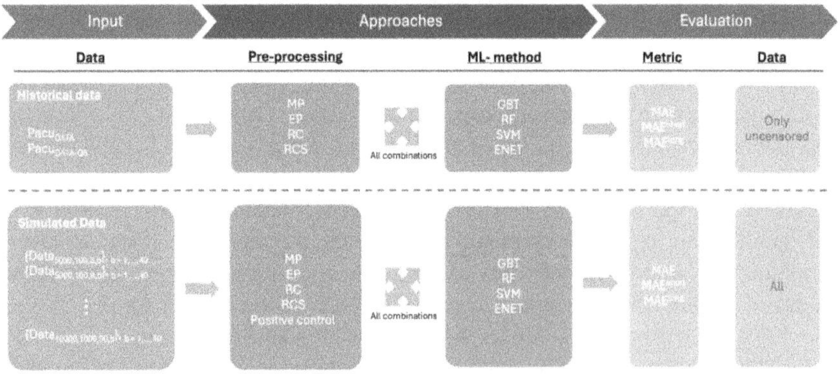

Fig. 1. Combinations of pre-processing strategies and ML-methods.

3 Results and Discussion

Preliminary results show that the commonly used EP-strategy performs considerable worse than the alternative strategies MP, RC, and RCS regardless of ML-method. For simulated data the gain of using alternative strategies over EP was at least 30% reduced MeAE. The same trends were observed in the PACU data although the differences were smaller. A comparison between the alternative strategies suggests that RC offers a robust, well performing solution, independently of ML-method and length of the true CTs. The performance of the strategies was further investigated by varying the number of observations, explanatory variables, and influential variables. Increasing the number of observations and explanatory variables had no noticeable impact on the performance, but increasing the number of influential variables resulted in increased MeAE values.

4 Conclusions

The results suggest that selecting an appropriate preprocessing strategy when performing ML-modelling in the presence of interval-censored observations can have a major impact on predictive performance. Particularly, ignoring censoring when modelling CT, and applying the EP-strategy, is likely to result in poor performance, whereas the RC-strategy provides a robust alternative that performed well across different data sets and ML-methods.

Acknowledgments. This study was funded by the industrial doctoral school (IDS) at Umeå University and Region Västerbotten.

Disclosure of Interests. The authors have no competing interests to declare.

References

1. M Fairley D Scheinker ML Brandeau 2019 Improving the efficiency of the operating room environment with an optimization and machine learning model Health Care Manag. Sci. 22 4 756 767
2. Cho, H., Jewell, N.P., Kosorok, M.R.: Interval censored recursive forests. J. Comput. Graph. Stat. **31**(2), 390–402 (2022)
3. J Sun 2014 Interval censoring, Encyclopedia of Biostatistics 3 Wiley New York
4. J Friedman T Hastie R Tibshirani 2000 Additive logistic regression: a statistical view of boosting (with discussion and a rejoinder by the authors) Ann. Stat. 28 2 337 407
5. Breiman, L.: Random forests. Mach. Learn. **45**(1), 5-32 (2001)
6. Vapnik, V., Golowich, S., Smola, A.: Support vector method for function approximation, regression estimation and signal processing. In: Advances in Neural Information Processing Systems. vol. 9 (1996)
7. H Zou T Hastie 2005 Regularization and variable selection via the elastic net J. R. Stat. Soc. Ser. B Stat Methodol. 67 2 301 320

WoMED: Designing a Clinical Tool to Aid in Diagnosis, Assessment, and Decision-Making by Utilizing Women's Health Data

Riikka K. Arffman(✉), Marko Arffman, Janne Wäli, Elisa Hurskainen, and Terhi T. Piltonen

Faculty of Medicine, University of Oulu, Research Unit of Clinical Medicine, MRC Oulu, Oulu, Finland
riikka.arffman@oulu.fi

Keywords: Women's Health · Healthcare · Clinical Decision Support System · Health applications · User Needs

1 Introduction

The impact of women-specific health issues on overall health remains insufficiently recognized. Even though they have been shown to impair quality of life, work ability, and fertility, many women's health issues remain underdiagnosed, with long diagnostic delays. In addition, despite many women's health issues having a broad health effect that extends beyond reproduction, they are often not considered important risk factors or utilized in risk assessment algorithms. One of the reasons is that key information (e.g., menstrual history, contraception, fertility and pregnancy events, screening results, relevant lab results, and diagnoses such as PCOS or endometriosis) is fragmented across sectors and formats, limiting holistic risk assessment and delaying diagnosis, intervention, and prevention.

2 Methods

WoMED is a proof-of-concept initiative to design a nationwide clinical decision-support tool that integrates women's reproductive, gynecological, obstetric, and metabolic health data into a single, usable view for both clinicians and patients. The project will define user needs and data standards, align with medical device and regulatory requirements, and plan for integration with Finland's national Kanta Services. The application will combine patient-reported inputs with health record data, present them in a structured graphical profile, and provide risk alerts, suggested follow-up tests, and links to Current Care Guidelines. WoMED aims to enable earlier recognition of conditions and long-term comorbidity risks (e.g., cardiometabolic risks after gestational diabetes or preeclampsia).

Work proceeds through three packages: data and usability (WP1), Kanta-based women's health profile and questionnaires (WP2), and prototype development and sandbox testing (WP3) in collaboration with university hospitals, patient organizations, and digital health/AI experts.

M. Särestöniemi et al. (Eds.): NCDHWS 2026, CCIS 3010, pp. 746–747, 2026.
https://doi.org/10.1007/978-3-032-28819-6

3 Conclusion

Health professionals recognize a lack of effective tools for collecting data on women's health. The WoMED tool can provide a solution. The implementation of all work packages is ongoing. In 2026, the project will focus on developing the platform into a sandbox version that will be by a focus group.

Acknowledgments. This research was supported by the Research Council of Finland (365592).

Disclosure of Interests. The authors have no competing interests.

Artificial Intelligence-Assisted Decision Support in Nursing: A Qualitative Descriptive Study

Suonnansalo Petra[1,2], Härkönen Henna[1,2], Alastalo Mika[3], Zhou Wentao[4], and Jansson Miia[1,2,5](✉)

[1] Research Unit of Health Sciences and Technology, Faculty of Medicine, University of Oulu, Oulu, Finland
miia.jansson@oulu.fi
[2] Medical Research Center Oulu, Oulu, Finland
[3] Master School, Laurea University of Applied Sciences, Vantaa, Finland
[4] Alice Lee Center for Nursing Studies, University of Singapore, Singapore, Singapore
[5] Royal Melbourne Institute of Technology (RMIT University), Melbourne, Australia

Abstract.
Introduction. Registered nurses play a central role in clinical decision making [1]. This process is often challenged by organisational, professional, and environmental factors that can complicate nurses' ability to make timely and informed decisions [2]. Recent evidence indicates that integrating artificial intelligence into nursing practice can improve decision-making, strengthen the quality of patient care, and enhance workflow efficiency, underscoring the importance of understanding nurses' perspectives on artificial intelligence-supported tools [3]. Although the potential of these tools is well recognised, research to date provides only limited insight into how registered nurses experience decision-making in everyday clinical settings and which factors influence this process. Thus, this study aimed to describe registered nurses' experiences of clinical decision making to identify opportunities for artificial intelligence-assisted clinical decision support systems in nursing.

Materials and Methods. Data were collected in Finland between 2022 and 2025 through 16 semi-structured individual interviews with registered nurses working on inpatient wards in a Finnish university hospital. The interview guide was developed using the clinical reasoning model [4]. Data were analysed using inductive content analysis [5], enabling categories and themes to be derived directly from participants' experiences.

Results. Nurses described a range of challenges influencing their decision-making, including organisational issues, multiprofessional collaboration, nurse-patient interactions, professional factors, and availability and trustworthiness of data. Artificial intelligence–assisted clinical decision support systems could potentially ease some of these challenges by optimising health information management, streamlining clinical workflows, and elevating the overall quality of nursing care.

Conclusions. Nurses experienced diverse challenges and needs in clinical decision-making, shaped by organisational, professional, relational, and

M. Säreströniemi et al. (Eds.): NCDHWS 2026, CCIS 3010, pp. 748–749, 2026.
https://doi.org/10.1007/978-3-032-28819-6

information-related factors. Integrating artificial intelligence–assisted decision support systems may enhance decision-making, improve patient care quality, and enhance workflow efficiency. Achieving these opportunities requires coordinated efforts at individual, organisational, and societal levels, including competence development, workflow redesign, strong data governance, and a culture that fosters trust in technology. Overall, the results imply that well-designed artificial intelligence–assisted decision support systems may enhance nurses' clinical decision-making and contribute to safer and higher-quality care.

Keywords: Artificial intelligence · clinical decision support systems · nursing

Acknowledgements. We would like to thank the RNs who participated in the study, the study nurse who helped with the participant recruitment and PhD (blinded for review) for partici-pating in the conduct of the interviews.

No funding was received for this research.

References

1. C Thompson N Cullum D McCaughan T Sheldon P Raynor 2004 Nurses, information use, and clinical decision making—the real world potential for evidence-based decisions in nursing Evid. Based Nurs. 7 3 68 72
2. Bijani, M., Abedi, S., Karimi, S., Tehranineshat, B.: Major challenges and barriers in clinical decision-making as perceived by emergency medical services personnel: a qualitative content analysis. BMC Emerg. Med. **21**(11), (2021)
3. Mikkonen, K., et al.: Artificial intelligence technologies supporting nurses' clinical decision-making: a systematic review. J. Clin. Nurs. Epub ahead of print (2025)
4. T Levett-Jones 2010 The 'five rights' of clinical reasoning: an educational model to enhance nursing students' ability to identify and manage clinically 'at risk' patients Nurse Educ. Today 30 6 515 520
5. Kyngäs, H., Kääriäinen, M., Elo, S.: The trustworthiness of content analysis. In: Kyngäs, H., Mikkonen, K., Kääriäinen, M. (eds.) The Application of Content Analysis in Nursing Science Research, pp. 41–48. Springer, Cham (2019). https://doi.org/10.1007/978-3-030-30199-6_5

A Discrete Event Simulation Framework for Analysing and Optimising Emergency Medical Service Workflows

Kean Tang[1,2(✉)] and Patrik Rydén[1]

[1] Department of Mathematics and Mathematical Statistics, Umeå University, Umeå, Sweden
kean.tang@umu.se

[2] Umeå Centre for Gender Studies, Umeå University, Umeå, Sweden

Abstract. Simulating sequential events becomes challenging when the underlying dependency structure is complex. Traditional statistical or mathematical models often fall short in capturing the intricacies of such systems, particularly when priority-queues and task interruptions are involved. In this paper, we propose a framework of constructing a discrete event simulation model (digital twin) which aims to predict the performance of Emergency medical service (EMS) workflows under various scenarios. We evaluated the model in a case study of EMS care chain activities in Umeå municipality, Sweden. The results show that our model can effectively capture the dynamics of the EMS system and provide insights into resource allocation optimisation. We believe that the proposed framework can easily be adapted to EMS systems outside Sweden.

Keywords: Discrete event simulation · Emergency medical service · Scenario analysis · Data-driven optimisation

1 Introduction

Discrete event simulation (DES) is a powerful tool for modelling and analysing complex healthcare systems [1]. In the context of Emergency Medical Services (EMS), DES offers a practical decision-support tool for analysing operational workflows, such as resource dispatch, travel to patients, on-site treatments and transport to healthcare facilities. In this study, each operational component was modelled using dedicated statistical distributions or machine-learning-based functions to capture process durations and dispatch decisions. By integrating these components into a unified simulation framework, the digital twin captures how emergency calls, ambulance availability, and dispatch decisions interact over time under realistic workload and capacity constraints.

The digital twin was designed as a policy-testing environment. Previous studies [2, 3] have demonstrated that by repeatedly running a DES model under alternative staffing schedules, different alarm distributions, or decision-making guide-

M. Säreströniemi et al. (Eds.): NCDHWS 2026, CCIS 3010, pp. 750–753, 2026.
https://doi.org/10.1007/978-3-032-28819-6

lines, decision-makers can assess how organizational changes propagate through the system.

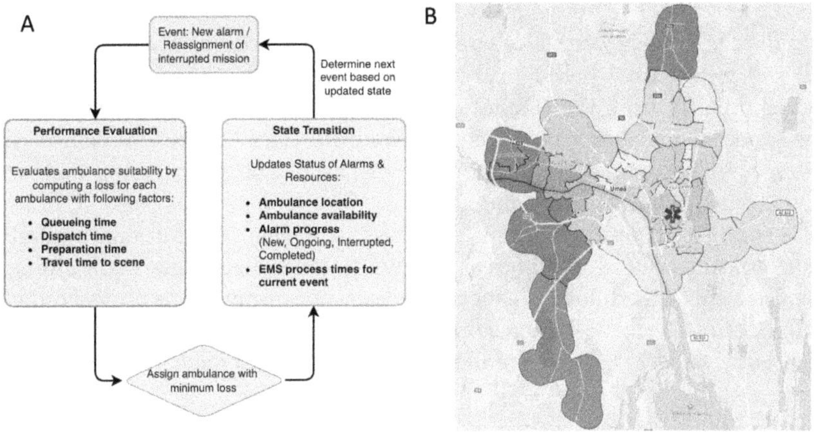

Fig. 1. A: Simulation flowchart; B: Median response time in Umeå municipality with one ambulance station (blue Star of Life symbol) under historical allocation

2 Methods

The DES framework consists of two main modules: the performance evaluation module and the state transition module, see Fig. 1A. The performance evaluation module is a proxy of healthcare decision-making guidelines which evaluates the suitability of each resource (ambulance) for a given emergency alarm based on various factors, such as dispatch time, preparation time, travel time, and queueing time. The state transition module, on the other hand, manages the dynamic state of the system by updating the status of alarms and resources after each assignment decision.

The simulation processes one event at a time, starting with either the arrival or reassignment of an emergency alarm. For each event, the performance evaluation module calculates a loss for each ambulance based on the current state of the system and the characteristics of the alarm. The ambulance with the minimum loss is then assigned to the alarm. Following the assignment, the state transition module updates the status of the assigned ambulance and the alarm, reflecting changes such as the ambulance's real time location, availability, and the alarm's progress (e.g., new, ongoing, interrupted, completed). The simulation then determines the next event to process based on the updated system state and continues this cycle until the end of the simulation period.

2.1 Study Scenario

We evaluated our framework by modelling EMS operations in Umeå, Sweden, using alarm and mission data between 2022 and 2023. Umeå has a single ambulance station with five ambulances serving roughly 130,000 residents.

Predictive models were developed to estimate the dispatch time, preparation time, and travel time based on historical data, while the queueing time was observed directly from the simulation. The loss for each ambulance was defined as the expected *response time* (time interval from alarm call to ambulance arrival at the scene.), estimated by summing the dispatch time, preparation time, travel time to scene, and queueing time.

We conducted multiple simulation runs in which an additional ambulance station was introduced at different candidate locations, while maintaining the original staffing schedule by reallocating existing resources (e.g., assigning two ambulances to the new station and keeping three at the original station). For comparison, we also ran the simulation using historical allocation, see Fig. 1B.

3 Results and Discussion

Preliminary results indicate that introducing a second station would substantially improve median response times across the municipality. For most candidate locations, median response times decreased, with the largest reductions approaching 10%. Equally important, the additional station reduced disparities in response times between urban districts within Umeå municipality. Some placements were particularly beneficial for elderly patients, whereas other locations showed neutral or even adverse effects for this group. This illustrates the value of simulation-based evaluation, as it can reveal varying effects across locations and population groups which would not be apparent from overall performance.

4 Conclusions

We have presented a DES framework that mirrors real-world EMS workflows. By applying the model in Umeå, we demonstrated its utility in evaluating organizational changes. The framework can be expanded to incorporate learning components for adaptive parameter calibration and optimisation loops. This transforms the digital twin from a one-off analytical model into a platform for continuous evaluation and policy testing.

Acknowledgments. This study was funded by Kempe Foundations (JCK-2022.2), VINNOVA-UDI (2021-03970) and Umeå Centre for Gender Studies.

References

1. Mahdiraji, S.A., et al.: A framework for constructing discrete event simulation models for emergency medical service policy analysis. Procedia Comput. Sci. **210**, 133–140 (2022)
2. Bozorgmanesh, H., Ryden, P.: Optimal placement of ambulance stations using data-driven direct and surrogate search methods. Int. J. Med. Inform. **196**, 105790 (2025)
3. Ridler, S., Mason, A.J., Raith, A.: A simulation and optimisation package for emergency medical services. Eur. J. Oper. Res. **298**(3), 1101–1113 (2022)

Author Index

M. Särestöniemi et al. (Eds.): NCDHWS 2026, CCIS 3010, pp. 755–757, 2026.
https://doi.org/10.1007/978-3-032-28819-6